P9-EEN-622

DATE DUE

DEMCO 38-296

Space Biology and Medicine

Joint U.S./Russian Publication
in Five Volumes

Series edited by

Arnauld E. Nicogossian, Stanley R. Mohler (U.S.)
Oleg G. Gazenko, Anatoliy I. Grigoryev (Russia)

Co-Editors

United States

L. F. Dietlein
C. L. Huntoon
S. R. Mohler
J. D. Rummel
F. M. Sulzman

Russia

V. V. Antipov
S. A. Bugrov
A. M. Genin
A. I. Grigoryev
A. A. Gurjian
M. V. Ivanov
V. A. Kotelnikov
I. D. Pestov

**American Institute of Aeronautics
and Astronautics**
Washington, DC

Nauka Press
Moscow

Riverside Community College
Library
4800 Magnolia Avenue
Riverside, CA 92506

RC1135 .S62 1993
Space biology and medicine

American Institute of Aeronautics and Astronautics, Inc.
370 L'Enfant Promenade, SW, Washington, DC 20024-2518

Library of Congress Cataloging-in-Publication Data

Space biology and medicine / edited by Arnauld E. Nicogossian . . . [et
al.].
        p.   cm.
    Simultaneously published in Russian.
    Includes bibliographical references and index.
    Contents: v. 1. Space and its exploration / editors, J.D. Rummel
and V.A. Kotelnikov, M.V. Ivanov
    1. Space medicine. 2. Space biology.   I. Nicogossian, Arnauld E.
    RC1135.S62   1993   616.9'80214--dc20   93-26189
        ISBN 1-56347-061-6 (v. 1)

Copyright © 1993 by the American Institute of Aeronautics and Astronautics, Inc. All rights in the English language reserved, except that no copyright is claimed within the territorial jurisdiction of the United States of America for separable contributions of U.S. Government employees included in this volume. The U.S. Government has a license for Governmental purposes under the copyright claimed herein. For permission to translate from the English or Russian version, contact the NASA Scientific and Technical Information Division or the Russian Academy of Sciences Scientific Publishing Counsel.

Data and information appearing in this book are for informational purposes only. AIAA is not responsible for any injury or damage resulting from use or reliance, nor does AIAA warrant that use or reliance will be free from privately owned rights.

ISBN 1-56347-061-6

*This series is dedicated to the men and women who have devoted their lives
to the exploration and conquest of space.*

Series Preface

The appearance of this work has an entire history behind it. As early as the mid 1960s Hugh L. Dryden and Dr. Anatoliy Arkadevich Blagonravov signed a number of agreements on collaboration in space research between the National Aeronautics and Space Administration of the U.S. and the U.S.S.R. Academy of Sciences. One of them was an agreement to publish a joint scientific work—"Foundations of Space Biology and Medicine"—in both Russian and English.

The material in that book, published in 1975, was based on the results of observations and research that had been conducted mainly on short-term flights of approximately 50 manned spacecraft carrying more than 70 crew members, and also of dozens of space flight experiments conducted on dedicated biosatellites or "hitch-hiking" on unmanned spacecraft. The 1975 edition was generally well received by readers and reviewers, and for some time satisfied the need for information in space biology and medicine.

However, since that time, human space flight has made extensive use of space shuttle systems and long-term orbital space stations. New empirical data—the results of numerous, often unique flight and simulation experiments—have accumulated rapidly. The scope of biological experiments in space has expanded significantly. Thus by the mid 1980s it had become clear that it was time to summarize and analyze the knowledge we have gleaned in this area.

In 1987 a new intergovernmental agreement, Concerning Cooperation in the Exploration and Use of Outer Space for Peaceful Purposes, was signed (the first one was signed in 1971). Item 16 of the Addendum to this Agreement stipulated publication of a new edition of the joint U.S./U.S.S.R. scientific work, "Foundations of Space Biology and Medicine." A joint editorial board was formed to implement this project within the framework of the U.S./U.S.S.R. Joint Working Group on Space Biology and Medicine.

After considering the complexity of preparing and publishing a work covering the knowledge and experience acquired by both countries, the editorial board concluded that given the enormous amount of new material, and the new set of authors who would be preparing the chapters, the new edition would not simply be an updated version of the 1975 book, but in essence a whole new work. The goal of this new work would be to provide access for specialists, physicians, biologists, and engineers involved in space flight planning and management and the general scientific community to concise and systematic information about space biology and medicine that has accumulated during the last 25-30 years.

The five-volume work will be published in authenticated Russian and English versions. The editors of Volume 1, *Space and Its Exploration*, are Dr. J. D. Rummel of the U.S. and Academicians V. A. Kotelnikov and M. V. Ivanov of the Russian Federation. This volume covers the history of space exploration, the space environment, life in the universe, and spacecraft technology.

Volume II, *Life Support and Habitability*, has two parts: Part 1—*The Spacecraft Environment*, and Part 2—*Life Support Systems*. The editors are Dr. F. M. Sulzman of the U.S. and A. M. Genin of the Russian Federation. This volume addresses major issues and requirements for safe habitability and work beyond the Earth's atmosphere.

Volume III, *Humans in Space Flight*, is edited by Dr. C. L. Huntoon of the U.S. and Professor V. V. Antipov and corresponding member of the Academy of Sciences, A. I. Grigoryev of the Russian Federation. This volume has two books, which provide in-depth discussions of physiological adaptation to the space environment.

Volume IV, *Crew Health, Performance, and Safety*, is edited by Dr. L. F. Dietlein of the U.S. and Professors I. D. Pestov and S. A. Bugrov of the Russian Federation. This volume presents a concise description of systems and preventive measures necessary to assure crew health.

Volume V, *Reference Material*, is edited by Professor S. R. Mohler of the U.S. and Dr. A. A. Gurjian of the Russian Federation. This volume includes extensive reference material relevant to the major topics discussed in the previous volumes.

With only a few exceptions, volumes are being written by chapter authors who did not contribute to the 1975 version, and the editors had to devote considerable effort to ensure the consistent organization of the book as a whole, avoid contradictions, and link individual chapters. Nevertheless, we are aware that in spite of all our efforts, we have not been able to produce a work that is homogeneous with respect to consistency of presentation, being written by scientists of two countries.

Thus, this five-volume edition represents another successful completion of a collaborative project between the Russian Academy of Sciences and the U.S. National Aeronautics and Space Administration in the area of space biology and medicine. We hope that this work will be a useful reference to the reader. We would like to officially express our gratitude for the efforts of the Joint Editorial Board and the many individuals who provided invaluable help in the preparation of this work for publication.

In addition, on behalf of the Joint Editorial Board we wish to express our sincere appreciation to the publication staff.

Arnauld E. Nicogossian, U.S.
Oleg G. Gazenko, R.F.
Editors-in-Chief

Foreword

The National Aeronautics and Space Administration and the Russian Academy of Sciences are once again pleased to introduce a joint work devoted to "Space Biology and Medicine."

The first such work, "Foundations of Space Biology and Medicine," appeared in both English and Russian versions in 1975 on the eve of the historic first international space mission, the Apollo-Soyuz Test Project. This classic work provided an exhaustive overview of fundamental and applied knowledge in space medicine, biology, exobiology, radiobiology, and environmental medicine, written by leading experts, and acquired painstakingly by the scientists of both countries over the first 15 years of space exploration. For many years this edition provided sound reference material to the serious students and specialists involved in the exploration of the final frontier—space.

Since that time, many changes have occurred in space exploration. New discoveries have been made, new spacecraft and laboratories have been flown. More men and women have flown in space, some for extended periods of time in low Earth orbit. Robotic spacecraft landed on Mars, ventured beyond the solar system, and opened windows on worlds never before seen so closely. Many of the engineering and medical advances in space biology and medicine have found application in the practice of terrestrial medicine and public health.

The joint U.S. and Russian editorial board, established under the 1987 Agreement between the United States of America and the Union of Soviet Socialist Republics Concerning Cooperation in the Exploration and Use of Outer Space for Peaceful Purposes, has made significant efforts to bring the reader this up-to-date treatise, renamed "Space Biology and Medicine." Significant revisions and rewrites occurred in the process of reviewing the first treatise. This second edition, in essence, can be considered a totally new publication.

Daniel S. Goldin
Administrator
U.S. National Aeronautics
   and Space Administration

Yuriy S. Osipov
President
Russian Academy of
   Sciences

Космическая Биология и Медицина

Совместное российско-американское издание в пяти томах

под общей редакцией

Олега Г. Газенко, Анатолия И. Григорьева (РФ)
Арнольда Е. Никогоссяна, Стенли Р. Молера (США)

ТОМ I

КОСМОС И ЕГО ОСВОЕНИЕ

Редакторы

В.А. Котельников, М.В. Иванов (РФ)
Д.Д. Раммел (США)

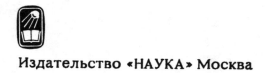

Издательство «НАУКА» Москва

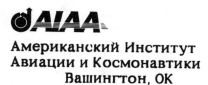

Американский Институт
Авиации и Космонавтики
Вашингтон, ОК

Volume I

Space and Its Exploration

Editors

J. D. Rummel (U.S.) and V. A. Kotelnikov, M. V. Ivanov (Russia)

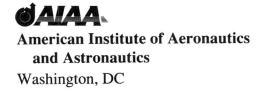

**American Institute of Aeronautics
and Astronautics**
Washington, DC

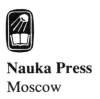

Nauka Press
Moscow

Acknowledgments for Volume I

In addition to the authors and editors, many people have contributed to the preparation of this volume. The U.S. and Russian editors would like to acknowledge the contributions of Sergey I. Aksenov, Lyudmila B. Buravkova, Aleksandr P. Drozshilov, Tatyana B. Kasatkina, Igor V. Khatuntsev, Sergey O. Nikolayev, Eleonora F. Panchenkova, Aleksandr V. Rodin, Dmitriy V. Titov, Aleksey A. Vasilyev, and Yuriy I. Yefremov on the Russian side, and Derek Buzasi, Ronald Dutcher, Kim Ellsworth, Glenn Ferraro, Karen Gaiser, Elizabeth Hess, Natalie Karakulko, Witalij Karakulko, Paul Makinen, Michael Meyer, Natalie Owen, Carl Pilcher, Terri Ramlose, Edward J. Stone, and Ronald Teeter on the U.S. side. Galina Ya. Tverskaya was an asset to both sides.

The editors would also like to thank the Lockheed Engineering and Sciences Corporation for their assistance with the preparation of the English manuscripts for publication, and particularly Dr. Lydia R. Stone, who was responsible for translations for the U.S. side. Marc Shepanek was invaluable in managing the editorial process on the U.S. side.

Finally, the editors would like to thank Dr. Sylvia Fries of NASA for her work on the historical section of this volume, and Dr. James Oberg for his careful reading and correction of an earlier version of the current section. The final version published here owes much to their efforts, but the view of history expressed in the final version is that of the authors.

Introduction to Volume I:
Space and Its Exploration

Perhaps one of the greatest gifts that has been given to the people of the world in the last few hundred years has been an emerging sense of the place of our planet and its inhabitants within the context of the vast universe. Our knowledge of the rest of the universe has not come quickly, nor was the process of attaining it only recently begun; however, the unprecedented acceleration of that process has benefitted from a fundamental new aspect of our species that has only manifested itself in the last 30 years or so, the ability to travel in space.

Before the space age, the Universe was studied only through observations from the Earth. All that has changed with the beginning of the space age. Machines built by humans have flown to all but one of the nine planets that revolve around our Sun, have ventured billions of miles from the Earth and looked back, and have landed on three other worlds. Spacecraft in orbit around the Earth have viewed the sky at a vast number of electromagnetic wavelengths, detecting the shape of the galaxy and the universe, and even measuring the remnants of the universe's beginning. Human explorers have ventured forth, first for short stays in orbit, then, later, walking upon the Moon and living for long periods in space. As they did so, billions of people on the Earth came to view the Earth in a fundamentally different way, not just as the familiar day-to-day backdrop for their lives, but as a small oasis suspended in the night sky above an alien landscape.

It is this new view of the Earth that is the true gift of space exploration. Space exploration has at once given us a new perspective on the value of our world, and a new perspective from which to understand how it operates. It has shown us that the Earth is by far the most precious place in the solar system in terms of supporting human life, while revealing that other destinations may still be compelling. The exploration of space has at once become a challenge for humanity to overcome and a path to our common future.

But for humanity to embark on this path, we need to understand ourselves in a new environment. As such, an understanding of the biological consequences of and opportunities in space flight is essential. In this, the first volume of a joint U.S./Russian series on space biology and medicine, we describe the current status of our understanding of space and present general information that will prove useful when reading subsequent volumes.

Since we are witnesses to the beginning of a new era of interplanetary travel, a significant portion of the first volume will concentrate on the physical and ecological conditions that exist in near and outer space, as well as heavenly bodies from the smallest ones to the giant planets and stars.

While space exploration is a comparatively recent endeavor, its foundations were laid much more than 30 years ago, and its history has been an eventful one. In the first part of this volume, Rauschenbach, Sokolskiy, and Gurjian address the "Historical Aspects of Space Exploration" from its beginnings to a present-day view of the events of the space age.

The nature of space itself and its features is the focus of the second section of the volume. In the first chapter of the part, "Stars and Interstellar Space," the origin and evolution of stars, and the nature of the portions of space most distant from Earth are described by Galeev and Marochnik. In Chapter 2, Pisarenko, Logachev, and Kurt in "The Sun and Interplanetary Space" bring us to the vicinity of our own solar system and provide a description and discussion of the nearest star and its influence on the space environment that our Earth and the other planets inhabit.

In our solar system there are many fascinating objects, remnants of the formation of a rather ordinary star in a rather obscure portion of the galaxy. Historical accident has caused us to be much more curious (and knowledgeable) about "The Inner Planets of the Solar System" than about any of these other objects. In Chapter 3, Marov describes the planets Mercury, Venus, Earth, and Mars, their history and origin, and their environmental conditions, and in Chapter 4 Owen provides similar information about Jupiter, Saturn, Uranus, Neptune, and Pluto, "The Outer Planets of the Solar System." Morrison provides a thorough discussion of "Asteroids, Comets, and Other Small Bodies" in Chapter 5. The understanding of these relics of the formation of the solar system may form the center of our ability to understand the origin of solar systems in general, and of the critical role that the beginning of the solar system had on the prospects for the origin of life and its continued survival and evolution in the face of their recurrent impacts on Earth.

In Chapter 6, the first chapter of the third part, Rummel describes the area of "Exobiology," the study of the origin, evolution, and distribution of life in the context of the origin and evolution of the universe. The same processes that have given rise to life on Earth may have given rise to life elsewhere. In Chapter 7, the "Earth and the Biosphere," the nature and function of the Earth are discussed as a specific instance of planetary and biological evolution. The effects of biological processes on the Earth under the influence of human activities are also addressed by Moore and Bartlett in Chapter 7. The final chapter in this section concerns the prospects that life in the universe may be widespread; "SETI," the Search for Extraterrestrial Intelligence, by Billingham and Tarter, presents the arguments for conducting a search for evidence of life elsewhere in the galaxy, and describes the various methods proposed for conducting such a search.

While SETI has a distinctly explorational character, more direct means are available for exploring the solar system around us. The fourth part of the volume addresses this subject of space exploration. Considering the prospects for research on space biology and medicine, the means of providing "Access to Space" are described by Feoktistov and Briggs in Chapter 9. This chapter addresses carriers and launch systems, the unmanned and manned spacecraft that they loft into space, and the task of mission operations by which these precious vessels are monitored, navigated, and controlled.

Despite the successes of the past and the capabilities of the present, it is clear that the study of space biology and medicine will be even more rewarding in the future than it has been to date. The work of the next few years that will be undertaken by the U.S. and Russia, both independently and jointly, will focus first on enabling greater capabilities in the exploration of space, and then on using the unique characteristics of the space environment to provide insight and greater understanding into biological systems, their behavior, development, and origin.

The chapters of the first volume were written by leaders in their fields from the U.S. and Russia. The material presented summarizes our current understanding of space and its exploration. We understand that the first volume will be of interest not only to medical personnel and biologists, but also to general readers who want information about space beyond their own particular fields of expertise.

Mikhail V. Ivanov, Vladimir A. Kotelnikov, and John D. Rummel
Moscow and Washington

Table of Contents

Volume I
Space and Its Exploration

Part I:

Historical Perspective

Historical Aspects of Space Exploration

B. V. Rauschenbach, V. N. Sokolskiy, and A. A. Gurjian

I. Origins to World War II

For centuries, humanity has speculated about reaching other worlds. Up until very recently, however, designs for interplanetary vehicles have been fanciful, even fantastic. Designs for air and spacecraft with some empirical basis (e.g., giant catapults or cannons) began to appear with the rise of technology over the last 150 years. Nevertheless, it was not until the end of the 19th century that a feasible means of space travel was proposed—the use of flight vehicles based on reactive propulsion.

A. First Designs of Reactive Flight Vehicles

It should be noted that the idea of using reactive propulsion for flight vehicles is several centuries old.[1] Indeed, during the 19th century more than 30 designs for flight vehicles using reactive principles were proposed (see Table 1).

Designs proposed in the 19th century for flight vehicles operating by reactive propulsion can be divided into three groups, depending on how altitude is achieved. The first group works on the balloon principle. The flight vehicle is lighter than air; altitude is achieved through the use of lighter-than-air gas. In the second group (reactive aircraft), the flight vehicle is heavier than air; altitude is achieved through the motion of air over supporting planes (wings). In the third group (rockets), the flight vehicle is also heavier than air; altitude is achieved through reaction to an exhaust jet.

However, unlike jet-propelled aircraft, which draw oxygen for combustion from the surrounding atmosphere, the rocket carries its own oxygen—indeed, its entire fuel supply—with it. The difference between vehicles of the second and third groups is that vehicles in the second group require an atmosphere to act as an aerodynamic medium and (in the case of jet-propelled aircraft) source of fuel, while for vehicles of the third group an atmosphere is not only not required, but is actually an impediment to motion, since it creates additional resistance.

Rocket-powered flight vehicles are central to the history of astronautics because they do not require an atmosphere for acceleration, altitude, or directional motion, and can thus theoretically be used for flight in the vacuum of space. However, although their vehicles did not require an atmo-sphere to act as a supporting medium, not one of the 19th century inventors, including Arias, Kibalchich, Nezhdanovskiy, and Fedorov, considered the possibility of using these vehicles for interplanetary flight.

This idea was first proposed and justified by one of the leading scientists of the time, Konstantin E. Tsiolkovskiy, whose name is inextricably linked with the early development of space flight theory. Tsiolkovskiy began to be interested in the challenge of interplanetary flight in the 1870s and 1880s. In 1883, in a manuscript entitled "Free Space," he explored what it would be like for humans to be in an environment without gravity or resistance, and also proposed a spacecraft design (Fig. 1).

Late in the 19th century, H. Ganswindt (Germany) began to deliver lectures on the possibility of interplanetary flights, in which he described his own spacecraft design (Fig. 2).

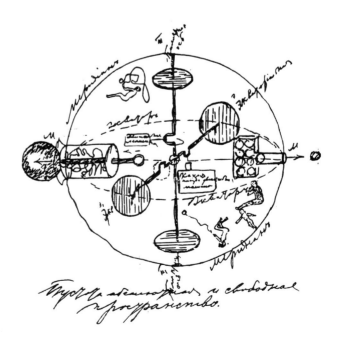

Fig. 1 Sketch of K.E. Tsiolkovskiy's spacecraft (sketch 1883)

Table 1   Designs for flight vehicles using reactive propulsion proposed in the 19th century

Aircraft Type	Energy Source			Combustion Products	
	Compressed Air or Other Gas	Water or Alcohol Vapor	Single Component Propellant	Liquid Propellant+ Air Oxygen	Liquid Propellant+ Liquid Oxidizer
Lighter than air (reactive aerostats)	Treteskiy (1849) Sokovnin (1866) Nezhdanovskiy (1882) Thayer (1884)	Treteskiy (1849)	Italia (1831) Treteskiy (1849) Maclaret (1852) Petersen (1892) Battey (1893)	Lebedev (1892)	
Heavier than air (jet planes)	Nezhdanovskiy (1882)	Golightly (1841) Butler & Edwards (1867) Nezhdanovskiy (1884) Geshvend (1887)	von Siemens (1845-1855) Maffiotte (1858) Ewald (1886)	Teleshev (1867) Nezhdanovskiy (1889)	
Heavier than air (rocket aircraft)	Nezhdanovskiy (1882) Fedorov (1896)	Geshvend (1887)	Arias (1872, 1876) Nezhdanovskiy (1880) Kibalchich (1881)	Arias (1872, 1876)	Nezhdanovskiy (1882-1884)

This table does not include designs of Ch. De Louvier, Emil Jira, S. M. Nemirovskiy, V. D. Spitsin, and certain other inventors, since information about the technical characteristics of their designs is insufficient.

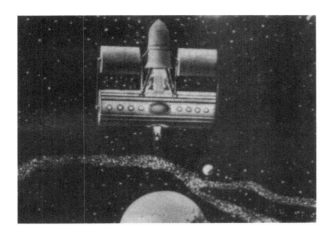

Fig. 2 H. Ganswindt's spacecraft (drawing 1891)

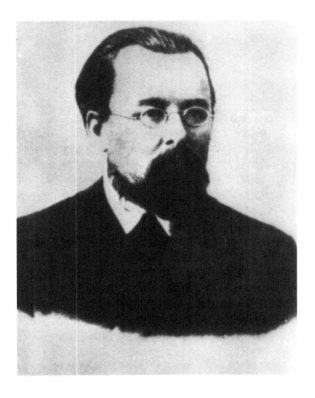

Fig. 3 K.E. Tsiolkovskiy (1957-1935)

B. Development of the Theory of Space Flight

Starting in 1896, Tsiolkovskiy (Fig. 3) began to work on the development of the theoretical bases for space flight. In May 1897 he derived the now famous formula of rocket dynamics that bears his name.[2] This formula establishes the association between speed of rocket flight, jet exhaust velocity, propellant mass, and the mass of the rocket vehicle.

At the beginning of the 20th century, scientists and inventors in a number of countries, generally working independently and often unaware of similar work being conducted by others,

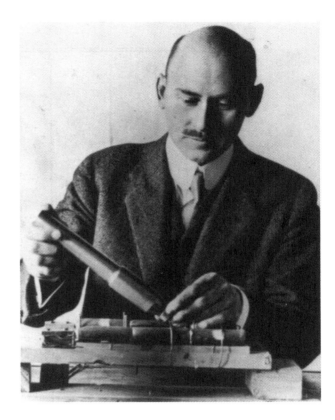

Fig. 4 R. Goddard (1882-1945) (NASA 74-H-1050)

began to take an interest in the problem of space flight. In addition to Tsiolkovskiy and Ganswindt, who had begun their work at the end of the 19th century, individuals working on the problem included R. Goddard (U.S.), R. Esnault-Pelterie (France), H. Oberth and W. Hohmann (Germany), F.A. Tsander and Yu.V. Kondratyuk (Russia), F. Ulinski, G. von Pirquet, F. von Hoefft (Austria) and others (Table 2, Fig. 4, 5, 6). Proposals made in space flight theory in the late 19th and first third of the 20th century, include a striking variety of power sources—from solid propellants (sticks of dynamite and smokeless powder) to electric and nuclear energy and light pressure.

The most effective way to increase the velocity of rocket flight is to increase the jet exhaust velocity. For this reason the efforts of scientists were focused on selection of the highest energy propellants, i.e., those with the greatest heat value. The use of liquid rocket propellant not only provided high thrust per unit mass, but, even more important, enabled ignition and combustion to be controlled. As early as 1903 Tsiolkovskiy proposed the use of liquid hydrogen and oxygen as rocket propellants.[3] Subsequently liquid propellants were considered by other researchers.

However, the energy requirements for the propellant were frequently incompatible with operational requirements and the use of liquid oxygen and hydrogen as reactants was associated with major operational problems. Furthermore, in the first quarter of the 20th century the technology for producing liquid hydrogen—a desirable fuel because of its high exhaust

Table 2   Space flight proposals, end of the 19th, beginning of the 20th centuries

Power Source	Attainment of Space Velocities		Launched from an Aircraft	Orbital Launch
	One-stage Rockets	Multi-stage Rockets		
Solid propellant	Ganswindt /1893/ Oberth <1909>	Goddard (1919)	Ganswindt /1901/ Hoefft (1928)	
Liquid propellant: hydrocarbon + oxygen	Oberth <1912>(1923> Tsiolkovskiy (1914)	Oberth <1918>(1923) Tsiolkovskiy (1929)		
Liquid propellant: hydrogen + oxygen	Tsiolkovskiy (1903) Goddard (1907) Oberth <1912> (1923) Kondratyuk <1917-19> Tsander /1923/ (1924)	Oberth <1918> (1923) Hoefft /1924- 28/ Tsiolkovskiy (1926-29)	Tsiolkovskiy (1911-12) Oberth (1923) Hoefft (1928)	Hoefft (1928)
Use of spacecraft material	Tsander <1909-12>	Kondratyuk <1920 > (1929)	Tsander (1924)	
Nuclear power	Goddard <1907> Tsiolkovskiy (1912) Esnault-Pelterie /1912/ (1913) Tsander /1925/			
Electric power				Goddard <1906> Tsiolkovskiy (1912) Ulinski <1915-16>(1920-27) Kondratyuk <1917> Tsander /1926/ Glushko /1928-29/ Oberth (1929)
Light pressure				Tsiolkovskiy <1921> Tsander (1924)
No power source indicated		Goddard <1909>	Ganswindt <1901> Goddard <1907>	Goddard /1913/ Pirquet (1928)

Note: (...) - Dates of proposals published in books, articles, patents
/.../ - Dates of proposals published in reports, applications or demonstrated on exhibitions
<..> - Dates of proposals from unpublished manuscripts of working notebooks of author

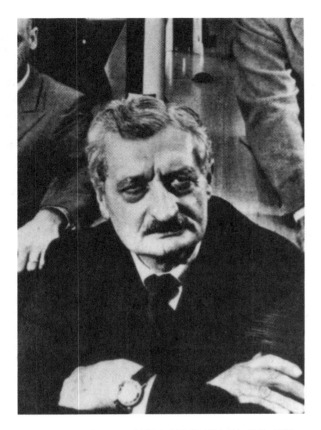

Fig. 5 H. Oberth (1894-1989) (NASA CC-417)

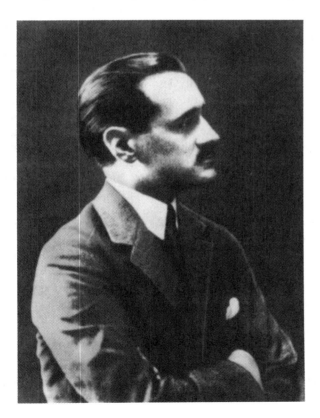

Fig. 6 R. Esnault-Pelterie (1881-1957)

and reaction rate—for use as a rocket fuel was still rudimentary. Thus some designers settled for propellants that produced less energy but were safer, more available, and easier to handle, e.g., various hydrocarbons (such as alcohol, benzene, kerosene, etc.). However, it soon became clear that there existed propellants that could produce more heat than the combination of hydrogen and oxygen. In 1909, F.A. Tsander of Russia conceived of the possibility of using the material of the interplanetary vehicle itself as the combustible material,[4] and in 1912 he specifically proposed using a metal propellant.[5] In 1917 Tsander began to experiment with burning molten metal and soon obtained numerical values for the heat value of magnesium oxide and other materials.[6] In 1920-1924, Tsander's countryman Yu. V. Kondratyuk also wrote of the possibility of using high energy metals as propellants.[7,8] However, calculations showed that one-stage rockets using chemical propellants could not (given a feasible ratio of propellant to structural material) reach even orbital velocity. For this reason, scientists and inventors continued to search for other forms of energy having significant advantages over chemical propellants.

One of these forms of energy was nuclear energy. In an unpublished manuscript, Tsiolkovskiy suggested using the energy of decaying atomic particles, since disintegrating atoms "emit particles of various masses, moving with astonishing, incredible speed, not far from the speed of light."[9] A similar proposal appeared in Goddard's writings from 1907.[10-12] Tsiolkovskiy published his proposal in 1912.[13] That same year R. Esnault-Pelterie also proposed the use of nuclear energy for space flight.[14]

Another promising form of energy for space flight was electric energy, which can be used to achieve very high exhaust velocities. As early as the first decade of the 20th century, the idea of building electric rocket engines occurred independently to Tsiolkovskiy[15] and Goddard.[16] This idea was first published by Tsiolkovskiy in a 1912 issue of the Russian journal *Bulletin of Aeronautics*.[13]

In 1916-1917, Robert Goddard conducted experiments on creation of an ion-powered rocket engine. In 1920, he obtained a patent for "Method of and Means for Producing an Electrofied Jets of Gas."[17] Meanwhile, the Austrian F. Ulinski wrote of building an electronic spacecraft[18]; according to a number of authors [e.g. Ref. 19], this was an idea he had conceived as early as 1915-1916. Subsequently, Goddard (1916-1929), Kondratyuk (1917-1919), Tsiolkovskiy (1921-1925), Tsander (1926), Ulinski (1927), Glushko (1928-1929), and Oberth (1929) all continued to explore the use of electric rocket engines.

Notwithstanding these efforts to advance alternatives to liquid chemical rocket propulsion fuels, the necessary technologies were not sufficiently developed to build actual engines for use on flight vehicles. During the first third of the 20th century proposals for using these forms of energy for space flight could only be considered as long-term exploratory development. Moreover, the engines being proposed were low-thrust and could operate only after overcoming Earth's gravity and entering orbit. Researchers were faced with finding a technique for reaching orbital velocity that could be implemented given the technology available at that time.

Identifying and developing optimum rocket propellants was one approach to the technological challenge of space travel; minimizing the passive mass of space vehicles during flight was another. Analysis of the major forces controlling rocket dynamics in Tsiolkovskiy's formula showed that to increase the speed of a rocket's flight as propellant combustion progresses, the portions of the rocket that had become unnecessary should be discarded as quickly as possible, leaving only those portions essential to the continued nominal functioning of the rocket. The application of this principle to modern rocketry was proposed by Goddard as early as 1909.[20] In 1911, A. Bing obtained a patent[21] for an "apparatus for studying the upper layers of the atmosphere, including the most rarefied," which also made use of these ideas. In 1912, Tsander similarly concluded that individual components of rockets should be jettisoned when no longer needed.[5] The same ideas can also be found in works by Kondratyuk of 1917-1919.[22-24]

The most advanced design for a multistage rocket was proposed in 1914 by Goddard, who also obtained a patent for a two-stage rocket.[25] In 1919, Goddard expressed the idea that a two-stage rocket could be used for sending projectiles to the Moon.[10] Subsequently, ideas concerning the use of multistage rockets for space flight were developed by Oberth, who in his 1923 work considered in detail the possibility of creating a two-stage spacecraft,[26] and by Tsiolkovskiy, who in 1926-1935 developed the foundations for a mathematical theory of multistage rockets.[27, 28, 29]

Use of the multistage rocket principle accelerated the solution of the problem of attaining orbital velocity. By 1946, the United States was able to launch a small two-stage rocket, and achieved an altitude on the order of 400 km. Finally, the first manmade object successfully orbited. The Soviet Union's Sputnik, was inserted into orbit in 1957 by a one and one-half stage rocket (one stage assisted by "strap-on" booster rockets). Today multistage rockets are used extensively.

However, the use of the multistage principle does not fully solve the problem of minimizing the detrimental effect of passive rocket mass. Components of the rocket are simply jettisoned as they become unnecessary, but do not provide any additional benefit. This led scientists to consider the possibility of using these rocket components as combustion material. First Tsander (1909),[5] and then, somewhat later, Kondratyuk (1920)[7] raised this possibility, proposing to use the material of the rocket as additional propellant. This proposal was not published until the 1920s[8,31] and has still not been implemented. Although even today scientists and engineers do not agree on whether it will be ever be attempted, in the 1920s this proposal was considered seriously and evoked substantial interest.

A third proposed approach to achieving orbital and escape velocity, and one that attracted much attention, especially during early work on space flight theory, was to launch space rockets not from the Earth's surface, but from the air—from bases ranging from mountains to air ships. The first such proposals were made in the early 20th century by H. Ganswindt, who proposed that his projected spacecraft be lifted by helicopter to as great an altitude as possible, after which the rocket engine would be ignited. Analogous proposals (only using lighter-than-air craft) were advanced in the first quarter of the century by Goddard (1907)[32] Tsiolkovskiy (1911),[33] Oberth (1923),[26] and von Hoefft (1928).[34] This proposal was particularly attractive to inventors, because it eliminated the need to overcome the resistance of the densest layers of the atmosphere and would thus certainly decrease energy demands. However, the actual implementation of this proposal presented difficulties; it was totally impossible during this period, and even today is not in use.

The most farsighted of these proposals was the notion of launching rockets from platforms already orbiting in space—manmade space stations. This idea occurs in the works of a number of scientists. In 1928 the issue of using a satellite as an intermediate interplanetary station was considered in comparatively great detail in the work of von Pirquet.[35] Kondratyuk had the interesting idea of using not a manmade satellite, but the Moon itself as the intermediate base.[8,22] The idea of using manmade stations as intermediate bases is highly promising and has been incorporated in a number of modern projects for reaching remote celestial objects. In spite of this, it has still not been implemented, due to its complexity. In the period being considered here its implementation was completely out of the question.

Launching rockets from the Moon—or, conceivably, from other planetary bodies—had the additional advantage of offering possibilities for mining materials for rocket propellants.[22-24,36] Researchers were also influenced by the significantly lower (compared to Earth) weight of objects on these bodies, which would make it possible to attain lift-off speed using substantially less propellant. None of these researchers, however, thoroughly examined how one might obtain and process the essential material, build the launch complex, or undertake the other relatively complex technical operations associated with preparing and launching spacecraft from the Moon or other celestial bodies.

During the first quarter of the 20th century, scientists working on solution of the problems of space flight proposed one more very interesting idea—to use light pressure for interplanetary flights.[22,37,38] These scientists displayed correct understanding of when each of the different types of rocket engines would operate. When leaving or returning to Earth, they reasoned, i.e., at times when the Earth's gravity had to be overcome and significant acceleration imparted to the spacecraft, chemical propellants would have to be used; after injection into orbit at significant distances from Earth, i.e., during flight in interplanetary space, light pressure would be used as energy.

Thus, by the mid-1920s, at a point in time when no nation had yet created a reliable rocket engine or rocket-powered spacecraft, theoreticians had already solved in principle all the major problems associated with development of the theory of space flight.

C. Practical Development of Liquid-Propellant Rockets

After World War I, interest in the potential for interplanetary rocket flights increased. Beginning in the 1920s, under the influence of the work of Tsiolkovskiy, Goddard, Oberth and others working on problems of space flight, an increasing number of individuals began to think about the possibility of space flight. Clubs, associations, and scientific societies were established in various countries, bringing together people interested in this area. An increasing number of researchers began to work on scientific problems associated with interplanetary flight.

During this period practical work to build liquid propellant rockets began. The first liquid propellant rocket in the world was built by R. Goddard in the mid-1920s (Fig. 7) and successfully flight tested in March 1926.[10] Subsequently, Goddard continued to work on liquid propellant rockets and created a number of successful designs (see Table 3). During the 1930s, he worked to improve their control systems, and also on issues related to welding, insulation, and pumps. His later rockets achieved altitudes of 2286 m above the launch pad in New Mexico.

J. Winkler of Germany was responsible for the first European launch of a liquid-fueled rocket in 1931. From 1933 to 1941 about 30 different liquid-fueled rockets were developed in the U.S.S.R. Fourteen of them were tested in flight. Work on the "A" series of liquid-fueled rockets was started in Germany under the supervision of W. von Braun in 1934. This work concluded with the creation of the "A-4" rocket (Fig. 8) —the most advanced rocket of the period—in the early 1940s. This rocket would come to be known by another name, the V-2.

In addition to work on ballistic rockets, researchers began to consider the development of rocket-powered aircraft; winged rockets were developed and used fairly extensively in the 1930s for performing various experiments and flight studies (see Table 3). They served as a kind of intermediate link between ballistic rockets and rocket gliders. The idea of combining rockets and aircraft to meet the challenges of space flight is first encountered in the work of the early space flight theoreticians. The first mention can be found in 1913 in R. Esnault-Pelterie.[14] Tsander began to work on the development of an "Interplanetary Air-Spacecraft" and in 1921 he presented this idea to an inventors conference in Moscow. In 1924 he presented a completed design (Fig. 9) to the Committee on Inventions.[24]

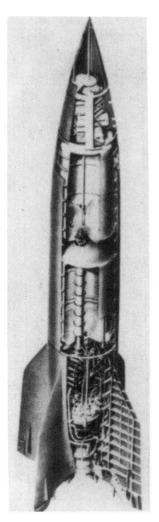

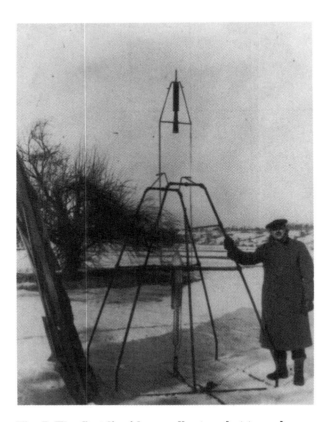

Fig. 7 The first liquid propellant rocket to undergo flight testing (Goddard, 1926) (NASA 74-H-1065)

Fig. 8 German liquid propellant A-4 (V2) rocket (1942) (Reprinted from Marbarger, J.P. (Ed.) *Space Medicine*. The University of Illinois Press at Urbana, 1951, p. 16.)

Table 3 Ballistic and winged rockets, flights tested prior to the 1940s

Type of propellant	Ballistic Rockets			Winged Rockets		
	<50 kg	50 - 500 kg	>500 kg	<50 kg	50 - 100 kg	>100 kg
Solid	RS-82 (1932-33) RS-132 (1932-33) Damblanc (1935) ARS (1935-39) M-8 (1939) M-13 (1939)	Damblanc (1938-39) R-604 (1940) R-521 (1940)		Tilling (1932) 48/I (1934-35) 48/II (1934-35)	217/I (1936) 217/II (1936)	803 (1940)
Liquid Benzine kerosene + oxygen	Goddard (1926, 1929, 1932) Repulsor (1931) ARS No 2-4 (1933-34)	Goddard* *A(1935) *L-6 (1936) *L-II (1937) *P-15 (1940)				
Liquid Ethanol + oxygen	GIRD-X (1933) GIRD-07 (1935) RBD-01/2 (1936) R-03 (1936-38) R-06 (1936-38) ANIR-5 (1939)	A-2 (1934) Aviavnito (1936)	A-3 (1938) A-5 (1939)		06/III (1936-37)	
Liquid propellants Kerosene (benzine) + nitric acid (nitric oxides)		R-604 (1940) R-521 (1940)				212/603 (1940) 803 (1940)
Hybrid	GIRD-09 (1933) GIRD-13 (1933-34)			06/1 (1934) 06/II (1935-36)		
Ram-jet engine using chemical propellants	Merkulov's rocket (1939)					

Starting in the 1920s, the Austrian rocket enthusiast Max Valier worked on the issue of installing a rocket engine on aircraft. Valier[19] saw the rocket-powered aircraft as the starting point for development of spacecraft. Another Austrian scientist, von Hoefft,[34] worked on development of interplanetary spacecraft using aerodynamic lift. E. Saenger made a valuable contribution to the theory of rocket powered aircraft. In 1933, he published *The Technology of Rocket Flight*,[40] in which he considered rocket-spaceplanes as a means of attaining high altitudes and flight velocities. Subsequently, with his collaborator, Irene Bredt, he continued to work in this area. The results of their work were summarized in a project report, "On the rocket-spaceplane," which was published later in 1944, with some additional military chapters, as "On the rocket engine for long-range bombing".[41]

Practical development of winged rockets began in the 1930s in Germany (Tilling, 1932) and the U.S.S.R. (RNII/ Reactive Propulsion Research Institute, 1934-1939). Later (during World War II), the A-7 (1941), A-9 (1943-44), and A-4B (1944) rockets were developed in Peenemunde.

Work on long-range guided missiles in the 1930s and 1940s led to the solution of a number of research problems in the area of rocket flight dynamics, including supersonic aerodynamics and strengthened structures and materials for flight vehicles. Engineers were also able to design more reliable liquid-fueled engines with thrusts of 25-27 tons, and develop a variety of propellant combinations as well as guidance and control systems, without which further progress in rocket technology would not have been possible.

Scientific research centers were established in virtually all the larger countries to conduct research in the area of rocket technology. At the end of the 1930s and beginning of the 1940s, such developments as multistage rockets for studying the upper atmosphere and for intercontinental missiles, liquid propellant rocket engines with thrusts of up to 100-200 tons and a number of very promising systems of control and guidance had reached the stage of long-range development in Germany, the U.S.S.R. and the U.S.

However, as was the case with space flight theory, theoretical engineering designs outstripped practical capacities, so that these extremely interesting projects were not implemented before the end of World War II. At the same time World War II persuasively demonstrated the enormous potential of solid- and especially liquid-propellant rockets. This made it possible to turn to building of long-range and then space rockets immediately after the war ended.

II. Development of Rocket and Space Technology and Space Biology After World War II

A. Work on Rocket-Powered Flight Vehicles After 1945

After the end of World War II, a number of industrially developed countries, especially the U.S. and U.S.S.R, resumed their work on liquid-propellant rockets, making extensive use of experience accumulated in the prewar and postwar years in various countries (Germany, U.S.S.R., U.S.A., and others). The complex international situation that developed in the mid 1940s, including the Cold War and military conflicts between countries representing different social systems, encouraged increased attention to liquid-propellant rockets.

The ways in which rocket technology was developed in the U.S. and U.S.S.R. were somewhat different. In the U.S, along with work on ballistic missiles (MX-774, Viking, and others), from the very beginning great attention was devoted to winged missiles (explosive robot aircraft) and also the "X-series" of experimental hypersonic rocket-powered aircraft. Engineers at the National Advisory Committee on Aeronautics (NACA) were encouraged in their work by material on a proposed hypersonic rocket-aircraft developed in 1944 by E. Saenger and I. Bredt.[41] This work eventually led to the ambitious X-20 Dyna-Soar project, which was ultimately cancelled because of excessive costs.

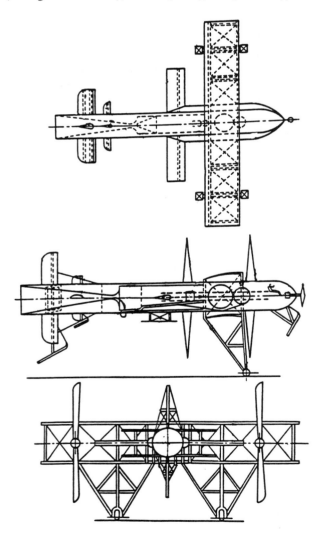

Fig. 9 Design of F.A. Tsander's high-altitude air-spacecraft (1926)

In the U.S.S.R. attention was focused from the very beginning on the development of long-range ballistic missiles. This goal was approached systematically, involving gradual increases in flight range, payload weight, engine thrust, and other rocket performance parameters. A 1946 resolution officially inaugurated a state rocket industry. Organizations were created and given the responsibility for developing missiles with automatic control, manufacture of rocket engines, systems of radio and internal control of rocket flight, and ground-based equipment and gyroscopic systems.

It should be noted that by the time extensive work began on rocket technology, the Soviet Union already had substantial experience from prewar and wartime work. This included the design of rockets and their systems, the building of powerful and relatively reliable rocket engines, and to a lesser extent, but still important, experience with automatic flight control systems. All this made it possible to use captured technology [in particular, the German A-4 (V-2) rocket] to accelerate rocket development. Development of the first Soviet long-range ballistic missile, the R-1, began in 1947; the first flight tests had been conducted by the fall of 1948 and in 1949 work on the R-1 was completed. Aside from its military uses, this missile was used to study thermal conditions during flight and to verify methods of ballistic and strength calculations as well as methods for analyzing flight stability. Production methods for technology of this type were developed, systems and machinery for production were assembled, and supporting materials research was conducted.

While the R-1 was being manufactured and tested, the staffs of various design bureaus, supported by institutes of the U.S.S.R. Academy of Sciences, conducted in-depth research on ways to make radical improvements in missiles. As a result, a completely new design configuration was developed for a ballistic missile involving integral fuel tanks and a nose cone that was jettisoned at the conclusion of the active portion of the trajectory. With a somewhat increased specific impulse and substantially increased engine thrust, the flight range of these missiles significantly exceeded that of the V-2. A great deal of research was conducted on the gas-dynamics of the reentry of the nose cone into the atmosphere and on related problems of thermal protection for the hulls of flight vehicles.

The R-2, developed under the direction of Sergey Korolyov, followed the R-1. With a flight range twice that of its predecessor, the configuration of the R-2 featured a nose cone that separated after the active portion of the trajectory and a partial replacement of structural steel by aluminum alloys. Today, the integral design configuration with a separable nose cone is considered standard for both one- and two-stage rockets and launch vehicles. Designers from other countries have also adopted this configuration.

B. Upper Atmosphere Research

Advances during the 1940s in long-range ballistic missile development allowed scientists to use rockets to study the upper atmosphere, a use forecast earlier by Tsiolkovskiy,

Goddard, Oberth, Esnault-Pelterie, and others. Indeed, during the 1930s, S.P. Korolyov, M.K. Tikhonravov, T. von Kármán, F. Malina, and scientific conferences in several countries explored practical proposals to use rockets to study the stratosphere. In 1934 in the U.S.S.R. (Leningrad), an All-Union Conference on the study of the stratosphere was held, at which several papers were devoted to the possibility of using rockets for that purpose. These proposals were included in the resolutions of the conference.[42] In 1935 in Moscow, there was a conference totally devoted to this issue,[43] at which V.P. Vetchinkin, V.P. Glushko, S.P. Korolyov, Yu.A. Pobedonostsev, M.K. Tikhonravov, and other scientists and engineers read papers. In the U.S. in February 1936, researchers at the Guggenheim Aeronautical Laboratory of the California Institute of Technology began a program to develop a high-altitude research rocket. The group's efforts, which required the development of a reliable engine and computation of flight characteristics, were halted at the beginning of World War II. Work was resumed in 1943-44, resulting in 1945 in successful flight tests of the WAC-Corporal, which attained an altitude of approximately 250,000 feet (over 70 km).

Comparable progress occurred concurrently in the Soviet Union, where in 1943 the Physics Institute of the U.S.S.R. Academy of Sciences proposed building a rocket equipped with scientific instruments that could reach an altitude of 40 km. In 1945, a stratospheric three-stage solid-propellant rocket was developed in the Laboratory of M.K. Tikhonravov under the direction of P.I. Ivanov. In 1946, tests were performed with generally positive results. However, by this point it was clear that liquid-propellant rockets had significantly greater potential.

Rocket-based study of the upper atmosphere was relatively extensive in the U.S. as well. As early as January 1946, the Artillery and Logistics Command issued an announcement concerning the use of rockets in research. In April of the same year, the U.S. Air Force conducted a vertical launch of a captured A-4 (V-2) rocket, which reached a height of approximately 100 km. After this, rocket-based upper atmosphere research progressed rapidly in the U.S. V-2 rockets were used (from 1946 to 1951 there were 70 vertical launches of such rockets), as well as the specially designed high-altitude Aerobee (manufactured by the Aerojet firm) and Viking (Glenn-Martin) rockets. The highest altitude (approximately 400 km) was attained using Bumper two-stage rockets (first stage–V-2, second stage–a solid-propellant WAC-Corporal rocket built in 1945 at the California Institute of Technology) (Fig. 10).

From 1947-1949, the Soviets launched six liquid fueled ballistic missiles based on V-2 rockets, to carry out high-altitude research. By May 1949, the U.S.S.R. had reached an altitude of 110 km with V-1A (Fig. 11) liquid-fueled upper atmosphere research rockets based on the R-1 rocket.

During the initial period of high-altitude research, scientists focused primarily on such questions as the change in the composition of the atmosphere with altitude, the density of meteor dust, ambient temperature and pressure, ionospheric

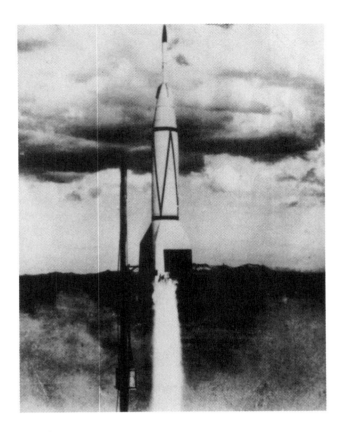

Fig. 10 American Bumper high altitude rocket (1949) (NASA 67-H-1452)

investigations, study of solar radiation, intensity of cosmic rays, and other issues associated with the physics of the upper atmosphere. Subsequently, the range of issues studied expanded considerably.

C. Biomedical Research

In addition to the scientific and technological aspects of space flight, early theoreticians also focused on biomedical problems associated with the need for humans to live and work in space and endure high acceleration on take-off and landing.

If humans were to travel through space, the kinds and degrees of physiological risks to which they might be subjected—whether those risks were tolerable, and how they might be minimized—had to be understood and countermeasures developed. As early as the 1870s, K.E. Tsiolkovskiy conducted experiments on the effects of acceleration on animals,[44] and in the early 1890s he proposed possible techniques for protecting humans from high levels of acceleration.[45] Oberth, too, wrote about the possible consequences of acceleration and reduced gravity on humans. At the end of the 1920s and beginning of the 1930s, experiments with animals under conditions simulating space flight were conducted by N.A. Rynin, A.A. Likhachyov[46] (U.S.S.R.), and C.D. Generales (U.S.).[47] As noted above, a conference on the

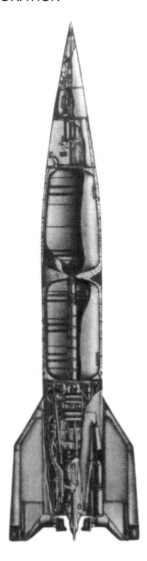

Fig. 11 Soviet V-1A geophysical rocket (1949)

stratosphere was held in Leningrad in 1934, where a number of papers were devoted to various aspects of biomedical study of the stratosphere and space flight.[42]

High-altitude rockets also made it possible in the late 1940s and early 1950s to begin research associated with preparation for the first flights of animals in the upper atmosphere and space. As early as 1946-1947, at the White Sands testing grounds, V-2 rockets carried fungi spores and *Drosophila* to an altitude of approximately 100 km.[48] A systematic biological research program was conducted in the United States between 1948 and 1951, involving flights of monkeys and mice on V-2 and Aerobee rockets. The first passenger to fly on the V-2 rocket was the rhesus monkey called Albert. The first time a monkey and mice were returned successfully was the 1951 flight of the Aerobee rocket.[49] Telemetric recording of physiological measurements enabled scientists to study the influence of dynamic flight factors (including weightlessness of up to 2-3 minutes in duration) on the cardiovascular system. In addition, the behavior of mice was recorded with movie cameras.

In 1948-1950, the first two symposia on biological problems of space flight were organized in the United States by Harry G. Armstrong. The proceedings of the second of these symposia were edited by J.P. Marbarger and published in 1951, becoming the first book to bear the title *Space Medicine*.[50] This encouraged the treatment of this field as a new medical discipline.

In 1950 the Soviet Union established a special group for the study of the biomedical problems of flight on high-altitude rockets.within the Institute of Aviation Medicine. This group, headed by V.I. Yazdovskiy and staffed by flight surgeons, physiologists, and other biomedical personnel, as well as engineers, was made a department of the Institute in 1956. During the early 1950s the Soviet Union flew dogs and other biological subjects on vertical launches of rockets at altitudes on the order of 100-220 km. The first dogs to attain an altitude of 100 km (in June 1951) on the R-1B (V-1B) rocket were called Tsygan and Desik.

These studies showed that animals (dogs and monkeys) could satisfactorily endure the dynamic phases of flight and a period of weightlessness (3-6 minutes). They also showed that the life support, ejection, and parachute landing systems, as well as the methods used for recording physiological functions and filming the animals, operated effectively.[49, 51] (See Fig. 12.)

Of all the biomedical disciplines, none was as important to the pioneering days of human space travel as aviation medicine. From its unique perspective at the juncture of medicine and technology, this discipline had revealed a great deal about the physiological effects of flight factors, the interaction of man and machine, life support and flight safety systems, flight certification, medical selection, and monitoring of the health of flight crews. It was thus natural for flight surgeons to be among the first medical personnel to help prepare the first astronauts and cosmonauts for space.

It is noteworthy that space medicine began to develop as a discipline 10 years before the first manned space flight (1951 vs. 1961); in contrast, aeronautical medicine did not get started until more than 90 years after the first manned balloon flight (1783 vs. 1875), and aviation medicine not until 10-20 years after the birth of aviation (1903 vs. 1910-1920).

D. Further Development of Ballistic Rockets

In the late 1940s and early 1950s, work on ballistic missiles entered a new phase, surpassing all that had been achieved before the end of World War II. In the U.S.S.R., during the second half of the 1940s, work began on the R-3 long-range ballistic missile project (with projected flight range up to 3000 km) and then (after 1951) work began on designing the R-5 and R-7 missiles. During this period, intensive research was conducted on the development of propulsion systems, flight control systems, and ground launch and command complexes. A great deal of work was also performed on the mechanics of rocket flight, the problem of providing thermal insulation, and other issues associated with the development of rocket and

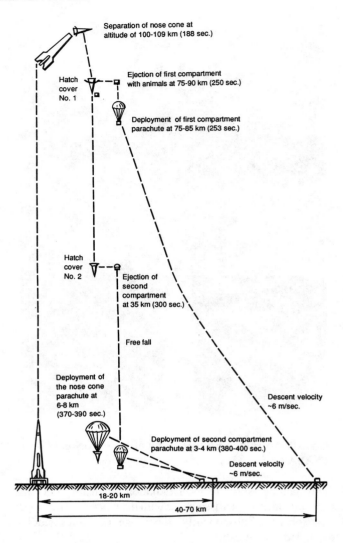

Fig. 12 General plan of flight of dogs on R-1E (V-1E) high-altitude rockets

space technology. These investigations were conducted by selected design bureaus, as well as by scientific research institutes of the U.S.S.R. Academy of Sciences. A major role was played by M. V. Keldysh.

In the U.S. during the early and mid-1950s, work was conducted on short-range (Redstone) and mid-range (Jupiter and Thor) ballistic missiles and intercontinental rockets (Atlas and Titan). In 1950 the United States established the Army Ordnance Guided Missile Center at its Redstone Arsenal, transferring to the new organization the team of German rocket scientists, under the leadership of Wernher von Braun, who had been flying captured V-2 rockets at the White Sands, New Mexico, test range since emigrating to the United States in 1945. Taking a conservative, systematic approach, the von Braun team developed the Redstone missile which, in 1961, would launch the first U.S. astronaut into a suborbital flight. These missiles could launch ballistic payloads over distances ranging from 280 km (Redstone) to 9650 km (Titan 1). The Atlas (first successfully flown in 1958), when combined with the Centaur upper stage, could lift over 1100 kg to Earth orbit; with the Agena upper stage the Atlas could lift over 2500 kg.

By 1952 one of the most serious problems confronting missile and spacecraft designers—aerodynamic heating on reentry—was solved in the United States by H. Julian (Harvey) Allen. Up until that time, researchers had assumed that the slender needle-nosed shape was the best aerodynamic shape for a missile nose cone, and they had dealt with the reentry problem by concentrating on improved ablative materials. Allen, observing that "meteors get through the atmosphere," proposed a blunt-nosed shape.[52] Allen tested the blunt-body concept in a special wind tunnel he had designed, and confirmed that a blunt body moving at extreme speed generates a bow shock wave that dissipates heat to the air; only a small portion of the total heat remains in the boundary layer near the body. Combined with ablative heat shields, the blunt-nose principle became a part of the design of essentially all U.S. reentry vehicles—intercontinental ballistic missiles (ICBMs), early manned spacecraft, and the Space Shuttle.

Work was done in the United States in the late 1940s and early 1950s on the development of winged cruise missiles powered by air-breathing turbojet engines. Most remarkable among these vehicles was the Navaho surface-to-surface guided missile, which weighed 136,000 kg and demonstrated through three successful flights that it was capable of carrying a warhead over a maximum range of 10,000 km, reaching speeds of Mach 3.

The United States was able to transfer some of the technological experience it had acquired in its cruise missile work to the development of intercontinental ballistic missiles. The Navaho's all-inertial guidance system could be used for ICBMs, and the heavy vehicle was initially lifted into the air by three liquid-fueled rocket engines with 54,000 kg of thrust each. Developed by the commercial firm of Rocketdyne, variants of the Navaho booster-engines were developed for the Thor, Atlas, Redstone, and Jupiter rockets; the engines developed for the Jupiter were instrumental in the evolution of the engines for the Saturn rocket that carried the first humans to the Moon.

The extremely rapid development of rocket technology in both the United States and Soviet Union made it possible for the first flight of a manmade satellite to occur in a matter of a few years.

E. Preparations for the First Satellite Flight

In the mid-1950s (1954-1955) work to develop rocket technology reached a new level, making the task of creating a booster rocket to launch a manmade satellite an attainable one. It should be noted that exploratory work in this area had begun as early as the mid-1940s, when individual groups of researchers began to study the practical possibility of building manmade satellites. In the U.S. during this period (1945-1946) specialists of the Aeronautics Bureau of the U.S. Navy and the "Project Rand" group of the U.S. Army began to work on this problem.[53]

Beginning in 1947 in the U.S.S.R. a group of researchers under the direction of M.K. Tikhonravov began to work on developing a theoretical rationale for the possible construction of compound (multistage) rockets, including wrap-around configuration rockets. The solution of this problem made it possible to achieve orbital velocity using existing rocket technology. Subsequently the scientists in this group continued to work in this area, concentrating (starting in 1953) on in-depth study of the problem of building a manmade satellite.

In 1955, the U.S. officially announced the forthcoming launch of a manmade satellite within the Vanguard project[54] using a three-stage rocket of the same name. Meanwhile the U.S. was also working on the Jupiter-C four-stage rocket, developed under the direction of W. von Braun.

In 1954, S. P. Korolyov proposed to the Soviet government that practical work be begun on a manmade satellite based on the R-7 two-stage intercontinental ballistic missiles that were being developed at that time.[55] This work represented a major advance in the development of rocket technology—a completely new rocket system, which presented scientists and engineers with broad potential and which led to the creation of a completely new form of technology—space rockets.

In 1957, the work being conducted in the U.S.S.R. to design and manufacture the R-7 rocket was completed successfully. On August 21 of that year the first launch of a two-stage intercontinental ballistic missile took place, and on October 4, 1957, using a modified booster rocket, later named the "Sputnik" booster rocket (Figs. 13 and 14), the first manmade satellite was launched into orbit around the Earth. This outstanding event made an enormous impression on the world community and marked the beginning of a new epoch—the space era—in human history.

III. Dawn of the Space Era

A. Early Satellites

After the first manmade satellite was launched, work to study and explore space continued at an accelerated rate. Only a month after the start of the space era, the U.S.S.R. placed a second manmade satellite in orbit. This was also the first biological satellite—carrying the dog Layka.

Less than 4 months after the launch of Sputnik, in January 1958, the United States used a Jupiter-C booster to launch Explorer 1 to an orbital altitude of 2876 km. Because of the United States' early success in miniaturizing instruments and electronics, Explorer 1's scientific instruments weighed only 8.24 kg, yet made one of the most important discoveries of the International Geophysical Year: the Earth's Van Allen radiation belts. Explorer 1 was followed on March 17 by Vanguard 1, which contained the first solar-powered batteries and whose geodetic observations showed that the Earth was actually pear shaped. Nine days later a Jupiter-C launched another Explorer satellite into orbit, which provided further information on the

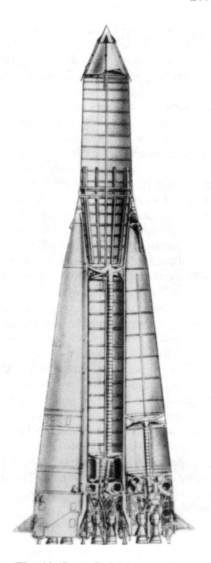

Fig. 13 Sputnik booster rocket

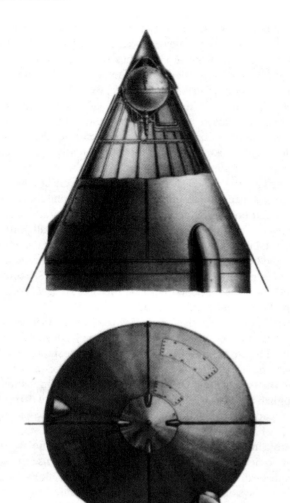

Fig. 14 First manmade Earth satellite under the nose cone of the rocket (October 1957)

Earth's radiation belts. The momentous possibilities of space travel were already becoming apparent in these first months of the space age.

The third Soviet satellite, launched on March 15, 1958, was actually a kind of space laboratory. It weighed 1327 kg and carried more than 10 different scientific instruments, which were used to perform a rather extensive program of research on near-Earth space.

By the close of 1960 the United States had successfully launched 35 satellites, including the Explorer, Pioneer, and Discoverer series. These launches not only increased knowledge of the physical and electromagnetic environment of near-Earth space, but also resulted in the first transmittal of a human voice from space (Score, launched December 1958), the first polar orbit (Discoverer 1, launched February 1959), a record for space communication of 41.1 million km on June 26, 1960 (Pioneer 5, launched March 1960), the first global cloud-cover photographs from orbit (Tiros 1, launched April 1960), and the first successful recovery of a manmade object

from orbital flight (Discoverer 13, launched August 1960).

After the launch of the first manmade satellites, marking the start of the space era, researchers were confronted with the need to select further directions for the development of rocket and space technology. At the time it was thought that three major directions were possible: 1) improvement of robotic, unmanned satellites for the study and utilization of near-Earth space; 2) development of unmanned spacecraft for the study of the Moon and the neighboring planets of the solar system; 3) development of spacecraft for manned flights in space.

In both the U.S. and U.S.S.R., work proceeded simultaneously in all three directions. By the end of the 1950s and the beginning of the 1960s, a large number of manmade satellites had been placed in orbit around the Earth. These satellites facilitated the study and exploration of space and the solution of a number of research and applied problems. During these years progress in Earth orbit continued, and both the U.S. and U.S.S.R. launched unmanned probes to the Moon, Venus, and Mars. Scientists and designers also began to prepare for the flight of humans in space, and work on manned spacecraft began. In the U.S.S.R. this work was conducted under the general direction of the Council of Chief Designers, including at that time S.P. Korolyov, V.P. Glushko, N.A. Pilyugin, V.P. Barmin, V.I. Kuznetsov, and M.S. Ryazanskiy.

B. Use of Satellites to Solve Applied Problems

During the first years of the space era, when robotic or manned spacecraft (manmade Earth satellites, interplanetary probes, or space vehicles) were launched, their chief mission was typically neither to solve a serious scientific problem nor to produce a direct practical benefit. During this period, scientists, engineers, and other experts working in this area considered their chief mission to be proving that it was possible to achieve some concrete goal: launching a satellite; flying living creatures in space; landing a vehicle built on Earth to another celestial body (the Moon); launching fly-by probes to Venus and Mars; performing extravehicular activities (EVAs), etc. In all these cases, everything was being done for the first time, and the chief objective was to achieve the goal that had been set. Of course, some scientific and applied problems were solved along the way, but at this stage they represented subordinate, and not major, goals. However, as early as the middle of the first decade in space (around the beginning of the 1960s), the relationships between these two very different aspects of space exploration began to change gradually—the importance and complexity of the scientific and applied tasks addressed by space researchers began to increase.

In this context, the launch of the first manmade satellite marked the beginning of the systematic study of near-Earth space. Although the spacecraft launched during this period were experimental, even during the first years of the space era they generated a considerable amount of new information on the composition of the upper atmosphere, the ionosphere, and magnetosphere. For example, Explorer 1's discovery of Earth's radiation belts convincingly demonstrated the efficacy of manmade satellites as a new and powerful means of scientific study of near-Earth space.

Experience with manmade satellites in the late 1950s and early 1960s also demonstrated their potential for solving applied problems. The best example was the extensive use of communications and meteorological satellites. Subsequently satellites were also used for geodesy and cartography, understanding environmental change and the use of natural resources, tracing land use patterns, and for navigation.

C. Communications Satellites

As World War II drew to a close in the spring of 1945, British scientist Arthur C. Clarke proposed, before the British Interplanetary Society and in the pages of *Wireless World*,[56] a system of three geostationary satellites positioned at equal distances on a circular equatorial orbit at a height of approximately 36,000 km. At this orbital distance the period of Earth-satellites matches the rotation rate of the Earth. Such a system could provide virtually simultaneous global radio communications. However, in the mid-1940s this proposal could not be implemented, since it was 10 years ahead of its time and the technology for putting satellites into orbit was only developed in the late 1950s.

Sputnik, the first manmade satellite to orbit the Earth, launched in October 1957, was equipped with a radio-transmitter whose signals were received by ground stations. Slightly more than a year later in December 1958, the United States, with its experimental communications satellite Score, transmitted the first human voice from space as U.S. President Dwight D. Eisenhower sent a personal recorded Christmas message to the Earth.

The initial stage in the development of communications satellites (1958-1964) was marked by theoretical exploration and field tests of manmade satellites for retransmitting radio signals (passive and active). Echo 1 and Echo 2, passive satellites flown by the United States in 1960 and 1964, respectively, were large reflective balloons (31 m and 42 m in diameter). Two months after the launch of Echo 1, the United States successfully demonstrated the possibility of active global communications with the Courier 1-B satellite. The potential of global communications satellites was also amply demonstrated by communications satellites in the Soviet Union's Cosmos series and by the United States' Telstar 1 (the first active-repeater comsat, launched July 1962), Relay (a medium-altitude active-repeater comsat), and others. The first live transatlantic telecast was relayed by Telstar 1, inaugurating global television communications from medium-Earth orbit.

Among the most successful communications satellites during this period were the Telstar (mass 77 kg) satellites launched by the United States in July 1962 and May 1963. These satellites provided 20 minutes of television communications between opposite shores of the Atlantic Ocean (U.S. and Europe), marking the beginning of global television communications based on satellites in low Earth orbit. The global nature of satellite communications made it necessary to deal with practical issues. In 1963 an Extraordinary Administrative Conference of the International Telecommunications Union was convened in Geneva. The Conference adopted a resolution reserving a special frequency band (in the range 3.4-8.4 GHz) for satellite communications and regulating the parameters and operating procedures of ground stations. Affirming the truly international nature of communications for the future, Syncom 3, launched into an equatorial orbit in August 1964, transmitted the opening ceremonies of the XVIII Olympic Games in Tokyo to viewers all over the globe.

During the same month, the International Telecommunications Satellite Organization (INTELSAT) was created as an international corporation to produce, manage, and operate a global satellite communications system. In April 1965, this organization launched the first commercial geostationary communications satellite, Early Bird (INTELSAT 1). At virtually the same time, the U.S.S.R. put the Molniya 1 automated communications satellite into synchronous orbit. This satellite was launched by the four-stage Molniya booster rocket developed by S.P. Korolyov's Experimental Design Bureau. This satellite was designed for long-distance telephone and phototelegraphic communications. Using this satellite as a base, the U.S.S.R. developed the Orbita satellite communications system, designed to serve extensive regions of the country, especially its more remote and inaccessible areas. The launch of Syncom 3, INTELSAT 1, and Molniya 1 marked the beginning of a new stage in the development of space communications—the gradual development of internal and regional systems of satellite communications based on satellites in geostationary orbit.

D. Meteorological Satellites

Another direction in the history of applied satellite systems in the late 1950s and early 1960s was the development of meteorological satellites designed for operational observations and transmission to ground stations of cloud-cover images and information about thermal emissions of the Earth to provide meteorological data for weather prediction.

Upper atmospheric research with instrumented rockets in the late 1940s and early 1950s inaugurated the era of global climate study from space. Meteorological satellites extended capacities in this area, enabling the routine and systematic study of processes occurring in the upper atmosphere. This challenged scientists to further increase the use of satellites for atmospheric observations. Tiros 1, the first of 10 satellites transmitting data from above the clouds, was launched by the United States in April 1960. The flight was successful and demonstrated the practicality of weather satellites. The Nimbus and ESSA satellites, first launched in 1964 and 1966, respectively, increased the coverage of global weather patterns.

Between 1963 and 1964 the U.S.S.R. developed meteorological satellites of the Cosmos 23 type. In June 1966, the Cosmos 122 satellite, carrying a set of instruments for meteorological research, was launched and, in February-April 1967, Cosmos 144 and Cosmos 156 were put into orbit. These two satellites formed the Meteor experimental space meteorological system, which provided essential meteorological data on a global scale with very little delay.

E. Lunar and Planetary Exploration

Advances in rocketry during the post-World War II period enabled the rocket-powered vehicles of the late 1950s and 1960s to attain sufficient velocity to escape Earth's gravity so that work could be begun to send unmanned spacecraft to the closest celestial bodies—the Moon, Venus, and Mars. As early as 1959, using the Vostok three-stage booster rocket, the Soviet Union successively launched (in January, September, and October) the three unmanned spacecraft Luna 1, 2, and 3. The first approached within 5000 to 6000 km of the Moon's surface and, overcoming Earth's gravity, went into orbit around the Sun, becoming the first manmade satellite of the Sun. The second collided with the surface of the Moon, and the third flew past the Moon and photographed the far side (which cannot be seen from Earth), and transmitted the images back to Earth. This flight subsequently made it possible to draw the first map and atlas of portions of the far side of the Moon.

In March 1959, the American unmanned probe Pioneer 4 was the first U.S. spacecraft to achieve Earth escape velocity. It flew to within 60,000 km of the lunar surface, and went into solar orbit (with an aphelion of 148 million km and a perihelion of 120 million km). With the flight of Pioneer 5 in 1960, communications were maintained up to a distance of 36.2 million km from the Earth. In April 1962, the Ranger 4 probe (weighing approximately 365 kg) impacted the surface of the Moon. The most successful spacecraft in the Ranger series was Ranger 7. During its high-speed approach to lunar impact, Ranger 7's 6 television cameras obtained more than 4000 photographs of the lunar surface which improved the effective magnification of available images of the Moon by a factor of 2000, making it possible to see lunar craters with diameters as small as approximately 1 mile. Ranger 8 and Ranger 9, launched during February and March of 1965, transmitted more than 7000 and 6000 images, respectively.

An important benchmark in lunar exploration was achieved when the Soviet Luna 9 probe made it possible to land a 100 kg instrument capsule on the Moon (February 1966). This enabled direct experimental investigations of the surface of the Moon, and for the first time provided reliable information about the structure of the lunar soil. Cameras transmitted panoramic photos of the lunar surface near the Ocean of Storms.

The next spacecraft to make soft landings on the surface of the Moon were Surveyor 1 (U.S., May-June 1966), Luna 13 (U.S.S.R., December 1966), and Surveyors 3, 5, 6, and 7 (U.S., April 1967-January 1968). These probes investigated the mechanical and chemical properties of lunar soil. A large number of photographs were obtained and transmitted to Earth. In addition, one of the probes (Surveyor 6) relocated to another point on the lunar surface (a distance of approximately 2.5 m) using three vernier liquid-propellant rocket engines.

The mid-1960s also witnessed the first manmade satellite in orbit around the Moon. The Soviet Union's Luna 10 spacecraft was placed into lunar orbit in April 1966. Weighing 245 kg, it carried instruments that gathered data (transmitted back to Earth over a period of 2 months) on near-Moon space as well as on the Moon's magnetic and gravitational fields, the composition of its rock, infrared and gamma radiation at the lunar surface, radiation and meteor conditions, and other phenomena. Active radio communications with the spacecraft were maintained for approximately 2 months (until the on-board power supply was exhausted). During this period there were more than 200 communications sessions, and a significant amount of scientific information was obtained.

The United States' 380 kg Lunar Orbiter followed in August of that same year, photographing possible sites for an

American manned Moon landing and obtaining the first view of Earth from the Moon. Subsequently, more than 10 manmade lunar orbiters were launched by the U.S. and U.S.S.R. (Lunar Orbiter 2, 3, 4, 5, and Luna 11, 12, 14, 15, 18, 19, 22).

Research was begun on the planets of the solar system using robotic probes in the early 1960s. In May 1961 the U.S.S.R.'s Venera 1 probe, launched in February and weighing 643 kg, passed within approximately 100,000 km of the surface of Venus after traveling on the order of 270 million km. Eighteen months later, in December 1962, the United States' Mariner 2 probe, which weighed over 200 kg, passed within 35,000 km of the venusian surface and returned the first data about the planet's magnetic field, its heavily clouded atmosphere, and its mass.

In November 1962, the U.S.S.R. used the four-stage Molniya booster rocket to dispatch the Mars 1 probe (mass 898 kg) to within 197,000 km of the martian surface, although no data were returned. The U.S. Mariner 4 and U.S.S.R. Zond 2 probes followed in 1964. Mariner 4 passed within a comparatively small distance (approximately 10,000 km) from Mars and returned the first data about that planet, transmitting more than 20 photographs of its surface and additional data about the composition of its atmosphere. The Soviet Union launched two spacecraft toward Venus in November 1965—Venera 2 and Venera 3. Four months later Venera 3 became not only the first spacecraft to enter the venusian atmosphere, but the first to make a hard landing on the planet's surface.

Development of interplanetary probes designed to fly to Mars and Venus raised a number of new issues, which had never before been confronted by the developers of space technology. These issues included:

• The absence of reliable information about physical conditions on these planets (the composition of their atmosphere, their pressure and temperatures, etc.), which compelled development of equipment capable of withstanding a relatively wide range of environmental parameters

• The significant distance between these planets and Earth (on the order of hundreds of million km) and the relatively long duration of the flights (up to 7-8 months) made it necessary to ensure reliable control of spacecraft flight at great distances, sufficient power resources for the probes, increased reliability of operation of on-board systems, and improved temperature regulation systems

• The impossibility of ensuring in advance (at the time of launch) that the interplanetary probes would hit their target on the planet required midcourse correction of interplanetary flight trajectories, and thus development of a special engine capable of being turned on more than once during space flight

All of these goals were essentially attained during the first half of the 1960s, resulting in the launch of the probes enumerated above (Venera 1, 2, 3; Mariner 2, 4; Mars 1; Zond 2). The flight of these probes yielded the first experimental data on the characteristics of interplanetary space, and made it possible to test the operation of various systems during long-term space flight and to improve long-distance radio communications.

During the first half of the 1960s new basic data on the neighboring planets of the solar system had not yet been obtained by the interplanetary probes, since during this period not one had been able to achieve a soft landing on the surface of these planets and transmit information to Earth about their physical conditions and the composition of their atmospheres.

However, in October 1967, the Venera 4 probe travelled over 350 million km and entered the atmosphere of Venus with escape velocity. Next, a descent module carrying scientific instruments and two radio transmitters separated from it and began a 1 and 1/2 hour parachute descent into the atmosphere of Venus, while measuring pressure, density, temperature, and chemical composition, and transmitted this information to Earth.

These measurements showed that temperature and pressure increased as the apparatus descended into the planet's atmosphere. After slightly more than 90 minutes of descent (at an altitude of approximately 22 km), radio communication with the apparatus stopped. By this time atmospheric pressure had reached 18 atmospheres and temperature had reached 277 °C, unexpected pressure and temperature values for which the descent module and its equipment had not been designed. In general, the flight of Venera 4 provided extremely interesting scientific results, which significantly altered existing scientific ideas about this planet. For the first time scientists could study experimental data on the venusian atmosphere at a pressure interval of 0.5-18 atm. They also learned that the planet's atmosphere is primarily (more than 90 percent) composed of carbon dioxide, and not nitrogen, as was believed previously.

Two days after the launch of Venera 4, a U.S. Atlas-Agena D booster lifted the 245 kg Mariner 5 on its journey to Venus. Designed to fly by the planet at 4000 km, Mariner 5 was instrumented to gather data on its way to Venus about the interplanetary environment during a period of increased solar activity. With the spacecraft's instruments, scientists learned that the solar wind interacts with Venus, which has no radiation belts or atmospheric oxygen. The Mariner 5 mission was flawless; the spacecraft returned intelligible telemetry from as far as 320 million km and was still operating 36 months after launch.

Thus, the flights of robotic spacecraft to the planets of the solar system during the first decade of the space era enabled direct study of the planets through fly-by spacecraft or landers.

F. Animals in Orbit: Biological Research on Rockets and Orbital Spacecraft

The first orbital flight of a living creature (the dog Layka) (Fig. 15), on the nonrecoverable satellite Sputnik 2, enabled testing of the life support system, methods of selecting and training animals, and methods for monitoring and transmitting physiological data during flight. The experiment demonstrated that it was possible for higher animals to survive flights in near-Earth space.[57]

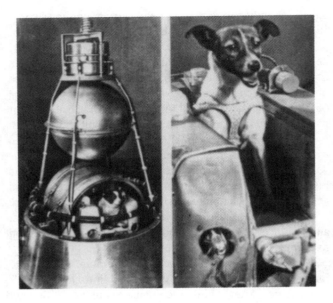

Fig. 15 The first living creature in near-Earth orbit—the dog Layka (November 1957)

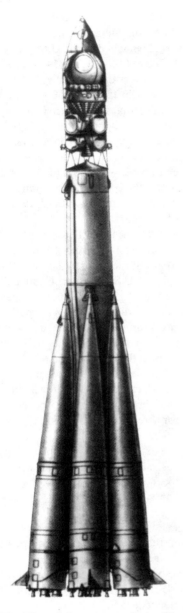

Fig. 16 The Vostok booster rocket with manned spacecraft

After Sputnik 2 was launched, biomedical studies in space developed rapidly. In 1958, the U.S.S.R. conducted experiments with dogs (ascending in rockets to altitudes up to 473 km) and other animals (mice, rats, rabbits). From 1958 to 1961, the U.S. performed biological experiments with monkeys and other biological subjects on high-altitude and ballistic rockets, and in 1960 on three Discoverer satellites (carrying microorganisms and grain). This program culminated in November 1961 with the two-orbit flight of the chimpanzee Enos aboard the Mercury spacecraft.[49] In France, the rat Hector flew to an altitude of over 150 km on the Veronique rocket in 1961, while the cat Felicette completed a similar flight in 1963.

To enable future manned space flight, means of safe recovery after orbital flight had to be developed. This was accomplished on flights of recoverable orbital spacecraft, such as the important flight in August, 1960 of the dogs Belka and Strelka and other biological subjects (of various species and at various phylogenetic levels) with full instrumentation and a thermally insulated descent module. The animal passengers were safely recovered close to the scheduled landing site after completing 17 orbits over the course of a day. In the spring of 1961, there were two more successful launches of orbital satellites carrying dogs and other biological subjects.[58] Flights of orbital spacecraft as well as biological experiments on rockets, supported the conclusion that human beings could safely fly in space and return to Earth.

G. Preparations for Manned Space Flight

Before any nation could hope to send humans into space it had to develop a booster rocket capable of carrying the weight of the spacecraft, the crew, and their supplies and support systems (in excess of 4.5 tons). Accordingly, under the direction of S.P. Korolyov, the Soviet Union added a third stage to its Sputnik launch vehicle, which became known as the Vostok booster (Figs. 16 and 17).

The creation of a reliable booster rocket allowed serious work to begin on the development of the Vostok spacecraft, intended for the first manned flight in space. The booster and spacecraft were developed virtually simultaneously and in a parallel fashion. The developers of the spacecraft confronted many complex and completely unprecedented problems without analogs in work on Earth.

Development of a "man-ratable" spacecraft required the design and production of systems for air regeneration, water supply, and maintenance of normal temperature conditions. It

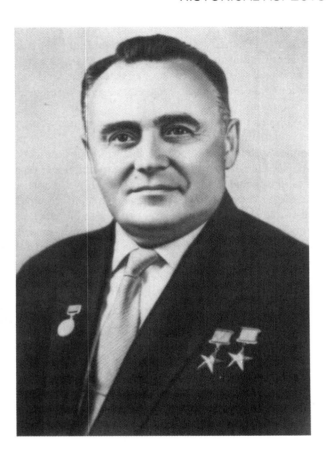

Fig. 17 S.P. Korolyov (1907-1966), chief designer of Soviet rocket and space systems

was also essential to return the crew to Earth safely, and to ensure that landing occurred in the preselected area, that acceleration was limited, and that thermal insulation of the spacecraft operated reliably upon entry into the dense layers of the atmosphere.

In designing its Vostok spacecraft, the Soviet Union chose to separate the craft into two principal modules, a descent module (containing the crew cabin with systems necessary for various stages of the flight up to and including landing) and a module containing instruments and equipment essential only for orbital flight and therefore not requiring thermal protection. Limiting thermal protection to the crew module reduced the weight of the total payload, a decided advantage, since it increased the weight available for additional equipment, instruments, and the life support system. This design also made the task of the designers and builders significantly easier, and was subsequently used in the design of the majority of Soviet spacecraft.

The United States took a different approach in the design of its first manned spacecraft, Mercury, which was begun in 1958. Mercury's integrated design combined the crew compartment with flight and life-support systems in a single spacecraft weighing 1832 kg. The design employed the "blunt-body" concept, which resulted in a sleek, conical

shape. Reentry heating was dissipated by the large flattened base of the conical capsule, which was slightly over 2 meters wide.

Meanwhile, the United States in summer 1959 began a series of 19 flight tests (ending in November 1961) of individual systems necessary for the first U.S. manned space flight. These systems included the escape tower, the instrumented capsule itself, the Redstone and Atlas booster rockets, and parachute landing, ocean surface recovery, telemetry, and tracking systems. The United States chose to conduct two suborbital test flights with astronauts before attempting a manned orbital flight.

At approximately the same time as these engineering developments were going on, the Soviet Union and the United States began to select and prepare their first contingents of cosmonauts and astronauts. This represented a considerable challenge to the physicians, psychiatrists, and flight training personnel in both countries during the first decade of human space travel. Both countries devoted considerable attention to the selection of space crews; candidates underwent a painstaking medical examination. Selection criteria included exemplary health, psychological stability, capacity to endure physical and psychological stress, physiological potential, etc. During preparation for flight, emphasis was placed on biomedical preparation, including conditioning of the muscle, cardiovascular, and vestibular systems. The main goal was to prepare candidates for the combined effects of such unfamiliar factors as acceleration, weightlessness, vibration, vehicle motion, psychological stress, and isolation.[59] The program made extensive use of thermal and barochambers, centrifuges, anechoic chambers, training simulators, vibration platforms, and other equipment.[60]

After a great deal of preparatory work, in the spring of 1960 the final stage of preparations for human space flight began in the Soviet Union—the flight of five unmanned Vostok orbital satellites to test their designs and systems for a manned space mission. The results showed that development of a spacecraft suitable for manned flight was virtually complete and that manned space flight using available technology was possible in principle and could be achieved without unacceptable risk. This made it possible to advance to the final stage of preparation for manned flight.

H. First Manned Flights

On April 12, 1961, only 3 1/2 years after the launch of Sputnik 1, a remarkable event occurred—cosmonaut Yuriy Gagarin (Fig. 18) rode Vostok into a 301 km by 174 km orbit of the Earth. After 108 minutes and nearly one orbit, a journey of 40,000 km, he reentered the atmosphere and landed safely. A new era—the era of humans in space—had begun.

This momentous flight was followed by a large number of manned flights by U.S. and Soviet astronauts and cosmonauts. In May 1961, Alan B. Shepard Jr. completed a suborbital flight in a Mercury 3 capsule (Freedom 7); in August of that year G.S. Titov orbited the Earth 17 times on Vostok 2. John

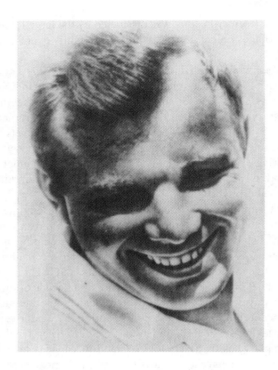

Fig. 18 Yu.A. Gagarin (1934-1968)

H. Glenn, Jr. (Fig. 19) became the first U.S. astronaut to orbit the Earth on February 20, 1962, in a 5-hour flight on Mercury 6. These initial manned flights demonstrated that human beings could survive and function in space. How well and for how long were difficult questions, requiring years of biomedical investigation.

With this tentative assurance, both the United States and the Soviet Union began to investigate empirically the more complex systems and procedures that would be necessary for sustained human scientific and exploratory activities in space. Questions included whether humans could live and work in space for extended periods, whether women could be astronauts and cosmonauts, along with issues related to the functioning of multi-person crews, rendezvous and docking of spacecraft in space, and extravehicular activity. Both the United States and the Soviet Union began a series of missions to answer these questions and acquire experience in anticipation of their major human space flight undertakings in the following decade.

The first two-man crew (A.G. Nikolayev and P.R. Popovich) flew in August 1962. In June 1963 the first woman in space, Valentina Tereshkova, completed a 3-day flight. In September 1964 a three-person crew, consisting of a professional cosmonaut, a researcher, and a physician, spent slightly over 24 hours in space on the first flight of Voskhod 1. Voskhod 2 carried cosmonauts P.I. Belyayev and A.A. Leonov in March 1965 on a flight during which Leonov performed a program of

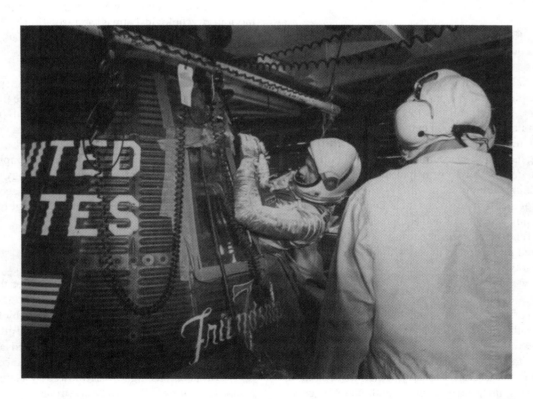

Fig. 19 U.S. Astronaut John H. Glenn, Jr., climbs into the Mercury Friendship 7 spacecraft before his February 20, 1962, flight (NASA-62 MA6-108-A)

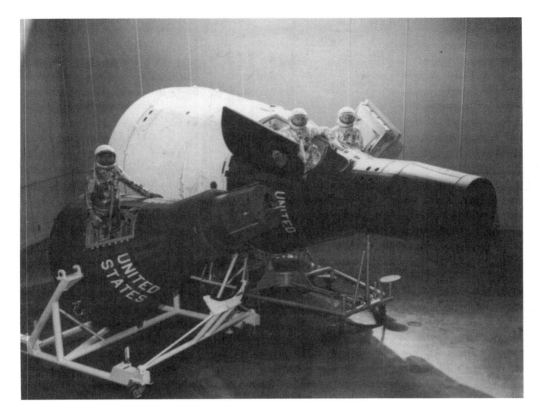

Fig. 20 One-man Mercury and two man-Gemini (NASA 63-Gemini-24)

activities outside the spacecraft. In August of that same year, American astronaut Edward H. White successfully completed a "space walk."

Between March 1965 and November 1966 the United States flew 10 Gemini two-man spacecraft (Fig. 20). Gemini flights pioneered manually controlled maneuvers in space (Gemini 3), piloted rendezvous (Gemini 6), docking, and joint flights (Gemini 11 and Agena). Five Gemini flights included extravehicular activity, with one (Edwin E. "Buzz" Aldrin Jr. on Gemini 12) lasting over 5 hours.

The Gemini series of flights was designed in part to test rendezvous, one of the more critical procedures required for the Apollo Program. The United States, in planning its lunar landing mission, knew that it would have to fly two separate lunar spacecraft—a lunar orbiter and a lunar lander. Confidence that the lander could separate from and return to the orbiter was essential.

The next important step in the development of manned space flight involved the development of the Soyuz spacecraft in the Soviet Union. Soyuz was a multipurpose vehicle intended for autonomous navigation, transport operations (delivery of cosmonauts to a space station), and biomedical and other scientific and applied investigations in near-Earth space. Soyuz was in essence a wholly new type of spacecraft, differing from its predecessors (Vostok and Voskhod) not only by virtue of its substantially greater mass (about 6.5 metric tons), but by its capacity to maneuver, rendezvous, and dock with other vehicles in orbit. The Soyuz spacecraft cabin

consisted of two modules—a descent module for the return of cosmonauts from orbit and an orbital module for habitation and research.

The design, development, construction, and testing of the Soyuz spacecraft, which was begun in mid-1962, required 5 years. At the end of 1966 and beginning of 1967 it was flight-tested in an unmanned mode, and in April 1967 V.M. Komarov piloted Soyuz 1 on its first manned test flight. The flight lasted 27 hours and orbited the Earth 19 times. On its return from orbit the spacecraft's deceleration and atmospheric braking system operated successfully, but a malfunction in the parachute system caused the spacecraft to crash upon landing, taking Komarov's life.

The first decade of space exploration (1957-1967) witnessed 25 manned space flights, on which 30 individuals flew in space (11 in the U.S.S.R., 19 in the U.S.), including 8 who flew twice. That humans could live and work in the vacuum and microgravity environment of space for periods of at least 2 weeks was amply demonstrated.

IV. Second Decade in Space (1967-1977)

A. Continued Spacecraft Development

The second decade of the space era was marked by intensified work in the area of manned cosmonautics. Both the duration and remoteness of human space flight underwent an historic increase between 1967 and 1977, as important in its own way as the initial human ventures into space that marked the first decade in space. The Soviet Union continued work on its Soyuz program (see Fig. 21 and Table 4) of manned space flights, accumulating experience and conducting biomedical research into the effects of the space environment on humans. In October 1968 the Soviet Union successfully launched

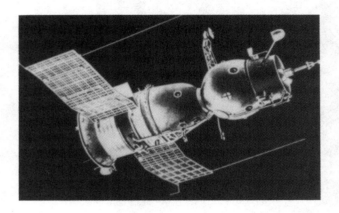

Fig. 21 Soyuz spacecraft

Soyuz 3 (cosmonaut G.T. Beregovoy), followed in January 1969 by the joint missions of Soyuz 4 (V.A. Shatalov) and Soyuz 5 (B.V. Volynov, A.S. Yeliseyev, Ye.V. Khrunov). A group flight of three spacecraft (Soyuz 6-8), involving seven cosmonauts, took place in October 1969.

The flight of Soyuz 9 (A.G. Nikolayev and V.I. Sevastyanov) was of great significance for the further development of manned space flight, including the solution of biomedical problems. This flight, which continued for approximately 18 days (425 hours), set an endurance record for human space flight. While the crew had difficulty enduring such a relatively long-duration exposure to weightlessness, the experience gained yielded valuable material for studying the possibility of long-term habitation of orbital stations and interplanetary spacecraft. Soyuz 9 provided data on the response of the cardiovascular and musculoskeletal systems to prolonged exposure to weight-lessness. The role of physical exercise was investigated, as were the characteristics of the postflight recuperation period. The cosmonauts displayed significant muscle atrophy and orthostatic intolerance, requiring an 11-day period of medical rehabilitation.

Between April and June of 1971, Soyuz 10 and 11 were launched with the mission of docking with Salyut. Cosmonauts V.A. Shatalov, A.S. Yeliseyev, and N.N. Rukavishnikov

Table 4   Soyuz missions (1967-77)

Mission Designation	Crew	Flight Dates
Soyuz 1	Komarov, V.M.	4/23-24/67
Soyuz 2	Unmanned	10/25-28/68
Soyuz 3	Beregovoy, G.T.	10/26-30/68
Soyuz 4	Shatalov, V.A.	1/14-17/69
Soyuz 5	Volynov, B.V., Yeliseyev, A.S., Khrunov, E.V.	1/15-18/69
Soyuz 6	Shonin, G.S., Kubasov, V.N.	10/11-16/69
Soyuz 7	Philipchenko, A.V. Volkov, V.N., Gorbatko, V.V.	10/12-17/69
Soyuz 8	Shatalov, V.A., Yeliseyev, A.S.	10/13-18/69
Soyuz 9	Nikolayev, A.G., Sevastyanov, V.I.	6/1-19/70
Soyuz 10	Shatalov, V.A., Yeliseyev, A. S., Rukavishnikov, N.N.	4/23-25/71
Soyuz 11	Dobrovolskiy, G.T., Volkov, V.N., Patsayev, V.I.	6/6-30/71
Soyuz 12	Lazarev, V.G., Makarov, O.G.	9/27-29/73
Soyuz 13	Klimuk, P.I., Lebedev, V.V.	12/18-26/73
Soyuz 14	Popovich, P.R., Artyukhin Yu.P.	7/3-19/74
Soyuz 15	Sarafanov, G.V., Demin, L.S.	8/26-28/74
Soyuz 16	Philipchenko, A.V., Rukavishnikov, N.N.	12/2-8/74
Soyuz 17	Gubarev, A.A., Grechko, G.M.	1/11-2/9/75
Soyuz 18I	Lazarev, V.G., Makarov, O.G.	4/5/75
Soyuz 18	Klimuk, P.I., Sevastyanov, V.I.	5/24-7/26/75
Soyuz 19	Leonov, A. A., Kubasov, V.N.	7/15-21/75
Soyuz 20	Unmanned	11/17-2/16/75
Soyuz 21	Volynov, B.V., Zhelobov, V.M.	7/6-8/24/76
Soyuz 22	Bykovskiy, V.F., Aksenov, V.V.	9/15-23/76
Soyuz 23	Zudov, V.D., Rozhdestvenskiy, V.I.	10/14-16/76
Soyuz 24	Gorbatko, V.V., Glazkov, Yu.N.	2/7-25/77
Soyuz 25	Kovalenok, V.V., Ryumin, V.V.	10/9-11/77

rendezvoused with Salyut in the Soyuz10, docked and separated, but were unable to enter the station. In June cosmonauts G.T. Dobrovolsky, V.N. Volkov, and V.I. Patsayev arrived at the space station in the Soyuz 11. After completing a 23-day mission and flight program, they returned to Soyuz 11, separated, and prepared to return to Earth. However, during the crew's descent from orbit the descent module depressurized and the cosmonauts perished.

Subsequently, during the second decade of the space era, 14 Soyuz spacecraft were launched (Soyuz 12-25). They were used primarily to exchange Salyut crews. In addition, various spacecraft systems were evaluated and tested, astrophysical observations were conducted, and methods for studying the Earth from space were developed. The Apollo-Soyuz mission (discussed in more detail in the section on international collaboration) was performed by Soyuz 19.

The Soviet Union's series of Soyuz space flights featured an extensive program of biomedical research, including in-, pre-, and postflight studies . The effects of weightlessness on the central nervous system, fluid-electrolyte balance, metabolism, and blood chemistry were studied. Methods and regimens of physical exercise, special exercise machines, and prophylactic countermeasures against the adverse effects of weightlessness (e.g., the "Penguin" suit) were developed. In addition, orthostatic tolerance, sensitivity to pain, hand strength, and other functions were studied.[61]

B. To the Moon

Meanwhile, the late 1960s brought the United States closer to the Apollo Program's goal of sending a man to the Moon within the decade and returning him safely. During summer of 1962, after much discussion, the United States had decided that the fastest and most feasible way of achieving the manned Moon landing was to launch a command and service module (CSM) and lunar landing module (LM) combination to lunar orbit, carry out the lunar landing itself with the LM, while the CSM waited in orbit, return the astronauts to the CSM in the LM, and after jettisoning both the LM and service portion of the CSM, return the astronauts to Earth in the command module. Thus the Apollo Program consisted of work on three major elements: the launch vehicle (a Saturn 5), the Apollo spacecraft (command and service modules), and the LM. One of the heads of this project was Wernher von Braun (Fig. 22).

First and foremost the program had to develop a powerful booster rocket able to put a payload weighing not less than 300 metric tons into Earth orbit and one weighing 100 metric tons into lunar orbit. Such a booster would require three stages. The technology for what became the Saturn 5 rocket, which ultimately carried the Apollo spacecraft to the Moon, was tested with an earlier Saturn 1 stage (weight on the order of 500 metric tons) and two-stage Saturn 1B (weight 590 metric tons) rocket. The most powerful rocket in the series, the three-stage Saturn 5, had a launch weight of almost 3000 metric tons.

Work on the Apollo spacecraft, with the mission of manned flight to the Moon, was conducted concurrently with development of the Saturn booster. This spacecraft, weighing up to 47 metric tons, consisted of a main module (which delivered the crew to lunar orbit) and a lunar module (for descent of two crewmembers to the surface of the Moon and return to lunar orbit).

Between 1961 and 1965, NASA conducted 10 test flights of the Saturn 1, including 5 tests (starting in May 1964) involving orbital insertion of an Apollo mock-up. In February 1966 the Saturn 1B successfully completed a suborbital flight with the Apollo command and service modules. The Apollo spacecraft underwent an unmanned orbital insertion, reentry, and landing test in February 1966. Flight tests of an experimental prototype of the main module and a mock-up of the LM and its experimental prototype were conducted during the next 2 years.

However, just as the Soviet space program experienced reverses in the dangerous undertaking of space flight, so also did the U.S. Apollo Program. During the evening of January 27, 1967, a crew of three (Edward H. White II, Roger B. Chaffee, and Virgil I. Grissom) perished in a flash fire in the spacecraft during a pre-launch test. After an investigation and elimination of the causes of the fire, flight tests resumed and increased in complexity as the first manned test of the Apollo spacecraft (Apollo 7) was carried out during an 11-day orbital flight in October 1968. The flight, which was launched by a Saturn 1B, successfully demonstrated the command/service vehicle's rendezvous capability, crew/vehicle support systems, and the Apollo heat shield.

In December 1968, Apollo 8 (without the LM) was put into lunar orbit and returned to the atmosphere of the Earth with escape velocity. This was a manned flight to the Moon

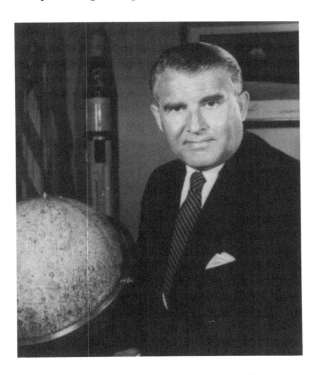

Fig. 22 W. von Braun (1912-1977)

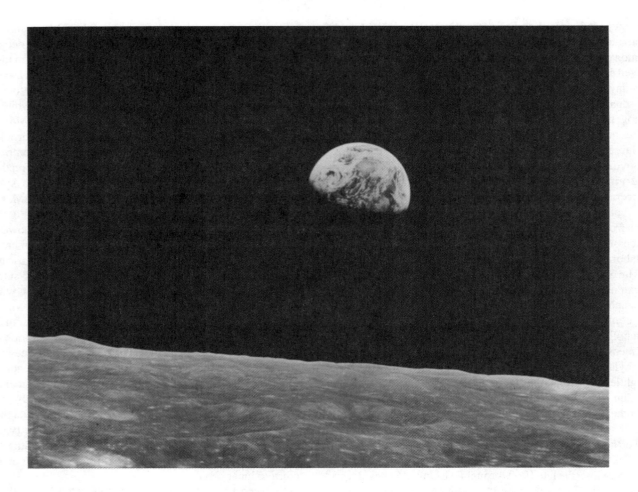

Fig. 23 View of Earth from Apollo-8 (NASA-68-1401)

(astronauts William Anders, James A. Lovell Jr., and Frank Borman). Television and photography not only confirmed the lunar landing sites, but provided the first manmade photographs of the Earth from the vicinity of the Moon (Fig. 23). Photographs of the Earth as a whole, with brilliant blues, whites and browns illuminated by the Sun, dramatized the unity of the planet and intensified the concern of many that humanity protect and preserve its planetary home.

In March 1969 Apollo 9 (carrying the LM) was tested in near-Earth orbit. Tests involved redocking the modules and autonomous flight of the LM carrying two astronauts. Individual life support systems were tested by EVAs. In May 1969 Apollo 10 was put into orbit around the Moon and the LM with astronauts aboard separated and orbited the Moon at an altitude of 14-15 m, but did not land.

After successful completion of these flights, preparations began for the launch of Apollo 11 (Neil A. Armstrong, Michael Collins, and Edwin E. Aldrin Jr.), which was destined to serve as the culmination of the efforts of thousands of engineers and scientists and finally land human beings on the Moon (Fig. 24). On July 16, 1969, Apollo 11 was launched and on July 19 inserted into circular lunar orbit. On July 20, 1969, Armstrong and Aldrin entered the LM, which soft

landed on the Moon, and on July 21 Armstrong (and later Aldrin) left the module, and descended to the surface of the Moon to begin a program of scientific investigations.

This was an outstanding achievement in the history of space exploration, matched only by the beginning of the space era or the first manned space flight. For the first time, humans reached the surface of another celestial body in a manmade vehicle and spent more than 2 hours walking on it.

The American astronauts took a series of photographs of the lunar surface, collected more than 20 kg of samples of lunar material, which were returned to Earth and taken to the Lunar Receiving Laboratory in Houston, and set up solar wind detection and other instruments. Two billion inhabitants of our planet watched their exploits on the Moon on television.

During the next 3 1/2 years (until December 1972) the United States sent six expeditions to the Moon (Apollo 12-17), five of which were completely successful (Fig. 25 and Table 5). After that, lunar flights were cancelled. A total of 12 astronauts landed on the surface of the Moon, some remaining several days, and traversed lunar terrain in the Lunar Roving Vehicle (nicknamed the "Moon Buggy") over as much as 22 km during a single mission. They conducted a large number of scientific studies and collected more than 380 kg of samples of lunar rocks and soil, which were studied in laboratories in the U.S. and other countries. The Apollo Program also yielded valuable biomedical information.[62]

While the U.S. missions to the Moon ceased in 1972, Apollo/Saturn systems were used for two further U.S. programs: transport to and from the first U.S. space station, Skylab (operated from May 1973 through February 1974),

and the first rendezvous and docking of the spacecraft and crews of the two principal spacefaring nations, the United States and the Soviet Union, in July 1975.

During the time frame of the Apollo Program, work on a manned lunar flight program was also conducted in the U.S.S.R.[63] After the first manned space flight, in late 1961 the S.P. Korolyov Experimental Design Bureau was assigned the

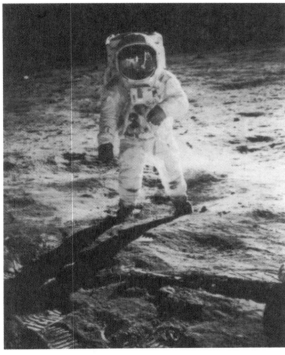

Fig. 24 Astronaut Edwin Aldrin, Jr., walking on the Moon (NASA 690 HC-684)

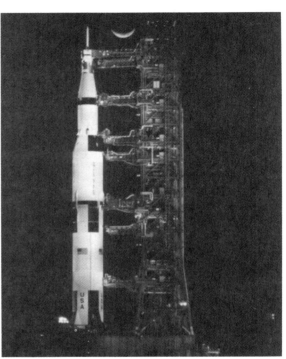

Fig. 25 Apollo 14-Saturn V complex (NASA 108-KSC-71P-74)

Mission Designation	Crew	Flight Dates
Apollo 1	-	2/26/88
Apollo 2	-	7/5/66
Apollo 3	-	8/23/66
Apollo 4	-	11/9/67
Apollo 5	-	1/22-2/11/68
Apollo 6	-	4/4/68
Apollo 7	W. Schirra, D. Eisele, W. Cunningham	10/11-22/68
Apollo 8	F. Borman, J. Lovell, W. Anders	12/21-27/68
Apollo 9	J. McDivitt, D. Scott, R. Schweickart	3/3-13/69
Apollo 10	T. Stafford, J. Young, E. Cernan	5/18-26/69
Apollo 11	N. Armstrong, M. Collins, E. Aldrin	7/16-24/69
Apollo 12	C. Conrad, R. Gordon, A. Bean	11/14-24/69
Apollo 13	J. Lovell, J. Swigert, F. Haise	4/11-17/70
Apollo 14	A. Shepard, E. Mitchell, S. Roosa	1/31-2/9/71
Apollo 15	D. Scott, J. Irwin, A Worden	7/26-8/7/71
Apollo 16	J. Young, C. Duke, T. Mattingly	4/16-27/72
Apollo 17	E. Cernan, R. Evans, H. Schmitt	12/7-19/72

Table 5 Apollo missions

task of developing two new booster rockets, with payloads of from 40 to 80 metric tons. In the same year, the V.N. Chelomey Design Bureau was assigned to develop a rocket-spacecraft complex for a manned lunar fly-by.

At the end of 1964, the Korolyov Experimental Design Bureau developed the preliminary design of the N1-L3 Lunar Rocket-Spacecraft Complex for landing a man on the surface of the Moon. A second cosmonaut was to stay in the main spacecraft in circumlunar orbit. The payload weight of the N1 booster rocket was to be increased to 90-95 metric tons.

The UR 500K-L1 program to conduct a lunar fly-by with two cosmonauts was adopted in late 1965. The booster rocket was to be the updated Proton rocket, along with rocket pod "D"

from the N1-L3 complex. The manned spacecraft (7K-L1) for this program was also based on the lunar orbital spacecraft from this complex.

Practical work on these two programs (UR 500K-L1 and N1-L3) began in the second half of the 1960s. From March 1968 to October 1970, five spacecraft (Zond 4-8), unmanned analogs of the manned 7K-L1 spacecraft, were launched with the four-stage Proton rocket.

At the end of the 1960s, flight-design testing was begun on the N1 three-stage booster rocket (Fig. 26), which, with an initial mass of 2700 metric tons had to inject the L3 Lunar

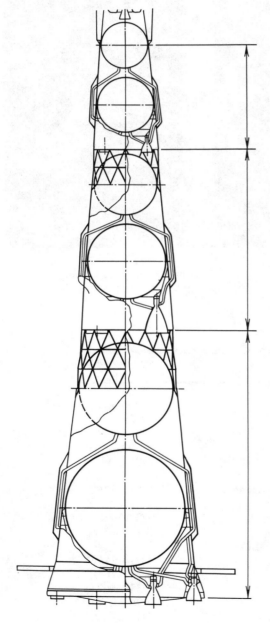

Fig. 26 N1 booster rocket

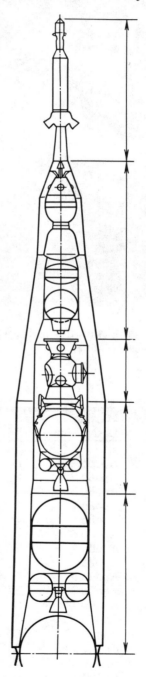

Fig. 27 L3 Lunar Complex

Complex (Fig. 27), initially weighing 92 metric tons (and subsequently increased) into Earth orbit. From February 1969 to December 1972 there were four experimental launches of the N1 booster rocket with a mock-up of the lunar spacecraft; all were unsuccessful.

Soon after this, despite the experience with the new booster rocket accrued in the testing process (including the identification of problems with individual systems and units and planned measures for eliminating them), the U.S.S.R. decided to terminate work on the lunar program as a whole, and on the N1 booster rocket. It should be noted that the issue of the program's cost was relevant to the decision to terminate it.

C. Orbiting Space Stations

While practical development of orbiting space stations only started in the late 1960s, the idea of orbiting permanent facilities or "stations" in space can be found in the visionary writings of previous decades. The idea can be traced back at least to the 19th century, when the U.S. author Edward E. Hale (1822-1909) wrote of an imaginary "brick Moon" in space in an 1869 issue of the *Atlantic* magazine.[64] Early 20th century space visionaries and pioneers such as Tsiolkovskiy, Oberth, H. Noordung, and the British Interplanetary Society also imagined a permanently orbiting human outpost in space. As developments in rocketry in the 1940s and 1950s made human space travel even more likely, space station proposals began to proliferate.[65] Actual development of such orbiting outposts, however, did not begin until the late 1960s and early 1970s, i.e. after the development of relatively advanced spacecraft (Apollo, Soyuz) and study of their use as means of transportation.

In late 1969, work to design the Salyut orbital station (Fig. 28) began in the U.S.S.R. In 1970 ground-based tests of

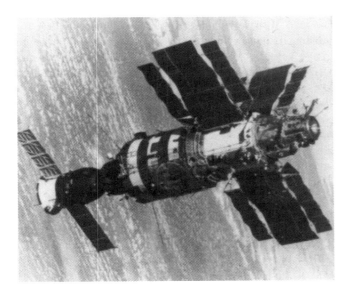

Fig. 28 Salyut Space station with docked Soyuz (exterior view)

individual systems were performed and the first flight prototype of the station was manufactured. By April 1971 the Soviet Union was able to insert the station into orbit. The Salyut station met the requirements essential for long-duration inhabitation by cosmonauts. Its weight, after injection into orbit, was 18.9 metric tons (docked with Soyuz it weighed 25.6 metric tons). The length of the station was 16 m (23 m when docked with Soyuz). The station consisted of two—the orbital and transport—modules connected by permanently opened hatches, for a total pressurized volume of 100 m³.

The first station was in orbit for 175 days, from April 19 until October 11, 1971. During this time, as mentioned above, two spacecraft (Soyuz 10 and 11) docked with it. In April 1973 Salyut 2 was inserted into orbit. During its almost 4-week flight, the design of the station and on-board apparatus were tested. There was no docking with another spacecraft.

The American long-term orbiting station, Skylab (Fig. 29), was an important step in the development of manned space flight. It was developed in the United States and injected into orbit in May 1973 at an altitude of approximately 450 km. Work on this project was conducted over a relatively long period of time and went through a number of phases. Skylab provided a favorable living and working environment for astronauts (its habitable volume was over 280 m³, and it had separate modules for working, sleeping, recreation, and exercise) (Fig. 30).

The 28 m long, 75 metric ton laboratory was outfitted with an Apollo telescope mount, the most powerful astronomical observatory ever put in orbit, which enabled experiments covering the entire range of solar physics. Skylab was highly successful, resulting in an unprecedented number of man-days in orbit for the U.S. space program, and returning a wealth of images of the Earth and solar phenomena. Between May 1973 and February 1974 Apollo spacecraft transported three crews to Skylab, for missions of 28, 59, and 84 days. A significant amount of scientific and biomedical research was conducted by the crews, and the first crew contained the first American astronaut-physician, Joseph Kerwin. During the Skylab flights, investigations were conducted into the dynamics of changes in fluid electrolyte metabolism in various bones and muscles, total body weight and tissue dehydration, orthostatic intolerance, physical endurance, and the dynamics of postflight recovery. Evidence was gathered about those parameters that continue to deteriorate and those that stabilize during the flight. Factors determining the severity of space motion sickness symptoms, as well as potential predictive indicators and prophylactic countermeasures (particularly drugs) were studied.[66,67] Meanwhile, due to a launch mishap, Skylab crews had to perform EVAs to repair the station prior to occupying it. The most important tasks involved repairing the solar panels, which did not operate properly at first, and providing additional thermal protection on the station's exterior.

Between 1974 and 1976, the Soviet Union launched three additional Salyut space stations (Salyut 3, 4, and 5). The crews of six spacecraft (Soyuz 14, 15, 17, 18, 21, and 24) were able to dock and carry out research, spending a total of 176

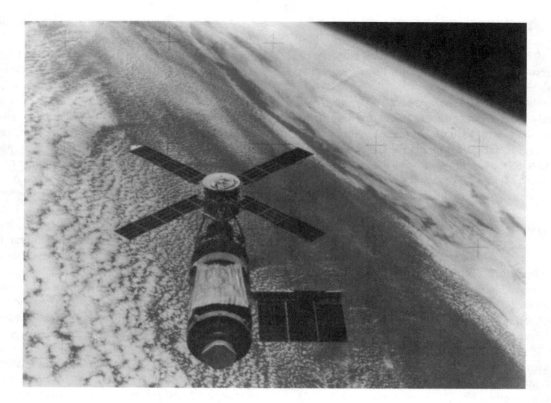

Fig. 29 An overhead view of the U.S. Skylab space station in Earth orbit as photographed from the Skylab 4 Command and Service Modules (NASA 74-H-98)

days in orbit. During these flights cosmonauts conducted an extensive set of scientific, technological and biomedical investigations. Special attention was given to regimens of physical exercise on exercise machines, and adjustment of the work/rest schedules to improve cardiovascular tolerance to gravity after return to the Earth. For example, the Chibis apparatus, similar to the Skylab lower-body negative pressure device (LBNP), which simulates the effects of the Earth's gravity on blood and thus counteracts excessive flow of blood to the head, was used for the first time on Salyut 4. A rotating chair for the study of vestibular functions and a bicycle ergometer (to supplement the already installed treadmill) were installed on the station. Another new apparatus was the Tonus, developed for electrical stimulation of individual muscle groups. In addition, the crew transported on Soyuz 18, which flew for 8 days during December 1973, consumed a diet with increased levels of salt and a great deal of fluid. These countermeasures have proved to be highly effective in increasing crew tolerance to conditions after return to Earth.[69]

Experience with the Salyut 3, 4, and 5 stations was critical to the development of the second-generation long-term orbital station—the Salyut 6, which was put into orbit in September 1977. While its weight and dimensions were virtually the same as those of previous Salyuts, it incorporated a number of important improvements, and was intended for missions of up to several months and multiple crew exchanges.

D. Lunar and Planetary Exploration

Study of the Moon and planets with automated spacecraft also continued during the second decade of the space era. Between March 1968 and October 1970 five automated spacecraft, Zond 4-8, were launched by the U.S.S.R. These probes differed significantly from Zond 1-3 and were much heavier. The goal of these launches was to develop technology for unmanned flight around the Moon and return to the Earth with escape velocity. In addition, scientific experiments were performed, including the study of radiation conditions and the level of cosmic rays on the flight path, and experiments with various biological subjects (tortoises, insects, plants, bacteria).[70]

During this period the Soviet Union also experimented with automated, remotely controlled lunar probes. In September 1970 Luna 16 became the first unmanned spacecraft to land on the Moon and return to Earth with hermetically sealed lunar samples. The spacecraft made a soft landing on the Moon in the region of the Sea of Fertility. Remotely controlled drilling and soil collection equipment collected more than 100 grams of lunar material, which was returned to Earth for study.

In November of that year, the first automatically controlled vehicle to explore the Moon's surface, the Lunokhod 1 (Fig. 31), soft landed on the Moon by Luna 17, was deployed on the Moon in the area of the Sea of Rain. Lunokhod 1, weighing more than 750 kg, travelled over 10.5 km, exploring more than 80,000 m^2 within the next 10 months.

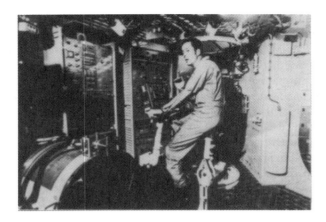

Fig. 30a J. Kerwin on bicycle ergometer (Reprinted from: Nicogossian, A.E., Huntoon, C.L, and Pool, S.L. Space Physiology and Medicine, 2nd edition. Philadelphia, Lea and Febiger, 1989, pp. 12.)

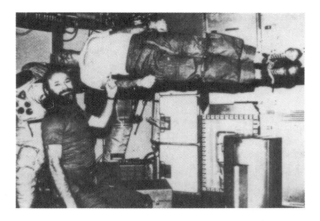

Fig. 30c Skylab 4 astronauts demonstrate weightlessness (Reprinted from: Nicogossian, A.E., Huntoon, C.L, and Pool, S.L. Space Physiology and Medicine, 2nd edition. Philadelphia, Lea and Febiger, 1989, pp. 51. Reprinted with permission.)

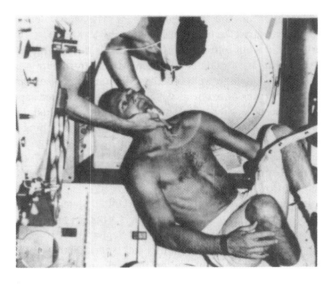

Fig. 30b Dental exam (Reprinted from: Johnston, R.S and Dietlein, L.P. (Eds.), Biomedical Results from Skylab, Washington, D.C., NASA, 1977.)

The Soviet Union and the United States also explored our neighboring planets—especially Venus—with automated planetary probes. Between January 1969 and March 1972, the U.S.S.R. sent to Venus four Venera probes (Venera 5, 6, 7, and 8), which incorporated improvements suggested by results from earlier Venera probes. These included a strengthened shell on the descent module to better resist the planet's higher temperatures and pressure. The Venera 5-8 missions produced additional and more precise data about the composition and properties of the venusian atmosphere down to the surface. The descent module of Venera 7 was the first to successfully reach the surface of this planet and for 23 minutes transmitted information about it to the Earth. Venera 8's descent module was the first to achieve a soft landing on the sunlit side of the planet.

In November 1973, Mariner 10, a Venus-Mercury probe, was launched into a heliocentric orbit. Mariner 10 was the first spacecraft to use gravity assist in a dual-planet mission and the only one yet to explore Mercury. In June 1974, as it flew past Venus, Mariner 10 transmitted the first television images of that planet to Earth from a distance of 5800 km. The spacecraft confirmed the high-speed circulation of Venus' upper atmosphere and revealed a long tail of charged particles trailing behind the planet and away from the Sun; it verified the presence of a bow shock wave created by the solar wind acting upon the dense atmosphere; detected hydrogen, helium, and argon in the venusian atmosphere; and discovered temperature-inversion zones suggestive of deeper stratiform cloud layers. During its three encounters with Mercury, Mariner 10 came within 327 km of it to take the closest photographs ever made of that planet; the probe also revealed that Mercury's crust was lunar-like at the surface and Earth-like at the interior, and found an unexpected magnetic field a hundredth the strength of the Earth's.

During the early 1970s the Soviet Union also developed a second generation of Venera probes, which were significantly heavier (on the order of 5 metric tons) than their predecessors and had much greater observational capabilities. In June 1975, Venera 9 and Venera 10, which included descent modules (1560 kg), were launched toward Venus. In October of the same year, these probes soft landed on the surface of the planet and for 53 and 65 minutes transmitted panoramic photographs of the landing site. After the descent modules separated, the probes were put into highly elliptical orbits around the planet (with a rotation period of approximately 2 days), becoming the first manmade satellites of Venus. Their scientific instruments collected and transmitted a good deal of data about the venusian atmosphere and space environment.

Through the use of the planetary exploration spacecraft discussed above, much was learned about Venus during the second decade of the space era. More precise data on the

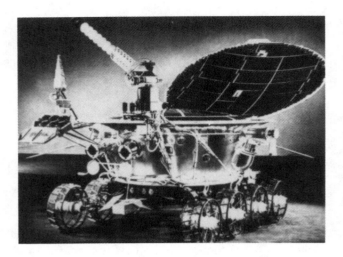

Fig. 31 Lunokhod 1—the first Earth-controlled vehicle for locomotion on the Moon

composition of its atmosphere and new information on the temperature and pressure at the planet's surface were obtained. These results, obtained over a comparatively short period of time, significantly altered ideas about Venus that had been based on many years of astronomical observations.

During the period under discussion, there was an increase in the amount of attention devoted to Mars, which, as the most similar to the Earth of all our planetary neighbors, has always aroused special interest. Between 1969 and 1976 the United States and the Soviet Union sent more than 10 probes to this planet.

In February and March 1969, the U.S. launched Mariner 6 and Mariner 7 (mass of over 400 kg). These spacecraft, which passed within 3400 km of the planet, returned scientific data including more than 2000 ultraviolet spectra and more than 400 infrared spectra of the atmosphere and surface. An infrared radiometer returned more than 800 near-encounter and 100,000 far-encounter surface and atmospheric measurements. Television cameras produced 198 high-quality analog pictures of the martian surface.

In May 1971, during a period when conditions were optimal (when the distance between the Earth and Mars was close to minimal), the U.S.S.R launched Mars 2 and 6 and the U.S. Mariner 8 and 9 to Mars.

In November of that year, the Mariner 9 spacecraft became the first manmade satellite of Mars. Mariner 9 transmitted a great deal of scientific information back to Earth, and also more than 7000 images of Mars and its moons, Deimos and Phobos. These photographs revealed higher mountains and deeper valleys than any found on Earth.

During the same period, the Soviet Union dispatched its Mars 2 and Mars 3 spacecraft (weighing more than 4.5 tons), which consisted of orbital and descent modules. They approached Mars in late November and early December 1971, and Mars 2 became the second manmade satellite of this planet; the descent module of Mars 3 entered the martian atmosphere and reached its surface (though no data were

returned), while the orbital module became the third manmade satellite of Mars.

During the Mars missions launched in 1971, scientific interest in the U.S. and U.S.S.R. focused on the composition of the martian atmosphere and the proportion of water vapor it contained, measurement of the temperature on the surface, study of the magnetic field in the vicinity of Mars and the physical characteristics of the planet. The investigations conducted on Mariner 9 and Mars 2 and 3 were complementary, enabling planetary scientists to complete an extensive set of experiments.

The Soviet Union continued its investigation of Mars in 1973 with the launch of four probes (Mars 4-7) in July and August. The first two, Mars 4 and 5, were to go into orbit around the planet, and the second—Mars 6 and 7—to land descent modules. The Mars 5 and 6 probes successfully performed their flight missions. Mars 4 failed to orbit but passed within 2200 km of the surface of the planet, photographing and transmitting to Earth images of the surface of Mars by means of a television camera. The Mars 7 descent module went past the planet at a distance of 1300 km from the surface and went into solar orbit. Mars 6's descent module returned important data about the martian atmosphere—for example, that it underwent broad oscillations of pressure and contained traces of ozone as well as much more water vapor than supposed earlier. The spacecraft also transmitted data that showed that Mars had a hydrogen corona reaching to 19,300 km in altitude, a magnetic field 7 to 10 times greater than the interplanetary field, and eroded "riverbeds" that provided evidence that the now-dry martian surface had once seen the flow of liquid water.

In August and September 1975, the United States launched on a martian journey the orbiter/landers Viking 1 and Viking 2 (mass 3.4 metric tons). In July and September 1976, both landers (mass 577 kg) successfully soft landed on the martian surface. During descent and on the surface, they gathered information about the composition of the atmosphere and properties of the soil. A great deal of effort was devoted to searching for evidence of rudimentary life forms on the planet; however, no definitive answer to the question of life on Mars was produced during this period.

Flights of robotic interplanetary probes to Mars produced much new information about the physicochemical properties of the atmosphere and surface of this planet and substantially expanded scientific understanding of its nature. During the second decade of the space era, humanity learned more about Mars than it had during the entire period of study of the planet prior to the space era.

By the early 1970s, accumulated skills and experience with automated spacecraft enabled the exploration of the outer planets as well. In March 1972, the United States launched Pioneer 10 toward Jupiter. The spacecraft completed a "fly-by" of that planet in late 1973, transmitting a large number of photographs from a distance of 130,000 km. Three years later, Pioneer 10 intercepted the orbit of Saturn. As it continued on to the edge of the solar system, the spacecraft returned valuable data on the nature of the interplanetary medium and the unexplored space beyond Jupiter. Pioneer 10, as of 1991, is still operating over 7 billion km from Earth.

In April 1973, Pioneer 11 was also sent towards Jupiter and in 1974 passed at a distance of approximately 43,000 km from the planet. The spacecraft continued on in the direction of Saturn, which it first encountered in 1979. Both probes gathered data about interplanetary space, the radiation field of Jupiter, its cloud cover, and also its satellites. In August and September of 1977, the United States launched a new generation of space probes, Voyager 1 and Voyager 2, designed to explore the planets of the outer solar system. Their accomplishments belong to the third decade of space exploration.

V. Development of Rocket and Space Technology and Space Biology and Medicine 1977-1992

By the beginning of the third decade of the space era, humanity had already gained considerable experience in the study and exploration of space and in application of the results obtained to practical problems. By this time, work in this area was already being conducted on a rather extensive basis. Research on near-Earth space and the planets of the solar system continued; the use of spacecraft for applied objectives had expanded considerably; second generation long-term space stations were beginning to be flown, and the number and duration of manned space flights continued to increase.

Fundamental technologies in rocketry, communications, telemetry, and other basic systems had been developed and used successfully. What remained were incremental improvements or new approaches to well established objectives. Most importantly, space technology and space exploration ceased to be dominated by two countries—the United States and the Soviet Union. And, as space exploration became a truly international endeavor, international law evolved to include principles to assure some degree of order and harmony in the new regime of outer space.

A. Further Development of Spacecraft

During the period under consideration, spacecraft continued to fly and additional work was conducted on their development. In the U.S.S.R., 15 Soyuz series spacecraft were launched between 1977 and 1987 (see Table 6). The increasingly extended periods spent by space stations in orbit required designers to develop new spacecraft to increase these stations' operational duration and efficiency. Accordingly, the Soviet Union in the late 1970s developed the Progress unmanned cargo vehicles. The launch weight of Progress exceeded 7 metric tons, including 1.3 tons of dry cargo and water in containers, and 1 ton of propellant and compressed gas. The first flight of a Progress transport vehicle occurred in January 1978; 3 days later it docked with the Salyut 6, forming a new orbital complex consisting of Salyut 6, Soyuz 27, and Progress 1. This flight was successful and confirmed that it was possible to deliver materials needed by life support systems and other equipment to stations in orbit using unmanned cargo vehicles. Subsequently the unmanned vehicles were used rather extensively for delivery of cargo in space—during the next 10 years more than 30 Progress vehicles were launched.

During the 1970s the Soviet Union developed an advanced Soyuz spacecraft, Soyuz T, to be used for crew transport operations in near-Earth space, that is, to carry crews to, from, and between orbiting stations. The first flight (in an unmanned mode) occurred in December 1979. It was a success and demonstrated the reliability of the new spacecraft. Manned flights of the Soyuz T began in June 1980 (Table 7). In all, during the period between 1977 and 1987, more than 50 cosmonauts flew on Soyuz and Soyuz T, including cosmonauts from 13 other nations. These spacecraft were used to deliver crews to orbiting stations, for joint flights of Soviet and non-Soviet cosmonauts, and for flights from one station to another.

Table 6 Soyuz missions

Mission Designation	Crew	Flight Dates
Soyuz 26	Romanenko, Yu.V., Grechko, G.M.	12/10/77-1/16/78
Soyuz 27	Dzhanibekov, V.A., Makarov O.G.	1/10-3/16/78
Soyuz 28	Gubarev, A.A., Remek, V. (Czechoslovakia)	3/2-3/10/78
Soyuz 29	Kovalenok, V.V., Ivanchenkov, A.S.	6/15-9/3/78
Soyuz 30	Klimuk, P.I., Germashevskiy, M. (Poland)	6/27-7/5/78
Soyuz 31	Bykovskiy, V.F., Jaehn,Z. (GDR)	8/26-11/2/78
Soyuz 32	Lyakhov, V.A., Ryumin, V.V.	2/25-6/13/79
Soyuz 33	Rukavishnikov, N.N., Ivanov, G. (Bulgaria)	4/10-4/12/79
Soyuz 34	Unmanned	6/6-8/19/79
Soyuz 35	Popov, L.I., Ryumin, V.V.	4/9-6/3/80
Soyuz 36	Kubasov, V.N., Farkash, B. (Hungary)	5/26-7/31/80
Soyuz 37	Gorbatko, V.V., Fam Tuan (Vietnam)	7/23-10/11/80
Soyuz 38	Romanenko, Yu.V., Mendez A. (Cuba)	9/18-9/26/80
Soyuz 39	Dzhanibekov, V.A., Gurragcha, Zh. (Mongolia)	3/22-3/30/81
Soyuz 40	Popov, L.I., Prunariu, D. (Romania)	5/14-5/22/81

Table 7   Soyuz T missions

Mission Designation	Crew	Flight Dates
Soyuz T	Unmanned	12/16/79-3/26/80
Soyuz T-2	Malyshev, Yu. V., Aksenov, V. V.	6/5-9/80
Soyuz T-3	Kizim, L. D., Markov, O. G., Strekalov, G. M.	11/27-12/10/80
Soyuz T-4	Kovalenok, V. V., Savinykh, V. P.	3/12-5/26/81
Soyuz T-5	Berezovoy, A. N., Lebedev V. V.	5/13-8/27/82
Soyuz T-6	Dzhanibekov V.A., Ivanchenkov A.C., Chretien, J.L. (France)	6/24-7/2/82
Soyuz T-7	Popov, L. I., Serebrov, A. A., Savitskaya, S. Ye.	8/19-12/10/82
Soyuz T-8	Titov, V.G., Serebrov, A. A., Strekalov, G. M.	4/20-22/83
Soyuz T-9	Lyakhov, V. A., Aleksandrov, A. P.	6/27-11/23/83
Soyuz T-10	Kizim, L.D., Solovyov V.A., Atkov, O.Yu.	2/8/84-10/02/84
Soyuz T-11	Malyshev, Yu.V., Strekalov, G.M., Sharma, R. (India)	4/3/84-4/11/84
Soyuz T-12	Dzhanibekov, V.A., Savitskaya, S.E., Volk, I.P.	7/17/84-7/29/84
Soyuz T-13	Dzanibekov, V.A. Savinykh, V.P.	6/6/85-11/21/85
Soyuz T-14	Grechko, G. M.,	9/17/85-9/26/85
	Volkov, A. A., Vasyntin, V.V.	9/17/85-11/21/85
Soyuz T-15	Kizim, L. D., Solovyov, V. A.	3/13/86-7/16/86

B. Advanced Space Transportation Systems

In the third decade of the space age, the idea of a reusable transport spacecraft or Space Shuttle was finally implemented. Designers had been working on conceptual precursors to a Space Shuttle since the 1960s, when they had attempted to develop a successor program to Apollo.

However, a combination of political and economic considerations (the war in Vietnam, expensive social programs) made the United States Congress reluctant to allocate funds for this new space program. Because of budgetary pressures, in the early 1970s, the U.S. was unwilling to undertake another space station program beyond Skylab.

Anxious to reduce the costs of launching space missions, U.S. space planners proposed developing a wholly reusable two-stage launch system improving upon ideas first proposed in the 1920s. Development of the new Space Transportation System (STS) was approved in 1970, and by 1972 work had begun to develop a system designed for injecting spacecraft vehicles into orbit, for conducting scientific and technological research, performing various operations in space, including servicing and repair of spacecraft in near-Earth orbit, and returning to Earth research results and spacecraft in need of repair or modification.

As many as eight crewmembers have flown on a single mission of the STS. Crew cabin atmosphere is 79-percent nitrogen and 21-percent oxygen at a sea-level pressure. The assembly is launched by two solid rocket boosters, which after separation (at an altitude of approximately 40 km) descend by parachute into the ocean. The three main engines also fire at launch and are fueled by LOX/hydrogen carried in the external tank, which is strapped to the hull. To maneuver through the vacuum of space, the Shuttle orbiter uses 46 rocket thrusters in its nose and tail. It is able to safely land itself and a payload of up to 29,500 kg carried in the 18 × 4.5 m cargo bay, on a 3000 m runway without engine power and with the help only of rudder, elevons, body flaps, and the Shuttle's own aerodynamic design.

The first prototype system, Enterprise, was completed in 1976. The system was successfully flight-tested in the atmosphere by 1977, which confirmed that orbital flights could be implemented by reusable spacecraft of the Shuttle type.

The first manned flight of Columbia took place in April 1981 (J. Young and R. Crippen). By January 1986, the STS had flown 24 successful missions lasting as long as 10 days. More than 100 astronauts in crews containing up to 8 individuals had flown, including citizens of the Federal Republic of Germany, Canada, France, Saudi Arabia, the Netherlands, and Mexico. See Table 8.

The crews of the Shuttle orbiters Columbia, Challenger, Discovery, and Atlantis have conducted an extensive program of scientific research and experiments on these spacecraft. Astronauts have performed EVAs using the Manned Maneuvering Unit backpack system for locomotion, performed work with a remote manipulator arm, and recovered, repaired, and redeployed satellites in space. Numerous scientific and technological research experiments have been carried out on the Shuttle (Fig. 32).

Repeated trips into space have also increased opportunities for biomedical research (Fig. 33). Flight studies, combined with laboratory and postflight studies, have produced valuable data on the effects of microgravity, space radiation, and other flight factors on fundamental biological processes, vestibular function, cardiovascular, hematological, immunological, electrolyte, hormonal and other parameters.[67] The dynamics of adaptation of individual physiological systems to flight conditions, and also the process of medical rehabilitation postflight, have been tracked, providing useful indicators for improving life support systems, training, and prophylactic countermeasures.

Table 8   Space Shuttle flights

Mission-Shuttle	Crew	Flight Dates
STS-1 Columbia	J. Young, R. Crippen	4/12-14/81
STS-2 Columbia	J. Engle, R. Truly	11/12-14/81
STS-3 Columbia	J. Lousma, C. Fullerton	3/22-30/82
STS-4 Columbia	T. Mattingly, H.Hartsfield	6/27-7/4/82
STS-5 Columbia	V. Brand, R. Overmyer, J. Allen, W. Lenoir,	11/11-16/82
STS-6 Challenger	P. Weitz, K. Bobko, D. Peterson, S. Musgrave	4/4-9/83
STS-7 Challenger	R. Crippen, F. Hauck, S. Ride, J. Fabian, N. Thagard	6/18-24/83
STS-8 Challenger	R. Truly, D. Brandenstein, G. Bluford, D. Gardner, W. Thornton,	8/30-9/5/83
STS-9 Columbia	J. Young, B. Shaw, R. Parker, O. Garriott, B. Lichtenberg, U. Merbold (FRG)	11/28-12/8/83
41-B Challenger	V. Brand, R. Gibson, B. McCandless, R. Stewart, R. McNair,	2/3-11/84
41-C Challenger	R. Crippen, F. Scobee, T. Hart, J. van Hoften, G. Nelson	4/6-13/84
41-D Discovery	H. Hartsfield, M. Coats, R. Mullane, S. Hawley, J. Resnik, C. Walker	8/30-9/5/84
41-G Challenger	R. Crippen, J. McBride, D. Leestma, S. Ride, K. Sullivan, P. Scully-Power, M. Garneau (Canada)	10/5-13/84
51-A Discovery	F. Hauck, D Walker, J. Allen, A.Fisher, D. Gardner	11/8-16/84
51-C Discovery	T. Mattingly, L. Shriver, E Onizuka, J. Buchli, G. Payton	1/24-27/85
51-D Discovery	K. Bobko, D. Williams, J. Hoffman, S. Griggs, R. Seddon, C. Walker, J. Garn	4/12-19/85
51-B Challenger	R. Overmyer, F. Gregory, D. Lind, N. Thagard, W. Thornton, T. Wang, L. van den Berg	4/29-5/6/85
51-G Discovery	D. Brandenstein, J. Creighton, J. Fabian, S. Nagel, S. Lucid, P. Baudry (France), S. Al-Saud (Saudi Arabia)	6/17-24/85
51-F Challenger	C. Fullerton, R. Bridges, S. Musgrave, A. England, K. Henize, L Acton, J. Bartoe	6/29-8/6/85
51-I Discovery	J. Engle, R. Covey, J. van Hoften, W. Fisher, J. Lounge	8/27-9/3/85
51-J Atlantis	K. Bobko, R. Grabe, D. Hilmers, R. Stewart,W. Pailes	10/3-7/85
61-A Challenger	H. Hartsfield, S. Nagel, J. Buchli, G. Bluford, B. Dunbar, R. Furrer (FRG), E. Messerschmid (FRG), W. Ockels (Netherlands)	10/30-11/6/85
61-B Atlantis	B. Shaw, B. O'Connor, M. Cleave, J. Ross, S. Spring, C. Walker, R. Neri-Vela (Mexico)	11/26-12/3/85
61-C Columbia	R. Gibson, C. Bolden, G. Nelson, S. Hawley, F. Chang-Diaz, B. Nelson, R. Cenker	1/12-18/86
51-L Challenger	F. Scobee, M. Smith, E. Onizuka, J. Resnik, R. McNair, G. Jarvis, C. McAuliffe	1/28/86
STS-26 Discovery	F. Hauck, R. Covey, J. Lounge, G. Nelson, D. Hilmers	9/29-10/3/88
STS-27 Atlantis	R. Gibson, G. Gardner, R. Mullane, J. Ross, W. Shepherd	12/2-6/88
STS-29 Discovery	M. Coats, J. Blaha, J. Buchli, R. Springer, J. Bagian	3/13-18/89
STS-30 Atlantis	D. Walker, R. Grabe, N. Thagard, M. Cleave, M. Lee	5/4-8/89
STS-28 Columbia	B. Shaw, R. Richards, D. Leestma, J. Adamson, M. Brown	8/8-13/89
STS-34 Atlantis	D. Williams, M. McCulley, S. Lucid, E. Baker, F. Chang-Diaz	10/18-23/89
STS-33 Discovery	F. Gregory, J. Blaha, M. Carter, S. Musgrave, K. Thornton	11/22-27/89
STS-32 Columbia	D. Brandenstein, J. Wetherbee, B. Dunbar, M. Ivins, D. Low	1/9-20/90
STS-36 Atlantis	J. Creighton, J. Casper, D. Hilmers, R. Mullane, P. Thuot	2/28-3/4/90
STS-31 Discovery	L. Shriver, C. Bolden, S. Hawley, B. McCandless, K. Sullivan	4/24-29/90
STS-41 Discovery	R. Richards, R. Cabana, B. Melnick, W. Shepherd, T. Akers	10/6-10/90
STS-38 Atlantis	R. Covey, F. Culbertson, C. Meade, R. Springer, C. Gemar	11/15-20/90
STS-35 Columbia	V. Brand, G. Gardner, J. Hoffman, J. Lounge, R. Parker, S. Durrance, R. Parise	12/2-10/90
STS-37 Atlantis	S. Nagel, K. Cameron, J.Apt, L. Godwin, J. Ross	4/5-11/91
STS-39 Discovery	M. Coats, B. Hammond, G.Bluford, G. Harbaugh, R. Hieb, D. McMonagle, C. Veach	4/28-5/6/91

Table 8 (continued) Space Shuttle Flights

Mission-Shuttle	Crew	Flight Dates
STS-40 Columbia	B. O'Connor, S. Gutierrez, J. Bagian, T. Jernigan, R. Seddon, D. Gaffney, M. Hughes-Fulford	6/5-14/91
STS-43 Atlantis	J. Blaha, M. Baker, S. Lucid, D. Low, J. Adamson	8/2-11/91
STS-44 Atlantis	F. Gregory, T. Henricks, S. Musgrave, M. Runco, J. Voss, T. Hennen	9/12-18/91
STS-42 Discovery	R. Grabe, S. Oswald, N. Thagard, W. Readdy, D. Hilmers, R. Bondar, U. Merbold (FRG)	1/22-30/92
STS-45 Atlantis	C. Bolden, B. Duffy, K. Sullivan, D. Leestma, M. Foale, D. Frimout, B. Lichtenberg	3/23-4/1/92
STS-49 Endeavour	D. Brandenstein, K. Chilton, R. Hieb, B. Melnick, P. Thuot, K. Thornton, T. Akers	5/7- 16/92
STS-50 Columbia	R. Richards, K. Bowersox, B. Dunbar, E. Baker, C. Meade, L. DeLucas, E. Trinh.	6/25-7/9/92
STS-46 Atlantis	L. Shriver, A. Allen, C. Nicollier, M. Ivins, J. Hoffman, F. Chang-Diaz, F. Malerba (Italy)	7/31-8/892
STS-47 Endeavour	R. Gibson, C. Brown, M. Lee, J. Davis, J. Apt, M. Jemison, M. Mohri (Japan)	9/12-20/92
STS-52 Columbia	J. Wetherbee, M. Baker, T. Jernigan, C. Veach, W. Shepherd, S. McClean	10/22-11/1/92
STS-53 Discovery	D. Walker, R. Cabana, G. Bluford, J. Voss, M. Clifford	12/2-12/9/92

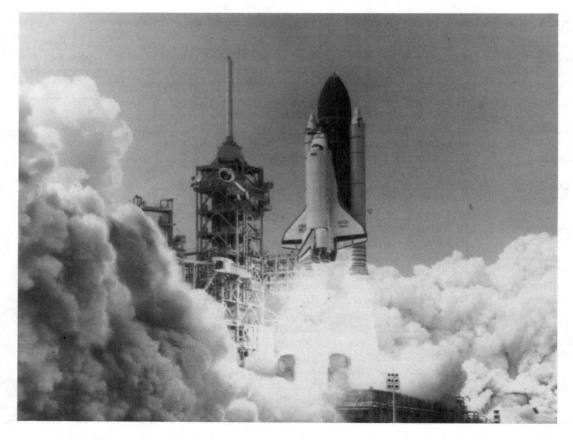

Fig. 32 Space Shuttle Atlantis is launched from Kennedy Space Center carrying the spacecraft Magellan into low Earth orbit (May 4, 1989). (NASA 89-HC-301)

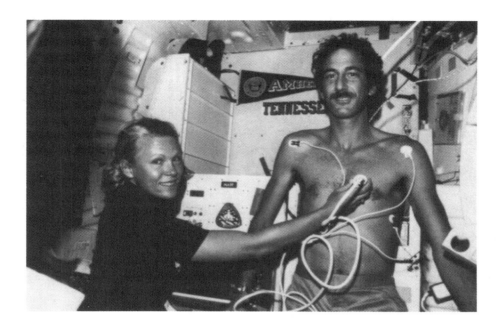

Fig. 33 Mission Specialist Rhea Seddon performs biomedical experiment on Mission Specialist Jeffrey A. Hoffman during Space Shuttle Mission STS-51-D (May 10, 1985). (NASA 85-H-141)

Unfortunately, the launch of Challenger on January 28, 1986, ended in tragedy. Due to a structural defect, almost immediately after lift-off there was an explosion at one of the joints in the casing of the solid rocket booster and the astronauts perished. This catastrophe led to a significant delay in implementation of the Space Shuttle Program to allow time to identify and eliminate the cause of the disaster. The U.S. resumed flights of its Space Shuttle in September 1988 when Discovery successfully deployed a Tracking and Data Relay Satellite (TDRS), which was then boosted into geosynchronous orbit. Space Shuttles Atlantis, Columbia, and Discovery subsequently carried into space the Magellan and Galileo spacecraft (see below), another TDRS satellite, and the Hubble Space Telescope (April 1, 1990). On one Space Shuttle mission (January 1990), the Columbia brought a spacecraft back from space. The Long Duration Exposure Facility (LDEF), which had spent almost 6 years in space, provided scientists an opportunity to test the effects of weightlessness and the space environment on various materials and biological samples.

An important stage in the history of Soviet rocket and space technology was the development of a new multipurpose heavy lift launcher, Energiya.[68] Its development was shaped by the requirements of the new Soviet space launch system that would include the Buran, and also anticipated future Soviet space transportation (both manned and unmanned) needs for the next two to three decades, including possible manned flights to the Moon and Mars. As a result of detailed analysis of current and potential future requirements and the technical capabilities of the Soviet rocket-space industry, the major specifications for this system were formulated precisely, and its major characteristics derived. The launch weight of the Energiya booster rocket is approximately 2400 metric tons,

and it can inject into orbit a payload weighing approximately 100 metric tons (length up to 40 m, and diameter up to 7 m). A critical requirement was that it be multipurpose, i.e., that it be capable of carrying a variety of cargoes differing in size and weight.

Another Energiya requirement was that it be useful as a basis for developing future medium- and heavy-lift rockets, from 10 to 200 metric tons. This would enable standardization of the design of these boosters, minimizing the number of new sustainer engines and rocket modules that would need to be developed for their construction. As a result, the Energiya booster rocket was designed to be built on the modular principle from components used in other booster rockets.[68]

After ground-based optimization of the component parts of the booster rocket, complex firing tests of full-sized first and second stage modules, and flight tests of the first stage modules (as components of another booster rocket), Energiya was scheduled for an experimental launch with a large-sized mock-up of a spacecraft. The first such launch, which took place in May 1987, verified the adequacy of work performed on the ground to optimize the booster rocket, as well as the readiness of ground-based facilities for flight tests of the new booster rocket with an orbital station, and showed how it would be affected during actual launch and flight. The only exception to the success of this test was the failure of the mock-up of the spacecraft (due to a malfunction in its on-board systems) to enter the scheduled orbit. On the whole, the successful launch of the Energiya booster rocket signified its readiness for flight tests of the Energiya-Buran space transportation system (Fig. 34).

The first launch of the Energiya booster rocket with the unmanned Buran space vehicle occurred on November 15,

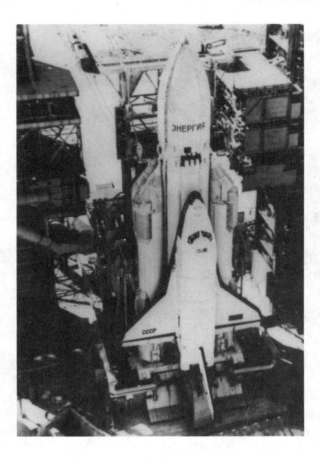

Fig. 34 Energiya-Buran system

1988. It was successful, and the return to Earth and precise landing of the Buran spacecraft convincingly demonstrated the reliability of the systems of the booster rocket as well as the space vehicle. More than 1200 research, development, and engineering groups were involved in the design and development of Energiya. Their work produced significant advances in several areas of technology development; for example, structural materials with newer and greater tolerances, new varieties of high-strength steel, new aluminum and titanium alloys, and new thermal insulating and protective coatings—not to mention advanced technological processes.[68] The successful development of Energiya opened up many new possibilities for the future, such as the construction of major scientific research laboratories in near-Earth orbit, as well as space factories for the manufacture and processing of super-pure substances, alloys, optical materials, vaccines, and drugs.

C. Orbiting Space Stations

During the late 1970s and early 1980s work continued in the U.S.S.R. to develop and utilize orbiting research space stations. In September 1977, Salyut 6, a member of the second generation of Soviet stations, was put into orbit. The new Salyut had an integrated propulsion system with a single power system, as well as new engines and a new control system.

It also had not one, but two docking ports, which enabled it simultaneously to receive two transport vehicles that could be flown manned or unmanned. Because of this development, unmanned cargo spacecraft of the Progress type could be used for the first time, substantially increasing the duration of active functioning of the station and its crews through delivery of additional propellant, materials for crew life support (including a special crew shower), and other needed materials. Salyut 6 spent more than 4.5 years in orbit. During this time, it was inhabited by 27 cosmonauts of 16 crews (5 prime and 11 visiting crews). Twelve Progress vehicles delivered approximately 20 tons of cargo during Salyut 6's time in orbit. A large number of scientific/technological and bioastronautic studies were performed, including more than 1600 biomedical and biological experiments.[69]

In April 1982, the last orbiting station in the Salyut series, Salyut 7, was put into orbit. It was essentially analogous to the previous station. The major differences lay in the expansion of scientific and technological research facilities and improvement of crew living and working conditions. Salyut 7 was operational in space for more than 4 years. The more than 10 crews that worked there (both prime crews, staying as long as 237 days, and a number of visiting crews) consisting of more than 30 cosmonauts, including the second female cosmonaut, S.Ye. Savitskaya; the French cosmonaut, J.L. Chretien; the Indian cosmonaut, R. Sharma; and the second Soviet cosmonaut-physician, O.Yu. Atkov, who conducted a large number of ultrasound studies of the crewmembers' cardiovascular systems, studied their mineral and carbohydrate metabolism, and determined the optimal schedules of physical exercise and exertion.

In 1982, work began on a manned Spacelab module developed by the European Space Agency (ESA). The module was designed to be carried as a Shuttle payload. The Spacelab module was first flown in November 1983 and carried a crew of six, including West German payload specialist Ulf Merbold. The pressurized Spacelab module provided extensive opportunities for various types of biomedical and physiological research. A number of new research methodologies were used on Spacelab (Fig. 35), which flew 24 times in 6 years.

In February 1986 the Soviet Union placed into orbit the core module (weighing more than 20 tons) of its third generation long-duration space station, Mir. Mir will be the core module for future multi-module designs. In addition to two docking ports (located along the vertical axis as on Salyut 6 and Salyut 7), Mir has four more berthing ports located along the sides for attaching scientific research modules. Mir has provided significantly improved crew living and working conditions. The living quarters, in the center of the module, are more spacious and the life support system has been improved; there are many robotic devices on the station.

In March 1986, cosmonauts L.D. Kizim and V.A. Solovyov were transported to the Mir where they remained for 125 days.

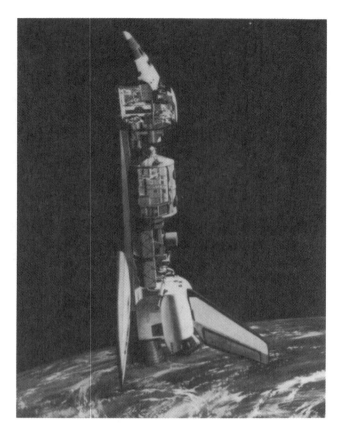

Fig. 35 Spacelab, inserted into orbit by Space Shuttle (NASA 78-H-105)

Then, in May, they flew to the Salyut 7 station on the Soyuz-T 15 vehicle, where they remained for another 50 days before returning to Mir in June. This was the first time crewmembers had ever been transported from one space station to another and back.

The multipurpose astrophysical science module Kvant, designed for extra-atmospheric astronomical research and other scientific experiments, was sent to and docked with the Mir in April 1987 (Fig. 36).

Subsequently, the station continued to operate in a virtually uninterrupted manned mode. From 1987 to 1992, more than 14 crews (over 30 cosmonauts) worked on Mir, including cosmonauts from Afghanistan, Austria, Bulgaria, France, Germany, Great Britain, France, Japan and Syria. (See Fig. 37, Table 9). In November, 1989 the Kvant 2, which substantially expanded the scientific capacity of the Mir complex, was delivered to the station.

D. Planetary Exploration

During the third decade of the space age the United States and Soviet Union continued to explore our planetary neighbors in the solar system with interplanetary probes. While the primary objects of this exploration continued to be Venus and Mars, probes also began the systematic investigation of the

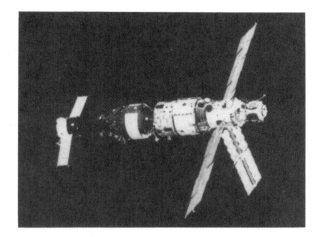

Fig. 36 Mir with Kvant and Soyuz TM

more distant planets of the outer solar system. During 1978 both the Soviet Union and the United States launched further missions to explore the planet Venus. In December the U.S. Pioneer-Venus 1 began to orbit Venus and transmit information about the space surrounding the planet and results of radar sounding of its surface. In November during approach to the planet, four of Pioneer-Venus 2's five probes separated and entered the planet's atmosphere and two survived after reaching the planet's smoldering (480 °C) surface, one continued to transmit information for 67 minutes.

In September 1978 the Soviet Union sent Venera 11 and 12 spacecraft to Venus, and in October and November Venera 13 and 14 followed. Instruments on these probes added to our store of knowledge about the atmosphere of the planet and the chemical composition of its surface materials. Telephotometry from the descent modules of Venera 13 and Venera 14 returned panoramic images of the landing site. Some of the photographs were taken through light filters, providing the first color images of the venusian surface. In June 1983, Venera 15 and 16 were launched and eventually entered venusian orbit. Taking remote sounding and radar surveys (using a side looking radar) of the planet's surface, Venera 15 and 16 were able to map a significant portion of the surface, from the north pole to 30° north latitude with resolution of 1-2 km, providing information for the first detailed atlas of this area of Venus.

The Soviet Union's Vega 1 and Vega 2 were dispatched in December 1984 to Venus and to a rendezvous with Halley's Comet. In June 1985 they reached the vicinity of the planet and studied the atmosphere, cloud layer, and surface with descent modules carrying aerostat probes and other instruments, which had been developed through the combined efforts of scientists and technicians from the Austria, Bulgaria, Czechoslovakia, the Federal Republic of Germany, France, the German Democratic Republic, Hungary, Poland, and the Soviet Union. Study of the planet continued and new scientific data were obtained.

a)

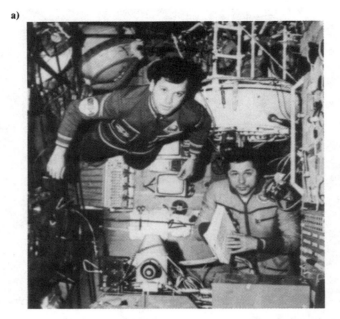

b)

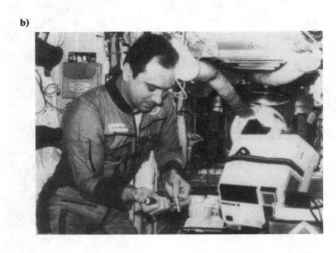

Fig. 37 Study of the effects of weightlessness on Salyut and Mir: a) V. Savinykh (U.S.S.R.) and D. Prunariu (Romania) on Salyut 6; b) cosmonaut-physician V. Polyakov on Mir performs a blood analysis

After the Venus flyby, the gravity of the planet put Vega 1 and 2 into a flight trajectory to Halley's Comet. For their rendezvous with Halley's Comet in March 1986, Vega 1 and Vega 2 approached to within 8000-9000 km of the comet's core. During this very interesting experiment, a cometary research program produced new information, especially about the nucleus.

The Vega spacecraft rendezvous with Halley's Comet was well coordinated with the rendezvous mission jointly mounted by the ESA. Launched by an Ariane launcher, ESA's 340 kg Giotto spacecraft measured the atmosphere, ionized particles, and dust from the coma boiling off Halley's nucleus under the effect of solar heating, photographed the nucleus with an onboard camera to a 50-m resolution, and measured atomic composition with spectrometers. Other spacecraft in the

flotilla that encountered Halley's Comet during its historic close approach (700 million km) to the Earth were Japan's Sakigake and Planet A. Meanwhile, the United States' ICE (International Cometary Explorer) spacecraft, which had first been launched as the International Sun-Earth Explorer 3 on September 11, 1985, conducted an historic encounter with the comet Giacobini-Zinner 71 million km from Earth, the first comet intercept in history. ICE entered the 22,000-km wide tail of the comet 8000 km from its core, where it spent 20 minutes gathering data on cometary materials.

During this third decade of the space age, the use of automated space probes gradually expanded. Whereas during the first part of this period their use was limited to study of the Moon and closest planets to the Earth (Venus and Mars), beginning in the second half of the 1970s, probes were also

Table 9   Manned flights on Mir

Spacecraft	Crew	Launch Date
Soyuz TM	Unmanned	5/21/86
Soyuz TM-2	Romanenko, Yu.V., Laveykin, A.I.	2/6/87
Soyuz TM-3	Viktorenko, A.S., Aleksandrov, A.P., Mukhammed, F. (Syria).	7/22/87
Soyuz TM-4	Titov, V.G. Manarov, M.Kh., Levchenko, A.S.	12/21/87
Soyuz TM-5	Solovyov, A.Ya., Savinykh, V.P., Aleksandrov, A.P. (Bulgaria)	6/7/88
Soyuz TM-6	Lyakhov, V.A., Polyakov, V.V., Mohmad, A.A. (Afghanistan)	8/29/88
Soyuz TM-7	Volkov, A.A., Krikalev, S.K., Chretien, J.L. (France)	11/26/88
Soyuz TM-8	Viktorenko, A.S., Serebrov, A.A.	9/6/89
Soyuz TM-9	Solovyov, A.Ya, Balandin, A.N.	2/11/90
Soyuz TM-10	Manakov, G.M., Strekalov, G.M.	8/1/90
Soyuz TM-11	Afanasyev, V.M., Manarov, M.Kh., Akiyama, T. (Japan)	12/2/91
Soyuz TM-12	Artsevarskiy, A.P., Krikalev, S.K., Sherman, H. (United Kingdom)	5/18/91
Soyuz TM-13	Volkov, A.A., Aubakirov, T.O., Viehboeck, O (Austria)	10/2/91
Soyuz TM-14	Viktorenko, A.S.Kaleri, A.Yu., Flade, K.D. (Germany)	3/17/92
Soyuz TM-15	Solovyov, A.Ya., Avdeyev, S.V., Tonini, M. (France)	7/27/92

used to study Jupiter and Saturn, and in the 1980s, Uranus and Neptune also came under scrutiny by automated space probes. The range of use of the probes was also extended to study of planetary moons.

By 1982, the United States' Voyager 1 and Voyager 2 spacecraft, launched in September and August of 1977, respectively, had completed their primary missions—further reconnaissance of the planets Jupiter and Saturn. Each of the spacecraft had traveled more than 2.4 billion kilometers and their instruments had investigated seven major bodies of the solar system. They made comparative studies of the Jupiter and Saturn systems, including their satellites, rings, and fields and particle environments, from distances as close as 4000 km. They also measured characteristics of the interplanetary medium from Earth to Saturn. During their relatively trouble-free journey the spacecraft acquired more than 62,000 images from the outer solar system, including images of the jovian and saturnian moons, and discovered rings around Jupiter and unusual braiding, spokes, ringlets, and shepherding satellites in the rings of Saturn. The Voyagers also discovered new satellites of Jupiter and Saturn, lightning on Jupiter, eight active volcanoes on Io, and new sources of radio emissions in the Jupiter and Saturn systems. While making these discoveries, the spacecraft measured the atmospheric composition, temperature, pressure, dynamics, magnetospheres, and particle environments of Jupiter, Saturn, and Titan and also the distribution of microparticles in their field.

In January 1986, Voyager 2 approached the planet Uranus. As it sped by Uranus, using the gravity of that planet to "slingshot" it on its way to Neptune, the spacecraft discovered 10 new uranian moons and imaged the 5 already known. Miranda, the smallest of the previously known moons, was found to have an especially tortured surface, while the others displayed every possible geological phenomenon. Uranus also revealed some curiosities: an offset magnetic field, an ultraviolet sheen called an "electroglow," and erratic atmospheric patterns. The slingshot maneuver succeeded, and in 1989 Voyager 2 approached within 4900 km of Neptune. The spacecraft returned data and photographs of that brilliant blue planet, revealing its great dark spots and the features of its moon, Triton. In February 1990 this "Grand Tour" of the outer solar system culminated in the creation of a composite family portrait of the planets in our solar system taken by Voyager 1 (Fig. 38). This photograph gives visual testimony to civilization's progress through the age of space exploration since the Earth was first photographed "rising" over the horizon of the Moon by an Apollo spacecraft in 1968. Both Voyagers continue their missions as they fly outward, seeking the edge of the heliopause, where the particle field of the Sun gives way to interstellar space.

In 1989 the U.S. launched additional missions to Venus and Jupiter, using the Space Shuttle to carry the Magellan and Galileo spacecraft into near-Earth orbit, where they were launched on their interplanetary trajectories. Equipped with

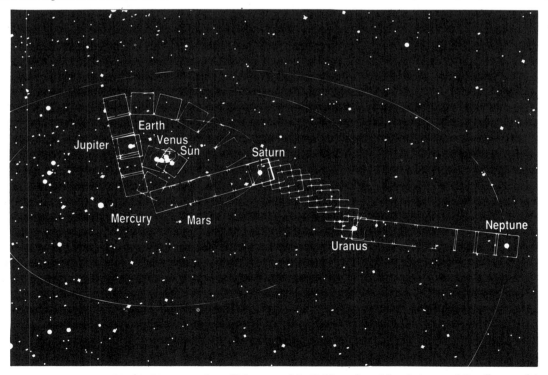

Fig. 38 The cameras of U.S. Voyager 1 on February 14, 1990, pointed back toward the Sun and took a series of pictures of the Sun and the planets, making the first ever portrait of our solar system as seen from the outside. In the course of taking this mosaic, consisting of a total of 60 frames, Voyager 1 made several images of the inner solar system from a distance of approximately 7 billion km and about 32 degrees above the ecliptic plane (1990). (NASA 90-H-401)

instruments for high resolution radar mapping, altimetry, and microwave radiometry, the Magellan spacecraft reached Venus in August 1990 and is completing a detailed radar map of the surface of Venus, revealing numerous new features and evidence of extensive volcanic activity. Galileo is taking advantage of the opportunity for three planetary gravity-assist swing-bys (one at Venus and two at Earth) in order to reach Jupiter in December 1995. For the first time we will be able to examine one of the outer planets with an atmospheric probe. Galileo is equipped to conduct long-term observations of Jupiter and its moons as it orbits the planet, and it is also expected to return information about Venus, the Earth and the Moon, and two asteroids encountered on its long journey.

E. Biology and Exobiology

After the start of manned space flight, and in addition to human medical research, biological experiments using a variety of organisms were continued both on manned and unmanned spacecraft and orbital stations. These included the Gemini, Soyuz, Apollo, and Space Shuttle spacecraft and the Salyut, Skylab, and Mir stations, as well as special Soviet and U.S. biosatellites. Biological research was performed on 11 Soviet Cosmos series biosatellites (1966-1989), and the Soviet Zond 5 (1968) and Zond 7 (1969) spacecraft. U.S. research was conducted on OV1-4 (1966), high-altitude rocket Aerobee-150A (1967), OFO-1A (Orbiting Frog Otolith, 1970), and Biosatellites 2 and 3 (1967 and 1969). Life scientists from many nations have participated in biological investigations on Soviet and U.S. spacecraft.

During these missions, experiments in space biology were performed on a broad range of biological subjects and experimental animals: microorganisms, tissue cultures, lower and higher plants, fish, amphibians, insects, reptiles, mice, rats, dogs, and primates. Research was conducted at various levels of biological organization—from the molecular level to the level of the population.

In one of the earliest Cosmos flights (1966), two dogs were flown for 22 days in a study of the effects of weightlessness on the functions of the cardiovascular system. In the U.S., the flight of the high-altitude rocket Aerobee 150A was used to determine the level of artificial gravity preferred by rats, while the activity of the vestibular nerve of a frog was studied on the biosatellite OFO-1A. In 1968 and 1969 tortoises and other organisms made a 7-day flight around the Moon on Zond 5 and Zond 7 and in 1972 five mice flew to the Moon on Apollo 17.[49]

The biological effects of artificial gravity and the combined effects of weightlessness and a source of ionizing radiation were studied on the U.S. Biosatellite 2 (1967), and the U.S.S.R. Cosmos (1974 and 1977). Those missions demonstrated that weightlessness did not significantly alter the biological effects of ionizing radiation. Genetic and radiobiological studies were also conducted on Apollo 16 and 17 (1972).

Physiological, biochemical, morphological, population, and embryological investigations on a number of Cosmos series biosatellites (1978, 1983, and others) identified adaptive changes in rats in physiological systems that are subject to static gravitational loading on Earth (leg bones, spine, muscles). Changes were also found in fluid-electrolyte metabolism and hormonal regulation. Embryological experiments have studied the effects of weightlessness on the course of mammalian development.

Because of the physiological similarity between monkeys and humans, experiments with monkeys were used in the U.S. and U.S.S.R. to study the effects of flight on psychoemotional behavior, the central nervous and cardiovascular systems, the sense organs, vestibular and eye movement reactions, and the performance of elementary operator (instrumental) tasks, and on chronobiological and other parameters (Biosatellite 3,

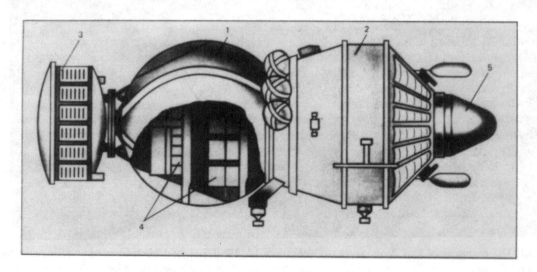

Fig. 39 Configuration of Cosmos biosatellites; Legend: 1—descent module with pressurized cabin for biological subject; 2—instrument/equipment module; 3—pressurized container with power sources; 4—scientific equipment; 5—retrorocket

1969; Cosmos, 1983, 1985, 1987, 1989, 1992; Space Shuttle). Finally, an experiment on biosatellite Cosmos (1989) (Fig. 39) and associated laboratory studies investigated pathological and regenerative processes in the healing of injuries and wounds, and revealed quantitative and qualitative changes in the course of regeneration in space.

Biological experiments in space provide an opportunity to obtain scientific material for the in-depth study of the mechanisms of biological and physiological adaptation to flight conditions, and thereby also shed light on the operation of biological systems in general. Results of space biology experiments combined with ground simulations and laboratory studies have served as the basis for biological insights and medical recommendations. Biological research in space has done a great deal to elucidate the role of gravity in the formation and development of biological systems, demonstrating that microgravity can be used as a tool to study biological phenomena such as morphogenesis and reproduction. These experiments have also revealed the extensive potential of systemic physiological adaptation to space flight conditions.[71-74]

Current and future manned and unmanned space exploration calls for systematic progress in the theoretical and experimental aspects of exobiology. Researchers are focusing on the age-old philosophical and fundamental biological and chemical issues of the origin of life in the universe, the routes and factors of biological evolution, the evolution of organic substances—particularly carbohydrate compounds—and the study of carbon meteorites. Laboratory studies have simulated the physiological effects of extreme ambient conditions and examined theoretical and methodological issues related to the search for extraterrestrial life and the defining criteria for living systems, including protobiological forms.[75-77] Numerous specialists have examined the principles, methods, and problems of planetary quarantine to prevent the contamination of celestial bodies by terrestrial life forms, and vice versa, the unpredictable consequences of bringing alien life forms to Earth.

Observations of the surface of Mars made from orbit by Mars, Mariner, and the Viking orbiters played an important role in the investigation of the possibility of life on Mars. Data from the Viking 1 and Viking 2 landers, equipped with physical, chemical, and biological instruments and video cameras, have proved particularly critical. Valuable information was obtained about the planet's atmosphere (nitrogen was discovered), landscape, and composition and mechanical properties of the soil. The major conclusion of exobiological research on Viking was that there were no definitive signs of life or evidence of organic compounds found in the martian soil.[67, 78]

Most researchers tend to believe that these conclusions cannot be considered final and that work should go on with continuous improvements in the methodology for searching for signs of life elsewhere in the solar system.[79]

The celestial body closest to Earth, the Moon, has received especially intensive study by exobiologists. Soviet and American probes have transmitted images of the lunar surface,

and collected samples of lunar soil from various regions and returned them to the Earth for laboratory analysis and study of their biological effects. Extremely valuable information about conditions on the Moon was obtained by the crews of Apollo 11-17, who worked on the Moon's surface for many hours, travelling a considerable distance in lunar rovers and collecting samples of lunar soil for return to Earth.[62, 67] The results of these studies are consistent: no signs of life have as yet been detected on the Moon.

F. Work on Rockets in Other Countries

Only the Soviet Union and the United States survived World War II with the ability to launch spacecraft for research and applied purposes. Soon, however, it became possible for other countries to participate more actively in the exploration of space.

During the first half of the 1960s, the first British satellite, Ariel (April 1962), the first Canadian satellite, Alouette 1 (August 1962), and the first Italian satellite San Marco 1 (December 1964) were inserted into near-Earth orbit. The first two satellites were launched by the American booster rocket, Thor-Delta, and the third by the U.S. booster rocket, Scout. U.S. booster rockets were used because neither the United Kingdom, Canada, nor Italy yet had rockets capable of putting spacecraft into orbit.

France became the third spacefaring nation when, using its own booster rocket (Diamant), it launched the first French satellite, Asterex 1, in November 1965. Japan in February 1970, China in April 1970, and the United Kingdom in October 1971 used their own booster rockets to insert into orbit the first Japanese satellite Osumi, the first Chinese satellite China 1, and the British Prospero.

Since the mid-1970s, ESA has increased its space activities. The agency includes 13 West European countries: Austria, Belgium, Denmark, France, Germany, Ireland, Italy, the Netherlands, Norway, Spain, Switzerland, Sweden, and the United Kingdom. ESA cooperates actively with the U.S., Canada, and other countries. ESA's main activities have consisted of independent space launches provided by the Ariane (developed mainly by France and Germany) and the development of commercial satellites.

Work has continued in other countries as well. In February 1975 the flight testing program began for the Japanese booster-launcher "N," manufactured on a contract basis by McDonnell Douglas (and based on the Delta rocket). In April 1975 the first Indian satellite, Ariabhata, was placed in orbit by a Soviet booster-launcher, and in July 1975 the Indian satellite Rohini was placed in orbit by an Indian rocket.

In 1981 the Japanese launched the N-2 rocket, capable of placing a 350-kg spacecraft in geostationary orbit. January 1984 saw the first flight tests of China's Long March 3 (CZ3) rocket. In 1988, the Long March 4 rocket lifted the first Chinese weather satellite to orbit.

In August 1986 the Japanese completed the first experimental launch of the H-1 rocket. The rocket had an oxygen/hydrogen liquid-fueled engine, and was able to lift 550 kg into geostationary orbit. Since then it has replaced the N-2, and Japanese scientists are currently working on the most up-to-date version of the H-2 rocket.

G. Evolution of International Space Law

Soon after the start of the space age, especially after manned space flights had begun, society had to confront legal issues associated with this new area of human endeavor, including regulation of the activities of nations and international organizations in the exploration and use of space. The first work toward development of a theory of international space law was accomplished in the late 1920s and early 1930s.[80] An early discussion of the need for "interplanetary transportation laws" in association with the approach of the era of high-altitude flights and interplanetary communications appeared in the work of the Soviet scholar V.A. Zarzar,[81] while the Czechoslovak jurist V. Mandl published a book completely devoted to space law in Germany in 1932.[82] In 1933 the Soviet jurist Ye.A. Korovin produced a report at the Conference on Air Law in Leningrad concerning legal questions associated with exploration of the upper atmosphere.[83] Several theses of the report anticipated legal problems to appear later during space exploration.[80]

After the launch of the first manmade satellites, interest in legal aspects of space exploration increased. A number of works on space law were published in the U.S.S.R., most notably the review by the eminent Soviet jurist Ye.A. Korovin.[84] A number of works on this area were also published in the United States.[85]

Among the many novelties produced by space exploration has been a new body of international law. As with the Law of the Sea, the opportunity to travel and trade over geographic areas beyond the limits of individual sovereign territories has required that nations agree on common principles to minimize conflicts and protect common interests.

Unlike the Law of the Sea, however, space law does not derive from codified principles elaborated to cover all conceivable circumstances; rather, the development of space law has been incremental and pragmatic in character, describing general principles based on experience and political as well as technological realities. International space law embraces two categories of laws and conventions: those formulated within the United Nations, and those arrived at through bilateral and multilateral treaties and agreements. National legislation bearing on space activities (which are beyond the scope of this chapter) both help to shape and are shaped by international space law.

When the Soviet Union launched Sputnik in 1957 the first question to be resolved was whether space travel should be subject to an international regime. It could be argued, for example, that the sovereignty of the nation launching a space object reached upwards indefinitely (an extension of that nation's air space), and that the fact that the object launched passed over other sovereign nations was simply incidental to the fact of the Earth's revolution.

An even larger question than the location of the boundary between sovereign "air space" and "outer space" was that of the legal status of outer space. If no nation can claim sovereignty over space, is space res nullius—simply unexplored territory subject to claims? Or is it res extra commercium, under the jurisdiction of the United Nations? Or is it res communis omnium, the heritage of all mankind to be protected by the international community as a whole?

That the principal organization to oversee a new international order for outer space should be the United Nations was a natural development. The most critical issue initially before the United Nations was twofold: what general principles should govern the use of outer space, and what kind of entity should the United Nations establish to oversee members' use of space?

The question of the kind of United Nations organization that should be established to identify and resolve the legal issues arising from space exploration was answered in December 1958 when the United Nations General Assembly created an Ad Hoc Committee on the Peaceful Uses of Outer Space, or COPUOS. The Ad Hoc Committee was created amid the reluctance of the great powers to commit to formal restrictions against military uses of space or requirements for international cooperation. For this reason, immediately after it was formed, COPUOS limited its discussions to such issues as the registration of spacecraft, the liability of their owners, exchange of scientific information and allocation of radio frequencies.

The United States' policy on the general issues initially posed by the dawn of space exploration was and remains expressed in The Space Act (Public Law 85-568, July 29, 1958), which declares that activities in space should be devoted to peaceful purposes for the benefit of all mankind. What such peaceful purposes might be were surveyed by the Ad Hoc COPUOS, which reported in July 1959 that satellites could be expected to improve weather forecasting, global communications, mapping, navigation, and the human exploration of space. Shortly thereafter, the United Nations General Assembly agreed to the creation of a permanent COPUOS composed of 24 members, with 2 permanent subcommittees, a legal subcommittee, and a scientific and technical subcommittee.

UN Resolution 1721 (December 20, 1961) outlined an extensive program for comprehensive collaboration of the member nations in the area of exploration and use of space. In this document COPUOS was tasked, among other things, to consider legal issues. The resolution extended international law to the realm of outer space and celestial bodies, and declared that this realm was not subject to national appropriation.[86] The COPUOS provided the initial forum in which consensus could be built around principles that would then became the basis of UN Resolutions, which themselves might become the basis of international draft treaties.

Subsequently, for almost two decades international agreement on legal aspects of space exploration was crafted within the United Nations. In December 1963, the UN adopted a "Declaration of the legal principles governing the activity of states in the exploration and use of outer space." Although this document did not have the force of an international treaty, it did a great deal to facilitate further work in the area of space law.

An important milestone in the development of the legal principles of space exploration was the Treaty on Principles Governing the Activities of States in the Exploration and Use of Outer Space, Including the Moon and Other Celestial Bodies, which became effective in October 1967. The Outer Space Treaty of 1967 provided that: 1) international law and the Charter of the United Nations shall apply to space activities; 2) outer space and celestial bodies are the province of mankind and shall be used only for peaceful purposes and for the benefit of all mankind; 3) nuclear weapons, weapons of mass destruction, military bases, and military maneuvers are banned from space; 4) outer space shall be free for exploration, use, and scientific investigation; 5) there can be no claims of sovereignty or territory by nations over locations in space, by means of use or occupation or by any other means; 6) jurisdiction over space objects launched from Earth shall be retained by the launching state; 7) private interests are recognized as having freedom of action in space, so long as a government or group of governments on Earth authorizes and exercises continuing supervision over their activities. Signatory nations are therefore under a duty to oversee the activities of their citizens and commercial ventures in space; 8) governments are liable for damage caused on Earth by their space objects; and 9) astronauts are Envoys of Mankind and are entitled to noninterference and all necessary assistance in distress.

Several articles of the Outer Space Treaty have themselves become the basis for separate treaties. These include the Agreement on the Rescue of Astronauts, the Return of Astronauts and the Return of Objects Launched into Outer Space (1968), the Convention on International Liability for Damage Caused by Space Objects (1972), and The Convention for Registering Objects Launched in Outer Space (1975). A fourth treaty, the Agreement Governing the Activities of States on the Moon and Other Celestial Bodies (Moon Treaty), was adopted by the United Nations General Assembly in 1979 and entered into force in July 1984.

Individual spacefaring nations have also formulated agreements outside of the United Nations framework. One of the oldest of these is the agreement to abide by the International Telecommunications Convention creating the International Telecommunications Union (ITU). The ITU allocates and registers radio frequencies, as well as limited slots in the geosynchronous orbit required by telecommunications satellites. The International Telecommunications Satellite Organization (INTELSAT) agreement, effective 1973, established an international organization to operate a global commercial communications system. Following the pattern set by INTELSAT, INMARSAT—the International Maritime Satellite Telecommunications organization, was established in 1978 to operate a global system of maritime satellites to serve the commercial maritime safety needs of its signatories.

Institutional arrangements to oversee and regulate the communications satellites of the Soviet Union, Bulgaria, Cuba, Czechoslovakia, the German Democratic Republic, Hungary, Mongolia, Poland, and Rumania were created by the INTERSPUTNIK agreement of 1971. Similar arrangements for the regional (multinational) administration of a system of communications satellites, ground stations, and equipment were created with the 1976 Agreement of the Arab Corporation for Space Communications and, in 1977, with the agreement creating EUTELSAT (the European Telecommunications Satellite organization).

International law treaties arising out of the needs of the new era of space exploration are the first known such documents to speak not primarily of the rights of sovereign nations, but of the world's people or all mankind. Thus they perpetuate the concept of natural law as the proper foundation for laws between states. Similarly, they have fostered cooperation rather than competition among nations in the exploration of space.

H. International Scientific Collaboration

International scientific collaboration has played an important role in the history of space exploration. Indeed, this subject was even considered in the works of the first theorists of space flight.[87]

While major work in rocket and space technology was being conducted in the late 1940s in the U.S. and U.S.S.R., similar studies were going on in other countries as well. In these smaller nations, attempts were made to focus on issues that did not require a great deal of design, and also on theoretical work on principles of interplanetary flight. By the late 1940s, there began to be interest in uniting the efforts of large and small nations for the study and use of space for peaceful purposes and in the establishment of international scientific collaboration in this area. For this purpose, an International Astronautical Conference was held in 1950 in Paris. Its main result was the establishment of the International Astronautical Federation (IAF) to reinforce contacts among participants in the space activities of many countries. The International Council of Scientific Unions created a special committee in 1952 to plan and coordinate the efforts of scientists during the International Geophysical Year (1957-1958), which was a watershed in the development of international scientific collaboration.

This coordinated program—involving scientists from over 60 countries—conducted geophysical observations and studies in accordance with a unified program and using a standardized methodology and was the first to create a planetary observation system for monitoring the Earth's physical fields and atmospheric circulation. The professional contacts between scientists from different nations that developed during this period facilitated the initiation of international collaboration in space research after the launch of Sputnik. This event, marking the beginning of the space age, pointed up the need for high-level scientific collaboration. In 1958, the National

Aeronautics and Space Act, the law that created NASA, charged the agency, among other things, to conduct its activities so as to contribute materially to cooperation by the United States with other nations and groups of nations.[88] In fulfillment of this mandate, NASA—over the past three decades—has entered into agreements with more than 130 countries and international organizations. These relationships have covered a broad spectrum of collaborative endeavors, ranging from the development of major elements of space infrastructure to the sharing of space data among scientists around the globe.

Experimental communications satellites provided one of the earliest opportunities for international cooperation in the arena of space applications. As early as 1959, the International Telecommunications Union first considered the issue of space communications and adopted a resolution concerning identification of a specific region on the radio frequency spectrum for this purpose. A program for comprehensive collaboration, adopted in 1961 by the UN General Assembly, stipulated that international collaboration be established in the area of scientific and technological aspects of the study and utilization of space. One specific recommendation was that initial emphasis should be placed on two research areas—space meteorology and space communications. It was emphasized that research in these areas should serve the peoples of the world on a global and nondiscriminatory basis.

Accordingly, in the Relay, Telstar and Syncom experiments (1962-1964), a dozen countries built ground terminals at their own expense to work with NASA on trans-oceanic testing of these communications satellites. The global INTELSAT consortium evolved from this early beginning. Space technology was also applied early and directly to terrestrial needs in meteorology. Following launch in 1960 of Tiros 1, the first polar-orbiting weather satellite, NASA and the U.S. Weather Bureau invited weather services around the world to make ground-based weather observations coordinated with satellite photography in order to assess the value of this new technology. Beginning in 1963, the incorporation in Tiros satellites of the Automatic Picture Transmission (APT) system permitted any country in the world to receive satellite cloud cover photographs for its own region on a routine, direct and daily basis using simple radio devices costing only a few thousand dollars. Ultimately APT direct-readout facilities were built in more than 120 countries around the world.

In June 1962, the first agreement was signed instituting collaboration between Soviet and U.S. scientists in research and utilization of space. This agreement, signed by NASA and the Soviet Academy of Sciences, called for a number of projects in space communications and meteorology, and also the exchange of research results. In 1965 an agreement was reached on collaboration in the area of bioastronautics and preparation of a joint multi-volume U.S.-U.S.S.R. work, "Foundations of Space Biology and Medicine," which was completed in 1975.[89]

The Intercosmos Council played a significant role in establishing and developing international contacts of Soviet scientists in the area of cosmonautics. Intercosmos was a council for international collaboration on the study and utilization of space under the auspices of the U.S.S.R. Academy of Sciences. Intercosmos was established in 1966 for coordination of work performed by various state and scientific and technological organizations in the space arena.

In November 1965 and April 1967, meetings of representatives of a number of Communist nations—Bulgaria, Hungary, the German Democratic Republic, Cuba, Mongolia, Poland, Rumania, the Soviet Union, and Czechoslovakia—were held in Moscow. A program of collaboration in space research (called the Intercosmos program) was developed at these meetings, as were the forms and directions this collaboration would take. The drafters of this agreement attempted to take into account the level of development of science and technology in each of the participating countries, as well as the particular interests of various scientific groups within each country.

During this period 25 Intercosmos satellites and 11 Vertikal geophysical rockets were launched and scientific apparatus produced by participant nations was installed on 8 Cosmos and 5 Prognoz satellites. Three Magion satellites manufactured in Czechoslovakia were also launched.

In 1966, an intergovernmental agreement between the U.S.S.R. and France concerning collaboration in the study and conquest of space was signed in Moscow. This agreement served as the basis for joint research and a number of joint experiments. In France, the practical work of implementing the scientific collaboration was performed by the Centre National d'Etudes Spatiales (CNES). Active collaboration of these two nations included: launch of the Soviet booster carrying the French Satellite for Research in Environmental Technology (SRET) for experiments in the area of technology; joint experiments in laser sounding of the Moon using the French laser-reflector on Lunokhod 1 and 2; launch of the French astrophysical satellite SNEG 3 by a Soviet booster rocket; conduct of the joint Arcad (Arc Auroral Density) project to study dynamic processes in the Earth's magnetosphere; and flights of French cosmonauts on Soviet spacecraft and space stations.

Because of the high cost of developing and operating space technology, European countries in the early 1960s formed the European Space Research Organization (ESRO) and the European Launch Development Organization (ELDO). The ESRO 1 experimental satellite was launched in 1967.

A number of nations took an active part in the U.S. Apollo scientific program. Participation in important space science and applications programs was not limited to providing flight hardware or conducting flight observations. Much valuable work was done on the ground. For example, the program to analyze Moon rocks and dust returned from the Apollo missions included more than 90 foreign scientists selected as principal investigators on the basis of the scientific merit of their proposals. In addition, more than 280 other foreign scientists were associated as co-investigators in scientific teams headed by U.S. scientists. Thus, researchers in countries from many nations were able to contribute to—and share directly in—the Apollo Program's scientific findings.

NASA by 1970 had entered into some 250 agreements for cooperative projects with 35 countries. Fifteen unmanned scientific satellites built by foreign partners had been launched on NASA rockets and some two dozen foreign-built scientific experiments had been flown on NASA missions (including a Swiss instrument placed on the lunar surface by Apollo astronauts to determine the composition of the solar wind and the German "Biostack" experiment).

As NASA began to plan for a permanently manned space station and a reusable space shuttle to build and service it as the major development programs of the 1970s to follow Apollo, it sought out international partners to share the costs—and the benefits. This U.S. post-Apollo initiative was welcomed in Western Europe and Canada, where space budgets, industrial capabilities and ambitions had reached levels that no longer excluded them from the challenging arena of manned space flight. Although NASA was forced by budget limitations to postpone plans for the space station, development of a partially reusable space shuttle went forward in 1972. Agreements were subsequently concluded with the European Space Agency and Canada to contribute, respectively, the Spacelab manned laboratory and the Canadarm remote manipulator system to the Shuttle-based Space Transportation System. In parallel, science cooperation expanded to include larger, more ambitious efforts such as the Helios solar probe project. In this mission two German-built spacecraft containing both U.S. and German scientific instruments were launched in 1974 and 1976 by U.S. rockets, and travelled closer to the Sun than any previous spacecraft.

The decade of the 1970s also saw an expansion of opportunities for Third World participation in cooperative space projects with NASA. One such project was the Satellite Instructional Television Experiment (SITE) conducted by India in 1975-76 using NASA's ATS-6 experimental communications/broadcast satellite.

The 1972 launch by NASA of the first Landsat satellite provided another major opportunity for developing nations (as well as industrialized countries) to gain a new perspective on their own renewable and nonrenewable resources. To determine the value of Landsat data for different purposes in various geographic settings, NASA provided satellite data to researchers from 46 nations and 4 international organizations. As the value of Landsat data became better understood, more than a dozen countries—including Brazil, China, India, Indonesia and Thailand—invested in ground stations to receive and process Landsat data directly from the satellites.

An agreement establishing an organization and system of international space communications (Intersputnik) to enable the participant nations to exchange radio and television programs, and also to support other forms of communications, was signed by the Soviet Union and others in 1971, ratified, and put into effect the next year.

In May 1972 in Moscow, during a U.S./U.S.S.R. summit meeting, a bilateral agreement was signed concerning collaboration in the area of research and utilization of space for peaceful purposes. It mandated a number of joint experiments, as well as exchange of information concerning research in various areas of space life science. Five working groups in various areas of space research, including one in space biology and medicine, were established pursuant to this agreement. This group holds annual meetings to initiate and coordinate plans for joint research and to discuss results. This agreement also mandated the creation of common docking interfaces to enable rendezvous and docking of Soviet and American spacecraft and manned orbital stations, including the experimental flight of the Apollo and Soyuz spacecraft (Fig. 40). After a great deal of preparatory work, this flight was successfully completed in June 1975. Soviet cosmonauts A.A. Leonov and V.N. Kubasov and the American astronauts T. Stafford, D. Slayton, and V. Brand participated in the flight.

Although the major objective of the Apollo-Soyuz Program was development and manufacture of a common interface for rendezvous and docking of spacecraft from different countries, the significance of this experimental flight was considerably broader. This was the first international flight of spacecraft from two nations. It was very successful and demonstrated that, with available technology, major international programs were fully feasible.

The difficulties of coordinating sophisticated technology management tasks and determining equitable funding became substantial, and in 1975 the new European Space Agency (ESA) was formed, absorbing ESRO and ELDO. ESA was built around three main projects: the MARECS marine navigation satellite system, for which the United Kingdom had primary responsibility; the sophisticated Spacelab laboratory module, funded and developed largely by West Germany and flown on the American Space Shuttle; and the Ariane heavy satellite launcher funded and built primarily by France.

At the time the successful flight of Apollo-Soyuz was expected to be the precursor of follow-on joint manned missions involving the U.S. Shuttle and the Soviet Salyut space station, but in the late 1970s the political climate turned chilly again. Due to the worsening of the relationship between the U.S. and the U.S.S.R. these negotiations were first suspended and then terminated, and plans for further flight cooperation were put on hold.

The manned flights of international crews within the framework of the Intercosmos program marked a new stage in the development of international collaboration. From March 1978 to May 1981 there were nine such flights, in which cosmonauts from the Intercosmos nations flew, along with Soviet cosmonauts, on Soyuz spacecraft. Starting in June 1982, cosmonauts from France, India, Syria, Afghanistan, England, Japan, and Austria flew with Soviet cosmonauts on Soyuz spacecraft. Throughout the 1970s and especially the 1980s, the Soviet Union concluded bilateral agreements for scientific collaboration in space research with a number of countries (the United Kingdom, Austria, India, Canada, the

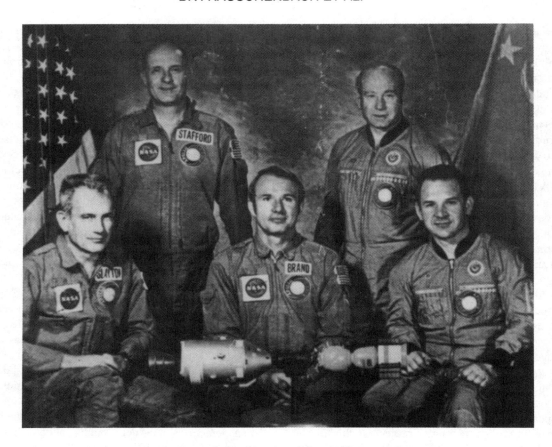

Fig. 40 Crew of the Joint U.S./U.S.S.R. flight, Apollo-Soyuz

Netherlands, Finland, Sweden, Argentina, China, Mexico, and others). The Soviet-Indian collaborative program accomplished the launch by Soviet rockets of five Indian satellites designed mainly for studying the Earth.

Starting in the early 1970s the Soviet Union began to collaborate with ESA—an organization comprising 10 European countries, including the United Kingdom, Spain, Italy, France, the Federal Republic of Germany, Sweden, and others. This collaboration was relatively broad and involved all major areas of space research. The agreement signed during the early 1980s between the U.S.S.R. Academy of Sciences and ESA on coordination of the Vega and Giotto missions is worthy of mention.

In the mid-1980s, the Kvant module of the Mir space station (equipped with X-ray telescopes developed in the U.S.S.R., Netherlands, F.R.G., and the United Kingdom) recorded the intense X-ray radiation of a Supernova, exploding in the Large Magellanic Cloud. The Phobos, Granit, and Gamma international projects were successfully implemented on Venera space probes.

In 1984-1986, an extensive international program was implemented to study Venus and Halley's Comet. The Vega and Giotto (ESA) projects were coordinated through a special agreement with ESA. In particular, Vega space probes were used to make accurate measurements of the ephemerides of Halley's Comet, measurements that were used to correct the flight of the Giotto spacecraft.

A space agreement between the U.S.S.R. and F.R.G. mandated collaboration in the study of Mars, high energy astrophysics, and solar-terrestrial physics, remote sensing of the Earth, and space biology and medicine.

It is noteworthy that recent U.S.S.R. fundamental space research projects all involve extensive international cooperation. Thus, for example, approximately 25 countries and ESA are participating in the Mars 94 and Mars 96 project. This is also true of other future projects: Interbol (study of solar-terrestrial linkages); Koronas (study of the Sun); Spektr (study of sources of radiation and their spectra in various wave bands, and also of astrophysical objects); Bion (study of effects of space flight factors on vital processes); and Priroda (remote sensing of the Earth).

International, nongovernmental scientific institutes created to unite space scientists from different countries have played a sound role in international cooperation in space exploration. The International Astronautical Federation (IAF), established in 1950, now unites scientists from 40 countries. The International Astronautical Congresses have been convened annually for more than 40 years to foster discussion of problems of space flight and space exploration. In 1958 the Committee on Space Research (COSPAR) was created by the International Space Unions Council. COSPAR discusses fundamental research and provides recommendations on Earth monitoring from space, space biology, exploration of the solar system, and space-based research in astrophysics. In 1960 the International Academy of Astronautics (IAA) was created by the IAF. World-renowned scientists with outstanding achievements in space science and technology are elected members of the Academy. The Academy has three branches: fundamental sciences, applied sciences, and social and human sciences. The IAA has international committees on space problems of relativity, space rescue, economic problems, the history of space and rocketry, rocket engines, etc., presents international awards in cosmonautics, and publishes the journal *Acta Astronautica*.

The INTELSAT (International Telecommunications Satellite Organization created in 1964) and the INMARSAT (International Maritime Telecommunications Satellite Organization) have fostered international contacts in space activity.

The Association of Space Explorers has done much to foster international collaboration in the area of cosmonautics. This organization was founded in 1985 after repeated (beginning in 1982) meetings of U.S. and Soviet astronauts and cosmonauts, and eminent scholars and scientists. Since 1985, the association has held regular congresses, with citizens of more than 20 nations participating. The espoused goal of this organization is to strengthen international scientific and technological collaboration, and provide favorable publicity on the role of space and space research.

In April 1987, a new intergovernmental agreement between the United States and the Soviet Union calling for collaborative efforts in the study and utilization of space opened up new opportunities to expand scientific contacts between the scientists of these two nations and others, increasing the international character of space exploration. While no space spectaculars such as the Apollo-Soyuz mission were initially adopted, 16 specific joint projects were called out for implementation by joint working groups established in five scientific disciplines: space biology and medicine, solar system exploration, astronomy and astrophysics, solar-terrestrial physics, and Earth sciences. Both sides consider that good progress has been made in the first few years in all five areas, laying the groundwork for more ambitious cooperation in flight projects in the 1990s, assuming the continuation of favorable political conditions.

Foreign contributions to joint programs with NASA over the first three decades of the space age include Europe's Spacelab, Canada's Remote Manipulator System for the Shuttle, and major foreign contributions to scientific spacecraft such as the Hubble Space Telescope and the Galileo Jupiter orbiter and probe. Overseas Shuttle emergency landing sites and Deep Space Network tracking stations provide vital operational support for NASA flight projects. With the exception of advanced technology development and applications projects with obvious commercial potential, virtually all areas of NASA's programs now have some international participation.

In 1988, the governments of the U.S., Canada, Japan, and the member nations of the ESA agreed to cooperate in the design, development, operation and utilization of Space Station Freedom, the largest and most complex international science and technology venture ever undertaken on a cooperative basis.

A number of milestones in U.S./U.S.S.R. collaboration occurred in 1991. The Progress cargo vehicle delivered American units (collectors) for studying heavy nuclei of cosmic rays to space station Mir. Russian cosmonauts installed these collectors on the station exterior during an EVA. The U.S. Total Ozone Mapping Spectrometer (TOMS) apparatus for ozone mapping was installed on board the Soviet Meteor 3 meteorological satellite. Data from TOMS are received regularly in ground stations in Obninsk (Russia) and Wallops Island (U.S.). Discussion of the results has demonstrated good correspondence of data recorded by both sides. In addition, data on the Earth's ozone layer from Nimbus 7 and the Upper Atmospheric Research Satellite (UARS) have been compared.

In parallel with the development of the U.S. Space Station Freedom, NASA has undertaken a Mission to Planet Earth aimed at achieving a better understanding of the interactions among the atmosphere, oceans, and the solid Earth that lead to global climate change. NASA's space-based contribution to this systematic study will be the Earth Observing System (EOS) based on the polar orbiting space platforms to be built as part of the Space Station Freedom Program. This study will involve scientists from the four corners of the Earth and will extend well into the next century. In 1988 Mission to Planet Earth was adopted by NASA and more than 20 of the world's space agencies as a major theme for the International Space Year (ISY) beginning in 1992.

VI. Conclusion

The mid-1950s of the 20th century were a watershed in the development of civilization. Just as, in their own time, living creatures left the water for the dry land and then spread across the surface of the Earth, so in the mid-20th century humanity developed the capacity to go beyond the boundaries of its planet and turn to the conquest of a completely new environment. However, while the first venture of living creatures into hitherto alien frontiers occurred over a long period of evolution and adaptation to new environments, in the 20th century humankind took another route; rather than adapting to the new environment it *created* an artificial environment to support life under new conditions.

Humanity's voyage to the stars (first ideas, development of theoretical principles, creation of actual spacecraft, work on the scientific, technological, and biological aspects of space flight) began several centuries ago. However, intensive work to achieve this goal has been going on for only the last 35 years.

During this period, significant advances have been achieved. As early as the first decade of the space age that opened in 1957, the first manmade satellite was launched and the first human being flew in space. A number of manned and unmanned spacecraft of various types and purposes were developed and flown, making it possible to begin to study near-Earth space. Along with scientific research, spacecraft were put to a number of practical purposes. Meteorological, communications, and navigational satellites were developed, as were satellites designed for the remote study of Earth from space.

Unmanned space probes began to explore the Moon and planets of our solar system. Much new information was acquired; more was discovered about these planets than had been learned during the entire previous history of mankind. An historic watershed was reached when the the the first humans to walk on the surface of another celestial body arrived at the Moon during the second decade of the space age and returned to Earth, bringing samples of the lunar soil and an experience unprecedented in human history. Robotic spacecraft also visited the Moon, obtaining additional material and generating new information.

Medicine and biology have made a significant contribution to the development of astronautics. Specialists in this area have studied the conditions necessary for survival during space flight, and participated in the development of regimens to enable optimum human performance under space flight conditions, prepared space crewmembers for flight, and provided them with operational medical support. As a result, a new discipline was born—space biology and medicine—which now has its own system of concepts and terms, research methodologies, specialized publications, and indeed a vast body of literature, and interacts closely with many technological, biomedical and psychosocial disciplines.

Rigorous, incremental work has enabled increases in the duration of space flights. Whereas the first space voyages were measured in days and hours, and later in weeks, they have now reached a year in duration.

An important and very promising direction has been the Soviet Union's development of orbital space stations designed for long-term human habitation and work in near-Earth orbit. During the last 2 decades approximately 10 such stations have been developed and have functioned successfully in space. The most advanced of these, the Mir, currently in orbit, is undergoing further improvement and a substantial expansion of capacities through the addition of new modules. In recent years, the first steps have been made to industrialize space—to create manufacturing concerns in near-Earth space, designed for the production of materials, devices, and drugs, including some that could never be produced on Earth. The development and utilization of the first orbital space stations created the prerequisites for achieving this objective.

Humanity's travel into space, and the significant successes attained along this route, have compelled us to rethink a number of ideas about the relationship of humanity to the cosmos and its home planet, the Earth. We have ceased to be constrained by the confines of our planet and increasing have begun to feel ourselves to be citizens of the universe.

The influence of astronautics on the development of society can be expected to increase in the future. Humanity has taken only the first steps on the road to study and conquer space—but the space frontier is still vast, and a greater understanding of our universe still beckons.

References

[1] Duhem, J. *Les Origines du Vol a Reaction*. Paris, 1943.

[2] Tsiolkovskiy, K.E. In: Archives of the U.S.S.R. Academy of Sciences, collection 555, inventory 1, file 32 (in Russian).

[3] Tsiolkovskiy, K.E. Exploration of space by reactive vehicles. *Nauchnoye Obozreniye*, 1903, no. 5, pp. 44-74 (in Russian).

[4] Zander (Tsander), F.A. *Die Weltschiffe (Aetherschiffe), die den Verkehr zwischen den Sternen ermoeglichen sollen. Die Bewegung in Weltenraum*. Archives of the U.S.S.R. Academy of Sciences, collection 573, inventory 1, file 26.

[5] Tsander, F.A. Space (ether) craft that enable interstellar communication. Motion in outer space. In: *From the History of Aviation and Astronautics*, 1971, vol. 13, pp. 3-36 (in Russian).

[6] Tsander, F.A. *The Problem of Jet Flight*. Moscow, 1932 (in Russian).

[7] Kondratyuk, Yu.V. Manuscript (third version), 1920-1924. Manuscript archived in the Institute of the History of Science and Technology, Russian Academy of Sciences (in Russian).

[8] Kondratyuk, Yu.V. *The Conquest of Interplanetary Space*. Novosibirsk, 1929 (in Russian).

[9] Tsiolkovskiy, K.E. Exploration of space by reactive vehicles. Archives of the U.S.S.R. Academy of Sciences, collection 555, inventory 1, file 7 (in Russian).

[10] Goddard, R.H. *The Papers of R.H. Goddard*, vol. 1, New York, 1970.

[11] Goddard, R.H. On the possibility of navigating interplanetary space, 1907. In: *The Papers of R.H. Goddard*, vol. 1, New York, 1970, pp. 85-87.

[12] Goddard, R.H. Memorandum in *Green Notebook Regarding the Use of Atomic Energy for Space Travel*, November 1907.

[13] Tsiolkovskiy, K.E. Exploration of space by reactive vehicles. *Vestnik Vozdukhoplavaniya* [Bulletin of Aeronautics], 1912, no. 9 (in Russian).

[14] Esnault-Pelterie, R. Consideration sur les resultats d'un allegement indefini des moteurs. *Journal Physique Theoretique et Applique* (Paris), 1913, Vol. 3.

[15] Tsiolkovskiy, K.E. Archives of the U.S.S.R. Academy of Sciences, collection 555, inventory 1, file 35, p. 10. (in Russian).

[16] Goddard, R.H. Reaction by streams of ions to furnish rocket propulsion. *R.H. Goddard's Green Notebooks*, 1906, pp. 82-85.

[17] Goddard, R.H., U.S. Patent No. 136303, *Method of and Means for Producing Electrified Jets of Gas*, December 21, 1920.

[18] Ulinski, F. Das Problem der Weltraumfahrt. *Der Flug*

(Vienna), 1920, S. 113-124.

19 Valier, M. Der Vorstoß in den Weltenraum. Munich, 1928.

20 Goddard, R.H. Multiple Rockets. *R.H. Goddard's Green Notebooks*, vol. 4, p. 24.

21 Bing, A. Belgian Patent No. 236477, June 10, 1911.

22 Kondratyuk, Yu.V. Manuscript (first version). 1917. Manuscript archived in the Institute of the History of Science and Technology, Russian Academy of Sciences (in Russian).

23 Kondratyuk, Yu.V. Manuscript (second version). 1918-1919. Manuscript archived in the Institute of the History of Science and Technology, Russian Academy of Sciences (in Russian).

24 *Pioneers of Rocket Technology: Kibalchich, Tsiolkovskiy, Tsander, Kondratyuk. Selected Works.* Moscow, 1964 (in Russian).

25 Goddard, R.H. U.S. Patent No. 1102653, Rocket Apparatus, July 7, 1914.

26 Oberth, H. *Die Rakete zu den Planetenraumen.* Munich and Berlin, 1923.

27 Tsiolkovskiy, K.E. *The Exploration of Space by Reactive Vehicles.* Kaluga, 1926 (in Russian).

28 Tsiolkovskiy, K. E. *Rocket-powered Space Trains.* Kaluga, 1929 (in Russian).

29 Tsiolkovskiy, K.E. The highest speed of rockets. Chapter in an unfinished manuscript. Archives of the U.S.S.R. Academy of Sciences, collection 555, inventory 1, file 105 (in Russian).

30 Tsiolkovskiy, K.E. *Papers on Rocket Technology.* Moscow, 1947 (in Russian).

31 Tsander, F.A. Flights to other planets. *Tekhnika i Zhizn*, 1924, 13, pp. 15-16 (in Russian).

32 Goddard, R.H. *The Papers of R.H. Goddard.* New York, 1970, vol. 1, p. 14; vol. 2, p. 693.

33 Tsiolkovskiy, K.E. Exploration of space by reactive vehicles. *Vestnik Vozdukhoplavaniya*, 1911, no. 21-22, p. 34 (in Russian).

34 Von Hoeft, F. Die Eroberung des Weltalls, *Die Rakete*, 1928, no. 3, pp. 36-42.

35 Von Pirquet, G. Fahrtrouten. *Die Rakete*, 1928, no. 9, pp. 137-140.

36 Goddard, R.H. Outline for paper on the navigation of interplanetary space. In: *The Papers of R.H. Goddard: Volume 1*, New York, 1970, p 122.

37 Tsiolkovskiy, K.E. Human settlement of space. Manuscript (1921). In: Archives of the U.S.S.R. Academy of Sciences, collection 555, inventory 1, file 246 (in Russian).

38 Tsander, F.A. Flights to other planets.(second communication). In: *Problems of Interplanetary Flights.* Moscow, 1988, pp. 10-17 (in Russian).

39 Goddard, R.H. Monthly Report to Smithsonian Institution. In: Goddard, R.H. *The Papers of R.H. Goddard*, New York, 1970, vol. 1.

40 Saenger, E. *Raketenflugtechnik.* Munich, 1933.

41 Saenger, E., and Saenger-Bredt, I. *Uber Raketenantrieb fuer Fernbomber.* Berlin Adlershof, ZWB, UM 3538, 1944.

42 Proceedings of the All-Union Conference on Stratospheric Research. Moscow and Leningrad, 1935 (in Russian).

43 All-Union Conference on the Use of Jets for Stratospheric Research (in Russian).

44 Tsiolkovskiy, K.E. Scenes from my life. In: *Tsiolkovskiy*, Moscow, 1939, pp. 28-29 (in Russian).

45 Tsiolkovskiy, K.E. How to protect fragile and delicate things from bumps and impacts. *Proceedings of the Divisions of Physical Sciences of the Society of Science Lovers*, vol. IV, no. 2, Moscow, 1891, pp. 17-18 (in Russian).

46 Rynin, N.A. and Likhachyov, A.A. The effect of acceleration on living things. *Proceedings of the Scientific Research Bureau of the Institute of Civil Aviation*, issue 1, Leningrad, 1931 (in Russian).

47 Generales. C.D. Recollections of early biomedical Moon-mice investigations. *AAS History Series*, vol. 6, San Diego, 1985, pp. 75-80.

48 Bushnell, D. History of research in space biology and biodynamics at the Air Force Missile Development Center Holloman AFB. 1946-1958. Office of Information, Holloman AFB, 1958.

49 National Aeronautics and Space Administration. *Biospex: Biological Space Experiments.* A compendium of life sciences experiments carried on U.S. spacecraft. Washington, D.C., 1979.

50 Marbarger, J.P. (Ed.) *Space Medicine.* Urbana, Illinois, University of Illinois Press, 1951.

51 Biomedical research on rockets. In: *Preliminary Conclusions of Scientific Research Using the First Soviet Satellites and Rockets.* Moscow, 1958, pp. 109-149 (in Russian).

52 Muenger, E.A. *Searching the Horizon: A History of Ames Research Center.* NASA SP-4304. Washington, D.C., National Aeronautics and Space Administration, U.S. Government Printing Office, 1985, p. 67.

53 Hall, R.C. U.S. satellite proposals. In Emme, E.E. (Ed.) *The History of Rocket Technology.* Detroit, 1964, pp. 67-93.

54 Emme, E.E. *Aeronautics and Astronautics: An American Chronology of Science and Technology in the Exploration of Space, 1915-1960.* Washington D.C., National Aeronautics and Space Administration, 1961, p. 79.

55 Korolyov, S.P. *The Creative Legacy of Academician S.P. Korolyov. Selected Works.* Moscow, 1980 (in Russian).

56 Clarke, A. *Wireless World*, October 1945.

57 Chernov, V.N., Yakovlev, V.I. Scientific research on animals flown on manmade satellites. *Manmade Earth Satellites*, issue 1, 1958, pp. 80-94 (in Russian).

58 Sisakyan, N.M. (Ed.) *Problems of Space Biology*, vol. 1, Moscow, 1962 (in Russian).

59 Link, M.M., Gurovskiy, N.N., Bryanov, I.I. Selection of astronauts and cosmonauts. In: Calvin, M., Gazenko, O.G. (Eds.) *Foundations of Space Biology and Medicine.* Washington D.C., National Aeronautics and Space Administration, 1975, vol. 3, pp. 419-438.

60 Link, M.M., Gurovskiy, N.N. Training of cosmonauts

and astronauts. In: Calvin, M., Gazenko, O.G. (Eds.) *Foundations of Space Biology and Medicine*. Washington D.C., National Aeronautics and Space Administration, 1975, vol. 3, pp. 438-453.

61 Gazenko, O.G., Kakurin, L.I., Kuznetsov, A.G. (Eds.) *Space Flights on Soyuz Spacecraft. Biomedical Studies*. Moscow, 1976 (in Russian).

62 Johnston, R.S., Dietlein, L.F., Berry, C.A. *Biomedical Results of Apollo*. Washington, D.C., National Aeronautics and Space Administration, 1975.

63 Mishin, V.P. *Why We Didn't Fly to the Moon*. Moscow, Znaniye, 1990, pp. 3-43 (in Russian).

64 Hale, E.E. Brick moon. *The Atlantic*, 1869-1870.

65 Ordway, F. The History, Evolution and Benefits of the Space Station Concept (in the United States and Western Europe). *Proceedings of XIII-th International Congress of the History of Sciences*, section XII, Moscow, 1974.

66 R.S. Johnston, L.F. Dietlein (Eds.) *Biomedical Results From Skylab*. Washington, D.C., National Aeronautics and Space Administration, 1977.

67 Nicogossian, A.E., Huntoon, C.H., Pool, S.L. (Eds.) *Space Physiology and Medicine*. Second edition. Philadelphia-London, Lea & Febiger, 1989.

68 Semenov, Yu.P. Energiya, a new multipurpose transport rocket system. Paper presented at the 15th Lecture Series Dedicated to the Memory of the Pioneers of Space Exploration. Moscow, January 1989 (in Russian).

69 Gurovskiy, N.A. (Ed.) *Results of Medical Research on the Salyut 6-Soyuz Scientific Research Complex*. Moscow, 1986 (in Russian).

70 Gaydamakin, N.A., Parfenov, G.P., Petrukhin, V.G., Antipov, V.V. Results of research on tortoises on certain flight vehicles. *Izvestiya AN SSSR. Seriya Biologicheskaya*. 1971, no. 3, pp. 451-453 (in Russian).

71 Ilyin, Ye.A., Parfenov, G.P. *Biological Research on COSMOS Biosatellites*. Moscow, 1979 (in Russian).

72 Dubinin, N.P. (Ed.) *Biological Research on Salyut Orbital Station*. Moscow, 1984 (in Russian).

73 Sanders, J.F. (Ed.) *The Experiments of Biosatellite II*. Washington, D.C., 1971.

74 Gazenko, O.G., Ilyin, Ye.A. Biosatellites: Adaptation to Weightlessness. *Nauka i Chelovechestvo*, Moscow, 1988, pp. 277-291 (in Russian).

75 Imshenetskiy, A.A. Biological effects of extreme environmental conditions. In: Calvin, M., Gazenko, O.G. (Eds.) *Foundations of Space Biology and Medicine*. Washington D.C., National Aeronautics and Space Administration, 1975, vol. 1, pp. 271-321.

76 Oparin, A.I. Theoretical and experimental prerequisites of exobiology. In: Calvin, M., Gazenko, O.G. (Eds.) *Foundations of Space Biology and Medicine*. Washington D.C., National Aeronautics and Space Administration, 1975, vol. 1, pp. 321-368.

77 Rubin, A.B. Search for and investigation of extraterrestrial forms of life. In: Calvin, M., Gazenko, O.G. (Eds.) *Foundations of Space Biology and Medicine*. Washington D.C., National Aeronautics and Space Administration, 1975, vol. 1, pp. 368-402.

78 Klein H.P. The Viking biological investigation. *General Journal of Geographical Research*, 1977, vol. 82, no. 28, pp. 4677-4680.

79 Aksyonov, S.I. On interpretation of data from Viking biological investigations. *Izvestiya AN SSSR. Seriya Biologicheskaya*, 1979, no. 3, pp. 389-394 (in Russian).

80 Zhukov, G.P. The history of Soviet international space law doctrines. *Research on the History and Theory of the Development of Aviation and Space and Rocket Science and Technology*, no. 6, Moscow 1988, pp. 31-48 (in Russian).

81 Zarzar, V.A. International public air law. In: *Questions of Air Law*, Moscow, 1927 (in Russian).

82 Mandl, V. *Das Weltraumrecht: Ein Problem der Raumfahrt*. Mannheim, 1932.

83 Corovine, E. La conquêt de la stratosphere et la droit international. *Rev. Gen, Droit. Internat. Publ.*, 1934, no. 6, pp. 675-686.

84 Korovin, Ye.A. On International space policy. *Mezhdunarodnaya Zhizn*, 1959, no. 1, pp. 71-80 (in Russian).

85 Jenks, C.W. *Space Law*. New York, Frederick A. Praeger, 1965, pp. 119-132.

86 Kopal, V. International collaboration in the development of space law. Paper presented at the Conference on the History of Aviation and Cosmonautics, Moscow, September 28-October 2, 1987 (in Russian).

87 Tsiolkovskiy, K.E. *Away from Earth*. Kaluga, 1920 (in Russian).

88 The Space Act (Public Law 85-56B, July 29, 1958).

89 Calvin, M., Gazenko, O.G. (Eds.) *Foundations of Space Biology and Medicine*. Washington D.C., National Aeronautics and Space Administration, 1975 (joint U.S./U.S.S.R. publication).

Part II:

The Space Environment

Chapter 1

Stars and Interstellar Space

Albert A. Galeev and Leonid S. Marochnik

I. The Universe

A. Hierarchy of Spatial Scales and Location of the Solar System

Space exploration with unmanned probes has traversed the distances between the Earth and the inner, and more recently, the outer planets of the solar system. The impressive Voyager missions provided data about Jupiter, Saturn, Uranus, and Neptune, which are situated at distances of 5, 10, 20, and 30 AU, respectively, from the Sun. (An astronomical unit, abbreviated as AU, is equal to the mean distance between the Earth and the Sun, that is, 1.49599 x 10^8 km or 1 AU $\cong 1.5 \times 10^{13}$ cm.) These are large distances in relation to the size of the planet Earth (the average radius of the Earth is $R_{SOL} \cong 6371$ km $\cong 4.3 \times 10^{-5}$ AU).

Pluto, the most distant planet, is at a distance of ~39.5 AU from the Sun.[1] However, Pluto's orbit does not form the outer boundary of the solar system. The periphery of the system is occupied by a giant cloud of comets, called the Oort Cloud, the aphelia of which are at distances of $r_{SOL} \cong 2 \times 10^5$ AU.[2] The Oort Cloud is important to an understanding of the large scale structure of the solar system.[3] It appears that the outer boundary of the Oort Cloud should be viewed as the outer boundary of the solar system.[2]

It is necessary to use different units of length upon leaving the solar system and entering galactic space. AUs are used for describing large-scale parameters within the solar system, but parsecs (pc) (derived from parallax-second) are a preferable unit for describing galactic scales. One parsec is the distance at which a star would have a parallax equal to 1 arc-second; 1 pc $\cong 2 \times 10^5$ AU $\cong 3 \times 10^{18}$ cm. In galactic terms, the size of the solar system is of the order of 1 parsec, which is approximately half of the mean distance between the stars in the circumsolar vicinity of the galaxy.

Infrared Astronomical Satellite (IRAS) data show that there are many stars with an excess of infrared radiation, implying the existence of extended dust disks in the circumsolar region. These disks are believed to be produced around these stars by comet clouds similar to the Oort Cloud. The linear size of such a disk surrounding the star Beta Pictoris is 1150 AU and its projective thickness is 50 AU. In other words, it can be postulated that systems similar to the solar system are not particularly uncommon, at least in the circumsolar vicinity of our galaxy.[3]

Distances between stars in the galaxy are measured in parsecs, whereas large-scale parameters of our stellar system are measured in kiloparsecs (1 kpc = 10^3 pc). Being inside our own galaxy, we obviously cannot observe it from the outside. However, there are physical indications (see below) and

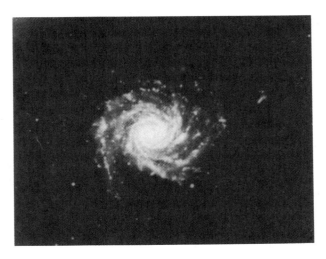

Fig. 1 Spiral galaxies NGC 4565 (view from the edge) and NGC 1232, analogous to the Milky Way

dynamic models suggesting that it can be regarded as a typical representative of the family of spiral galaxies, which compose about 80 percent of the known galaxies. The diameter of the galaxy is approximately 30 kpc. Figure 1 depicts spiral galaxies NGC 4565 and NGC 1232, which are believed to be very similar to the Milky Way.

The estimated distance from the Sun to the galactic center is 8 to 10 kpc, placing the Sun at the edge of the galactic disk. Current observations indicate that the Z-coordinate (i.e., altitude above the galactic plane) of the Sun is about 10-12 pc.

If we estimate the mass of the galaxy on the basis of number of stars it contains, we would obtain $M_G \approx 2 \times 10^{11} M_{SOL}$, where M_{SOL} is the mass of the Sun, since the galaxy consists of hundreds of billions of stars. The actual mass of the galaxy is an order of magnitude greater than this estimate, because it also includes the so-called missing mass, which can be derived from the curve of rotation (see below) but cannot be observed. Similarly, our estimate of the linear dimension of the galaxy is an order of magnitude greater if we take the halo into account.

Our galaxy (the Milky Way) is a member of the so-called local group of galaxies, whose brightest members are our galaxy and the Andromeda Nebula. Each of them has its own large family. The family of our galaxy includes 14 dwarf elliptical galaxies, several extragalactic globular clusters, and a few irregular galaxies, the largest of which are the Large and Small Magellanic Clouds. All these constitute a single gravitationally bound system.

As a rule, galaxies occur in clusters. Isolated galaxies, called field galaxies, are infrequent—no more than 10 percent of the total number of galaxies. Clusters usually include from several hundred to several thousand members and form gravitationally bound systems. Typically, their sizes are measured in megaparsecs (1 Mpc = 10^6 pc).

What are the largest presently known structural formations of matter in the universe representing the upper limit of the scale of its inhomogeneity? This question is part of a more general question, i.e., what is the hierarchy of structures in the universe? If we disregard planets, then the "smallest" structural formations are probably stars. Then come galaxies, which in turn aggregate to form clusters. Clusters aggregate in superclusters, a qualitatively new type of structure. Can this type of aggregation of structures go on indefinitely? Is it possible that superclusters will be found to aggregate into larger structural units, and so on?

Apparently, this is not the case. Astronomical observations show that superclusters of galaxies form the nodes of a network structure resembling a spider web. This implies that on a scale encompassing a large number of such elements, the properties of the universe should be uniform. In other words, beginning at the scale of these regions, the universe can be viewed as structureless or uniform and isotropic.

B. Evolution of the Universe

How can the hierarchy of the time scales of the universe be described? They must be related to evolutionary processes. Life on Earth is estimated to be 3.5×10^9 years old.[5] The age of the Earth—estimated using long-lived isotopes—is reported to be 4.6×10^9 years. The age of the Sun is estimated to be 5×10^9 years[1] and that of the universe, from 1×10^{10} to 1.5×10^{10} years (this value varies depending on the Hubble constant used) (see below).

In 1929, Edwin P. Hubble published his finding that the recessional velocity of the galaxies increases with distance from our galaxy (their red shifts increase with distance from the observer). This discovery, if we also abandon an anthropocentric bias, proves that the mean distance between galaxies continuously increases with time. This, in turn, suggests the expansion of the universe and consequently its evolution.

Like many other discoveries that have dramatically modified our understanding of the laws governing the world around us, Hubble's discovery introduced a new numerical factor, the Hubble constant H, which relates the speed of recession of a galaxy, v, to its distance, $r: v = H \cdot r$. Thus the unit of the Hubble constant H must be 1/time. H plays an important role in determining the major parameters of the current state of the universe.

As mentioned above, most galaxies are parts of larger structural units—clusters of galaxies bound together by gravitational attraction. The velocities of galaxies within their own cluster, controlled by their gravitational interactions, are superimposed on the Hubble field of galactic velocities. Clearly, the Hubble law, in its pure form, cannot be applied to galaxies. Are there then any bodies that have velocities describable by the Hubble law with some degree of accuracy?

The most recent estimates of the Hubble constant vary from 50 to 100 (km/s)/Mpc. We will use $H = 75$ (km/s)/Mpc here. Thus we assume that, due to the expansion of the universe, two clusters 1 Mpc apart are moving apart at a relative velocity of 75 km/s. The galaxies within the cluster have their own orbital motions at velocities of on the order of hundreds of kilometers per second, and can move in any direction. This means that galaxies within clusters can move closer together, which contradicts the Hubble law. In fact, this law holds true only for clusters of galaxies separated by distances greater than 10 Mpc. The clusters themselves do not expand, because they are gravitationally bound objects. Therefore, the smallest structural formation in the universe described by the Hubble law is the galactic cluster.

As noted above, beginning with those regions of the universe that contain a large number of supercluster network nodes, the universe can be considered to be structureless, i.e., on the average uniform and isotropic.

Using current data on the average density of matter, we can look into the future and try to answer the question of whether the universe will continue to expand indefinitely or begin to contract at some point. In order to do this, we need only compare the current density of matter with its critical density, which is a function of the gravitation constant $G = 6.687 \times 10^{-8}$ dyne cm^2/g^2, and the Hubble constant:

$$\rho_{cr} = 3H^2/8\pi G$$

At $H = 75$ (km/s)/Mpc, the critical density is approximately 10^{-29} g/cm^3. If $\rho > \rho_{cr}$ then expansion will give way to contraction; conversely, if $\rho \leq \rho_{cr}$ then expansion will continue to infinity. Which of these alternatives is correct? What is the ratio between the current density of matter in the universe to the critical density?

Let us consider the contribution of galaxies to the total density of matter in the universe. The ratio of the current density of matter and ρ_{cr} is represented by the parameter $\Omega = \rho/\rho_{cr}$. Assuming that members of each class of spiral and elliptical galaxies (which constitute the majority of observable objects) have the same ratio of mass to luminosity L, then the parameter Ω_G, reflecting the contribution of objects of this class to current density, will vary from 0.01 to 0.03.

However, there is reason to believe that galactic clusters contain a so-called missing mass, which must be postulated to account for their stabilization. What are the forms this invisible matter could take?

It is not impossible that a significant portion of the galactic mass could be concentrated in dim stars or massive bodies of relatively low luminosity (such as Jupiter). It is also possible that, during the formation of galaxies and galactic clusters, a substantial quantity of gas could have filled intergalactic space, remaining invisible because of its low luminosity. Both these hypotheses may be said to be based on our lack of detailed knowledge about the formation of the large-scale structure of the universe (i.e., galaxies, their clusters, and superclusters). However, they both assume that we can specify the matter from which these systems were formed. At the same time, we cannot exclude the possibility that the cosmological missing mass was produced by massive neutrinos, primary black holes, or other particles that originated in the early phases of expansion of the universe and are still present.

When we speak about the evolution of the universe we mean, among other things, evolution of its space-time metrics in conformity with the principles of Einstein's general theory of relativity. This occurs, for example, in the vicinity of black holes—which represent special space-time regions. What are black holes?

Assume a sphere of mass M and radius R. Any object can overcome the gravitational attraction of this sphere and escape from it if it moves with escape velocity, equal to

$$V = \sqrt{2GM / R}$$

If the mass M remains unchanged, but the radius is shortened (by compressing the sphere), then at $R = r_g = 2GM/c^2$, escape velocity equals the speed of light (c). The parameter r_g is called the gravitational radius. According to the theory of relativity, bodies cannot move with velocities exceeding the speed of light. If the sphere is compressed down to the gravitational radius, even light cannot leave it. (Obviously, this derivation of the gravitational radius is derived from Newton's laws, and thus, strictly speaking, is not valid for strong gravi-

tational fields. It is given here as an illustrative approximation.) This implies that no information can reach the observer from below the surface of the sphere, because the speed of light is the highest possible speed for transmittal of any information, and this is what produces the black hole phenomenon. In geometric terms, this means that the curvature of space in the black hole region is so high that particles of matter moving within it will never reach a remote observer.

Black holes can form through the natural evolution of sufficiently massive gaseous stars. In these stars, similar to our Sun, the pressure of gas, heated by thermonuclear reactions to high temperatures of about 10^6 K and thus in the form of plasma, is counteracted by gravity-induced compression. However, as the thermonuclear fuel (hydrogen, lithium, boron, etc.) burns itself out, the star begins to be compressed and is transformed into a compact object of an entirely different nature. In this situation, three types of transformation are possible. If the mass of a contracting star is not very great ($M \leq 1.4$ M_{SOL}), contraction will be terminated at the stage in which the plasma is compressed to the density of degenerate electron gas.

Stars of somewhat greater mass ($1.4 M_{SOL} \leq M \leq 2 M_{SOL}$) are transformed through compression into neutron stars with a radius on the order of 10 km, because the pressure of degenerate plasma is insufficient to counteract the gravitational forces. However, due to conservation of angular momentum and to the magnetic field frozen into the matter of the star, the star rotates rapidly (at an initial period of about 1 ms) and has a strong magnetic field of 10^{10}-10^{12} gauss. Rapidly rotating neutron stars were discovered as a result of observation of the periodic bursts of radio waves they regularly emit. These objects were named pulsars.

In the third case, that of more massive stars ($M \geq 2 M_{SOL}$), compression cannot be arrested at all, and the stars are transformed into black holes as soon as thermonuclear fuel burns out completely.

Another hypothesis, which cannot be refuted today, postulates that massive black holes ($M \cong 10^3 M_{SOL}$) exist in the central regions of some galaxies, and less massive black holes in the central regions of globular clusters. It is quite possible that the distant quasistellar objects, or quasars, that emit powerful radiation in a wide spectral range, are supermassive black holes.

Thus the problem of the future of the universe seems to be closely related to that of its past.

A discussion of the fine points of the evolution of the universe, or even of such basic issues as the origin of uniformity and isotropy of space-time or the prevalence of matter over antimatter is beyond the scope of this book. [Note that we are referring here to the current prevalence of the density of particles over that of antiparticles. Stars, galaxies, and other celestial bodies are composed of normal matter—protons, neurons, and nuclei of heavy elements. Observations have clearly shown that the universe contains no aggregates of antimatter (e.g., antistars, antigalaxies, etc.) in which particles are replaced by antiparticles.] We will note only that, according to current theories, the expansion of the universe obeys the law $\rho \cong \rho_{cr}$. In other words, expansion will go on forever. This prediction is associated with the role of the energy of the vacuum, which was the most important at earliest stages of evolution. We are referring here to the "inflationary universe theory."[6] If this theory is correct, then the age of the universe or the time elapsed since the onset of expansion can be derived from the equation.[7]

$$t = 2/3H$$

This equation refers to the extreme case in which the pressure of matter $P = 0$. This holds true, for example, for the phase of expansion of a universe composed of galaxies (the current situation).

The values of all these parameters are determined by H. Thus, an accurate empirical measure of this value is the fundamental problem in astrophysics today. Without going into further detail, we would like to note that many authors use $H = 55$ (km/s)/Mpc, which (using the equation above) produces an estimate of the age of the universe of 12 billion years.

C. Black Body Radiation

At present there are only two observational findings that enable us to look into the past of the universe: remnant electromagnetic radiation (black body radiation) and the abundance of light elements.

Let us consider the first of these. Evidence for the existence of microwave cosmic radiation was first encountered in 1964 by Bell researchers Penzias and Wilson while they were testing highly sensitive radio receivers. The high uniformity and isotropy of this cosmic radiation precluded its having been emitted by individual objects in the Milky Way or other galaxies. The lack of variation in the microwave background radiation suggested that it was of extragalactic origin. Calculations of radiation intensity in terms of the equivalent temperature of a black body yielded 2.7 K. Naturally, the data obtained at one wavelength were not sufficient to describe the entire spectrum of radiation. It was important to demonstrate experimentally that this radiation corresponded to an equilibrium quantum distribution over all wavelengths, since this would imply that the radiation source was formed at a period when radiation and matter were in thermodynamic equilibrium. This would have been possible only under condi-tions of very high temperatures and densities of cosmological plasma in a distant past.

However, cosmological conclusions could only be drawn from the existence of remnant radiation if it had a thermal black body spectrum. At present, it can be asserted with relatively high accuracy ($\sim 3 \times 10^{-5}$) that the background radiation has such a spectrum.·

It should be noted that the energy density of remnant radiation (equal to $\varepsilon_r = 4 \times 10^{-13}$ erg/cm³) dominates the remaining cosmic electromagnetic radiation with other energy densities over virtually the entire range of wavelengths.

At the same time, energy density $\varepsilon_r \gg \varepsilon_m$ where ε_m is energy density, including the missing mass.

For comparative purposes, we present the densities of different types of matter in the universe[8]:

$$\rho_v \cong 10^{-29}\, g/cm^3$$
$$\rho_{galaxies} \cong 3 \times 10^{-31}\, g/cm^3$$
$$\rho_{mm} \cong 3 \times 10^{-30}\, g/cm^3$$

where ρ_v corresponds to the energy density of a quantum vacuum, expressed in g/cm³, that would cause inflation of the universe within a time period of approximately 10^{-35}s from the onset of expansion; $\rho_{galaxies}$ is the mean density of matter concentrated in galaxies (luminous matter), and ρ_{mm} is the mean density of the missing mass.

Thus, comparison of the energy density of remnant radiation

$$\rho_r = \frac{1}{c^2} \cdot \varepsilon_r \cong 10^{-33}\, g/cm^3$$

to previous energy densities suggests that it cannot have any significant effect on the rate of expansion of the universe at the present time. However, this was not always the case.

Let us imagine that long before the present, some source of electromagnetic waves emitted a signal with wavelength of λ_i. Because of the nonstationarity of the universe, today this radiation would have the wavelength of λ_0. The discrepancy between λ_0 and λ_i is due to a Doppler shift in the frequency of quanta as they propagate from the source toward the observer. We can describe this shift quantitatively by using the red shift, Z_i, to stand for the following function of λ_i and λ_0:

$$Z_i = (\lambda_o - \lambda_i)/\lambda_i$$

The relationship between the wavelengths of emitted and recorded radiation $\lambda_0 = \lambda_i(1 + Z_{ij})$ derived from this equation shows that, as the universe expanded, λ_i increased by a factor $(1+Z_i)$ from the epoch with red shift Z_i to the modern epoch with $Z = 0$. The spatial dimensions associated with the kinematic characteristics of expansion will increase analogously, since we use electromagnetic radiation wave lengths to measure them. In particular, the radius of an arbitrary spherical region will vary as

$$R_{SOL} = R_i(1 + Z_i)$$

Since the volume of the sphere will increase as the red shift decreases in accordance with $(1 + Z)^{-3}$ the total density of matter in this region will diminish proportionally to $(1 + Z)^3$. However, the energy density of remnant radiation declines, as the universe expands, in accordance with

$$\varepsilon_r \sim (1 + Z)^4$$

This means that in the past the situation was just the opposite

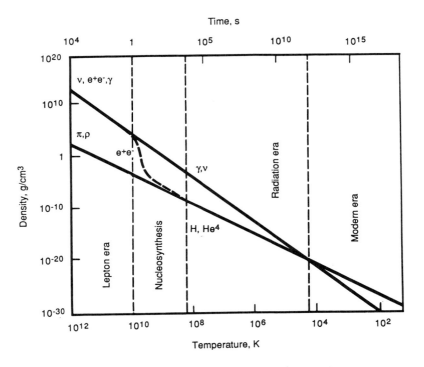

Fig. 2 Thermal history of the universe according to the Big Bang scenario and mass densities of various elements of matter and radiation as a function of time

of what we observe today; in other words, there was an epoch when $\varepsilon_r \gg \varepsilon_m$.

D. Big Bang Scenario

One of the working hypotheses of this Big Bang model is the proposition that the universe has been homogeneous and isotropic throughout its evolution. In addition, based on data on the spectra of microwave radiation, we postulate that in the past plasma was in a state of thermodynamic equilibrium with radiation at a high temperature. Finally, through extrapolating the principle of increasing density of matter and radiation energy into the past, we conclude that when the plasma reached temperatures of about 10^{10} K, it contained the protons and neutrons responsible for the formation of the chemical composition of cosmic matter.

Clearly, this set of "initial conditions" cannot be formally extrapolated to the earliest stages of expansion of the universe, when plasma temperature exceeded 10^{12} K, since under such conditions matter would have undergone qualitative changes related, among other things, to the quark structure of nucleons. This period, which preceded the stage at which $T \approx 10^{12}$ K, naturally occurred during the very earliest stages of expansion of the universe, our knowledge of which is, unfortunately, very poor.

As we explore the history of the universe, we inevitably will have to describe transformations of elementary particles with ever increasing energies, energies that exceed (by tens or even thousands of times) those that can be studied with even our most advanced accelerators. We will have to confront a

whole set of problems associated, first, with our lack of understanding of new types of particles originating in high density plasma, and second, with the lack of a reliable theory to help us derive the major parameters of the cosmological substrate of that period.

Nevertheless, even if we do not have a detailed understanding of the properties of super dense plasma at high temperatures, we can surmise that, beginning with temperatures slightly lower than 10^{12} K, these properties met the requirements listed above. In other words, at temperatures of approximately 10^{12} K, the matter in the universe consisted of electron-positron pairs (e^-, e^+); muons and antimuons (μ^-, μ^+); electron neutrinos and antineutrinos $(\upsilon_e, \bar{\upsilon}_e)$; muon neutrinos and antineutrinos $(\upsilon_\mu, \bar{\upsilon}_\mu)$; tau neutrinos and antineutrinos $(\upsilon_\tau, \bar{\upsilon}_\tau)$ (in nuclear physics these particles are called leptons; the stage in which these particles predominated is known as the lepton era); nucleons (protons and neutrons); and electromagnetic radiation.

Interactions of all these particles ensured thermodynamic equilibrium. However, as the universe expanded, this equilibrium changed for different types of particles at different stages. At temperatures less than 10^{12} K, muon-antimuon pairs, whose resting energies are about 10^6 MeV (plasma temperature of 1.16×10^4 K corresponds to a particle energy of 1 eV), were the first to undergo such changes. Later, at temperatures of about 5×10^9 K, electron-positron pairs were annihilated at a greater rate than they were generated through photon interaction. This ultimately brought about a qualitative change in the composition of plasma.

After that point in time, electromagnetic radiation played

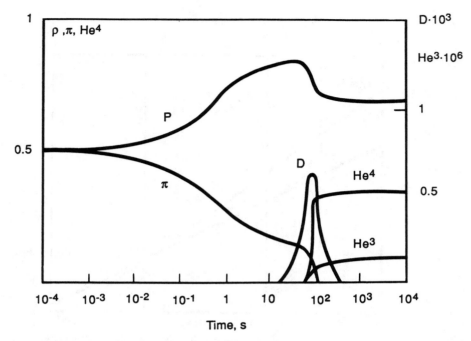

Fig. 3 Nucleosynthesis (in relative units) of light chemical elements as a function of time according to the Big Bang scenario (From: Zeldovich, Ya.B., Novikov, I.D. *Structure and Evolution of the Universe*, Moscow, Nauka, 1975, p. 209.)

the dominant role in the expansion of the universe, and the lepton era in the thermal history of cosmic plasma was superseded by the radiation era (Fig. 2). Indeed, it was during this period, when plasma temperatures were about 5×10^9 K, that the equilibrated spectrum of electromagnetic radiation was formed. This spectrum has reached us today in the form of microwave remnant background radiation.

At the end of the radiation era, when temperatures were approximately 10^4 K, interaction of free electrons and protons resulted in the formation of hydrogen atoms and decrease of free electric charge carriers. At that time, quantum-electron scattering became less effective, and, beginning with the period when the temperature dropped below 3000 K, photon propagation was essentially free. Decreases in the temperature of electromagnetic radiation after it decoupled from plasma were due only to the expansion of the universe, which caused the quantum spectrum to shift to the millimeter and centimeter bands.

This microwave background radiation is, therefore, a kind of vestige of early high-temperature stages in the evolution of the universe, or a remnant indicating that in the past this subsystem determined the major properties of cosmological plasma. However, in addition to the microwave radiation background, we should have received an "echo" of the radiation era in the expansion of the universe, in the form of nuclei and isotopes of light chemical elements. According to the Big Bang theory, these should have formed approximately a million years prior to the decoupling of matter and radiation.

Figure 3 illustrates the dynamics of cosmological nucleosynthesis and depicts mass concentrations of light chemical elements as a function of plasma temperatures. It can be seen

that at a temperature of 5×10^7 K, virtually all primary matter had already formed: ~ 23-26 percent of nucleons were bound, yielding nuclei of ^{4}He; hydrogen accounted for 74-77 percent of the mass and deuterium, helium-3 and tritium made up only 0.01-0.0001 percent of the mass. It should be noted, that the abundance of deuterium in the universe is very sensitive to the current density of matter. When ρ_m changed from 1.4×10^{-31} to 7×10^{-30} g/cm^3, relative concentration of deuterium (^{2}H/H) diminished by almost seven orders of magnitude. The mass content of ^{4}He is less dependent on baryon density, but it still increased by a factor of 2.

Figures 2 and 3 show the succession of epochs that occurred during the first 2-3 minutes after the Big Bang and the formation of primary (light) chemical elements. After the decoupling of radiation and matter at $Z < 1000$, and formation of hydrogen through recombination, the process of gravitational matter condensation began. Matter, which at that point consisted of approximately 75 percent hydrogen and 25 percent ^{4}He (with trace amounts of deuterium, tritium, ^{3}He, etc.), condensed into gravitationally bound gas clouds. There are a number of theoretical models of this process. In one these clouds are postulated to have a mass on the order of galactic protoclusters; in another they are hypothesized to be protogalaxies themselves.

As stated above, these structures formed during the epoch when matter dominated radiation, at a time, according to a number of theories, about 10^9 years after the Big Bang. After that point, gravitationally bound systems were no longer involved in the general Hubble expansion and evolved independently, according to different laws.

The next step in the development of the Big Bang model is

an explanation of the mechanism underlying the emergence of the large-scale structure of the universe.

E. Formation of a Large-Scale Structure of the Universe

All natural phenomena are controlled by four basic types of particle interaction: electromagnetic, strong (nuclear), weak, and gravitational. In the course of the entire "temperature" history of expansion of the universe, each of these interactions played a leading role in the particular processes that determined the present-day appearance of the universe.

The formation of the microwave radiation spectrum was due primarily to electromagnetic photon-electron interaction during the lepton era in the evolution of cosmological plasma. The key role in the thermonuclear synthesis of light chemical elements was played by the weak interaction of protons and neutrons with nucleons during their fusion into deuterium and helium nuclei. Finally, the weakest type of interaction—gravitational interaction—played the decisive role in the formation of the large-scale structure of the universe.

In contrast to the other three types of interaction of elementary particles on a scale comparable to the size of an atomic nucleus, gravitational interaction increases as a function of the number of particles. Because of this, the role of gravitational interaction is the most critical in such gigantic systems (compared with the atomic level) as galaxies and their clusters.

This assertion is incontrovertible with respect to the modern structural units of the metagalaxy—stars, galaxies, and galactic clusters. However, in the remote past the situation was vastly more complicated. During the era of the red shift $Z > 1000$, matter and radiation interacted with each other. At the same time, the pressure of radiation plasma was stronger than gravitational particle attraction in regions of increased (relative to the mean level) density of matter and energy. The size of these regions was on the order of hundreds of thousands times the diameter of the Sun.

Gravitational attraction of particles played the main role in the compression of these regions of increased density and further intensified their initial contrast with unperturbed matter. After decoupling of matter and radiation (at $Z < 1000$) this mechanism began to operate at virtually all scales. As a result, density fluctuations increased to such a degree that inhomogeneities were compressed by their own gravity, leading to the formation of gravitationally bound systems.

However, details of this process depend to a great extent on the specific type of small "seeding" fluctuations of density in the cosmological medium. Several types of protogalactic fluctuations were possible in the cosmological plasma. Although, this issue is beyond the scope of this chapter, the following important point should be noted.

We can obtain information about protogalactic perturbations of cosmological plasma by measuring variations of the intensity of microwave radiation in different directions. If, during the period of hydrogen recombination, when the radiation spectrum was "frozen," there were minor deviations from uniformity and isotropy of the distribution of matter in the

universe, they should have left an imprint on the microwave background spectrum causing fluctuations in its temperature $\Delta T/T$. Depending on the type of initial fluctuations, theoretical predictions are $\Delta T/T \geq 1 \times 10^{-4}$. Experts in this field have been waiting for more than 20 years for such variations to be found so that one of the most important problems of current cosmology can be solved. However, no fluctuations on the order of $\Delta T/T = 3 \times 10^{-5}$ have been detected so far. The situation remains intriguing and the question remains open.

II. The Milky Way Galaxy

A. The World of Galaxies

Regardless of how galaxies originated—as a result of gravity-induced condensation of primordial gas, gravity-induced fragmentation of protoclusters, or clustering of primordial stars—they are the second most numerous entities in the universe. Obviously stars are most numerous. As mentioned above, our galaxy consists of about 10^{11} stars; however, it is a medium-sized galaxy. Giant galaxies comprise 10^{12}-10^{13} stars. There are also many small galaxies with low luminosity, which are hardly detectable at great distances. For this reason, the exact number of galaxies in the universe cannot be determined; it can, however, be asserted that they number at least in the billions.

Both stars and galaxies are gravitationally bound systems. They are held together by their own gravity, which compensates for the gas pressure gradient in the case of stars, and for a similar force produced by dispersion of velocities of peculiar star motion in the case of galaxies. However, these systems are radically different. In particular, the stars in galaxies differ greatly in age—with the youngest being 10^7 and the oldest 10^{10} years old. Therefore, by observing stars of different ages in our galaxy we can verify our ideas about the evolution and, thus, the internal structure of stars.

The situation with galaxies is different. They all originated during approximately the same epoch ($t_G \cong 1$ - 2×10^{10} years); therefore, the difference in their ages must be less than t_G. Another important point is that the time scales for evolutionary effects for galaxies are comparable with the age of the universe. In order to study their evolution, we would have to observe galaxies at ever increasing distances from us. Because signals from these galaxies reach us at the speed of light, the farther away the galaxy is (the greater its red shift Z), the earlier is the stage of its evolution we are observing. Today's observable red shifts of galaxies are approximately $Z \sim 1$.

There are several classification schemes for galaxies. The simplest of these is the Hubble "tuning fork" diagram (Fig. 4). This diagram classifies regular galaxies (with clear morphology). As can be seen from Fig. 4 the galaxies are subdivided into elliptical (which in turn are subdivided into subclasses E0, E1, ...) and spiral. Spiral galaxies are subdivided into normal (upper branch) and barred galaxies. When Hubble proposed his classification scheme in the 1930s, he claimed that it represented the evolutionary sequence of galaxies.

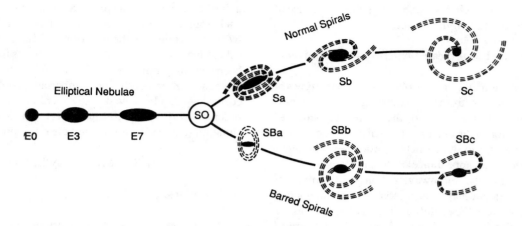

Fig. 4 Hubble diagram—The sequence of nebular types (From Hubble, E. *The Realm of the Nebulae.* **New Haven, Yale University Press, 1936, p. 45. Reprinted with permission from Yale University Press.)**

Today, it is clear that this is not the case. Irregular galaxies exist in addition to regular ones.

Elliptical galaxies are less flattened than spiral ones and this seems to be related to the original conditions under which they formed. The major properties of galaxies are their initial mass (or density of the protogalactic gas cloud) and their angular momentum. During gravitational compression, protogalaxies with high angular momentum must have compressed more along the axis of rotation than in the plane perpendicular to this axis. Ultimately, sufficiently rapid rotation of flat (younger) subsystems leads to the emergence of the spiral structure (see below) that is the defining feature of spiral galaxies.

The common evolutionary path of all galaxies evidently involved compression of the protogalactic gas cloud due to its own gravity. The gas energy dissipated through radiative loss. This means that the luminosity of earlier galaxies was greater than that of current ones.

B. Our Galaxy

Our galaxy is a complicated system consisting of several interrelated components; 93-97 percent of its mass is made up of stars and 3-5 percent of interstellar gas and dust. In addition, the interstellar medium is permeated with a magnetic field that exerts a strong effect on its dynamics as well as on the propagation of cosmic rays (energy particles) by extending their lifetime in the galaxy. The summary data presented here about the galaxy emphasize conditions in the vicinity of the Sun. More detailed information can be found in Marochnik and Suchkov.[4]

The evolution of our galaxy is usually described as follows. In the course of its condensation and radiative loss, the protogalactic hydrogen-helium cloud gave rise to the first and then to the subsequent generations of stars. If the random fluctuations in gas density in the protogalactic cloud exceeded a certain critical mass, the gas cloud collapsed and condensed due to its own gravity. Density increased and in central regions of the cloud reached a level which was sufficient to trigger the nuclear reactions that maintain star luminosity.

The evolutionary path of a star depends on its mass, rotation, magnetic field, and initial density. Evolution may result in the formation of ordinary stars belonging to various spectral classes as well as exotic high-density white dwarfs, neutron stars, and the black holes discussed previously. The equilibrium of a star (nonrotating and nonmagnetic) is maintained by the balance of two forces, its own gravity, which acts to compress the star, and a gas pressure gradient, which counteracts this force.

The mass of a white dwarf is comparable to that of the Sun, but its radius is one-hundreth that of the solar radius; its density is, therefore, 10^6 times greater than that of a normal star. A white dwarf represents one of the extreme possible equilibrated states in which gravitational forces are compensated for by the pressure of degenerate electron gas.

The radii of neutron stars (pulsars) are about 10-30 km, whereas their mass is comparable to that of the Sun. Consequently, due to an extremely high density of about 10^{11}-10^{15} g/cm³, the bulk of their matter is in the neutron state.

As a result of thermonuclear synthesis, heavier elements were formed in the stars. Massive stars of the first few generations exploded as supernovae, enriching the interstellar medium with metals. The process was repeated again and again: new generations of stars (already enriched with heavy elements) formed, and more heavy chemical elements (sometimes called metals) were generated in them. After the explosion of massive stars of subsequent generations, the interstellar medium became even richer in metals. Since this process developed in parallel to the condensation of the protogalactic cloud, the quantity of metals must have decreased along the Z-axis measured from the XY galactic plane, which is, on the whole, in agreement with observational data. A schematic model of our galaxy is presented in Fig. 5.

Actually, the entire situation was evidently much more complicated. We will cite only two of the circumstances that cloud this simple picture.

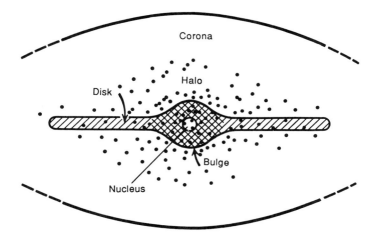

Fig. 5 Schematic diagram of the galaxy: view from the edge Points are globular clusters. (From Syunyayev, R.A. (Ed.). *Small Encyclopedia,* **Moscow, Sovetskaya Entsyklopedia, 1986, p. 63.)**

First, stars having the primary cosmologic (hydrogen-helium) composition and first-generation stars have never been detected in our galaxy. There are several possible explanations for this. For example, it may be argued that the most massive stars of the first generation were formed before the galaxies, and when they exploded, they enriched the pregalactic medium with heavy elements.

Second, there is no continuous transition from old objects containing only small quantities of heavy elements (old stars, globular clusters) to younger formations.[4] The transition occurs in a discrete manner suggesting that the evolution of the galaxy was not a uniform process, but included bursts of star formation, and, consequently, enrichment of the interstellar medium with heavy elements.

This in turn would mean that our galaxy would consist of subsystems with discrete differences in their kinematic and chemical properties (star orbit eccentricity, metallicity, etc.), since formation of these objects during condensation of the protogalactic gas cloud was a discrete rather than continuous process. Indeed, the kinematic parameters of the galactic subsystems do have the property of discreteness. Further details of this exciting issue can be found in Marochnik and Suchkov.[4]

Our galaxy is rotating. Two things must be remembered here. First, the different subsystems rotate differently. Second, this rotation is differential, i.e., the angular velocity of rotation, Ω, is a function of galactic distance R, i.e.,

$$\Omega = \Omega(R)$$

Figure 6 shows the rotational curve of the galaxy, i.e., its linear velocity ($v_\theta = \Omega(R) \times R$) as a function of distance from the galactic center.

The oldest subsystem in our galaxy is the so-called halo subsystem, with a virtually spherically symmetrical distribution of mass and weak rotation. The stars in the halo contain the smallest amounts of heavy elements, have high peculiar velocities (hundreds of kilometers per second in the circumsolar vicinity). In other words, the orbits of the stars of the halo are highly elongated (they are almost radial). This implies that they remain within the halo most of the time. The halo also contains globular clusters (Fig. 5) consisting of approximately 10^5-10^6 stars of low metal content.

C. Movement of the Sun in the Galaxy

Let us introduce the concept of the centroid of velocities of stars (in a certain region of the galaxy, e.g., near the Sun) or the local reference system. Using as large a sample of stars in this region as possible, we can determine the mean velocity of the local system (or centroid) relative to the Sun, i.e., the vector

$$<V> = N^{-1} \sum_{i=1}^{N} V_i$$

where i is the number of the star. Obviously, the velocity of the Sun relative to the centroid will be

$$V_{\text{SOL}} = -<V>$$

In a stationary cylindrical (galactocentric) reference system R, θ, Z, the centroid of the circumsolar vicinity moves with a circular velocity equal to $V_\theta^{\text{SOL}} \cong 220\,\text{km/s}$ at a distance of 8-10 kpc from the galactic center (in different models this velocity varies slightly). In the reference system connected with this centroid, the Sun has a random or peculiar velocity of approximately 20 km/s.

The variance of the peculiar velocities of stars in the circumsolar vicinity of the galaxy are related (in the reference system moving with the centroid) as follows:

$$\overline{V^2}_\theta \cong \overline{V^2}_Z \cong 0.4 \times \overline{V^2}_R$$

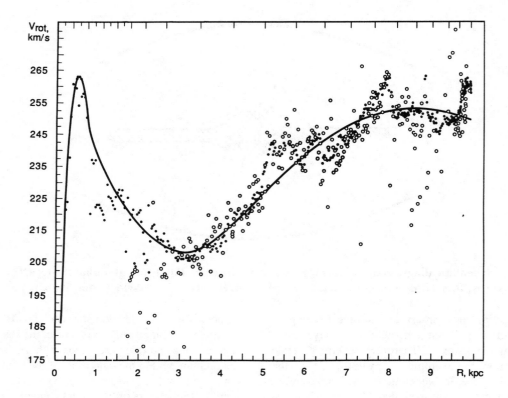

Fig. 6 Variation of the linear velocity of differential galactic rotation as a function of distance from the galactic center. The filled circles correspond to terminal velocities measured on HI profiles and the open circles correspond to terminal velocities measured on CO profiles. The black line represents a smooth approximation to the HI points (From: Burton, W.B, Gordon, M.A. Carbon monoxide in the Galaxy. III The overall nature of its distribution in the equatorial plane. *Astronomy and Astrophysics*, 1978, vol. 63, p. 7. Reprinted with permission of Springer-Verlag.)

Accordingly, the values

$$\sigma_\theta = \left(\overline{V_\theta^2}\right)^{1/2}, \sigma_Z = \left(\overline{V_Z^2}\right)^{1/2}, \sigma_R = \left(\overline{V_R^2}\right)^{1/2}$$

are termed the standard deviation of peculiar velocities of stars. By analogy with ordinary gas, these are their respective temperatures.

Here, two points should be made: 1) In the vicinity of the Sun, the distribution of stars with respect to peculiar velocities has the form of an anisotropic Maxwellian distribution (with temperatures that differ along coordinate axes); 2) As we saw above, the galaxy has many subsystems. When the standard deviations of peculiar velocities are determined separately for stars of different subsystems, the values are highly variable. The smallest standard deviation in peculiar velocities occurs for young stars and gas clouds of a flat subsystem and is on the order of:

$$\sigma = \left(\sigma^2_R + \sigma^2_Z + \sigma^2_\theta\right)^{1/2} \cong 10 - 20 \text{km} / \text{s}$$

The highest standard deviation is found for random velocities of stars in the halo and is an order of magnitude greater.

The first point implies that the distribution of stars with respect to velocity in the vicinity of the Sun is, to a high degree of accuracy, in statistical equilibrium; i.e., this is the distribu-

tion that must have developed due to star relaxation, star-star encounters, or other processes. (Actually, only Maxwellian isotropic distribution is in statistical equilibrium with respect to velocities with identical temperature in every direction. Anisotropic distribution of star velocities in the circumsolar vicinity is called the Schwarzschild distribution.) It is often assumed that since the vicinity of the Sun is not special in any manner, relaxation must have occurred in other areas of the galaxy as well. (This issue is discussed in Section III.C.)

The second point implies that rotation is the key parameter for disk-shaped subsystems. Compared to the linear velocity of these subsystems, the peculiar velocities of stars are low (an order of magnitude lower). For the halo it is just the opposite: systematic rotation is weak and linear velocity is a fraction of the standard deviation of peculiar velocities.

Before concluding this section about the position and motion of the Sun in the galaxy, several other points should be made.

Since the linear velocity of rotation of the centroid of the Sun is $V_\theta^{\text{SOL}} \cong 220$ km/s and the distance to the center of the galaxy is $R_{\text{SOL}} \cong 8$ - 10 kpc, the period of its revolution around the center is close to

$$T_{\text{SOL}} \cong 2\pi R_{\text{SOL}} / V_\theta^{\text{SOL}} \cong 2 - 3 \times 10^8 \text{years}$$

and the angular velocity of the Sun's rotation around the center of the galaxy is close to

$$\Omega_{SOL} = \frac{2\pi}{T_{SOL}} \cong 25 km/(s \cdot kpc)$$

At the same time, the Sun currently has a non-zero Z-component for peculiar velocity in a direction away from the galactic plane Z = 0. As the Sun moves away from the Z = 0 plane, it is increasingly strongly attracted by stars and other matter (molecular and diffusion gas clouds) that lie between it and the galactic plane. This leads to a sign change in V_Z^{SOL}. This process repeats itself many times; i.e, the Sun is oscillating with respect to the plane of the galaxy.

The altitude of the maximum ascent of the Sun over the plane Z = 0 (and, consequently, descent below the plane) is on the order of ± 100 pc, depending on the preferred model of the distribution of matter along the Z-axis. The period of the oscillation is on the order $T_Z^{SOL} \cong$ 32-33 million years. One hypothesis explaining the periodic extinction of plant and animal species on Earth[9] attributes it to the periodic passage of the solar system across the galactic plane.[10, 11]

Other specific features of the position and movement of the Sun in the galaxy are associated with its spiral arms. (See Section III.D.)

D. Stellar Dynamics

In accordance with Newton's laws of motion, all stars in the galaxy are attracted to each other with force $F = GM_i M_j/R_{ij}^2$ where M_i and M_j are the masses of the ith and jth stars, and R_{ij} is the distance between them. Since force F acts at long range, analogous to Coulomb interaction in plasma, any self-gravitating stellar system, including the galaxy, is a self-consistent system with collective properties. A gravitational field is generated by the particles within it. Because of the long-range interaction of forces, the effective cross-section of star interactions is very great (several orders of magnitude greater than the geometric cross-section required for collision of stars as elastic spheres).

The relaxation time for star-to-star encounters is given by the formula[4]:

$$\tau_R = \beta \frac{\sigma^3}{\pi G^2 M^2 n\Lambda}$$

where β is a coefficient close to unity, σ is the absolute value of the mean standard deviation of peculiar velocities of stars of mass M (for the sake of simplicity we will assume that the standard deviation of velocity and mass are the same for stars of every type, because the differences do not change the order of magnitude of the result), and $\Lambda = \ln N$; where N is the number of stars in the system, and n is their concentration.

Using typical values for the parameters for stars in the circumsolar vicinity of the galaxy

$$\sigma = 20 km/s, \quad n \cong 0.1 p\sigma^{-3}$$

we find

$$\tau_R \cong 10^{13} - 10^{14} \text{ years}$$

an enormous number. This suggests that in the circumsolar vicinity of the galaxy, star-to-star encounters will not occur throughout the entire lifetime of the galaxy (1-2 × 10^{10} years). Similar estimates of τ_R for other regions of the galaxy show that star-to-star encounters may occur only within its central parsec, where the star concentration is eight orders of magnitude greater than near the Sun. (Other regions where star-to-star encounters may take place are central regions of globular clusters.) Thus, the galaxy is a collision-free stellar system, with the exception of the central parsec and globular clusters, and is analogous (in many aspects, but not all) to an electron plasma.

Here, the following should be noted:

1) Stellar populations that belong to different subsystems have different kinematic characteristics; specifically, they rotate about the symmetry axis (0Z) of the galaxy with different angular velocities. Being collision-free, these subsystems form streams that pass through one another, like mutually penetrating beams of charged particles in an electron plasma. The basic difference is that plasma contains charged particles with both signs, so that both forces of attraction and repulsion operate in it, whereas stellar systems have only forces of attraction. This circumstance (different rotation of subsystems) is very important for a proper understanding of the nature of the spiral structure of the galaxy.[4]

2) Since the galaxy (and its circumsolar vicinity) is a collision-free stellar system, at first there appears to be nothing that could have led to establishment of the quasi-equilibrium Schwarzschild distribution of stars with respect to velocities. This is even more interesting because, as observational data show, the standard deviation of star velocities increases with their age. The so-called problem of relaxation pertains to the nature of this effect and the origin of the Schwarzschild distribution of star velocities.

This problem remains unsolved because there are good arguments in favor of two alternative points of view. According to the first view, the age-related increase in the standard deviation of peculiar velocities of stars of different populations is associated with the initial conditions under which they formed. According to the second view, relaxation did indeed occur, as a result of collisions of stars with interstellar gas clouds and the spiral arms of the galaxy. Because of the tendency toward equipartition, the kinetic energy (standard deviation of velocity) of stars colliding with massive clouds should increase with time (age).

3) In a rotating star subsystem, collective movements can arise in the form of waves of stellar density. The elasticity necessary for propagation of waves in a collision-free stellar system (in an ordinary gas, sound waves are propagated due to the elasticity caused by molecular collisions) is created by Coriolis forces acting on stars that have peculiar velocities in the reference system associated with the rotating subsystem.

E. Spiral Structure of the Galaxy

As noted above, in the plane view our galaxy resembles NGC 1232 (Fig. 1), i.e., it has a well-developed spiral structure. In other galaxies, the spiral structures are clearly delineated by young stars and interstellar gas, which for a long period of time have been considered to be the main objects forming the spiral arms in our and other galaxies.

It should be recalled that a flat subsystem, of which young stars and gas are examples, rotates differentially. For this reason, any structural formation that may have evolved as a result of one or another phenomenon (e.g., condensation) should with time be transformed into a segment of a spiral arm, since various portions rotate (due to the differential rotation of the galaxy) with different angular velocities; those located closer to the center rotate faster, whereas those located at greater distances rotate more slowly (Fig. 6). However, it has been clear for a long time that the differentiality of rotation is actually too high: $\Omega(R)$ is a rather steep function. This can be easily seen in Fig. 6 if one substitutes angular velocity for linear velocity $V(R)$ on the ordinate, i.e., $\Omega(R) = V(R)/R$, as this indicates that any structure would totally dissipate in 2-3 galactic years (revolutions of the galaxy). Therefore, the problem of explaining the spiral structure actually involves explaining why it has survived for so long (billions of years) despite the shearing effect of differential rotation.

Although new attempts have been made recently to explain the spiral structure phenomenon—the existence of an overall grand design—covering the galaxy as a whole, we maintain that this phenomenon, in principle, can be attributed to the star density waves mentioned above.

As the pioneering work of C. C. Lin and F. H. Shu (cited in Marochnik and Suchkov[4]) has demonstrated, the galaxy, when viewed as a differentially rotating disk that is not divided into subsystems, could have waves of stellar density whose front has a spiral shape. These waves would propagate at an angle of θ with constant angular velocity $\Omega p = const$. In other words, despite the variability (differentiality) of rotation of the disk ($\Omega = \Omega(R)$) simulating the galaxy, its spiral arms, which are actually density waves, would rotate at a constant angular velocity Ωp and thus would not be destroyed by the shearing effect of differential rotation.

Spiral density waves can be of two types: short-wave and long-wave modes, abbreviated as S- and L-modes. The main differences between them are that the S-mode has a radial velocity directed away from the periphery toward the center of the galaxy, while the L-mode acts in the opposite direction, and that their Ωp values are different. For the S-mode $\Omega p \cong$ 13 km/(s·kpc), while for the L-mode $\Omega p \cong$ 24 km/(s·kpc).

In our opinion, there are several important reasons why the L-mode offers a better explanation for the spiral structure of our galaxy. Considering that the galaxy consists of many subsystems, only the subsystem rotating at the highest velocity (the thin disk), the mean density of which is several times lower than the total density of the galaxy used in the Lin and Shu model, participates in the formation of the spiral structure. This assumption produces an estimate of $\Omega p \cong$ 24 km/(s·kpc), which is in best agreement with actual observations (as demonstrated by L. S. Marochnik and A. A. Suchkov). The reader can find further details about the origin of the spiral structure of the galaxy in Marochnik and Suchkov.[4]

Here we would like to note two important points. Spiral density waves propagate through the stellar population of a rapidly rotating flat subsystem, generating a spiral gravitational field, as a result of compression of the stellar gas, in addition to the regular axisymmetric gravitational field of the galaxy. The additional gravitational force is not large, only ~ 5-10 percent of the regular gravitational force of the galaxy; it is capable, however, of causing dramatic restructuring in interstellar gas of low mass. Specifically, the flow of the interstellar gas across the potential well of the gravitational potential of the interstellar gas gives rise to a powerful global shock wave (galactic shock wave), in which interstellar gas compresses and star formation is enhanced. Thus, the visible spiral structure (Fig. 1) delineated by interstellar gas and young bright stars is, in fact, an indicator of the "true" spiral structure formed by an invisible wave of stellar density, or more precisely, by its gravitational field.

Our second point may have direct bearing on the origin of the solar system and cosmogonic time scales measured on the basis of the extinct radioactivity of individual nuclides. This is associated with the fact that angular velocities of rotation of the Sun around the galactic center ($\Omega_{SOL} \cong 25$ km/(s·kpc)) and the L-mode of the spiral density wave are similar; in other words, their rotation is nearly synchronous (with respect to galactic measures).

F. The Interstellar Medium

As noted above, the interstellar medium is composed of interstellar gas and dust permeated by a magnetic field. The interstellar medium also incorporates cosmic rays, which are high-energy charged particles generated throughout the entire "lifetime" of the galaxy by explosions of supernovae and by pulsars (neutron stars).

Along with young stars, interstellar gas is localized primarily in the thin disk, whose half-thickness is close to 100 pc in the vicinity of the Sun. The major constituent of interstellar gas is hydrogen, which occurs in atomic (ionized and un-ionized) or molecular (H_2) forms. In addition, molecules of other elements, including organic compounds, have been detected (by their radiation lines) in the interstellar medium.

Traditionally, un-ionized hydrogen is denoted as HI and ionized hydrogen as HII. In terms of mass, molecular and atomic hydrogen occur in almost equal quantities in the galaxy although their distribution is completely different. Molecular hydrogen is concentrated, in the form of giant molecular clouds ($M \cong 10^4 - 10^6 M_{SOL}$), in the region of the so-called molecular galactic ring at 4-8 kpc from the center and inside the central kiloparsec of the galaxy. Cold atomic hydrogen HI, detectable at the 21 cm wavelength, is distributed more uniformly (Fig. 6). There is a "hole" in the gas

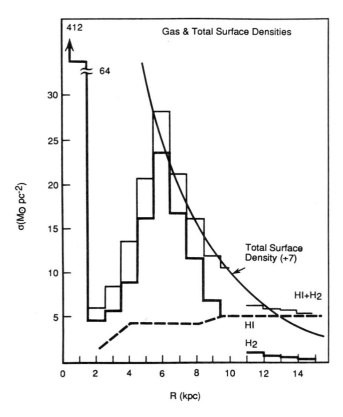

Fig. 7 Distribution of interstellar gas in the galaxy. The figures shows the surface densities of HI (broken line), H₂ (thick line), and H1 + H₂ (fine line). The smoothed curve represents an approximation to full gas density as a function of distance from the galactic center. The number 7 indicates the factor by which the total surface density of the stellar disk exceeds the total gas density in the area of the galaxy within ~ 10 kpc of the Sun, according to one model. (From: Sanders, D.B., Solomon, P.M., Scoville, N.Z. Giant Molecular Clouds in the Galaxy. I The Axisymmetric Distribution of He, *Astrophysics Journal*, 1984, vol. 276. p. 182. Reprinted with permission from *The Astrophysical Journal*.)

galaxy the distribution of the dust is highly nonuniform. It is concentrated in clouds of interstellar gas found primarily in the disk plane. In general in galaxies, dust occurs primarily in the spiral arms. Dust concentrated in the inner edges of spiral arms can be detected in other galaxies. This is interpreted as the result of strong compression of the interstellar medium in the narrow region of the front of the galactic shock wave.

The most important component of the interstellar medium is its magnetic field, which makes the most important contribution to energy balance and prolongs the lifetime of cosmic rays in the galaxy. Moving at just below the speed of light, cosmic ray particles should cover a distance on the order of the galaxy's diameter ($D \cong 30$ kpc) in time $t \sim D/c \sim 10^5$ years. It is, however, known that they spend $t_{cr} \sim 10^7$ years in the galactic disk, which can be ascribed to the effect of the magnetic field.

A charged particle moving at an angle to the line of force of the magnetic field begins to move in a spiral around that line; the radius of the orbital cross-section (the Larmor radius r_L) diminishes as the magnetic field intensity B increases:

$$r_L = mcV_\perp / eB$$

where m and e are the particle's mass and charge, and $V_\perp$ is the velocity component perpendicular to the vector B. In regions of convergence of lines of force (as the field intensifies), particles undergo repulsion. Magnetic traps have been constructed on the basis of this principle for use in experimental facilities for thermonuclear synthesis, and the same situation exists in nature. There are many instabilities of different types in both situations, leading to diffusion of charged particles across the magnetic field and their ejection from the retention area. For cosmic rays, this time period is ~ 10^7 years.

In the interstellar medium, magnetic field intensity is on the average close to $B \cong 3 \times 10^{-6}$ gauss = 3×10^{-10} T. The field has a chaotic and a regular component. The latter can be detected through use of synchrotron radio-frequency emission of electrons traveling in the magnetic field. The radio-frequency map of the synchrotron radiation of the galactic disk shows that a large-scale magnetic field is concentrated along the spiral arms.

In the interstellar medium, the magnetic field can be sustained only by internal electric currents since there are no other global sources of magnetization. Since λ, conductivity of the medium, is finite (its value differs in the clouds and in the medium between them, because it depends on level of ionization, temperature, and electron concentration), then, in theory, the magnetic field should dissipate. However, there is no question of dissipation of the large-scale field in the galactic disk because the interstellar medium behaves as a superconductor.

The time required for attenuation of a magnetic field in a volume with linear dimension L and conductivity λ can be derived from the well-known formula:

$$\tau_\beta \cong \frac{4\pi\lambda L^2}{c^2}$$

distribution in a region 2-4 kpc from the center. This region corresponds to the region in Fig. 6, where the curve of rotation has a minimum. HII regions are located around young hot stars, which ionize hydrogen with their ultraviolet radiation.

The distribution of HI in the disk is also nonuniform. The ionized hydrogen forms cold, diffuse clouds with typical density $n \cong 20$-40 cm^{-3}, linear dimension $L\sim10$-70 pc, and temperature $T\sim30$-70 K. Its global distribution throughout the galaxy is depicted in Fig. 7. The medium between the clouds has an extremely low density ($n \cong 0.1$ cm^{-3}) and a very high temperature $T \cong 10^4$ K. The interstellar medium possesses "corridors" or "tunnels" of very hot gas ($T \cong 10^6$ K), probably formed as a result of supernova explosions.

The interstellar medium contains substantial amounts of dust, which absorbs the light of stars and galaxies. In our

The reason why such a poor (in terrestrial terms) conductor as the interstellar medium ($\lambda_{ISM} \cong 6 \times 10^{12}$ CGSE for HII regions, compared for example to that of copper: $\lambda_{Cu} \cong 5 \times 10^{17}$ CGSE) acts as a superconductor is the huge cosmic scale of L. According to the above equation, the time that would be required for the field to attenuate in the spiral arms exceeds the age of the galaxy.

The superconducting properties of the interstellar medium are responsible for the fact that the lines of force of the magnetic field cannot move relative to the interstellar gas; in other words, a large-scale field becomes "frozen" into the medium. Because of this, when interstellar gas is compressed to form a galactic shock wave with spiral contours, the strength of the magnetic field also increases in the galactic shock wave region. (Since the magnetic field is "frozen in," gas compression causes the number of lines of force crossing a given area to increase, thereby increasing the strength of the magnetic field). This is the reason that the synchrotron radio-frequency radiation of the galactic disk has the same shape as the spiral arms.

Observations of the velocities of stars near the Sun are used to estimate the gravitational acceleration g_z along the Z-coordinate of the galactic disk. Poisson's equation relates gravitational acceleration to the density of the disk:

$$\frac{d^2\varphi}{dZ^2} = -4\pi G\rho$$

where

$$g_Z = \frac{d\varphi}{dZ} = -\lambda_z \times Z, \lambda_z = 10^{-29} / s^2$$

From this equation we can derive total density of matter in the vicinity of the Sun:

$$\rho_{to_t} \cong 0.15 M_{SOL} / pc^3$$

The densities of stars and gas can be calculated as follows:

$$\rho_{stars} \cong 0.064 M_{SOL} / pc^3$$

$$\rho_{gas} \cong 0.024 M_{SOL} / pc^3$$

The missing portion of the total density can be attributed to weak or extinct stars or another form of matter. In any case, it should be emphasized that there must be missing mass in the vicinity of the Sun. Evidently, there is missing mass both in the internal halo of the galaxy[4] and in its external halo, the corona.

What is to be said about the interstellar medium in the vicinity of the Sun? It is likely that the energy densities of the three basic components of the medium—interstellar gas, the magnetic field, and cosmic rays—are almost equal (to be precise, of the same order of magnitude). This implies that the pressures of the components of the medium are also nearly equal; i.e, in the vicinity of the Sun the interstellar medium must be in a state of thermodynamic quasi-equilibrium. Assuming a field intensity of $B \cong 3 \times 10^{-10}$ T, interstellar gas density = $0.024 M_{SOL}/pc^3$, standard deviation of velocities of gas clouds ~10 km/s, and cosmic ray energy density in the vicinity of the Earth $\varepsilon_{cr} \cong 10^6$ eV/m³, then the corresponding pressures are described by:

$$P_B \cong P_{cr} \cong P_{gas} \cong 5 \times 10^{-14} H / m^3$$

It should be noted that cold, dense clouds of HI and the hot

Table 1 Planets of the Solar System

Planet	Semimajor axis	Orbital eccentricity	Period of revolution, days	Equatorial radius (Earth = 1)	Mass (Earth = 1)
Mercury	0.387	0.206	87.969	0.380	0.055
Venus	0.723	0.007	224.701	0.950	0.815
Earth	1.00	0.017	365.256	1.00	1.00
Mars	1.524	0.093	686.980	0.532	0.107
Jupiter	5.203	0.048	4332.589	11.18	317.83
Saturn	9.539	0.056	10759.22	9.42	95.147
Uranus	19.182	0.047	30685.4	4.00	14.54
Neptune	30.058	0.009	60189	3.93	17.23
Pluto	39.44	0.250	90465	0.17	0.002

interstellar medium are also in a state of quasi-equilibrium, since their pressures are approximately equal to each other and to that of the magnetic field. We are using such terms as quasi-equilibrium, approximately equal, and the like because the measurement accuracy of the parameters of the interstellar medium is too low for greater certainty.

III. The Solar System in the Galaxy

A. Large-Scale Structure

The Sun is surrounded by nine planets and a belt of asteroids whose major parameters and distances are summarized in Table 1 and will not be discussed here.

The large-scale properties of the solar system, its mass and angular momentum, are distributed in a somewhat strange fashion. The bulk of its mass is concentrated in the Sun, which comprises 99.87 percent of the total (the Sun's mass M_{SOL} is 2×10^{33} g) and the mass of planets comprises 0.13 percent of the total. The total mass of the planetary system ΣM_p is 448.5 $M_\oplus$, where $M_\oplus = 6 \times 10^{27}$ g is the mass of the planet Earth. On the other hand, the major portion of the solar system's angular momentum is attributable to the planetary system. In fact, the total angular momentum of the planetary system is approximately $\Sigma J_p \cong 3.15 \times 10^{50}$ g $\times$ cm²/s. The angular momentum of the Sun is measured with respect to rotation of its surface is around $J_{SOL} \cong 1.6 \times 10^{48}$ g $\times$ cm²/s. Thus, approximately 99.5 percent of the total angular momentum belongs to the planetary system.

However, the Vega and Giotto missions to Halley's comet have provided evidence that this traditional picture of the large-scale distribution of mass and angular momentum in the solar system may need to be modified, since the Oort Cloud may prove to be more massive than was previously believed.[3]

Since the Oort Cloud may be important to our understanding of the large-scale structure of the solar system, we will describe it in greater detail.

B. The Oort Cloud

In 1950, existing ideas about the the solar system consisting of nine planets and their moons were further supplemented by a very significant hypothesis: that there was a cloud of comets at the periphery of the solar system. According to Oort,[2] comets occasionally escape from this cloud and enter the region occupied by the planets, where they are detectable by observers on Earth. The outer perimeter of this cloud of comets, sometimes termed Oort's bank or safe, is located at a distance of 1 pc or 2×10^5 AU from the Sun. Oort estimated the inner perimeter to be 4×10^4 AU from the Sun; the total number of comets in the cloud is estimated at on the order of 2×10^{11} (Fig. 8).

The distance of the outer perimeter of the Oort Cloud was estimated through a simple chain of reasoning. The distance to the nearest stars is about 2 pc. If the cometary reservoir belongs in the solar system (and no strongly hyperbolic

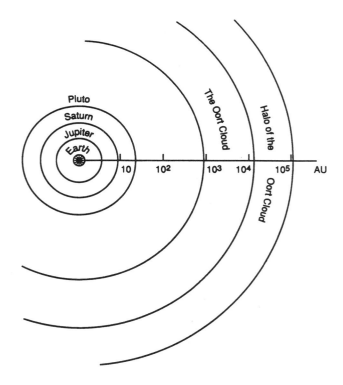

Fig. 8 Schematic structure of the solar system with Oort cloud at the periphery (From: Marochnik, L.S. *Encounter with a Comet*. Moscow, Nauka, 1985, p. 80.)

comets have been found), then it cannot extend beyond half the distance to the nearest stars, i.e., beyond 1 pc. The location of the inner perimeter (i.e., the one closest to the Sun) of the cloud of comets has not been determined precisely. The fact that the number of comets with $\alpha_o < 2 \times 10^4$ AU is severely diminished in distributions of the type shown in Fig. 9 places an upper limit on the estimate of the inner perimeter.

As a result of the tidal force of the galactic disk (along the Z-coordinate), the influence of giant molecular clouds in the galaxy, and gravitational effects of stars passing near the Sun, some comets from the Oort Cloud lose their angular momentum and enter the region of the solar system, where they have a short perihelion distance q, and consequently can be detected by observers on Earth. As mentioned above, the number of comets with semimajor axes $\alpha < 2 \times 10^4$ AU is severely diminished in the observable distribution $N(1/\alpha)$. Hence, they cannot enter the loss cone in the velocity space generated by the effects of near star transits. (The loss cone encompasses the velocity vectors of comets that, due to perturbations, are ejected into the planetary system and interstellar space.)

Giant molecular cloud complexes can also affect comet relaxation (scattering) in the Oort Cloud as a result of the scattering cone. Such complexes may be responsible for more than just thermalization and filling of scattering and loss cones. It is postulated that encounters with gigantic molecular complexes could have caused the solar system over the course its lifetime (approximately 4.6×10^9 years) to lose the entire

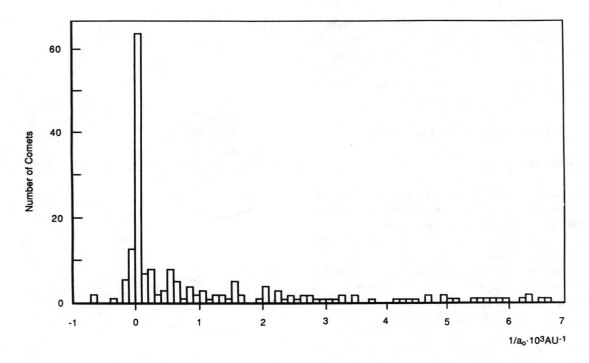

Fig. 9 Distribution of long-term comets with respect to the reciprocal of the initial semimajor axes of their orbits (From: Marochnik, L.S. *Encounter with a Comet*. Moscow, Nauka, 1985, p. 75.)

original population of the Oort Cloud. However, the opposite view is also held.

In 1981, on the basis of qualitative considerations, Hills[12] estimated the inner perimeter of the Oort Cloud to be $\alpha_H \cong 2 \times 10^4$ AU. He also concluded that the perimeter is well delineated because of the weak (power = 2/7) dependence of α_H on other parameters. As Hills demonstrated, comets with semimajor axes $\alpha < \alpha_H$ cannot always fill in the loss cone, which is in agreement with observational data. Hence, at distances shorter than α_H there may exist a dense and massive inner cloud of comets in a steady state. The detectable portion of the entire comet bank, i.e., the Oort Cloud *per se*, in all likelihood, comprises only the halo surrounding the inner cloud of comets, which comprises only a few percent of the total mass of the reservoir.

In his pioneering work published in 1950, Oort first hypothesized the existence of an internal comet cloud (ICC).[2] In 1964, Whipple showed that perturbations of Neptune's orbit may be associated with a circular belt of primary comets rotating around the Sun at a distance of no less than 50 AU.[3] The ICC concept may help to resolve several problems. For example, the postulated existence of a dense, massive ICC may help to explain the survival of the primary population of the Oort Cloud during the entire lifetime of the solar system. The ICC concept may be help to account for observed properties of distant objects that are seen through the ICC, for example, diffuse absorption bands in stellar spectra.

At the present time, there exist several approaches that could help detect the ICC. Geological data could become relevant, since the rare instances of star transit through the ICC

would have generated short-lived but powerful "comet showers," which might have fallen on the Earth.

Several years ago a hypothesis was put forward claiming strong evidence for the existence of the ICC. Extinction of certain biological species on Earth is also linked with comet showers that "bombarded" the planet in the past.[9-11] Another approach would try to locate the ICC through its gravitational effect, eclipses of distant stars and infrared radiation.[13]

The geometry and dimensions of the comet reservoir around the Sun are unknown. They may be influenced by cosmogonic factors (conditions under which the solar system was born) as well as by the physical conditions in the present-day Oort Cloud. There are arguments suggesting that the initial distribution of comets had the form of a flat ring or of a sphere. In either case, an ensemble of particles (the ICC comets) would form a collisionless system, in which collective fluctuations and low-amplitude waves would be possible.

If we could increase the sensitivity of infrared observations one order of magnitude above that required for measuring ICC background radiation, we should be able to detect angular flux variations associated with collective motion of a particle ensemble. Such movements are slow, with periods longer than those of ICC comets. Therefore, they may be observed as static inhomogeneities.

The temperature of the nuclei of primary comets in the Oort Cloud would be a function of the the presence or absence of internal sources of heat, distances between the nuclei and the Sun, and the ratio of their absorption capacity in the optical and long wavelength infrared spectral ranges. The initial temperature of comet nuclei cannot be higher than the melting point of ice and seems to lie in the range of 20-100 K. The extinct isotope [26]Al may have been an effective internal source of heating. It is estimated that comet nuclei with a radius R_c of about 100 km could have been sustained at a temperature of 120 K by the energy of radioactive decay of [26]Al for approximately 10^9 years.

The time required for the nuclei to cool through heat conduction is on the order of $t_c \cong R_c^2/æ$, where æ is the thermal conductivity of matter of the comet nucleus (for Moon rocks æ $\cong 10^{-3}$ - 10^{-4} cm²/s). If the half-life of [26]Al $= 0.72 \times 10^6$ years and $R_c \cong 5.5$ km for a comet nucleus whose dimensions are on the order of the nucleus of Halley's Comet ($16 \times 8 \times 8$ km[16]) and if æ $= 0.004$ cm²/s) we obtain $t_c \cong 2.5 \times 10^6$ years; consequently, comet nuclei should cool off as soon as the heating source [26]Al is exhausted. Since the cooling time is approximately three orders of magnitude less than the cosmogonic scale (4.6×10^9 years), it is clear that the relatively high initial temperatures of comet nuclei should rapidly drop to levels determined by the continuously acting heat sources.

As radioactive decay of normal amounts of long-lived nuclides (uranium, thorium, potassium-40) produces about 5 $\times 10^{-8}$ erg/(g·s), it can be demonstrated that a comet nucleus in the ICC must have a temperature of 10 K, the same temperature as the initial temperature of matter from which it was formed. This in turn means that comet nuclei in the Oort Cloud did not undergo chemical evolution due to their low temperature. Evidently neither did they evolve because of compression due to their own gravity, since the mass of comet nuclei is many orders of magnitude less than that of planets. It can therefore be concluded that comet nuclei "stored in Oort's safe" carry information about the primordial chemical composition and initial conditions of the formation of the solar system.

The hypotheses about the origin of the Oort Cloud can be roughly divided into two classes. The first class suggests that the cloud developed within the solar system, whereas those of the second class argue that it was captured from the interstellar medium. The lack of comets with strong hyperbolic orbits argues against their galactic origin. Nevertheless, the question of whether they are natives or outsiders is not absurd. It can be recast to ask whether Oort's bank in general can be of galactic origin. This question is based on the hypothesis that several times in the course of its existence the Sun could have crossed giant clouds of molecular hydrogen (containing dust or comet nuclei) with a mass of $M \cong (10^4$ - $10^6) M_{SOL}$. The galaxy contains many clouds of this kind, but they are mostly concentrated in a ring with an internal radius $R_1 = 4$ kpc from the center of our stellar system and an external radius $R_2 = 8$ kpc. According to different estimates, the distance between the Sun and the center of the galaxy varies from $R_{SOL} \cong 8.5$ to 10 kpc. At this distance there are essentially no giant molecular complexes [this is the term applied to the largest clouds with a mass of $(5 \times 10^5$ - $10^6) M_{SOL}$].

The assumption that the Sun has traversed (once or several times) such giant molecular clouds raises many questions: Would the Sun lose its hypothesized original comet reservoir totally or only partially? While traversing the region, could the Sun capture existing comet nuclei from the giant molecular cloud? If so, could it capture them in such a way as to give rise to Oort's bank with all the properties observed today? If yes, then how did these comet nuclei get into the giant molecular cloud? Or were they formed from gas and dust at a later time, when the solar system was already in existence? This is a far from exhaustive list of the questions that need to be answered.

An alternative explanation is that Oort's bank originated within the solar system itself through various mechanisms during the formation of the latter. One such mechanism involves comet nuclei originating in distant (and thus cold) parts of the solar system, or more specifically, the protosolar nebula. Under the perturbing effect of Jupiter, Saturn, Uranus, and Neptune, they would then have been ejected beyond the region of these planets. Another mechanism would involve comet nuclei forming in the protosolar nebula *in situ*, i.e., exactly where they occur now—in the region occupied by Oort's bank.

Thus, the solar system consists of nine planets revolving around the Sun plus a giant cloud of comets at its periphery, which is composed of a dense inner portion and an outer halo. Does this cloud make a significant contribution to the large-scale distribution of mass and angular momentum in the solar system?

In his pioneering work Oort[2] estimated the comet cloud mass to be $0.1 M_{\oplus}$. In other words, in spite of a huge population (2×10^{11} comets), the cloud appeared to be a dynamically insignificant formation. This followed from the assumption that the nuclear radius of an average comet was 1 km at a density of 1 g/cm³. (The shape of a nucleus may diverge greatly from spherical but, for the sake of simplicity, the idea of mean radius can be introduced. The mean radius is the radius of a sphere whose volume is equal to that of the irregular comet nucleus.) Currently the mass of the Oort Cloud is assumed to be much greater because 1) it must also include the mass of the comets in the inner cloud the number of which is a factor of 5-10 greater than those in the halo and 2) the dimensions and, hence, mass of comet nuclei are likely to be larger than thought previously. For example, the mean radius of Halley's comet $R_c \cong 5.5$ km[14]. If all this is true, then it is probable that the major portion of angular momentum of the solar system is concentrated not inside the planetary system, but in the cloud of comets, i.e., at the periphery of the solar system.[3]

C. Time Scales

A number of meteorites that have fallen to Earth have contained excessive amounts of [129]Xe as compared with the mean abundance of this isotope in the solar system. This stable isotope results from radioactive decay of short-lived iodine [129]I and plutonium [244]Pu isotopes. The half-lives of these isotopes are well known and are equal to 0.17×10^8 years and 0.82×10^8 years, respectively. Thus, if we know the amount of xenon, we can calculate the abundance of radioactive iodine and plutonium in the solar system at the time when the meteorites began to form in it. It was computed that at that instant the abundances of these radioactive isotopes were:

$$\alpha \cong {}^{129}I/{}^{127}I \cong 10^{-4} \quad \text{and} \quad \beta = {}^{244}Pu/{}^{238}U \cong 0.015$$

where ${}^{127}I$ is the stable iodine isotope, ${}^{238}U$ is the long lived uranium isotope, and α and β are the ratio of their abundances.

It is also known that thermonuclear synthesis of chemical elements in the galaxy is continuous. In particular, radioactive iodine and plutonium are formed during bursts of supernovae, which are accompanied by the extreme increase in temperature such synthesis requires. Computations show that in the course of galactic thermonuclear synthesis, these elements must have been formed in quantities so that $\alpha \cong 1$ and $\beta \cong 1$. Knowing the half-lives of iodine and plutonium, we can compute the period over which decay must have been occurring by the time meteorites were formed in order to produce values of $\alpha \cong 10^{-4}$ and $\beta \cong 0.015$, which correspond to the ${}^{129}Xe$ concentration detected in meteorites. This time T_1 was found to be 3×10^8 years.

Using theoretically derived formulas for the radioactive decay of long-lived isotopes of ${}^{238}U$ (half-life $= 4.5 \times 10^9$ years) and ${}^{232}Th$ (half-life $= 1.39 \times 10^{10}$ years), we can calculate the age of both terrestrial rocks and stone meteorites; the ages of the latter are very close to that of the solar system. The age of the solar system is thus estimated to be 4.6×10^9 years (T_2). This implies that about 300 million years before meteorites began to solidify, i.e., 4.9×10^9 years ago, iodine and plutonium must have penetrated the protosolar nebula. After that, and continuing until meteorites began to form, the continuous synthesis of chemical elements that occurs in the galaxy could not have been taking place in the solar system, or the quantities of radioactive iodine and plutonium in the protosolar nebula would have increased.

In 1974-76 it was reported that the protosolar nebula must have contained radioactive ${}^{26}Al$, which has a half-life of 0.72 $\times 10^6$ years. The meteorite Allende, which fell in Mexico, contained ${}^{26}Mg$ isotope in excess to its mean abundance in the solar system. This excess was attributed to radioactive decay of ${}^{26}Al$. As was done with the xenon measurements, magnesium abundance was used to calculate the quantity of radioactive aluminum that must have been in the material that formed the meteorites. Its abundance was estimated to be on the order of $\gamma = {}^{26}Al/{}^{27}Al \cong 5 \times 10^{-5}$, where ${}^{27}Al$ is the stable aluminum isotope.

Applying radioactive decay formulas, it is easy to demonstrate that ${}^{26}Al$ must have been decaying for several million years after it penetrated the cloud, so that its concentration would be 5×10^{-5} by the time the epoch of meteorite solidification occurred. Thus, in addition to the two aforementioned time scales $T_1 = 3 \times 10^8$ years and $T_2 = 4.6 \times 10^9$ years, cosmogonic theories of the solar system use a third time scale $T_3 = 10^6$ years.

When the T_3 scale was discovered, many astronomers believed that radioactive aluminum (${}^{26}Al$) entered the protosolar nebula as the result of a nearby supernova. This suggested the hypothesis that the solar system originated from a protosolar cloud stimulated by the supernova. However, today the hypothesis about a nearby supernova triggering the formation of the solar system is no longer widely held, because aluminum has been detected in the galactic interstellar medium.

Another time scale can be derived from the periodic extinction of certain biological species $T_4 = 26 \times 10^6$ years.[15] This scale was briefly discussed above and is associated with the tidal effects that comets in the inner regions of the Oort Cloud are subject to when the solar system crosses the galactic plane.[10, 11] The tides that arise when the solar system periodically passes through the regions with a large number of massive gas clouds, cause comets to escape from the inner Oort Cloud. Some of these bombard the Earth at intervals of 26 million years, as concluded from studying their craters.[11] Many astronomers agree that the extinction of certain species can be attributed to these events.[10, 11]

The major time scales of the solar system, derived from normal or "extinct" radioactivity of various nuclides and extinction of algae, require explanation. Below, we offer some speculations with regard to the position of the solar system in our galaxy.

D. Motion in the Galactic Space

T_3 requires no special comment because of the occurrence of aluminum in the interstellar medium. However, it should be noted that scales T_1, T_2, and T_4 are comparable to characteristic galactic time scales. We have already noted that the period of rotation of the circumsolar vicinity of the galaxy about its center is on the order 2.5×10^8 years $\sim T_2$, whereas the period of Sun's oscillations relative to the galactic plane is on the order 30×10^6 years $\sim T_4$. It is therefore logical to attempt to relate the time scales of the solar system to those of galactic processes.

We will discuss two approaches to the interpretation of scales T_1 and T_2. These approaches are similar in principle, but differ in the conclusions derived. Both relate the origin of the scales to the origin of the solar system via the spiral arms of our galaxy.

According to a hypothesis advanced by Reeves (cited in Marochnik and Suchkov[4]) the protosolar cloud, moving along the solar orbit within the galaxy, became "contaminated" with radioactive iodine and plutonium isotopes when it traversed a spiral arm or a density wave. When the cloud reached the region between the arms, the radioactive isotopes decayed freely (there are virtually no other sources of radioactive iodine and plutonium). This explanation of the abnormal abundance of the isotopes seems convincing, because the time T_1, during which iodine and plutonium must have decayed freely to produce xenon in the quantities detectable in meteorites, coincides with the time during which the protosolar cloud would have been moving between the spiral arms, if we assume that the S-mode of density waves is responsible for the spiral structure of the galaxy. Indeed, since the angular velocity of rotation of the spiral pattern in the galaxy should be $\Omega p \cong 13$ km/(s·kpc) and the angular velocity of rotation of the galaxy in the region where the Sun is located should be $\Omega_{SOL} \cong 25$ km/(s·kpc), the angular velocity of the Sun relative to the spiral pattern should be $\Delta\Omega = \Omega_{SOL} - \Omega p = 12$ km/(s·kpc). Since the spiral structure in our galaxy has, in all probability, two arms, the Sun will encounter another density wave (or spiral arm) at a time interval equal to $\Delta T = \pi/\Delta\Omega$. If we substitute 12 km/(s·kpc) for $\Delta\Omega$, we will obtain $\Delta T \cong 2.7 \times 10^8$ years.

There is nothing surprising about the cloud becoming "contaminated" with radioactive elements as it passed through the spiral arms. After all, these are the regions where supernovae occur and where thermonuclear synthesis, particularly of iodine and plutonium, takes place. The isotopes ejected by the explosion of the supernova could have penetrated the protosolar cloud. However, supernovae are rare in the region between the arms, and once they had entered this region iodine and plutonium would decay freely, with little likelihood of replenishment.

According to Reeves, the scenario of the early history of the solar system is as follows. The cloud crossed the spiral arms of the galaxy many times, becoming more and more "contaminated" with iodine and plutonium, which had had enough time to decay between encounters with the spiral structure. During the last encounter with the density wave prior to the beginning of the formation of the solar system, the cloud captured iodine and plutonium for the last time. This event occurred $T_1 + T_2 = (0.3 + 4.6) \times 10^9$ years ago. During the next 3×10^8 years, the radioactive isotopes underwent free decay and 4.6×10^9 years ago meteorites and other galactic objects of the solar system began to form.

The second approach to the interpretation of the scales T_1 and T_2 relates their origin to the L-mode of density waves in the galaxy.[4] As stated above, the angular velocity of L-waves is close to $\Omega p \cong 24$ km/(s·kpc). In this case, the angular velocity of the Sun relative to the spiral pattern is only $\Delta\Omega = (25-24)$ km/(s·kpc) $\cong 1$ km/(s·kpc). Thus, their rotation is nearly synchronous. The circle with radius R_c, in which the velocity of rotation of the galaxy and that of the spiral pattern are equal, is called the corotation circle. Every galaxy, including our own, has only one circle of this type, which makes it a special, unique place. The deviation of the Sun from the corotation circle is very small, reaching only

$$\Delta R / R_{SOL} = \left(R_c - R_{SOL}\right) / R_{SOL} = 0.03$$

In summary, the Sun (and, consequently, the protosolar nebula in the past) occupies an exceptional position in the galaxy: it is located near the unique corotation circle, in which the density wave and the galaxy are in synchronous rotation. Obviously, other galactic objects located along this circle are also in an exceptional position. It is clear that the physical conditions to which the interstellar gas and dust clouds that

enter this region would be subject, are different near the corotation circle than in the remainder of the galactic disk. This is an important observation because young stars originate in these clouds (which are typically molecular clouds composed primarily of molecular hydrogen). And if star formation proceeds under special conditions near the corotation circle that differ from those in the remainder of the galaxy, then this could mean that our own star—the Sun—was born under special conditions, which may have predetermined the specific features of the solar system (existence of planets, occurrence of life, etc.). If this is true, then systems resembling the solar system should be sought near the corotation circles of our and other galaxies.

What effect does the location of the Sun in the vicinity of the corotation circle have on interpretation of the cosmogonic time scales T_1 and T_2? Our knowledge of the value of Ωp is rather inexact. The best observational finding available yields $\Omega p = (23.6 \pm 3.6)$ km/(s·kpc).[4] For the sake of convenience, we will assume $\Omega p = 24.3$ km/(s·kpc). Substituting this value for ΔT, we can find the time during which the protosolar cloud remains in the galactic region between the spiral arms. This time is equal to 4.6×10^9 years, i.e., it coincides with the age of the solar system, T_2, derived from uranium and thorium radioactivity.

This is the reason for the convenient assumption of $\Omega p = 24.3$ km/(s·kpc). At this value of Ωp, ΔT is equal to the age of the solar system. We could also "reverse" the problem: assuming that, after all transformations of the protosolar cloud, the solar system could have ultimately formed only in a "calm" location, i.e., the region between the spiral arms, we can attempt to find Ωp, the numerical value of which is extremely important for solving problems of spiral structure theory. In other words, cosmogony may prove useful for solving problems of galactic astrophysics. So when we select Ωp to make ΔT and T_2 very similar, we have a good reason for doing so. The existence of life in the solar system may argue in favor of making just such an assumption.

References

[1] Allen, C.W. *Astrophysical Quantities*. London, Athlone, 1973.

[2] Oort, J. The structure of the cloud of comets surrounding the solar system and the hypothesis concerning its origin. *Bull. Astron. Inst. Neth.*, 1950, Vol. 11, pp. 91-110.

[3] Marochnik, L., Mukhin, L., and Sagdeev, R. The distribution of mass and angular momentum in the solar system. *Astrophysics and Space Physics Review*, 1989, Vol. 8, pt. 3, pp. 1-55.

[4] Marochnik, L. and Suchkov, A. *Our Galaxy*. Gordon and Breach, 1993 (in press).

[5] Laskano-Araucho, A. and Oro. G. The comet matter and the origin of life on the Earth. In: C. Ponnamperuma (Ed.). *Comets and the Origin of Life*. Dordrecht, Holland, Reidel Publ. Co., 1981.

[6] Linde, A.D. Inflating universe. *Uspekhi Fizicheskikh*

Nauk, 1984, Vol. 144, pp. 177-214 (in Russian).

[7] Zeldovich, Ya.B. and Novikov, I.D. *Evolution of the Universe*. Nauka, Moscow, 1975 (in Russian).

[8] Klapdor, H.V. and Grotz, K. Evidence of a nonvanishing energy density of the vacuum (or cosmological constant). *Astrophysical Journal*, Letters to the Editor, 1986, Vol. 301, pp. 39-43.

[9] Raup, D.M. and Spekoski, J.J. Periodicity of extinctions in the geologic past. In: *Proceedings of the U.S. National Academy of Sciences*, 1984, Vol. 81, pp. 801-805.

[10] Rampino, M.R. and Stothers, R. B. Terrestrial mass extinctions, cometary impacts and the Sun's motion perpendicular to the galactic plane. *Nature*, 1984, Vol. 308, pp. 709-712.

[11] Schwartz, R.D. and James, P.B. Periodic mass extinctions and the Sun's oscillation about the galactic plane. *Nature*, 1984, Vol. 308, pp. 312-313.

[12] Hills, J.G. Comet showers and the steady-state infall of comets from the Oort Cloud. *Astronomical Journal*, 1981, Vol. 86, pp. 1730-1740.

[13] Bailey, M.E. Theories of cometary origin and the brightness of the infrared sky. *Monthly National Royal Astronomical Society*, 1983, Vol. 204, pp. 47-52.

[14] Sagdeev, R.Z., Blamont, J., Galeev, A.A., Moroz, V.I., Shapiro, V.D., Shevchenko, V.I., and Szego, K. Vega spacecraft encounters with comet Halley. *Nature*, 1986, Vol. 321, pp. 259-262.

[15] Alvarez, W. and Muller, R.A. Evidence from crater ages for periodic impacts on the Earth. *Nature*, 1984, Vol. 308, pp. 718-720.

Chapter 2

The Sun and Interplanetary Space

N. F. Pisarenko, Viktoriya G. Kurt, and Yu. I. Logachev

I. The Sun and the Solar Corona

A. The Sun as a Star

Our galaxy includes more than 100 billion stars varying in size and luminosity. It is disk-shaped, thicker in the center, with disk diameter of 30,000 pc and disk width of 3000 pc (1 pc = 3.26 light years, i.e., 10^{13} km). If we were to view the galaxy from its poles, it would resemble an uncoiling spiral. Our Sun is located close to the plane of symmetry of the galactic disk, at the edge of one of the spiral arms, at a distance of $r \sim 9.2 \times 10^3$ pc from the center. The speed of rotation of the galaxy increases with distance from the center: at the distance of our Sun, the speed of rotation is $v \cong 250$ km/s, i.e., the Sun makes one revolution around the center in $t \approx 200$ million years. The age of the whole solar system, including the Sun, is currently estimated to be $t \sim 5$ billion years. The Sun is a yellow star and by virtue of its spectrum of electromagnetic radiation belongs to star class dG2. The mass of the Sun is $M_{SOL} \cong 2 \times 10^{33}$ g, 3.3×10^5 times the mass of the Earth. The mean density of the Sun is $\bar{\rho}_{SOL} \approx 1.41$ g/cm^3 or 0.256 times the density of the Earth. The acceleration of gravity at the surface of the Sun is $g_{SOL} = 273.8$ m/s^2, 28 times that of the gravity on the surface of the Earth. The Sun's radius is $R_{SOL} \cong 6.96 \times 10^5$ km, and its gravity escape velocity is 617.7 km/s. Data on the general properties of the Sun and solar atmosphere were taken from works by D.G. Menzel,[1] I.S. Shklovskiy,[2] and E. Gibson.[3] The mean distance of the Earth from the Sun (the semimajor axis of the ellipse of the Earth's orbit) is termed the astronomical unit (AU), 1 AU = 1.4953×10^8 km, or approximately 150 million km, or 215 R_{SOL}. The angular velocity of ratation of the Sun relative to the Earth, $\omega = (13.7 - 14.5)° - 2.7° \cdot \sin^2 \varphi$ per day, is a function of heliographic latitude φ, i.e., at the equator angular velocity is greater and equals approximately 1.72 km/s. The sidereal period of rotation of the Sun with respect to fixed stars is equal to 25.36 days at the equa-tor, 27 days at a latitude of $\varphi = 40°$, and 35 days at a latitude of $\varphi = 70°$. The synodic period of rotation, as determined from the Earth on the basis of passage of solar formations through the central meridian, is 27.27 days at the equator.

The axis of rotation of the Sun is inclined to the plane of the ecliptic so that the angle between the plane of the solar equator and the plane of the ecliptic is $i = 7.25°$, while the longitude (right ascension) of the ascending node of the equator is $\Omega = 73.667° + (T - 1850)\, 0.01396°$, where T is the date expressed in years. The Earth intersects the plane of the solar equator twice a year, at the beginning of June and at the end of December. During the first half-period the Earth is in the "southern" hemisphere, during the second it is in the "northern" hemisphere with respect to the plane of the ecliptic. The mean speed of revolution of the Earth around the Sun is $v = 30$ km/s.

B. The Solar Interior

Starting from the photosphere, the temperature, density and pressure, and strength of ionization of atoms of solar matter increase as one approaches the Sun's center. The gas inside the Sun is a high-temperature plasma and consists of a large number of free electrons, fully ionized nuclei of light elements, and significantly ionized nuclei of heavy elements.

Thermonuclear reactions, which transform light nuclei into heavier ones, are the major source of the Sun's energy. It has been proposed that as a result of one cycle of thermonuclear reactions, a single helium nucleus forms from four nuclei of hydrogen, releasing energy corresponding to a 0.7 percent decrease in mass of the reaction products, which corresponds to $\Delta\varepsilon = Mc^2 \cong 25$ MeV for one helium atom.

At the Sun's center, temperature reaches $T \cong 15 \times 10^6$ K, density $\rho = 150$ g/cm^3, and pressure $P \cong 250 \times 10^9$ atm.

Energy transfer from near the center to the surface of the Sun occurs as a result of absorption and emission of electromagnetic radiation; near the surface of the Sun convection is most important.

Figure 1 provides a diagram of the structure of the Sun and its atmosphere, and of outward energy flow. Readers may wish to refer to this diagram throughout their reading of this chapter.

C. The Solar Atmosphere

The solar atmosphere consists of three physically distinct zones: the photosphere, the chromosphere, and the corona. Between the chromosphere and the corona is a well-defined

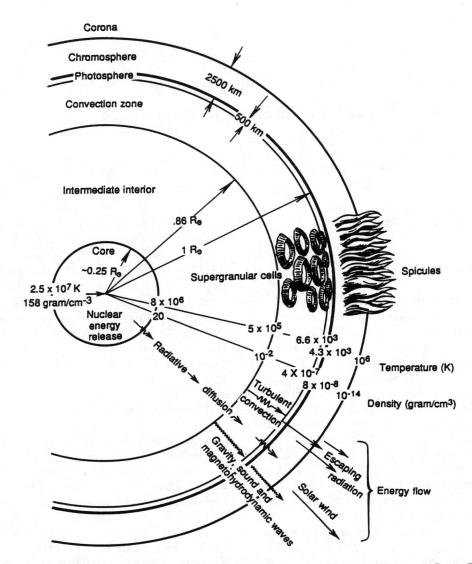

Fig. 1 Idealized picture of general solar properties, structure, and modes of outward energy flow. The features shown are not to scale and provide a qualitative picture only. (From: Gibson, E.G., *The Quiet Sun*. Washington, DC, Scientific and Technical Information Office, National Aeronautics and Space Administration, 1973.)

transition zone.

The visible surface of the Sun is the lower part of the solar atmosphere and is called the *solar photosphere*. It is the major source of radiation in the visible portion of the spectrum. The photosphere is a relatively thin layer, no more than 400 km thick. The temperature of the upper portion of the photosphere corresponding to the temperature minimum is $T = 4300$ K. If the radiation emitted by the Sun is considered to be in equilibrium, then the effective temperature of the radiating layer of the photopshere (a thin layer ~100 km thick) has the value 5780 K.[3] In the area near the temperature minimum, Mg, Si, Fe, Ca, Al, and Na atoms may be considered singly ionized, while H is in a neutral state. It is believed that the photosphere is in local thermodynamic and radiation equilibrium with the solar layers that surround it.

The density of the photosphere is from 10^{-9} to 10^{-8} g/cm^3 (the concentration of particles decreases from 10^{16} to 10^{15}/

cm^3). The lower layers of the solar photosphere are in direct contact with the convective zone of the Sun, giving the photosphere the appearance of a cellular structure called *granulation*. The mean size of each granule is approximately 700 km (from 200 to 2000 km); their lifetime is from 1 to 10 minutes. The granules themselves are the tops of convection cells in the Sun's convection zone. In the central portion of each granulation area, the solar gas below the photosphere rises to the surface, while at the outer edges the gas descends back down to the surface. This makes the temperature of the granules higher in the center than at the periphery. Evidently, granules are up to several hundred or even several thousand kilometers deep. Granulation of the Sun's photosphere reflects the turbulence, nonstationarity, and anisotropy of the convection process. It is virtually independent of heliocentric latitude and phase of solar activity cycle. Solar granules are of three sizes: granules proper (discussed above), super-

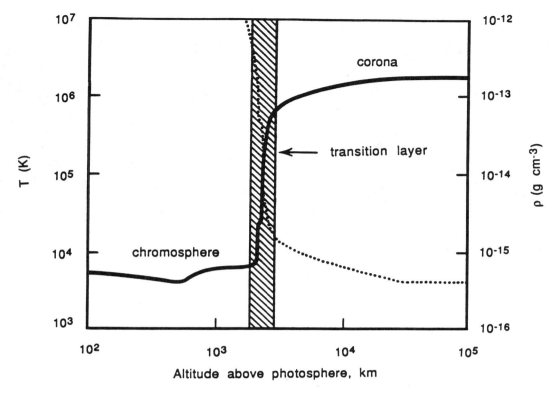

Fig. 2 Density (dotted line) and temperature (solid line) in the chromosphere, transition zone, and corona of the quiet Sun.

granules, and giant granules. The diameter of supergranules is on the order of 20,000-40,000 km, and that of giant granules 100,000-200,000 km. The smaller the diameter of the convective cell, the greater the speed of motion in the granules. Aside from the granules, the Sun's photosphere contains nonstationary formations associated with solar activity: spots, faculae, and flare effects, all of which are described below in the section devoted to solar activity.

In recent years, pulsation of the solar photosphere (fluctuation of the Sun's diameter) has been observed. The stability and periods of these pulsations are currently under intensive study. Among the large-scale fluctuations, the most probable are 5-min and 160-min fluctuations; fluctuations at intervals between 5 and 160 min have also been observed. Small-scale fluctuations in the Sun, inferred from observation of nonthermal widening of spectral lines and fluctuations in radiation intensity, have the greatest power in the range of approximately $t = 300$ s.

The layer directly above the photosphere is called the *chromosphere* and is about 15,000 km thick. The chromosphere has a lower particle density than the photosphere, decreasing from 10^{14} to 10^{10} cm^{-3}, and is inhomogeneous in temperature. The temperature in the chromosphere increases at a nonuniform rate with altitude, slowly in the lower portion, and rapidly in the middle and upper portions. The lower chromosphere has a temperature of $T = 4500$-4800 K; in the transition area, at the boundary with the corona, the temperature reaches $T \cong 10^6$ K (Fig. 2).

The increase in temperature as a result of the rapid decrease in density of matter with altitude and of the dissipation of energy due to absorption of acoustic and magnetoacoustic waves from the photosphere, as well as processes of magnetic dissipation of energy, reflects the lack of equilibrium in the chromosphere. When the limb of the chromosphere is observed for a quiet Sun, starting at an altitude of $h \cong 1000$ km, one sees a brushlike structure consisting of individual almost vertical jets, extending 10-15×10^3 km upward. These jets are called spicules. The lifetime of spicules is $t \cong 10$-20 minutes and their mean velocity of motion is $v \approx 20$ km/s. In equatorial regions they are frequently inclined, but at the poles they are radial. Observations of the disk frequently reveal the "chromosphere network": small dark and light mottles approximately 1000 km in diameter, dozens of which form larger units with diameters of 7000-10,000 km. These units are arranged on the disk in a honeycomb configuration. The lifetime of a network is 17-20 hours. At the boundaries of the cells is an intensified magnetic field, as well as increased density of matter. Frequently a filament structure is observed in the chromosphere, reflecting the nature of the magnetic fields carried by convection from the photosphere into the chromosphere. The appearance of many filaments accompanies the birth of a new active region on the Sun. During the active period, flares and flocculi are observed in the solar chromosphere.

The outermost and least dense area of the solar atmosphere is called the *corona*.

a)

b)

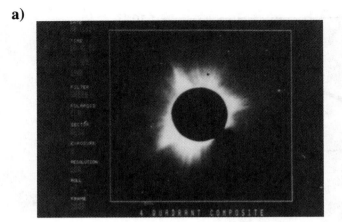
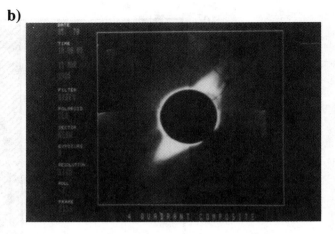

Fig. 3 Photographs of the corona during periods of maximum (a) and minimum solar activity (b), obtained in 1980 and 1985, respectively. The 1980 photographs show a typical sunspot maximum—bright streamers and rays appear at virtually all solar latitudes. The 1985 image shows the corona before the solar minimum. The bright helmet streamers and rays are confined to low latitudes. Coronal holes can be observed in the polar regions. (Courtesy of T.E. Holzer, High Altitude Observatory, National Center for Atmospheric Research.)

Between the chromosphere and the corona is the so-called *transition zone*, the density of which changes from 10^{-12} to 10^{-15} g/cm^3 (particle density from 10^{12} to 10^9/cm^3), while the temperature changes from 1×10^4 to 1.5×10^5 K. This area is characterized by high physical instability.

The corona may be divided into three zones: the inner ($r < 1.3\,R_{SOL}$), middle ($1.3 < r < 2.5\,R_{SOL}$), and outer ($r > 2.5\,R_{SOL}$). The mean temperature of the corona is 1.5×10^6 K. The temperature of the corona varies only slightly with altitude. The density of the corona bordering the transition zone is 10^{-15} g/cm^3 (the concentration of particles is 10^8/cm^3), and at a distance $3R_{SOL}$, $\rho \cong 6 \times 10^{-19}$ g/cm^3 (4×10^5/cm^3). The composition of coronal gas is similar to that of the photosphere; the ratio of concentrations of alpha particles to hydrogen is ~ 0.1. In the corona, hydrogen atoms and elements of the second period of the periodic table are almost completely devoid of electrons, i.e., the corona is a nearly totally ionized plasma.

The structure of the corona is rather complex, including large formations extending from the Sun in the shape of "fans" or "rays." The density of matter in these formations is evidently almost an order of magnitude higher than in the surrounding corona. On the other hand, the polar regions often contain "coronal holes," areas that may have abnormally low temperatures. Their total area reaches 15 percent of the entire area of the surface of the Sun; at lower latitudes, the area of coronal holes is less than 2-5 percent of the area of the solar surface. The lifetime of a single hole may exceed 5 rotations of the Sun (up to 20 rotations).

The rotation of such holes is close to that of a solid, while their density is an order of magnitude lower than the density of the surrounding corona.

The corona is spherical during years of maximum solar activity and oblate along the equator during years of minimal solar activity (Fig. 3).

The fundamentals and basic ideas of the hydrodynamic theory of the solar corona were proposed by E. Parker in 1958.[4] According to Parker, the solution of the hydrodynamic problem for the solar atmosphere suggests expansion of the corona into interplanetary space at supersonic speeds on the order of several hundred kilometers per second, the so-called "solar wind" (see below). The escape of coronal matter is relatively slight (several orders of magnitude lower than the loss of mass through radiation) and is balanced by the influx of substance from the chromosphere. Annual loss of solar mass constitutes $10^{-14}\,M_{SOL}$. Since the thermal energy of solar gas in the corona is comparable to its potential energy in the gravitational field of the Sun, the upper temperature boundary is determined by the rate of outflow of gas from the corona.

D. The Sun's Magnetic Field

The Sun's magnetic field plays an extremely important role, frequently the major role, in a whole series of physical processes on the Sun. Generally two variants of this field are considered.

The general magnetic field of the Sun is a poloidal field extending along the solar meridians and resembling a dipole field. Its field strength at the level of the photosphere is 1-2 G. Above the poles, the force lines of this field diverge more slowly than in the typical dipole and do not show a tendency to bend toward the equator. Measurements have shown that this general field consists of many small components varying in polarity and size. The field strength of individual components may be high, reaching values of 10-20 G. When field strength is averaged over a large number of measurements, a weak field of a single sign is typically found. The general field of the Sun reverses its polarity every 11 years (an 11-year cycle), producing a total period of $t \cong 22$ years, the 22-year cycle of solar activity.

Table 1 Major characteristics of plasma and magnetic field in the vicinity of the Sun

Region of Sun	Particle concentration η, cm^{-3}	Temp. T, K	Magnetic field strength B, G	Kinetic energy density of particles T, erg/cm^3	Energy density of magnetic field, $B^2/8\pi$ erg/cm^3
Photosphere (quiet)	10^{15}	6×10^3	1	800	0.04
Photosphere (active)	10^{15}	6×10^3	50	800	100
Chromosphere (quiet)	10^{13}	7×10^3	1	10	0.04
Chromosphere (active)	10^{13}	2×10^4	50	30	100
Corona	10^9	10^6	50	0.14	100

At latitudes of $|\varphi| < 50°$, there exist toroidal background magnetic fields extending along the direction of solar rotation. These are essentially the local magnetic fields of active formations on the Sun. They include large-scale bipolar (BM) and unipolar (UM) regions. Field strength in a bipolar region varies from one-tenth to several hundred G. The sign of the field differs in different portions of the BM areas and since these fields extend along east-west lines, one can always distinguish the leading (p) and following (f) polarities. These polarities differ in the northern and southern hemispheres and reverse sign at the beginning of each new 11-year cycle.

UM regions are closer to the poles than BM regions and have lower field strength, but are larger in area and have a longer lifetime. Field strength of a UM region is typically $\leq$ 2 G, $r \cong 0.1 R_{SOL}$, $\tau \cong$ 5-7 rotations of the Sun. The development of BM and UM regions precedes the appearance of active regions on the Sun and ceases after the latter's disappearance. BM and UM regions actually have a very complex multipolar structure, which can be detected when studying images produced by high resolution instruments. These small-scale fields are associated with granules, flocculi, pores, small spots, and other relatively small formations. Table 1 gives mean values for the major characteristics of plasma and magnetic fields close to the Sun.

II. Solar Activity

Solar activity (SA) comprises a variety of manifestations of nonstationary processes on the Sun: spots, active regions, prominences, coronal transients, flares, etc. All these phenomena are subject to periodic cycles. The most significant cycle has a period of ~11 years and is associated with nonstationary release of energy in the solar atmosphere. The phenomena themselves are accompanied by significant changes in many characteristics of the different layers of the solar atmosphere. For example, Table 2 cites estimates of electron densities at the maximum and minimum points of the 11-year cycle.

Let us consider certain important manifestations of solar activity within the 11-year cycle.

A. Sunspots

Sunspots appear to us as dark formations on the solar photosphere, consisting of an umbra and a penumbra.

A sunspot arises when a magnetic flux tube passes through the photosphere from the convective layer. The magnetic field in the center of the spot is almost vertical and is never below several hundred gauss in field strength. At the solar activity maximum, field strength increases to several thousand gauss. In the penumbra, the field is more nearly horizontal and field strength decreases toward the edge, where it does not exceed several hundred gauss. Within the sunspot itself, magnetic energy is a great deal higher than the kinetic energy of the plasma, which substantially depresses convection and leads to a decrease in the temperature of solar matter in the area of the spot.

There is granulation within the spot and the area of the penumbra includes radial flow lines. The umbra of the spot is below the level of the photosphere, while the penumbra forms

Table 2   Electron density in the corona η (cm^{-3})

Distance from center of the Sun (R_{SOL})	1.0	1.5	4.0
Phase of cycle and region on Sun			
Solar activity maximum	4×10^8	1.5×10^7	9×10^4
Solar activity minimum at equator	2.3×10^8	0.8×10^7	5×10^4
Solar activity minimum polar region	1.7×10^8	1.4×10^6	0.4×10^4

a kind of "funnel" around the umbra. The effective temperature of the umbra is $T_u \cong 4200$ K, and of the penumbra $T_{pu} \cong 5400$ K. Solar gas appears to rise in the area of the umbra and flow out of it in the area of the penumbra; at the edge of the penumbra this motion disappears. The rate of flow is $v \cong 2$ km/s. The rate of flow decreases with altitude and at the level of the chromosphere changes sign, i.e., the gas flows toward the center of the spot. The diameter of spots ranges from several hundreds to tens of thousands of kilometers. The smallest spots lack a penumbra and are called pores. Spots are rarely isolated and usually occur in groups, occupying large active regions, extending over tens of thousand of kilometers. The magnetic field strength in groups of spots may reach significantly higher levels, up to several thousand gauss.

A group of spots may persist from several hours to several months. The development of such a group begins with the appearance of pores, which subsequently develop into spots. Over the course of several days, their area and magnetic field increase markedly. Typically a group extends along a parallel with the leader closer to the equator. After 2-3 weeks, the group attains its maximum development and then begins to break up: first the follower spot and then other smaller spots disappear. At the completion of their development the group becomes unipolar. The leader itself persists until its diameter decreases to 30,000 km, after which it rapidly disappears.

The solar latitudes at which the spots are observed throughout a solar cycle, $5° < |\varphi| < 45°$, are frequently referred to in the literature as the activity belts.

B. Faculae, Prominences, and Coronal Condensations

Sunspots in the photosphere are always accompanied by light-colored filamentary formations called *faculae.*

Their diameter may reach 10,000 km, while the magnetic field strength in the most developed faculae equals hundreds of gauss. Faculae may exist in the absence of spots, typically appearing before the spots and disappearing after they do, sometimes "persisting" in the photosphere for several solar rotations. Faculae are difficult to detect in the center of the disk in white light, but they are easily seen near the limb.

The upper portions of the faculae in the chromosphere form *flocculi.* These formations are quite varied, and they are inhomogeneous in brightness, temperature, and magnetic field strength. The structure of flocculi reflects the structure of the local magnetic field; a large portion of flocular filaments are oriented along magnetic lines of force.

Prominences are masses of relatively cool ($T \cong 10^4$ K) and dense ($n \cong 10^{10}$-10^{11}/cm^3) gas, rising above the chromosphere into the corona up to altitudes of several hundred thousand kilometers (Fig. 4). On the edge of the disk they are seen in the form of light clouds or arches, and on the disk appear as dark filaments that extend along the meridians close to the equator and along the parallels at high latitudes.

Dynamic processes in prominences are the result of local and background magnetic fields in the solar atmosphere. Prominences typically occur in regions where the magnetic field is relatively stationary and oriented horizontally with respect to the surface of the Sun.

Formations also occur in the corona. These are called *coronal condensations.* Their density is greater by a factor of 3 than the density of the surrounding coronal plasma.

C. Solar Flares

Solar flares are the brightest manifestation of nonstationary processes in the solar atmosphere. The widely used term "flare" actually refers to a secondary effect of this phenomenon, appearing as an optical luminescence in a local area on the Sun.

Solar flares have been known for more than 100 years. Approximately 60 years ago, the nature of solar flares was studied by analyzing their spectra in the visible range. When, about 30 years ago, it seemed as if we were close to understanding the processes occurring in flares, we began to obtain data from extra-atmospheric observations and our understanding of flares became significantly more complex. Now it is known that the largest flares emit energy of $\varepsilon \cong 10^{32}$-$10^{33}$ erg (10^{25}-10^{26} J), with flare durations of 10^3-10^4 s. This corresponds to power of $<w> \sim 10^{29}$ erg/s, (10^{22} J/s). However, this rate is a factor of 10^4-10^5 below the power of full

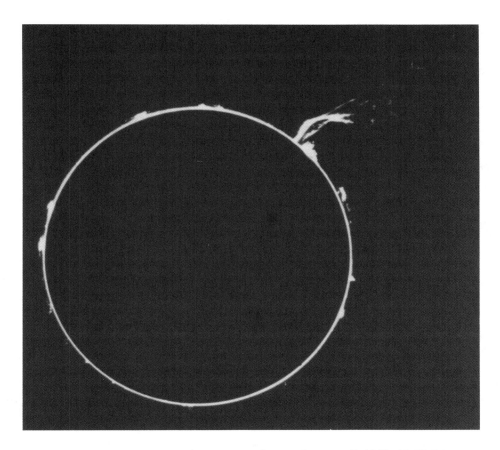

**Fig. 4 Spectacular prominence eruption on October 5, 1989, 17:55:01.
(Courtesy of R.C. Canfield, Institute for Astronomy, Honolulu, Hawaii.)**

solar radiation (full luminosity $L_{SOL} = 3.9 \times 10^{33}$ erg/s).

A solar flare arises as a consequence of a rapid outburst of energy in a certain area of the Sun's atmosphere. At the present time it is generally accepted that this energy accumulates and is stored as magnetic energy in the electric current systems that form in the solar atmosphere during convective upflow of mass from the interior of the Sun. The first energy outburst, which marks the beginning of the flare, is associated with a breakup of the current systems as a result of current instability or the effects of neighboring systems (for example, after intrusion of a new stream of matter carrying a magnetic field into an existing plasma-magnetic configuration). When current systems break up, strong electric fields arise and a portion of the magnetic energy is converted into energy of the charged particles (electrons, protons, and heavier nuclei) that are accelerated by these electric fields. The most probable altitude of the initial energy emission is from several thousand to tens of thousands of kilometers above the level of the photosphere, where plasma particle concentrations are 10^9-10^{10}/cm^3. Accelerated charged particles, propagating along the lines of force in the solar atmosphere, reach the dense layers of matter close to the chromosphere, heat the plasma, and induce the chain of secondary effects observed in interplanetary space and by observatories on Earth.

We have already stated that the magnetic field in the solar corona has two types of plasma-magnetic configurations: arch structures (Fig. 5) (closed systems) and "filamentous" (Fig. 4) jets, penetrating through the solar corona into interplanetary space. Particles accelerated in the flares may enter either type of magnetic field. In the first case they are captured, as in the radiation belts of the Earth, and in the second they escape into interplanetary space. Depending on the nature of the specific magnetic configuration, up to 1 percent of all accelerated electrons may escape and up to 50 percent of the accelerated protons (they are more difficult to trap). These escaping particles are called "solar cosmic rays." They present a danger to living things and spacecraft above the Earth's magnetosphere. The physics underlying the generation of penetrating (hard) radiation from solar flares will be considered in more detail below.

D. Coronal Transients

In recent years a number of phenomena, evidently directly associated with flares, have been observed in the solar corona. One of the most prominent of these phenomena is the ejection of enormous amounts of matter (10^{15}-10^{16} g) visible to heights exceeding 1-5 R_{SOL} at a velocity varying from several hundred km/s to 2-3000 km/s. These sporadic ejections have been termed coronal transients. Coronal transients may

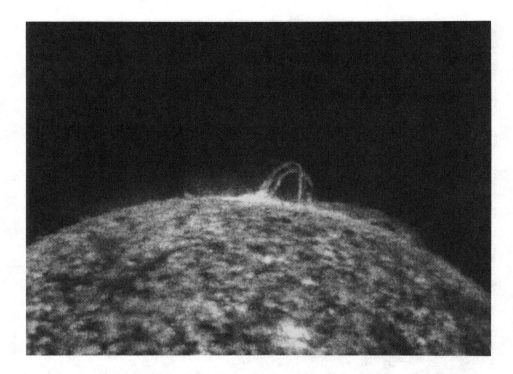

Fig. 5 Photograph of the Sun in the 304 Å emission line of He II showing the magnetic flux tubes in the solar corona, brighter than the surrounding corona. (Courtesy of Naval Research Institute.)

consist of a variety of structures of magnetized plasma. Sometimes they have the form of magnetic clouds, subsequently dispersing into interplanetary space. The kinetic energy of transients reaches 10^{31}-10^{33} ergs, which is comparable to the total energy of the most powerful flares. Observations have shown that sometimes transients begin their movement from the surface of the photosphere 5-30 min before energy emissions, leading to acceleration of particles and heating of the solar atmosphere, i.e., before occurrence of solar flares. It is very tempting to associate these two phenomena, arguing that the disturbances induced by movement of matter and the magnetic fields of the transient lead to restructuring of the magnetic field and the beginning of the flare. However, direct proof of such a causal connection has still not been obtained experimentally, and the mechanisms of the release of energy inducing coronal transients are still not understood.

E. Solar Activity Cycles

The development of various active formations in the solar atmosphere is a unified process, involving the development of active regions or centers of activity. Active regions consist of a certain number of sunspots surrounded by a background magnetic field. Active regions begin to appear and develop on the Sun when the 11-year solar activity cycle begins. At the beginning of the cycle, the number of active centers is small, then reaches a maximum that coincides with the solar activity maximum, then decreases as the phase of decline begins. At the beginning of the cycle rotation of active regions is close to that of a solid, while at the cycle maximum the differential rotation effect is significantly more pronounced.

The development of each active region may be divided into several phases.

During the first phase, small faculae and flocculi and an associated weak unipolar and complex magnetic field appear. Individual faculae become brighter and pores (dark spots) arise, which will subsequently develop into spots. The size of the region increases and it becomes bipolar. Coronal condensations form above this region. This phase lasts several days.

The next phase is the active one. It involves rapid, fluctuating development that continues for several weeks. The size and brightness of bipolar formations reach a maximum, the numbers of faculae and flocculi increase, and active prominences and flares appear. Transients appear in the corona. At the end of this phase, the spot group begins to break up and coronal effects begin to diminish.

During the third phase, which may continue for several solar rotations, the active region becomes more and more unipolar, spots gradually disappear, faculae and flocculi weaken, and quiet prominences appear.

During the last phase, which may last for several months, prominences disappear. The entire region becomes unipolar and by the end of the phase has been resorbed.

The position of spots on the disk of the Sun changes with the phases of cycle of solar activity: at the beginning of the cycle, spots occur at latitudes of $\varphi = \pm 35°$-$40°$; as the cycle continues, their latitude gradually decreases, and close to the

Solar Cycle 22 Compared to Previous Cycles

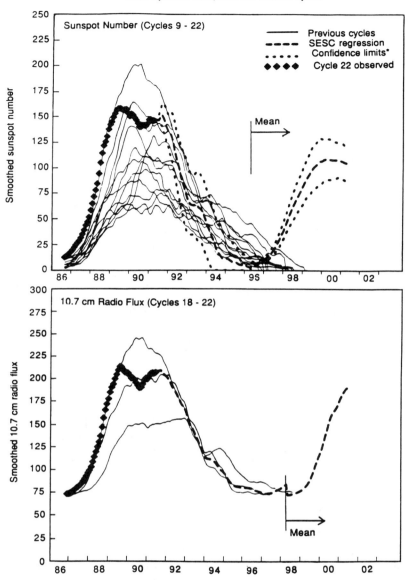

*90% Prediction interval or 90% confidence limit of the mean

Fig. 6a Mean number of sunspots as a function of phase for cycles 9-21 (upper panel). Mean flux of solar radiation at wavelength λ = 10.7 cm as a function of cycle phase for cycles 19-21 (lower panel) [Due to small sample size useful confidence limits cannot be provided for the radio flux precision]. (Courtesy of Space Environment Laboratory, National Oceanic and Atmospheric Administration.)

maximum the spots are located at latitudes of $\varphi = \pm 15°$. At the end of the cycle the spots lie at latitudes of $\varphi = \pm 5°\text{-}8°$.

Formation of spots in the northern and southern hemispheres of the Sun is frequently not symmetrical (i.e., there may be different numbers of spots in each hemisphere) and these differences may persist for several years, even to the extent that the maximum occurs at different times in the two hemispheres. The mean number of spots at a given phase of the activity cycle may change from cycle to cycle; this "strength" is the major quantitative parameter of the 11-year

solar activity cycle (Fig. 6a and b). Typically, the measure of the number of spots used in astrophysical statistics is the Wolf number, $R = K(10g + f)$, where g is the number of spot-groups, f is the number of individual spots, and K is a multiplier on the order of 1. The Wolf number is roughly related to the area of spots by the function $F = 16.7R$ where F is expressed in millionths of the area of the solar disk.

In the 1970s new formations were discovered on the surface of the Sun—coronal holes (see Section I.C).

During the declining phase of solar activity, large coronal

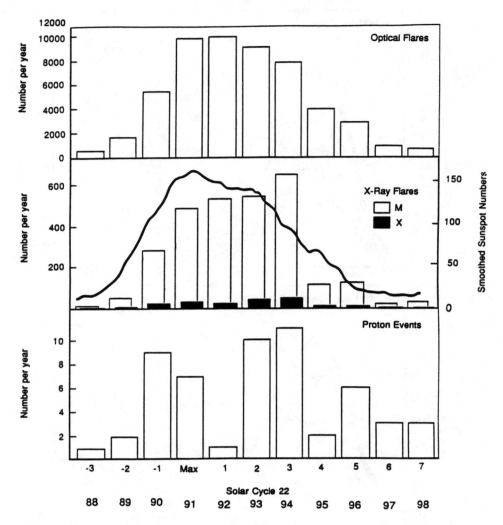

Fig. 6b Characteristics of cycle 21 of solar activity, and projections for cycle 22. The horizontal axis is also marked with reference to the maximum of the 21-year cycle of solar activity (December 1979). (Courtesy of Space Environment Laboratory, National Oceanic and Atmospheric Administration.)

holes are not only present at both poles, but also extend downward toward the equator. During the ascending portion of the cycle, polar holes decrease markedly in area and retreat toward the poles.

Close to the point of maximum activity, the holes are concentrated mainly at middle latitudes. This observation suggests that the solar cycle cannot be described only in terms of the number of sunspots. It has been established that the cyclical behavior of coronal holes is an important and fundamental part of the solar activity cycle.

Solar activity is marked by a large number of cycles of varying duration. The greatest interest for us lies in the 11-year (22-year) cycle and also in the 80-90 year cycle. Cycles with longer periods (160-200 years and 600 years) are also known.

The 11-year cycle of solar activity is defined on the basis

of Wolf numbers. Eleven-year cycles vary in duration from 7 to 17 years; their mean duration is 11.2 years. The cycles are asymmetrical, going from the maximum number of spots to their minimum (phase of decline) requires 6.7 years, while from the minimum to the maximum (growth phase) requires 4.6 years. The cycles also differ in the mean annual maximum Wolf number, which ranges from 46 to 190. As a rule, the intensity of the cycle is associated with duration: the more active a given cycle, the shorter it is, especially the growth phases, and the higher the solar latitudes at which the first active regions appear.

In any event, the most active manifestations of the maximum—large solar flares—occur most often not in the year of the maximum, but during the phases of growth and decline (Fig. 6a and b).

The roles of the northern and southern solar hemispheres

change from cycle to cycle; the times of their maxima are sometimes displaced by 1-2 years. During an 11-year cycle, the polarity of the magnetic field of all the leader spots within each hemisphere is usually the same, but those of the two hemispheres are opposite. During the next 11-year cycle the polarity of leaders reverses in both hemispheres. Thus we are actually talking about an overall 22-year cycle. There are indications that the mean area of active regions and also mean annual Wolf numbers are subject to 22-year cycles. Changes in the overall magnetic field of the Sun, as was noted above, also follow a 22-year cycle. There are also indications that there is a finer structure—that the 11-year cycle contains two peaks.

Numbering of 11-year cycles of solar activity begins with cycle 0 (arbitrarily starting in 1745). The 80-90 year cycle of solar activity is defined by quasi-periodic changes in the maxima of 11-year cycles. In general, throughout the history of study of solar activity several special periods are known: 1) 1645-1715—the Maunder minimum, when there were almost no spots on the Sun for 60 years; 2) 1410-1510, the Sporer minimum; and 3) 1120-1280—the medieval maximum.

It is hypothesized that the first of these minima was a superposition of the minima of the 600-year and 80-year cycles. Several catastrophes in the Earth's biosphere and the history of civilization are associated with these minima. Data exist that suggest that the Maunder and other solar activity minima coincided with periods of great attenuation or even the disappearance of the Sun's general magnetic field. While the 11-year cycle is a cycle of the frequency of appearance of active formations on the Sun, the 80-90 year cycle is a cycle of their mean duration. The asymmetry of solar activity in the northern and southern hemispheres is not pronounced in the 11-year cycle, but is very significant in the 80-90 year cycle. It is hypothesized that the north-south asymmetry of solar activity is associated with changes in the position of the Sun's core.

III. Electromagnetic and Corpuscular Radiation of the Quiet Sun

Almost all the electromagnetic radiation of the quiet Sun that reaches the external observer arises in the photosphere. The chromosphere and corona above the photosphere hardly attenuate this radiation at all. As a first approximation, the photosphere emits continuous thermal radiation like an absolute black body, heated to approximately 6000 K. (The effective temperature of the visible surface of the Sun T_{eff} = 5780 K.)

The upper portion of the photosphere and the transition zone between the photosphere and chromosphere are not transparent to certain frequencies (due to the atomic shell structure of the atoms forming this layer), causing lines of absorption, called Fraunhofer lines, to form in the spectrum. In the solar spectrum, more than 30,000 lines belonging to 70 chemical elements have been identified. The most abundant element is hydrogen; the amount of the second most abundant element—helium—is less than one-tenth that of hydrogen; and the atoms of all the remaining elements together amount to slightly more than one thousandth of the abundance of hydrogen atoms.

Radiation emitted by the upper layers of the solar atmosphere is one ten thousandth as strong as photospheric radiation.

In the chromosphere, the temperature increases to 10,000 K. For this reason, the chromosphere also displays, in addition to weak continuous luminescence, radiation lines similar in wavelength to the lines of photospheric absorption. Higher temperature lines, such as helium lines and lines of highly ionized iron, are also observed in the chromosphere. The transition zone is responsible for the majority of bright lines in the ultraviolet portion of the spectrum.

The flux of energy emitted by the corona is a millionth of the luminosity of the Sun. The hot corona ($T_c \approx 1.5 \times 10^6$K) emits bright emission lines that differ from those emitted by the chromosphere. The corona also emits a continuous spectrum, particularly in the wave band 10-100 Å (soft X-ray radiation).

Virtually all radiation energy of the quiet Sun is concentrated in the visible and infrared wave band (3500 Å to 500 μ). Extra-atmospheric and radio-astronomical methods have enabled measurement of the distribution of solar radiation in a broad wave band from 0.0001 Å (10^{-12} cm) to 1 km (Fig. 7). The total luminosity of the quiet Sun is L_{SOL} = 3.9 × 10^{33} erg/ s. The solar energy flux at a distance R = 1 AU is called the solar constant θ_{SOL}. The value of this constant is θ_{SOL} = 1.39 × 10^6 erg/cm²/s (2 cal/(cm²min)). It is hypothesized that, throughout the entire history of the Earth, variations in luminosity of the Sun have not exceeded 5 percent of the value of θ_{SOL}. Extra-atmospheric measurements of θ_{SOL} have made it possible to discover a systematic decrease during the last 8 years amounting to 0.01-0.02 percent.

Corpuscular radiation of the quiet Sun takes the form of continuous expansion of the corona and is called the "solar wind." The solar wind is a stream of solar plasma escaping continuously from the Sun and carrying the solar magnetic field with it.

The formation of the solar wind is associated with the flux of energy flowing from the Sun's core to its corona. The constant flux of energy to the corona is not entirely dissipated by its emission and thermal conduction. The excess energy is carried away by particles, which have thermal energy ("temperature") close to the temperature of the corona $T_\perp \approx 1.5 \times 10^6$ K ≈ 1-2 eV. Overcoming the gravitational attraction of the Sun, the particles move away ("escape") from the Sun with a constantly increasing velocity, since they are being "pushed by hot gas." At the base of the corona at an altitude of h = 2 × 10^3 km ≅ 0.03 R_{SOL} above the surface of the Sun, the velocity of directional motion of the particles is v_r = 100-300 m/s, while at an altitude of h = 4-5 R_{SOL}, this velocity becomes that of sound v = 100-150 km/s, and at a distance of 10-20 R_{SOL} the velocity of the directional motion of coronal plasma particles becomes supersonic and is equal to v = 300-350 km/s. This last

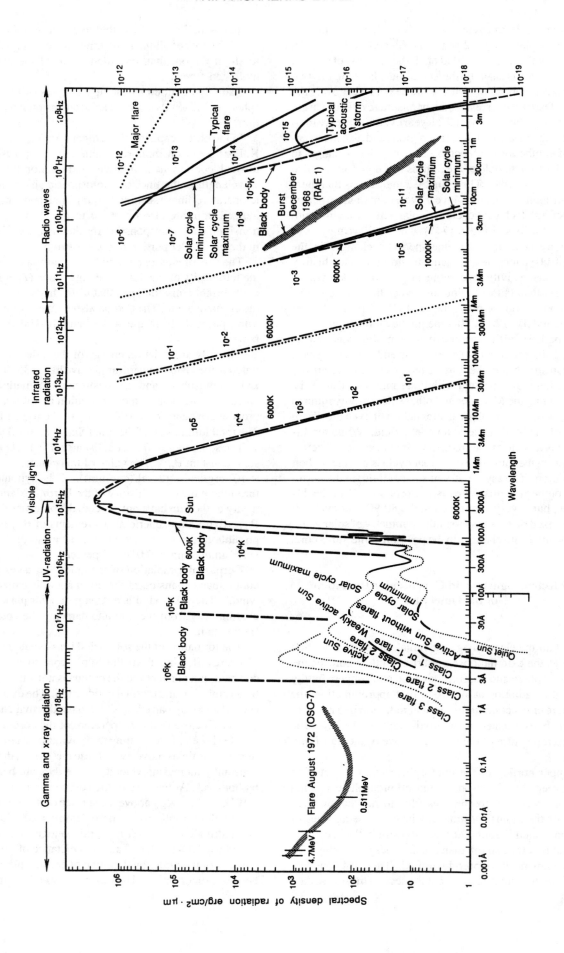
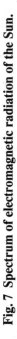

Fig. 7 Spectrum of electromagnetic radiation of the Sun.

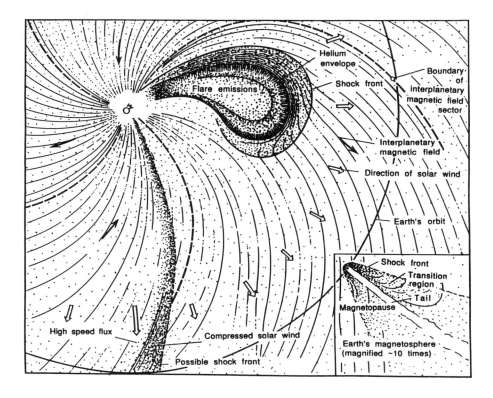

Fig. 8 Structural formations in the solar wind and their flow in the Earth's magnetosphere.

value is what is called the solar wind velocity. The velocity of the solar wind remains virtually constant up to 60-100 AU. The area occupied by the solar wind is called the heliosphere. The interaction of solar wind plasma, moving with supersonic velocity, with the atmospheres of the planets and the gas envelopes of comets leads to the formation of a standing shock wave from the daylight side of the planet (or comet) and a "tail" of rarefaction from the nightside (see Fig. 8).

The total energy flux carried by the quiet solar wind does not exceed $10^{-4} L_{SOL}$.

IV. Sporadic Solar Radiation

During the 30 years of the space era, it has been discovered that the nonstationary processes on the Sun resulting from its activity cycle have a strong effect on the geosphere. The following factors have been found to be particularly important to the Earth: 1) nonstationary phenomena in the solar wind, such as propagation of transients, shock waves, and outflows from the active regions with velocities of 350-2000 km/s; 2) high-energy particle emissions from solar flares—electrons, protons (solar cosmic rays) and hard neutral radiation (ultraviolet, X-ray, γ-radiation and neutrons). However, the flux of energy carried by these types of radiation is only a tiny portion of the energy flux of the quiet Sun. This paradox can be explained by the fact that energy fluxes carried by corpuscular and electromagnetic radiation are 10^3-10^8 times greater than

the normal background flux in this energy region and in the short time that they operate may become comparable to the constant radiation from the Sun. They effectively act on the Earth's magnetosphere and, particularly, on its geo- and biospheres.

A. Nonstationary Solar Wind

Nonstationary processes in the solar wind evoke various disturbances in the Earth's magnetosphere (e.g., magnetic storms or the aurora borealis) and evidently play some role in the formation of weather on the globe. We have already stated that the term "solar wind" was proposed by E.N. Parker in 1958.[4] An empirical description of the solar wind based on actual observations was made in 1966 by the Mariner spacecraft. Mariner studies were also the first to detect fast plasma fluxes. One year earlier the discovery of the interplanetary magnetic field had been made from this same spacecraft.

At present the solar wind is subdivided into the slow wind, with velocity of $v_{SW} \leq 350$ km/s and high speed solar wind streams ($v_{SW} \geq 600$ km/s). High speed wind streams are observed both in the form of long-lived structures that rotate with the Sun and in the form of sporadic, short-term emissions of "clouds" of plasma—transients—during major flares, after the collapse of prominences and other large-scale nonstationary processes in the chromosphere and solar corona. Table 3 presents mean plasma parameters in slow solar wind and in high-speed solar wind streams, and Fig. 8 shows the general pattern of propagation of the solar wind in the inner regions of

Table 3   Characteristics of solar wind plasma

Parameter	Fast fluxes	Slow solar wind
Flow rate, $<V_{sw}>$	700 km/s	300 km/s
Concentration of particles in flux	4 cm^{-3}	10 cm^{-3}
Magnetic field strength, $<H>$	10^{-4} G	5×10^{-5} G
Proton temperature, $<T_P>$	210×10^5 K	3×10^4 K

Table 4   Densities of chemical elements as compared to hydrogen

Element	Solar wind	Solar atmosphere
H	1	1
^{3}He	$(1.9 \pm 0.5)10^{-5}$	$(2.3 \pm 1.2)10^{-5}$
^{4}He	$(4.0 \pm 0.7)10^{-2}$	$(8.0 \pm 1.0)10^{-2}$
O	$(5.0 \pm 1.0)10^{-4}$	$(7.4 \pm 1.5)10^{-4}$
Ne	$(9.0 \pm 3.0)10^{-5}$	$(1.4 \pm 0.5)10^{-4}$
Si	$(1.3 \pm 0.7)10^{-4}$	$(3.6 \pm 0.2)10^{-5}$
Fe	$(1.1 \pm 0.5)10^{-4}$	$(3.3 \pm 0.1)10^{-5}$

the heliosphere.

The solar wind contains the same particles as the solar corona, i.e., mainly protons and electrons, as well as small quantities of α-particles (helium nuclei) constituting from 3 to 5 percent of the total, and small quantities of nuclei of various other elements. Electron density is identical to ion density within the limits of measurement error.

Table 4 presents the relative densities of nuclei of various elements in solar wind compared to their densities in the solar atmosphere. The mean values of solar wind parameters change periodically in accordance with the 11-year solar activity cycle. Figure 9 shows changes in density of helium as a function of cycle phase.

In the 1970s, X-ray observations from Skylab revealed that the structures in the corona from which the high speed wind streams come are coronal holes. Observations have shown that the large-scale structures observed in the photosphere persist when the inhomogeneous corona expands.

The source of the slow solar wind has not yet been completely established. There is reason to believe that the source regions on the surface are structurally similar to the regions responsible for the distribution of brightness in the continuous coronal spectrum and to the regions of the coronal magnetic fields with closed lines of force.

The same high- and low-speed solar wind streams are observed over the course of three to six rotations of the Sun. Streams with different velocities interact with each other, sometimes forming a shock front and an extended region of interaction, rotating along with the Sun. Figure 10 shows plasma parameters measured by Pioneer 10 up to 40 AU averaged for three solar rotations. The mean velocity v_{sw} is virtually constant between 1 and 40 AU, and the density decreases in proportion to the square of distance. The temperature decreases vastly more slowly than would be the case in a simple adiabatic expansion. It is possible that additional heating is due to the interaction (friction) among solar wind streams of different velocities.

B. Interplanetary Magnetic Field

The lines of force of the Sun's magnetic field are "frozen" into the plasma emitted by the corona and extended by the plasma into interplanetary space in the form of coronal loops. During time Δt, solar wind particles move away from the Sun

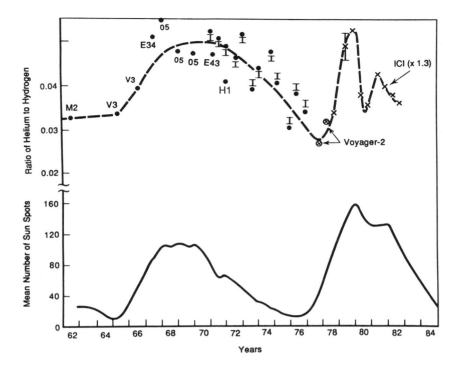

Fig. 9 Above: Variations of helium (He) abundance in the solar wind during solar cycles 20 and 21. Observations from: M2 (Mariner 2), V3 (Vela 3), E34 (Explorer 43), O5 (OGO 5), H1 (Heos 1), E43 (Explorer 43), I (IMP 6 and 8), Voyager 2 and ISEE-3/ICE (ICI=ion composition instrument). Below: Sunspot number for the same period as an indicator of solar activity (Ogilvie, K.W., Coplan, M.A., Bochsler, P., Geiss, J. Solar wind observation with the ion composition instrument aboard the ISEE-3/ICE spacecraft. *Solar Physics*, 1989, vol. 124, no. 1, pp. 167-184. Reprinted courtesy of Kluwer Academic Publishers.)

by distance $r = v_{sw}\Delta t$. During this time the Sun rotates by angle $\varphi = \Omega \times \Delta t$, where Ω is the angular velocity of solar rotation. As a result, in a system of coordinates fixed in relation to the Sun, the lines of the quasi-regular magnetic field assume the shape of an Archimedes spiral,

$$r = \frac{\sqrt{v_{sw}}}{\Omega} \times \varphi$$

the pitch of which for a given r is determined by the radial velocity of outflow, v_{sw} (Fig. 11). At $r = 1$ AU, the magnetic field is oriented at an angle of $\varphi = 45°$ to the direction to the Sun, and at the orbit of Jupiter ($r = 5.2$ AU), the magnetic field is almost perpendicular to this direction (Fig. 8). The strength of the magnetic field frozen in the solar wind, according to Parker's model, changes as follows: the radial component as $H_r \cong r^{-2}$, and the tangential and perpendicular to the plane of the ecliptic, H_φ and H_Z, as $\cong r^{-1}$.

The energy density of the frozen magnetic field—

$$\left[\frac{W = <H^2>}{8\pi} \quad << \quad \frac{\rho \times v_{sw}^2}{2} \right]$$

—is the density of the energy flux of the solar wind. The interplanetary field does not affect the majority of particles in the flux moving at velocity v_{sw}, but slows the faster particles,

accelerates the slower ones, and impedes displacement of particles across the field. This is reflected in thermal velocities of particles and leads to temperature anisotropy of the solar wind ($T_{II}/T_\perp \cong 10$) at a distance $\cong I$ AU. Here T_{II} and $T_\perp$ are the temperatures of the thermal motion of particles of solar wind along and across the magnetic field, respectively.

We have already stated that the first interplanetary measurements revealed that the large-scale structure of the magnetic field suggests the presence of a number of sectors in which the field is directed away from or toward the Sun. The number of these sectors changes during the solar activity cycle. Sometimes during periods close to the minimum there are only two or four such sectors. As solar activity increases, so does the number of sectors, and their structure becomes more dynamic.

Subsequently, it became clear that existing observations could be understood only if one postulated the following three-dimensional structure: the Sun's magnetic field is divided into a northern polar field and a southern polar field, extending into interplanetary space, but divided by a neutral flux layer, inclined toward the equator. This neutral layer stretches far out into the heliosphere (Fig. 12). This idea was confirmed experimentally only after measurements were made on Pioneer 11 in 1976, when, close to the solar activity minimum, it left the plane of the ecliptic by more than 15° north latitude by a distance of 3.8-4 AU and discovered a field

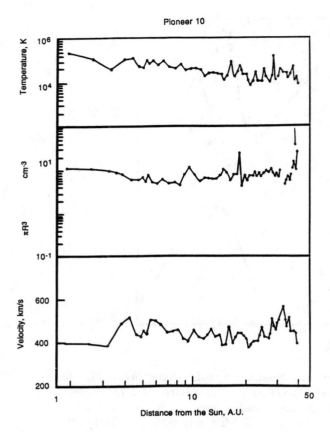

Fig. 10 Parameters of plasma, measured at various distances from the Sun on board Pioneer 10 (averaged over three solar rotations) (From Feynman J. The solar wind: Advances in our knowledge through two solar cycles. *Advances in Space Research*, 1989, vol. 9, no. 4., p. 95, with kind permission from Pergamon Press, Ltd.)

with only one sign. Measurements during Pioneer and Voyager missions made it possible to separate the spatial structure from temporal variations in magnetic field. A number of variations associated with the solar cycle were discovered.

The general agreement between Parker's prediction of magnetic field strength at 1 AU and the field measured by Pioneer 11 extrapolated back to 1 AU demonstrates that Parker's model is correct to a first approximation. However, there is a systematic difference of tenths of a percent. The angle of the helix also agrees rather well with Parker's model.

The interplanetary magnetic field undergoes variation over wide time and spatial scales. The nature of this variability may be described in terms of "waves," "magnetic inhomogeneities," and "turbulence."

The most general way to describe oscillations in any value is to decompose it into a power spectrum, which shows the contribution made by variations (in our case in field strength or direction) at various frequencies (or linear scales). When such power spectra are derived for the interplanetary field, they always show that the most powerful variations are the long-period ones associated with fluxes of various velocities.

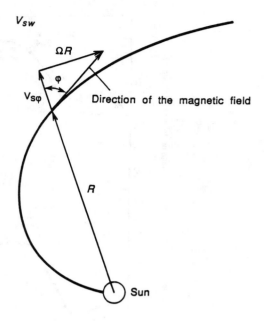

Fig. 11 Model of the formation of lines of force of the interplanetary field for the quiet solar wind.

The power spectrum covering the interval between 1 minute and 10 hours is associated with a definite type of oscillation in a plasma possessing a magnetic field. This oscillation is known as Alfven waves. Alfven waves essentially represent oscillations in the interplanetary magnetic field affecting the behavior of charged particles with energy ranging from tens of eV to hundreds of MeV.

The power spectrum in this frequency range has the form of a power function, i.e.,

$$\frac{dW(f)}{df} = A \times f - (1.7 - 1.9)$$

The level of oscillation between 1 and 5 AU decreases as $r^{-3/5}$ (Fig. 13).

We note here that oscillations in the interplanetary magnetic field play an essential role in propagation of particles of solar and galactic cosmic rays.[6]

C. Neutral Radiation from Solar Flares

An understanding of the nature of solar flares can be gained from studying the characteristics of the radiation they emit. In the exploration of space it is especially important to understand the characteristics of penetrating radiation. In this section we describe the nature of this radiation.

Measurements from Skylab have shown that magnetic loops must play a dominant role in the development of flares. For this reason it is not surprising that the current model of solar flares, depicted in Fig. 14, is based on a magnetic loop, extending into the corona. This figure shows only one loop; however, even in the simplest flares, whole arcades of loops are involved in the process (see also Fig. 5). The most intense

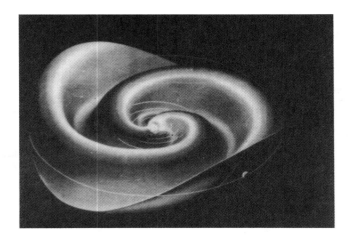

Fig. 12 Model of the neutral flow layer in the heliosphere (in two planes) [Artist: Werner Heil.] Wilcox, J.M., Hoeksema, J.T., Scherrer, P.H, Origin of the warped heliospheric current sheet. *Science*, August 1, 1980, vol. 209, p. 603. Copyright 1980 by the AAAS.

flares occur in complex magnetic regions.

The temporal course of the physical processes involved in flare development is depicted in Fig. 15 a, b. The process of primary energy release cannot be directly observed in the solar atmosphere; rather, a flare event is inferred on the basis of the emission of secondary effects, which occur in other regions and lag behind the primary release of energy by anywhere from a fraction of second to tens of seconds. As a result of dissipation of energy, the coronal plasma is heated, possibly up to temperatures of 10^8 K, while electrons, protons, and nuclei are accelerated impulsively to high energy. How the energy is distributed among the heated plasma and the accelerated particles is still not understood and this issue is currently under discussion. As Fig. 14 shows, different types of radiation occur in various regions of the loop.

Radiation from solar flares includes: 1) electromagnetic emissions, covering the wave band from several km (radio waves) to 0.0002 Å (hard γ-radiation with photon energy $\cong 40$ MeV); 2) accelerated (superthermal) protons and the nuclei of chemical elements and electrons escaping into interplanetary space during the development of flares; and 3) neutrons generated in nuclear reactions in the uncommon major flares.

The most important forms of radiation for understanding the acceleration of particles and, thus, the process of primary energy release are hard X-radiation, γ-radiation, radio waves, and neutrons. Most of these forms of radiation arise before accelerated particles lose all their energy in the surrounding atmosphere, and thus they carry important information about the processes of particle acceleration. Optical radiation, ultraviolet, and X-ray radiation with photon energy < 20 keV ($\lambda < 0.5$ Å) arise as a result of warming of the photosphere and the lower corona by fluxes of heat and accelerated particles. If heating is strong enough so that radiation losses and thermal

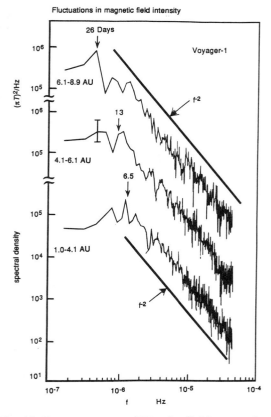

Fig. 13 Power spectra of H—the field strength of the interplanetary magnetic field—obtained on Voyager 1 for three different distances from the Sun. (Reprinted from Smith, E.J., Interplanetary magnetic field over two solar cycles and out to 20 A.U. *Advances in Space Research*, 1989, vol. 9, p. 164, with kind permission from Pergamon Press, Ltd.)

conductivity cannot compensate for it, then there is an explosion in the solar atmosphere. This explosion generates a shock wave, which has a number of effects (for example, additional acceleration of charged particles).

Radio waves from solar flares are not "dangerous" radiation; however, they are critical for understanding the "flare phenomenon" and thus we will begin our discussion of flare radiation with them. Radio waves arising during solar flares result from the development of turbulent motions in high temperature plasmas, and also from the motion of energetic electrons in magnetic fields (Fig. 14). Radio waves resulting from flares are very heterogeneous, have bursts varying in duration and amplitude, and have a complex frequency spectrum. Frequency of bursts of radio waves from flares fall in the meter and decameter wave bands (with the exception of microwave R_μ-bursts), i.e., they can occur only in the solar corona.

The difference in bursts of radiation measured at various frequencies (the form of dynamic spectra) have made it possible to construct a classification scheme of bursts, which is presented in Fig. 16.

Type III radio bursts, with fast drift from low to high

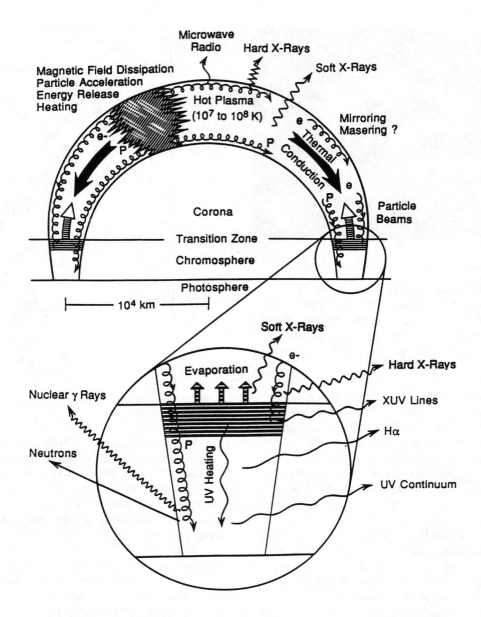

Fig. 14 Diagram of a simple flare showing flare phases and the areas of generation of various types of radiation. (Reprinted from: Dennis, B.R., Schwartz, R.A. Solar flares: The impulsive phase. *Solar Physics*, 1989, vol. 121, p. 77. Courtesy of Kluwer Academic Publishers.)

frequency (~ 10^{10} cm/s) and sometimes accompanied by a continuum in a narrow frequency band (Type V), are generated by a narrowly focused flux (beam) of electrons moving in the corona. The frequency of the burst decreases as the beam moves into a region of lower coronal density. Type III radio bursts are closely associated with the release of electrons along open lines of force and the escape of electrons into interplanetary space. Under certain conditions, the beams of electrons persist out to 1 AU and excite Type III radio bursts. We also note that sometimes Types U and J bursts occur (so named for their shape on dynamic spectra, with frequency defined as a function of time). In such cases the electron beams generating bursts move along the post-flare magnetic

loop. In Type U bursts, the return path is commensurate in length with the ascending path, in Type J bursts, the radio waves are dampened soon after the beam reverses.

Type V radio bursts are typically attributed to the capture of a portion of the accelerated electron beam in the arc of the magnetic field and its retention in the magnetic trap. A Type V burst often accompanies but lags slightly behind Type III bursts. Durations of Type V bursts are measured in minutes, whereas durations of Type III bursts (in the same frequency interval) are only a few seconds, and sometimes fractions of seconds.

Type II bursts show a slow drift in frequency with a velocity of 400-2000 km/s, and they sometimes have been ob-

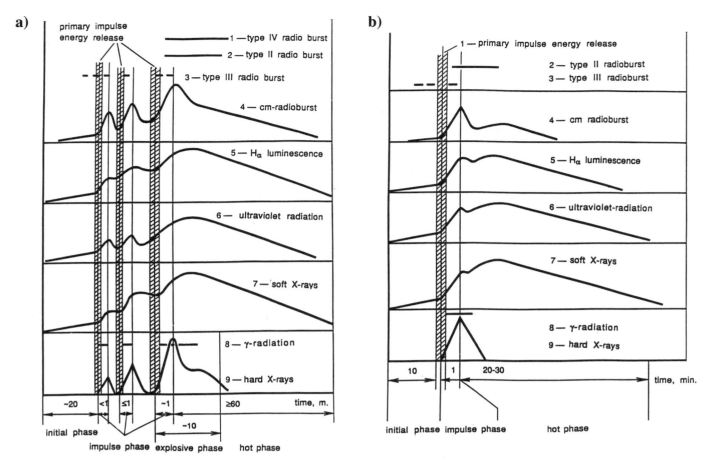

Fig. 15 Schematic representation of the development of a flare:
a) for a low power compact flare; b) for a powerful flare.

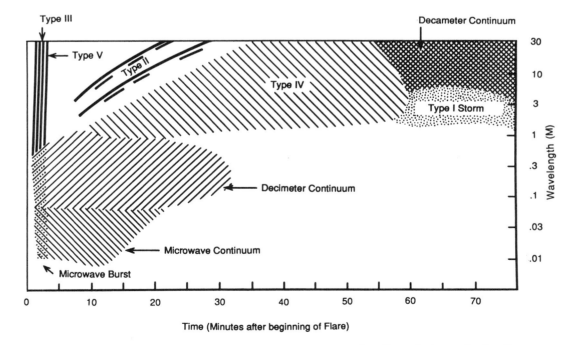

Fig. 16 Schematic representation of dynamic spectra of radio emissions of solar flares.
Behavior of radiation over time when various frequencies (wavelengths) are measured.

served as far as the orbit of Mars. A long-lasting continuum (Type IV burst) is often associated with these bursts. Durations of Type II bursts are on the order of 2-10 min, sometimes up to 20-30 min. These bursts occur only after powerful chromospheric flares and are vastly rarer events than Type III bursts.

Type IV radio bursts are complex and heterogeneous in structure. Many are closely associated with Type II bursts. The sources of Type IV bursts may move with a velocity of approximately 300 km/s, but may also be stationary. Observers have noted that Type IV bursts pass through a number of phases, which differ in time of occurrence, total duration (from tens of seconds to many hours), and frequency intervals.

The structural complexity and heterogeneity of Type IV radio bursts complicate their interpretation. It is usually assumed that long bursts occur if there is capture of fast electrons in magnetic traps, which may be stationary or moving at a slow rate. It is believed that the mechanism underlying emission of Type IV bursts is synchrotronic, i.e., the capture of electrons with energy of several hundred keV is hypothesized. Type II and IV bursts are often associated with powerful high-energy flares, after which energetic protons and electrons have been detected in interplanetary space. Moreover, the direct acceleration of protons and electrons on the fronts of shock waves generated in large flares have been established by *in situ* experiments. Type I noise storms constitute the decameter continuum and sometimes last for many hours after flares.

Microwave radiation (R_μ-radiation) at frequencies $f > 10^9$ Hz typically lasts as long as the flare in the hard X-ray radiation and is strongly correlated with the flare. Possible mechanisms underlying this radiation are: 1) emission of heated gas in the region of the flare; 2) emission of fast electrons moving in magnetic fields; and 3) excitation of radiation by the interaction of electrons with plasma turbulence developing in the flare loop.

Energetic electrons with energy of $E_e > 20$ keV arise in a flare either as a result of acceleration by some mechanism, or as a result of heating of the plasma in the flare to 2×10^8 K (20 keV = 2×10^8 K), hundreds of times the temperature of the lower corona at $T \cong 10^6$ K.

Energetic electrons interacting with the surrounding medium lose their energy, exciting *hard X-ray radiation* called Bremsstrahlung, in a broad energy interval starting nearly at the energy of electrons E_e. When they reach the chromosphere where $n = 10^{11}$-10^{12} cm^{-2}, the electrons lose their energy in ~1-2 s.

The loss of electron energy takes place so rapidly that the behavior of X-ray radiation reflects the temporal and energetic characteristics of the acceleration mechanism. The function linking the intensity of hard X-ray radiation (luminosity curves) to time in an energy interval of 20-1000 keV is complex in structure. The duration of X-ray bursts changes from several seconds to tens of minutes. By studying luminosity curves, scientists have been able to investigate and understand many aspects of the flare formation process. Compari-

son of X-ray luminosity curves with flare radiation in other wave bands (particularly R_μ-radiation) has made it possible to reconstruct an almost complete scenario of the flare events described in the beginning of this paragraph. This scenario is depicted in Figs. 14 and 15a and b.

In particular, luminosity curves have been used to classify flares according to duration. X-ray and R_μ flares are divided into impulsive (up to several minutes) and gradual (lasting from several minutes to tens of minutes) events.

It has proved possible to associate short (impulsive) events with compact active flare regions, and to associate long-lasting (gradual) events with elongated active regions, the magnetic field of which reaches altitudes of up to 0.1-0.3R_{SOL} above the photosphere and extends far into the corona.

The typical duration of hard X-ray bursts in large flares is $\Delta T \cong 10^3$ s, while short impulsive events typically last for $\Delta T \cong 5$-20 s. In flares, the flux of photons sometimes increases over a period not exceeding a fraction of a second in duration, reaching in the most powerful flares a magnitude of $I_X \cong 10^5$ phot/(cm^{2}s), which exceeds the background level of the quiet Sun by many orders of magnitude.

The shape of the energy spectrum of an X-ray burst—the distribution of the number of photons with respect to energy

$$\frac{dN}{dE_x} = f(E_x)$$

—has a one-to-one relationship with the electron spectrum and thus may be key to determining the type of acceleration mechanism in flares. Moreover, understanding the shape and dynamics of the spectrum in the flare makes it possible to correctly determine the total energy carried by the X-rays in one or another energy interval. Typically the shape of the spectrum in the burst can be approximated by a power law

$$\frac{dN}{dE_x} = AE_x^{-\varphi}$$

in the energy interval 20-300 keV. The parameter φ lies in the interval of φ values from 5 (soft spectra) to 2.5 (hard spectra). Events with high amplitude tend to have spectra with $\varphi < 3$, i.e., harder spectra, indicating greater effectiveness of the acceleration mechanism. The most likely value $\varphi_{prob} \approx 3.8$.

Frequency of occurrence of bursts of hard X-ray radiation is roughly comparable to the frequency of correspondingly large optical flares and alters with the solar activity cycle, as does the frequency of optical flares (see Fig. 6b).

Energetic protons and ions in flares with energy $E_p \geq 0.1$-1000 MeV/nucleon can arise only as a result of acceleration.

Energetic protons (ions), interacting with matter, lose their energy, and excite neutral radiation. This neutral radiation may be divided into three classes, the relative importance of which depends on the energy of the particles:

1) Radiation in narrow γ-lines arises as a consequence of interactions of accelerated protons, α-particles, heavy nuclei with He and other heavy nuclei of the solar atmosphere. The most intense lines arise during a transition from excited states of ^{12}C nuclei with energy of 4.438 MeV and of ^{16}O with

energy of 6.129 MeV. The most effective protons for excitation of these lines are those with energy $E_p \cong 10\text{-}30$ MeV. The lifetime of excited states is $\tau \cong 10^{-12}$ s or less, and for this reason the lines irradiate immediately without a visible delay and is thus called prompt radiation.

2) Neutron radiation arises during interaction between charged ions and matter of the solar atmosphere. The most important reaction is the interaction of protons with ^{4}He nuclei with an energy threshold of $E_p \cong 30$ MeV. The neutrons generated in this reaction may have a number of different fates:

• They may escape from the Sun and some of them may reach the vicinity of the Earth before decaying, as has been observed in an experiment on the Solar Maximum Mission Satellite. Some portion of the neutrons escape from the Sun and decay en route, according to the reaction n $\Rightarrow$ p + e$^-$ + γ. The protons created in this process then propagate in the interplanetary magnetic field.

• Neutrons remaining on the Sun may be captured by nuclei before they decay. The capture reaction, ^{3}He + n $\Rightarrow$ ^{3}H + p, occurs without photon emission, while the reaction H + n $\Rightarrow$ ^{2}H + γ causes photons with energy of $E_\gamma = 2.223$ MeV to be emitted. The 2.223 MeV emission is temporally delayed with respect to prompt flare emissions, due to the time required for neutrons to slow down to the thermal energies at which they can be captured by protons. Decay of this emission may be observed for 20 min.

Since time of capture of neutrons depends on the density of protons and ^{3}He nuclei, study of the temporal behavior of the 2.223 MeV line may yield information about the relative number of ^{3}He nuclei and the depth of the atmosphere at which the interaction occurs. Analysis of the decrease in intensity of lines in several flares has shown that capture occurs mainly in the photosphere where hydrogen concentration of $n_p \geq 1.3 \times 10^{17}$ cm^{-3}. The ^{3}He/H ratio obtained from the temporal behavior of the 2.223 MeV line in a flare on June 3, 1982, was $(2.3 \pm 1.2) \times 10^{-5}$. This value is close to the value that would be estimated if it is assumed that the turbulent displacement of solar matter does not significantly alter ^{3}He abundance from abundance estimated to have resulted from initial nuclear synthesis in the center of the Sun.

3) Gamma radiation from the decay of pions. The generation of pions (π-mesons), which requires protons with energy $E_p \geq 100$ MeV, leads to the appearance of photons with energy $E_p \geq 10$ MeV, either as a result of the direct decay of neutral pions or as a result of decay of charged pions into an electron and a positron, which are slowed through interaction with solar matter and which simultaneously excite radiation. This hard γ-radiation is recorded in powerful flares, in which protons have been accelerated up to energy of $E = 100\text{-}500$ MeV (Fig. 17).

After losing their energy, positrons annihilate with the surrounding electrons and emit two γ-quanta with energy of 0.511 MeV (or positronium breaks down into three photons with energy less than 0.511 MeV).

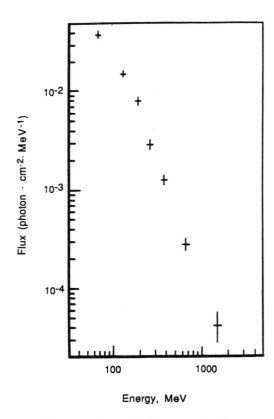

Fig. 17 Spectra of γ-radiation recorded in a powerful solar flare on June 15, 1991 using the "Gamma-I gamma-telescope." The figures shows that photon energy in this flare exceeds 1000 MeV, implying acceleration of protons to superhigh energies. (From: Akimov, V.V., et al., *Pisma v Astronomicheskiy Zhurnal* [Letters to the Astronomical Journal, 1992, vol. 18, no. 2, 167-172.)

D. Classification of Flares on the Basis of Energy and Comparison of the Energy of Different Kinds of Solar Flare Emissions

Recent comprehensive ground and space experiments have made it possible to measure and compare the proportion of energy carried by various forms of flare emissions. It has been demonstrated that on the average, the energy emitted in the optical wave band, soft X-ray ($E_x < 20$ keV) and hard X-ray ($E_x > 20$ keV) radiation, γ-radiation, and the energy of solar cosmic ray particles may be added to estimate the total energy in a solar flare.

In previous literature, the energy in flares was estimated from a form of secondary emission—by multiplying the area of luminescence in the H_α line (reflecting heating of the lower chromosphere) and the brightness of this luminescence (also associated with the power of the source) (Table 5). In recent years a classification scheme based on measurement of the amplitude of a thermal X-ray burst from the flare in the energy interval $\Delta E_x = 0.5\text{-}10$ keV has often been used (Table 6).

The latter classification scheme is clearly more exact and requires less subjective judgment on the part of the observer

Table 5   Classification of flares with respect to brightness and area of luminosity of H_α line (H_α importance)

[Reprinted from *Solar-Geophysical Data, Comprehensive Reports*, courtesy of Space Environment Laboratory, National Oceanic and Atmospheric Administration]

Relative intensity (brightness)	<2.0*	Area in square degrees			
		2.1-5.1	5.2-12.4	12.5-24.7	24.7
f - weak	S	1	2	3	4
N - normal	S	1	2	3	4
B- bright	S	1	2	3	4

* subflare

Table 6   Classification of flares on the basis of amplitude of X-ray bursts with energy 0.5-10 keV (GOES classification)

(Reprinted from *Solar-Geophysical Data, Comprehensive Reports*, Courtesy of Space Environment Laboratory, National Oceanic and Atmospheric Administration)

Flare importance	C	M	X
Amplitude of X-ray burst, erg/(cm²·s) at 1 AU	10^{-3}-9×10^{-3}	10^{-2}-9×10^{-2}	10^{-1}-5×10^{0}
	C1-C9	M1-M9	X1-X15

and fewer model assumptions. In Tables 5 and 6, we present both of these classification schemes. In Table 7 we cite the most probable values of the energy carried by various electromagnetic emissions of a solar flare and the total energy of fast electrons (determined from data on hard X-rays with energy 20-1000 keV) as a function of its H_α flare importance.

These relationships may be used to compute the energy balance in the flare and to assess the role of fast electrons in the flare process. We note that accelerated protons, the energy of which exceeds 100-200 keV, may contain approximately the same or even a greater proportion of energy than electrons.

The number of flares measured in a unit time is a function of their total energy ε (importance) as follows:

$$N_{\text{flare}}\left(\varepsilon > \varepsilon_o\right) \sim A\varepsilon^{-0.4\pm0.15}$$

The quantity A, the mean daily number of flares with energy ε_o, alters during the solar activity cycle (see Fig. 6b). The most powerful flares with importance $\geq$ 3B ($\varepsilon \sim 10^{32}$-10^{33} erg)

appear several times a year during the solar activity maximum. During such periods the frequency of the smallest flares—microflares with $\varepsilon \sim 10^{26}$ erg may be approximately one flare every 5 minutes.

E. The Charged Component of Solar Flares—Solar Cosmic Rays

"Solar cosmic rays" is a term referring to charged particles—electrons, protons, and the nuclei of heavy elements—that accelerate in the Sun during flares and then escape into interplanetary space. The energy of such particles lies in the interval from a few keV to tens and hundreds of MeV and sometimes even higher.

Solar cosmic rays have been studied intensively for the past 40 years. The first solar cosmic ray event was recorded in 1942. Since then instruments on the ground, on stratospheric balloons, and on spacecraft have been used to observe more than 350 increases in energetic particle fluxes associated with

Table 7   Estimates of solar flare emissions energy as a function of H_α importance (at $1\,R_{SOL}$)

Emission form	H_α importance			
	SN	SB	1N	1B
ε_{H_α}	$(2\text{-}6)10^{27}$	$(0.4\text{-}1.5)10^{28}$	$(2\text{-}5)10^{28}$	$(0.4\text{-}1.5)10^{29}$
ε_{opt}	1×10^{28}	2×10^{28}	1×10^{29}	$(2\text{-}3)10^{29}$
ε_{xt}	$(2\text{-}3)10^{28}$	$(0.8\text{-}2)10^{29}$	$(2\text{-}4)10^{29}$	$(3\text{-}10)10^{29}$
ε_e (>25 keV)	$(3\text{-}9)10^{28}$	$(1\text{-}2)10^{29}$	$(2\text{-}3)10^{29}$	$(3\text{-}10)10^{29}$

Emission form	H_α importance		
	2N	2B	3B
ε_{H_α}	$(2\text{-}5)10^{29}$	$(0.5\text{-}1.5)10^{30}$	$(9.3\text{-}2)10^{31}$
ε_{opt}	$(1.5\text{-}2.5)10^{30}$	$(3\text{-}5)10^{30}$	$(3\text{-}5)10^{31}$
ε_{xt}	$(1\text{-}3)10^{30}$	$(2\text{-}4)10^{30}$	$(1\text{-}3)10^{31}$
ε_e (>25 keV)	$(1\text{-}3)10^{30}$	$(2\text{-}4)10^{31}$	$(1\text{-}3)10^{31}$

solar flares.

During the past 15 years alone, approximately 200 of these events were recorded. This increase in the number of recorded solar events can be explained by the use of improved, more sensitive methods of detecting particles. The first solar cosmic ray events recorded were of enormous power, since only then could they be detected by ground-based instruments. Today, satellites can detect virtually all increases in solar cosmic radiation fluxes taking place in near-Earth space.

In the majority of flares, the maximum energy of accelerated protons does not exceed 50-100 MeV. Such flares occur rather frequently—twice a month during years of high solar activity. Less frequently—two or three times a year—the particles accelerate to 1 GeV. Especially powerful events, occurring five to six times in an 11-year cycle of solar activity, are marked by very large fluxes of accelerated particles, the maximal energy of which reaches 10 GeV and above. The charged particles accelerated in the flares are injected into interplanetary space and then propagate throughout the solar system. The process of propagation from the region of the flare to great distances from the Sun is very complicated, since the motion of charged particles takes place in a magnetic field having a number of sources. The motion of the charged particles is determined by this field, and their exit path can be only derived if one has exact knowledge of the field's structure. Certain lines of force in the magnetic field run from the region of the flare into interplanetary space so that the particles near these lines of force may leave the region of the strong field. Particles falling on the closed lines of force (into a kind of "magnetic trap") may remain there for a rather long time, sometimes until they lose all their energy. (It is these particles that emit Type I and IV radio bursts.)

Thus, the fates of particles accelerated during a flare and caught in a magnetic trap may differ: 1) While particles are in the magnetic trap, drift or diffusion may cause the particles to fall on open lines of force and to thus leave the flare region; 2) Particles moving in the magnetic field of a trap may fall into the dense layers of the atmosphere and lose their energy through collisions with ions and electrons of plasma matter, generating hard X-ray radiation ($E_x \geq 100$ keV), γ-continua ($E_\gamma \geq 300$ keV), γ-lines (for example, $E_\gamma = 2.223$ MeV), and neutrons; 3) Particles may pass from one arch-loop of the magnetic field into another, moving away from the site of the flare by large angular distances, until they fall on an open line of force or lose their energy through collision.

1. Propagation of Particles of Solar Cosmic Radiation in Interplanetary Space

After leaving the near vicinity of the Sun ($\approx 0.1\text{-}0.5\,R_{SOL}$, the particles fall into the interplanetary magnetic field. The particles conserve their magnetic moment when they move in the magnetic field, i.e., the ratio

$$\frac{\sin^2 \alpha(r)}{<H(r)>} = \text{const}$$

remains constant, in which α is the angle between the line of force of the interplanetary magnetic field and the velocity vector of the particles (pitch-angle of a particle), $<H(r)>$ is the field intensity, and r is the distance from the Sun. As a consequence, particle collimation should occur in the interplanetary magnetic field, which attenuates with distance from the Sun. On the path between the Sun and the Earth the magnetic field is attenuated by a factor of 100. Thus, theoretically, in Earth orbit the angle $a \Rightarrow 0$, no matter what the initial

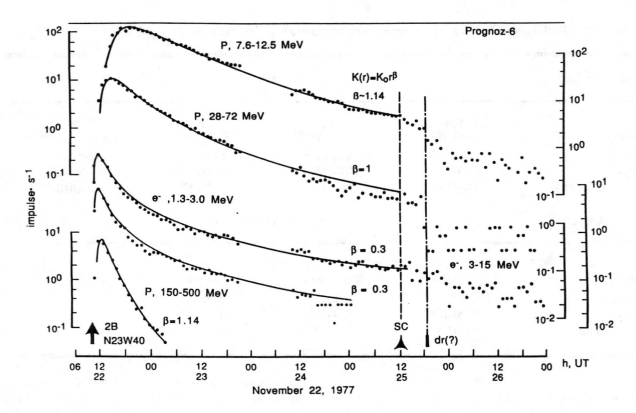

Fig. 18 Temporal profiles of charged particles fluxes during a flare on November 22, 1977.

angle of entry of the particle close to the Sun. However, nothing of the sort has ever been demonstrated experimentally. (Particle fluxes measured at $r \sim 1$ AU are observed at a broad interval of pitch angles; frequently they are distributed virtually isotropically with respect to the lines of force of the interplanetary magnetic field.) Scattering of the particles is caused by fluctuations (inhomogeneities of various sizes) of the interplanetary magnetic field (scattering particles of various energies) (see Section IV.B).

Motion of charged particles in this field would involve motion along the mean regular field $\langle H(r) \rangle$ with possible collimation of particles and their scattering on encountering magnetic inhomogeneities (turbulence). In interactions with magnetic inhomogeneities, particles are most effectively scattered by field inhomogeneities with dimension L close to the Larmor radius of the particle

$$R_L = \frac{cp}{z \langle H(r) \rangle}$$

where p is the momentum of the particle, z is its charge, and c is the speed of light. With $L \ll R_L$ the particles are scattered at a very small angle; with $L \gg R_L$ a particle moving along the line of force will skirt the inhomogeneity so that the angle of scattering is also small. When a particle interacts with a large-scale amplification of the field, mirror reflection from the inhomogeneity may also occur.

As a rule, the angular distribution of the particle relative to the line of force of the magnetic field has axial symmetry with the direction of the magnetic field as the axis.

Isotopic diffusion is the simplest model describing the process of particle propagation that allows for scattering by magnetic inhomogeneities. For an unbounded medium with a coefficient of diffusion $k(E)$ that is independent of r, this simple model provides the correct description of the flux of particles with energy E as a function of time, the time at which the maximum flux for a given energy is reached, and other characteristics, including, the rate of decrease of the flux with time. Experiments have shown, however, that events in which the propagation of particles follows the laws of simple diffusion are comparatively rare. As a rule, such events take place for particles with rather high energy, for example, protons with energy of $E_p > 100$ MeV. Particles of lower energy show significantly greater variety in time profiles of fluxes, suggesting that there are various possible modes of propagation in interplanetary space.

The differences observed experimentally in increases in solar cosmic rays are associated with the inhomogeneities and nonstationarity of physical conditions on the Sun and in interplanetary space.

Figure 18 shows a typical example of the time behavior of particle fluxes with different energy observed at 1 AU with a diffusive mode of propagation. This pattern is termed a diffusion wave and is always present to some degree.

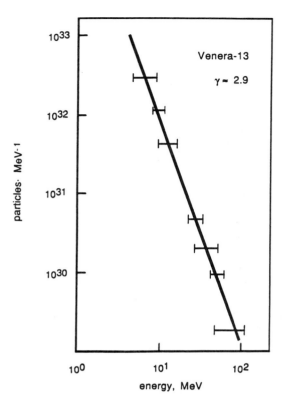

Fig. 19 Spectrum of injection of protons, obtained from measurements of proton fluxes on "Venera-13" on December 8, 1981 (full number of particles emitted by the Sun during the flare).

We have also said that charged particles accelerated in flares have a decreasing spectrum

$$\frac{dN}{dE} = f(E)$$

i.e., the greater the particle energy, the fewer particles there are. This is a universal law of all natural accelerated processes. What is important here is the shape of this spectrum, whether $f(E)$ is a power or an exponential decay function with respect to energy or momentum (hardness) of the particles. The hardness of the particles is considered the characteristic that determines the behavior of particles in regions with a magnetic field. Hardness $R = p/z$, where p is the particle momentum and z is its electric charge. Theoretical considerations of various mechanisms of acceleration suggest an exponential decay law of distribution of particles with respect to hardness.

We previously considered the energy spectrum of particles accelerated during a flare. Strictly speaking, the shape of the spectrum of particles accelerated in a flare can be determined only from observations of γ-quanta and neutrons for heavy particles, and from X-ray and radio emissions for electrons (see Section IV.C). However, there are few measurements to date of neutrons and γ-quanta and for this reason conclusions have been drawn about the proton spectrum based on mea-

surements of protons in solar cosmic rays. The spectrum of particles leaving the Sun can be determined from the value of the maximal amplitudes for fluxes of various energies. In practice, a power function is most often used, especially in the energy interval of 5-100 MeV:

$$\frac{dN}{dE} = AE^{-\delta}$$

The most probable value of the spectrum parameter, $<\delta> = 3$, has been obtained for the majority of flares of solar cosmic rays in which the maximal energy of accelerated particles does not exceed 100 MeV (Fig. 19). In very powerful flares, when the energy of accelerated particles exceeds 200-500 MeV, the spectrum of injection of protons and nuclei, as a rule, cannot be described by a simple power law. In these flares an exponential law (using a hardness representation of the spectrum) or Bessel function is used as the approximating function.

2. The Composition of Solar Cosmic Rays

The composition of particles accelerated in flares provides an idea of the atmospheric composition in the area of acceleration. As a rule, conditions supporting acceleration of particles (generation of quasistationary or induced electric fields) occur in regions of dynamic processes, of motion of solar material-plasma, and of changes in the magnetic field, i.e., in solar activity centers. In very powerful flares a large number of energetic particles appear, and it is usually assumed that here acceleration has been caused by a shock wave encompassing a very large area of the solar atmosphere. In this case, various anomalies of the solar atmosphere associated with the region of initial acceleration are smoothed over, allowing the composition of accelerated particles in a broad energy interval to provide a rather good picture of the mean composition of the solar atmosphere.

In flares of low power, a shock wave may not be generated, the area of acceleration is significantly smaller, and the chemical composition may differ from the solar average. On the other hand, it must be remembered that the particle acceleration mechanisms may differ in their efficacy in accelerating different nuclei and isotopes, notably the isotope ^{3}He and certain heavy nuclei.

In recent years low intensity solar cosmic ray flares enriched with ^{3}He and heavy elements have been detected. The coefficient of enrichment in these flares is

$$K = \frac{^3\text{He}}{^4\text{He}} \approx 1$$

Such flares, rich in ^{3}He, are usually also enriched with heavy elements (as compared with the elements on the Sun). Virtually all events enriched with helium with energy of $E = 1$ MeV/nucleon are associated with very weak flares occurring high in the corona and with fluxes of solar electrons with energy of $E_e \sim 2$-100 keV. The very high temporal correspondence for all components and the similarity of the shape of their spectra attest to the fact that the same acceleration process is respon-

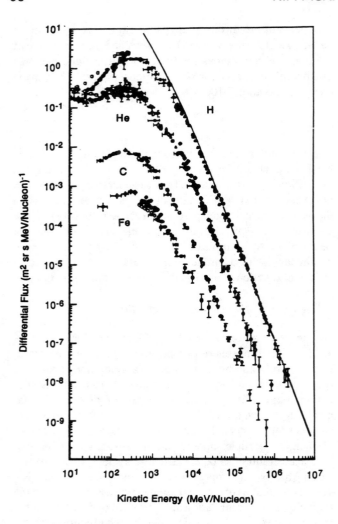

Fig. 20 Injection spectra of protons of He, C, and Fe nuclei. (Simpson, J.A. Elemental and isotopic composition of galactic cosmic rays. (Reproduced with permission from the *Annual Review of Nuclear Particle Science,* vol. 33, copyright 1983 by Annual Reviews, Inc.)

sible for acceleration of electrons, protons, and nuclei in these events.

Electrons are always present in solar cosmic rays, although the percentage of electrons entering interplanetary space is only 10^{-3} of the total number of accelerated electrons. Measurements of electron fluxes are an important aspect of the study of solar cosmic rays and the interplanetary medium. However, for understanding the flare process, it is much more informative to study X-ray radiation and the γ-continuum arising as a result of the deceleration of the electrons that were accelerated in flares (see Section IV.C). Solar flare processes are discussed in detail in works by Menzel, Kaplan, Svestka, and Priest,[1, 5, 6, 7] on which the preceding discussion was based.

V. Galactic Cosmic Radiation

Galactic cosmic radiation (GCR) is the name given to particles entering interplanetary space from outside the solar system, i.e., of galactic origin. GCR includes charged particles with energy greater than 10 MeV/nucleon for protons and other nuclei and greater than 1 MeV for electrons. [Particles with these energies are also generated in solar flares; such fluxes may exceed the flow of GCR particles by many times. For this reason the recording and study of GCR (except for particles with ultra high energy $\varepsilon > 10$ GeV) can be performed only during quiet periods of solar activity cycles in the absence of flares.] The first investigations of cosmic rays utilized ground-based instruments and instruments carried into the upper layers of the Earth's atmosphere by high altitude balloons and by sounding balloons during flights of high-altitude aircraft. These studies made it possible to establish the main properties of cosmic rays, determine their composition and energy spectrum in the high energy region, discover variations in the flux of cosmic rays, and study geomagnetic effects.

For the low energy ($E_z \leq 200$ MeV/nucleon for heavy particles and $E_e \leq 10$ MeV for electrons) regions, satellites and interplanetary probes were invaluable. These probes made it possible to determine the composition of particles in the low energy region, to study the spatial distribution of the particles, especially at great distances from the Sun, and to discover a number of other phenomena.

The flux of galactic cosmic rays in the inner regions of the heliosphere, including those within Earth orbit, varies strongly over the 11-year solar activity cycle, because penetration of the solar system by charged particles from interstellar space is impeded by the outflowing solar plasma and the solar magnetic field, which are also subject to 11-year cycles. As a result, the flux of near-Earth galactic particles, which is modulated by the solar wind, is considerably smaller than the interstellar flux.

Important characteristics of galactic cosmic rays are their composition and energy spectrum, which have been studied comprehensively in recent years.[8, 9, 10]

A. Energy Spectrum and Composition of GCR

Past research has firmly established that the energy spectrum of galactic cosmic rays in the energy region not subject to modulation processes (i.e., for energy $E > 10^{10}$ eV/nucleon) may be represented in the form $N(E) \sim E^{-\delta}$ with $\delta = 2.7$ (Fig. 20). This spectrum extends to very high energies, possibly up to 10^{15} eV. At very high energies, irregularities are observed in the particle spectrum; however, it remains sharply descending. The maximal energy of GCR particles reaches $10^{20}-10^{21}$ eV. Larger values of energy cannot exist due to loss through collision with relict radiation.

In the energy region below 100-1000 MeV/nucleon, the energy spectrum in interstellar space evidently undergoes a steep drop and the value of d decreases. Direct measurements

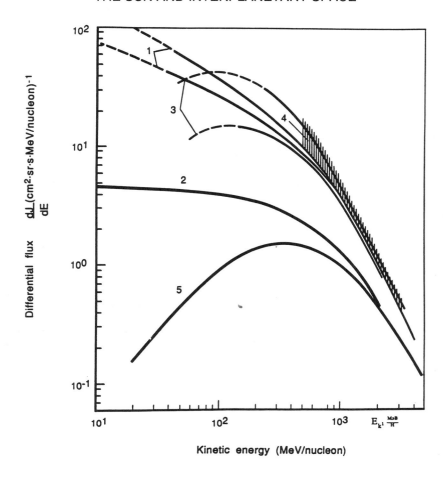

Fig. 21 Spectra of protons of galactic cosmic rays. Curves 1, 2, 3, and 4—nonmodulated computed spectra in interstellar space, obtained for various models. Curve 5—spectrum of protons in the minimum of solar activity (1965), measured close to Earth's orbit.

of the spectrum of cosmic rays outside the region of modulation (at the periphery of the solar system) have not been made and the spectrum in interstellar space, strictly speaking, remains unknown. However, on the basis of various considerations (for example, magnitude of the total energy contained in cosmic rays, which cannot greatly exceed the energy of the magnetic field) through indirect measurements, or from theoretical consideration of the motion of particles in the solar system, several authors have estimated the unmodulated spectrum of galactic cosmic rays. Figure 21 shows the energy spectra of galactic cosmic rays at 1 AU and outside the region of modulation.

Figure 22 presents a visual representation of the composition of galactic cosmic rays, which differs from the composition of elements of the Earth's crust and of the atmosphere of the Sun and stars.

It is possible that the predominance of heavy nuclei in cosmic rays can be explained by the fact that these particles are primarily accelerated in the sources.

The composition of heavy GCR particles with energy $E \geq$ 2.5 GeV/nucleon and electrons with the same energy is presented in Table 8. This composition is maintained up to energy of 10^3 GeV/nucleon. In the region of very high energy ($E \geq 10^3$ GeV/nucleon) the composition of GCR is much less well understood. Direct measurements have not yet been made for higher energies, and conclusions concerning the composition of the particles can be based only on indirect data, which suggest that the composition of GCR nuclei remains constant up to energies of $E = 10^8$ GeV/nucleon.

B. GCR Electrons

Loss of energy in the process of propagation in the interstellar medium is significantly higher for electrons than for heavy particles due to synchrotronic radiation and scattering by quanta of relict radiation. For these reasons the flux and spectrum of electrons also differ strongly from the flux and spectrum of protons. Figure 23 depicts the spectrum of galactic electrons in interplanetary space during quiet periods of solar activity.

Positrons, which differ from electrons only in the sign of the charge, may also be present in fluxes of electrons. The

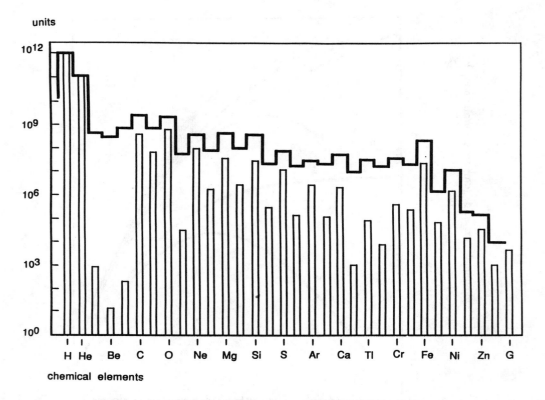

Fig. 22 Composition of galactic cosmic rays (solid line) and distribution of elements in the galaxy (bars)

Table 8   Composition and characteristics of galactic cosmic rays with energy $E_K > 2.5$ GeV/nucleon
[Petrov, V.M., Miroshenko, L.M. (Eds.), *Dynamics of Radiation* Conditions in Space. Moscow, Atomizdat, 1986]

Group	Particles in group	Nucleus charge	Mean atomic weight (AU)	Flux $(m^{-2} \cdot s^{-1} \cdot sr^{-1})$
P	Protons	1	1	1300
He	Helium nuclei	2	4	94
L	Light nuclei	3-5	10	2.0
M	Medium nuclei	6-9	14	6.7
H	Heavy nuclei	10	31	2.0
vH	Very heavy nuclei	20	51	0.5
eH	Super heavy nuclei	>30	100	10^{-4}
e	Electrons	1	1/1836	13

relative flux of positrons in the composition of light particles (electrons and positrons) are highly significant with respect to the origin of cosmic rays and the presence of antimatter in the universe.

Positrons in space where there is no antimatter may be generated as a result of the decay of positive ions forming through collisions of energetic particles. The number of positrons is vastly smaller than the number of electrons.

C. Modulational Effects in GCR

The flux of cosmic particles with energy below 5×10^2 MeV/nucleon, undergoes 11- and 22-year cycles of modulation. These modulational effects, as is now well known, are due to two causes. The first is associated with solar activity and involves the fact that particles of galactic cosmic rays are

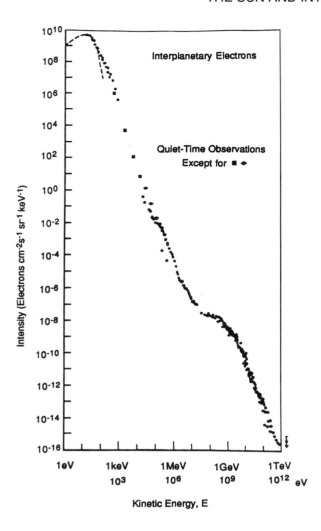

Fig. 23 Spectrum of electrons in interplanetary space in a quiet period. (From: Lin, R.P. Nonrelativistic solar electrons. *Space Sciences Review*, 1974, vol. 16, pp. 189-256. Courtesy of Kluwer Academic Publishers.)

propagated against the solar wind moving away from the Sun.

The region where modulation mechanisms operate has been termed the region of cosmic ray modulation. It is most likely shaped like an oblate ellipsoid with a radius in the plane of the solar equator of $r \sim 100$ AU, and a much smaller perpendicular dimension, perhaps only 10-25 AU. The size of the region of modulation determines the time delay for changes in the flux of cosmic rays with respect to the corresponding changes in solar activity, with its 11-year periodicity (which also controls the nature of the inhomogeneities in the interplanetary magnetic field). The magnitude of modulation and the time delay are a function of the point in space from which cosmic rays are observed, and of their energy and hardness.

Close to the Earth, but beyond the limits of its magnetosphere, the flux of particles of cosmic rays with energy $\varepsilon \geq 30$ MeV/nucleon changes from 5 to 2/(cm^2 s) between minimum and maximum solar activity. For particles with greater energy, this difference decreases.

Figure 24 presents results of recordings of mean monthly fluxes of GCR in the stratosphere, starting in 1957. Measurements were performed daily using sounding balloons launched in Murmansk and Mirnyy. The values cited correspond to the maximal rates of recording by cosmic ray detectors when the balloons ascended to an altitude of ≥ 20 km. The effective energy of the particles responsible for activating the detectors on the sounding balloons at these altitudes is 1 GeV. This same figure depicts the characteristics of solar activity, taking account of the latitude of sunspots. We see good agreement between the intensity of GCR and solar activity, with the exception of the periods 1971-1972 and 1983-1984.

A second factor explaining modulation of cosmic rays during these periods was discovered relatively recently, in the late 1970s. It is associated with the existence of a general solar magnetic field with lines of force in interplanetary space in the form of Archimedes' screws (see Fig. 11). In this magnetic field, the charged particles are subject to the effects of additional forces, which change their flux when the Sun's magnetic field changes sign. Computations performed by a number of authors have fully explained the effects observed in the measurement data.

Modulation effects lead to a situation where at 1 AU the energy spectrum of GCR particles differs strongly from the spectrum of particles beyond the boundaries of the modulation region.

Knowledge of the unmodulated spectrum is extremely important for solution of various astrophysical problems.

At the present time the Pioneer 10 spacecraft has reached a distance $r > 56$ AU from the Sun, but it still remains within the modulation region of GCR.

The periods of sharp decrease in particle intensity, which are clearly depicted in Fig. 10, are periods of propagation of shock waves from the Sun. The shock waves impede penetration of cosmic particles from the Sun into space. The shock waves, which act as expanding barriers to charged particles, are observed throughout the modulation region and are propagated with a velocity of $v \geq 500$ km/s, which leads to a pronounced delay in the corresponding decreases in intensity at points in space farther from the Sun.

Here, in the region where there is an expanding barrier, there is a strong radial gradient of particle flux, while between barriers there is virtually no gradient. During years of maximal solar activity, the number of shock waves is greater than during periods of weak activity, which leads to the observed decrease in the flux of galactic cosmic rays. Measurements on Pioneer 10 have demonstrated that shock waves are propagated up to $r \approx 56$ AU. It is not yet known whether the shock waves reach the boundaries of the heliosphere.

D. Nature and Sources of GCR

The spectrum of cosmic rays outside the region of modulation (see Fig. 21) makes it possible to determine the density of energy included in cosmic rays. This density equals ~ 1 eV/cm$^3 \approx 10^{-12}$ erg/cm^3. It is important to note that this same

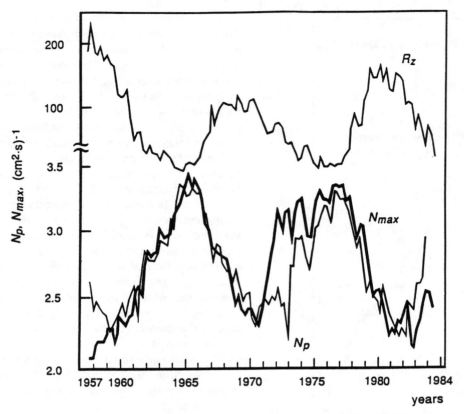

Fig. 24 Intensity of cosmic rays in the Earth's atmosphere ($h = 20$ km) and the number of sunspots (R_z) in the period from 1957 to 1984

N_{max} —experiment;

N_p—computation using the formula $N_p = 3.5^{-1.7}n^{0.8}\varphi^{-1.2}$,

    where n is the mean daily value of number of sunspot groups,

    $\varphi-$ is the mean heliolatitude of Sunspots.

energy density is involved in the kinetic motion of interstellar gas, in the interstellar magnetic field, and in the electromagnetic radiation from all stars throughout interstellar space. The identity of these energy densities attests to the important role played by cosmic rays in the development of the universe.

If the entire galaxy and the area surrounding it (the halo) were filled with cosmic rays, then the galaxy and halo, with a volume of $V \approx 5 \times 10^{68}$ cm^3, would contain a total energy of cosmic rays equal to 5×10^{56} erg. The galactic disk, with one hundredth the volume, contains energy equal to 5×10^{54} erg. What must be the power of the sources of cosmic particles to support the accumulation of the observed levels of energy? Over an infinitely long period, even weak sources are capable of emitting such energy. This raises the important question of the lifetime of cosmic ray particles in the galaxy.

The lifetime or age of the cosmic rays observed at present can be estimated from the composition of particles in cosmic rays and possible sources. It has been found that certain nuclei, for example group L (light nuclei Li, Be, B), are 6-8 orders of magnitude more abundant in cosmic rays than in the stars and, on the average, than in the solar system and in the galaxy (see Fig. 22). Such nuclei may enter cosmic rays as a result of decay (fragmentation) of heavier nuclei into parts

(fragments) during interactions with nuclei of the materials filling the medium through which the cosmic rays pass. It has been found that the lifetime of cosmic particles is equal to 2×10^7 years on the average and their sources must have power ~10^{41} erg/s. All the 10^{11} stars of our galaxy cannot supply such power.

A more powerful source of cosmic rays is explosions of supernova stars, which not only produce the necessary power for energy of cosmic rays, but are also capable of accelerating particles to the energy observed, at least, to energy of 10^{15} eV. Particles with greater energy may arise in certain rare events, and some of them may be of nongalactic origin.

Explosions of supernovae generate huge gas nebulae, reaching a size of ~5×10^{18} cm. One of the largest and most famous remains of a supernova, which exploded in 1054, is the Crab Nebula.

This short review of galactic cosmic rays has shown that our general understanding of sources of cosmic rays, how they are propagated, and the course of their existence in the solar system is relatively clear. More information is still needed, however, about certain important issues. These include the need for direct measurements of the energy spectrum of cosmic rays outside the modulation region, i.e., data about the spectrum in interstellar space and the need to obtain additional information about the mechanisms of modulation of cosmic rays and the composition of particles in a high-energy region. Superheavy nuclei in cosmic rays, like those in other objects of the universe, deserve particular attention on the part of researchers.

VI. Conclusion

The characteristics of near-Sun and interplanetary space, to which the majority of this chapter was devoted, are determined by the central body of the solar system—the Sun. There is only one exception—galactic cosmic rays, which reach us from outside the solar system—but the flux of galactic particles does depend on the Sun, on its magnetic field, and various manifestations of solar activity. All the remaining parameters of interplanetary space are directly determined by the Sun.

The most serious danger confronting living systems on interplanetary flights after weightlessness, the vacuum of space, and micrometeorites, is associated with solar and galactic cosmic rays. This danger will be considered in more detail in Volume III of this work; here we merely note that the most powerful flares on the Sun, which create a real hazard of radiation damage occur close to the solar maximum ($\pm$ 2 years), during the Sun's phases of growth and decline. At the same time, during the period of the solar maximum, the flux of galactic cosmic rays is one-half to one-third its magnitude during the period of the solar minimum. The absolute magnitude of the damaging factor from galactic cosmic rays during the solar activity minima is close to critical, and it is virtually impossible to obtain protection from such radiation.

These dangers compel us to conduct long-term interplanetary flights during periods closest to maximum solar activity and to select times with limited risk of receiving doses of radiation from powerful solar flares. This makes it especially important to be able to predict solar flares, if only a few days ahead, so as to interdict extravehiclular activity. Such warning would permit the crew to take measures to decrease the dose of radiation or neutralize it (by using a radiation shelter, turning the spacecraft to provide maximum shelter from particles and penetrating neutral radiation of solar flares, using pharmacological countermeasures, etc.). We will have to confront these and other difficult issues relating to space flight in the next few decades.

References

[1] Menzel, D.H. *Our Sun.* Cambridge, Massachusetts, Harvard University Press, 1959.

[2] Shklovskiy, I.S. *The Physics of the Solar Corona.* Moscow, Fizmatgiz, 1962 (in Russian).

[3] Gibson, E. *The Quiet Sun.* Washington, D.C., Technical Information Office, National Aeronautics and Space Administration, 1973.

[4] Parker, E.N. *Interplanetary Dynamical Processes.* New York, Interscience Publications, 1963.

[5] Kaplan, S.A., Pikelner, S.B, and Tsytovich, V.I. *The Physics of Solar Atmospheric Plasma.* Moscow, Nauka, 1977 (in Russian).

[6] Svestka, Z. *Solar Flares.* Dordrecht, Holland, D. Reidel, 1976.

[7] Priest, E.R. *Solar Flare Magnetohydrodynamics.* London, Gordon and Breach, 1981.

[8] Toptygin, I.N. *Cosmic Rays in Interplanetary Magnetic Fields.* Moscow, Nauka, 1983 (in Russian).

[9] Ginzburg, V.L., and Syrovatskiy, S.I. *The Origin of Cosmic Rays.* Moscow, Nauka, 1963 (in Russian).

[10] Ginzburg, V.L. (Ed.) *Astrophysics of Cosmic Rays.* Moscow, Nauka, 1987 (in Russian).

Chapter 3

The Inner Planets of the Solar System

M. Ya. Marov

I. Introduction/General Characteristics

The nine major planets of the solar system can be divided into the inner or terrestrial planets (Mercury, Venus, Earth, Mars) and the outer or giant planets (Jupiter, Saturn, Uranus, Neptune). The ninth planet, Pluto, is also classified as an outer planet, but it is more similar to the larger satellites of the giant planets in terms of size and properties (Fig. 1).

The main differences between the two categories of planets are their sizes, masses, and mean densities. These differences are due to differences among the ratios of the three main types of materials present in the planets: gases (primarily highly volatile gases with extremely low condensation temperatures, such as hydrogen and helium); ices (primarily water, ammonia, and methane); and rocks (iron, silicates, magnesium oxides, aluminum oxides, and calcium oxides, as well as oxides of other metals). These materials are frequently called the "light components" and "heavy components," respectively. While the terrestrial planets are solid bodies made up almost entirely of heavy components, the giant planets consist of gases and liquids, and the "heavy component" concentrated at the core makes up no more than a few percent of the planet's mass. None of the giant planets has a solid surface (in the accepted sense of the word).

The inner planets' basic mechanical characteristics, including orbital and rotational parameters, are presented in Table 1. Perturbations in these orbital and rotational motions are due to the mutual gravitational attraction of the planets and tidal interactions, causing the orbital parameters to deviate from a Keplerian ellipse. These interactions also affect the rotational parameters.

Mars has approximately the same rotation period as the Earth; the martian day is only 41 minutes longer than the Earth day (mean solar day). Venus and Mercury rotate extremely slowly, and Venus shows retrograde rotation. When observed from Earth, both Mercury and Venus show phases similar to those of the Moon, with a mean period of 584 days for Venus and 116 days for Mercury (synodic periods). In turn, the sidereal orbital period (i.e., the period relative to the stars) is 243.1 days for Venus and 88 days for Mercury.

Resonances due to tidal interactions and the asymmetric distribution of mass (i.e., deviations in the figure of a planet from strict sphericity) show their strongest effects in the rotational and orbital periods of Venus and Mercury. The sidereal rotation period of Venus is close to resonance with the Earth's orbital period, which means that Venus shows almost exactly the same face to the Earth at the superior and inferior conjunctions. Due to spin-orbit resonance in the motion of Mercury, its rotational period is exactly two-thirds of the sidereal orbital period (58.6 days).

The planet's oblateness (ε), determined by the difference between the equatorial radius (R_e) and the polar radius (R_p): $\varepsilon = (R_e - R_p)/R_e$, is one very important characteristic, which depends on the rotational period. Unlike the rapidly rotating giant planets, the inner planets exhibit small differences: for Earth the difference is 17 km ($\varepsilon = 1/298$), for Mars 25 km ($\varepsilon = 1/136$), and for Venus no more than a few hundred meters ($\varepsilon \sim 0$). The axial ratio in turn determines the distribution of gravitational potential energy in the planet as well as the internal structure of the planet and its figure. The Earth is nearly spherical (more precisely, an ellipsoid of revolution with axial ratio near unity, or a spheroid), while the northern hemisphere of Mars (with respect to a great circle inclined at ~35° to the equator) is more oblate than the southern hemisphere, i.e., shows more deviation from a spheroid. Venus has much less asymmetry of figure, while, unlike the Earth, it deviates strongly from hydrostatic equilibrium.

The parameters of orbital and rotational motion determine the thermal regime of the planet, including the daily and seasonal temperature variations at the surface and in the atmosphere. The effective (or equilibrium) temperature T_e, which is the temperature at which the energy incident from the Sun and the energy radiated by the planet into surrounding space are balanced, serves as a general energy parameter characterizing a planet. The bolometric spherical albedo (Bond albedo) A, which serves as a measure of the reflected flux of solar radiation and is given in Table 1 along with T_e, is also used for this purpose. As a consequence of the greenhouse effect, celestial bodies with atmospheres generally have temperatures greater than T_e.

Even a slightly elliptical orbit will cause noticeable seasonal variations due to the large energy input from the Sun at perihelion. For Mars, the difference is approximately 45 percent, while for Mercury the difference reaches 200 percent. However, the position of the rotational axis plays the most important role in seasonal variations and the duration of the

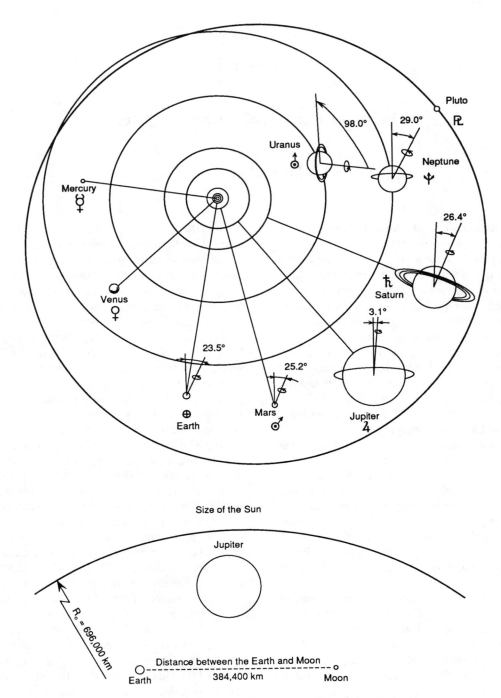

Fig. 1 Distance relationships in the solar system. (Reprinted from: Marov, M.Ya. *Planets of the Solar System*, **2nd edition, Moscow, Nauka, 1986, pg. 28.)**

seasons (especially when the rotational period is comparable to the period of revolution around the Sun).

Because of the low orbital eccentricity and insignificant deviation of the axis of rotation from the normal to the orbital plane, there are virtually no seasons on Venus. On Mars, however, both factors play a role, leading to seasons of different durations in the northern and southern hemispheres, as well as to marked differences among the seasons. Moreover, the inclination of the rotational axis for Mars probably under-

goes long-period variations, which, along with variations in the inclination of the plane of its orbit to the plane of the ecliptic and precession of the rotational axis itself, may lead to large variations in obliquity and thus in climate (Fig. 2).

Table 1 lists one additional important planetary characteristic—the strength of the equatorial magnetic field. Of the inner planets, Earth has the strongest magnetic field. Mercury also has a substantial magnetic field, while Venus has virtually no intrinsic field. Measurements from the Phobos 2

Table 1   Major characteristics of the inner planets

Planet	Mean heliocentric distance (orbital semimajor axis), AU[†]	Eccentricity	Inclination of orbital plane to ecliptic, deg	Sidereal period, yr	Sidereal rotation period, days	Equatorial radius, km	Volume[‡]	Mass[‡]
Mercury	0.387	0.206	7.0	0.24	58.6	2439	0.05	0.06
Venus	0.723	0.007	3.4	0.62	243	6051.5	0.90	0.82
Earth	1.000	0.017	0	1.00	1.00 ($23^h56^m 04^s$)	6378	1.00 (1.08×10^{12} km^3)	1.00 (5.98×10^{24} kg)
Mars	1.524	0.093	1.8	1.88	1.029	3394	0.15	0.11

Planet	Density, g/cm^3	Inclination of equator to orbital plane, deg	Direction of rotation	Number of satellites	Strength of magnetic field at equator, э	Albedo (integrated spherical)	Effective temperature, K
Mercury	5.44	7.0	Direct	none	0.0035	0.09	435
Venus	5.24	177	Retrograde	none	—	0.77	228
Earth	5.52	23.5	Direct	1	0.31	0.30	255
Mars	3.95	25.2	Direct	2	≤0.0006	0.20	216

[†]In astronomical units (AU); 1 AU is equal to the mean Earth-Sun distance ($\sim1.49598 \times 10^8$ km)

[‡]Relative to the volume and mass of the Earth

spacecraft suggest that, contrary to previous estimates, Mars probably also has no magnetic field, although the question remains open.

Only three of the rather large number of satellites in the solar system orbit inner planets. These include the Earth's Moon, which is one of the largest bodies in this class, and the two small asteroid-like satellites of Mars—Phobos and Deimos. The basic characteristics of the satellites of the inner planets are presented in Table 2. Mercury and Venus, the planets closest to the Sun, have no satellites.[1, 4, 5, 19]

II. Surfaces: Topography, Composition, and Properties

A. General Remarks

The features of a planet's topography and the physical and chemical characteristics of its different regions provide important information on the planet's past and present and the patterns and chronology of events responsible for its current appearance. Primordial structures frequently are camouflaged by later endogenous and exogenous processes, such as meteor bombardment, tectonic and volcanic activity, sedimentation, and various types of erosion. In addition to topography, comparative study of the elemental and mineral composition of the rocks that make up a planet is an extremely important way to interpret and understand its history, providing a chronicle "written in stone," which is essentially what

the surface is. Comparison of the characteristics of the solar radiation reflected by the surface of each planet with the reflection spectra of terrestrial minerals provides certain information about element and mineral composition. This method, first applied in the 1960s to the Moon, later underwent extensive development through research on Mars, Mercury, and the asteroids.

The sequence of processes involved in the formation of the surfaces of the terrestrial planets dates back to the final phase in the formation of the planets (i.e., the accretion phase), when the streams of bodies (planetesimals) falling to the surfaces of the planets were nearly exhausted. The large, partially modified craters on the lunar continents, the craters of similar morphology on Mercury, and the oldest, most highly eroded craters on Mars date back to this era. Traces of this stage have also been preserved on Venus; on Earth, not only the oldest structures, but also some later structures are generally either highly eroded or buried beneath deep sedimentary mantles.

B. Earth

Approximately two-thirds of the surface of our planet is covered by a thick layer of water, the oceans, under which there are extraordinary structures without parallel on the land. The heterogeneity of these structures is shown in the physiographic map of Fig. 3. Major features include the system of mid-oceanic ridges, a belt of deep ocean trenches and island

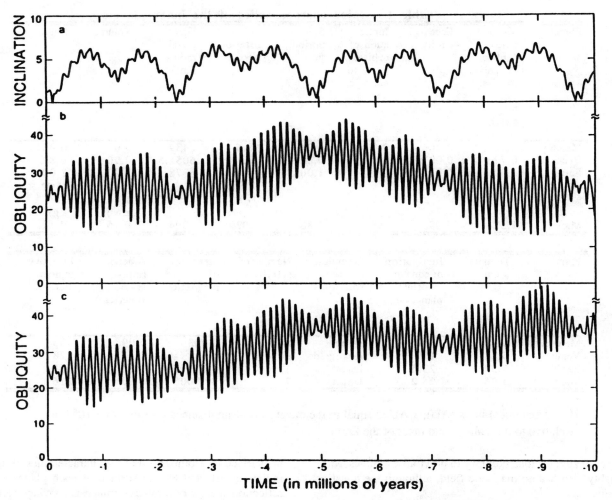

Fig. 2 (a) The orbital inclination for Mars with respect to the invariant plane of the solar system. The obliquity of Mars for the past 10^7 years for a precessional constant of **(b)** $\alpha = 8.26$ arcsec/year and **(c)** $\alpha = 8.32$ arcsec/year. (Reprinted from: Ward, W.R. and Rudy, D.J. *Resonant obliquity of Mars? Icarus,* 1991, vol. 94, page 161. Copyright 1991, Academic Press.)

arcs, and many individual seamounts and volcanoes.

The highly dissected topography of the mid-oceanic ridge system is global. This system forms a well-defined band that extends over the bottoms of all the oceans for approximately 60,000 km and even extends partially onto the continents. These ridges are best typified by the mid-oceanic ridges in the Indian and Atlantic Oceans, which have individual peaks rising some 3.5-4 km above the ocean floor. Large, tectonically active fault structures extend along the axis of each mid-oceanic ridge. These centers are called rift zones—narrow, steep-walled clefts up to 5 km deep with widths ranging from several kilometers to tens of kilometers. The rift zones are surrounded by mountain ranges (horsts), which are separated by intermontane graben valleys with relative differences in relief of 2-3 km. These rift zones show high seismicity and volcanism.

Island arcs and the associated deep ocean trenches are sites of current mountain formation on Earth. They are characterized by high seismicity and are the most frequent sites of

volcanic eruptions leading to landslides and the accumulation of material that partially smooths out the bottoms of the trenches. The system of volcanic island arcs includes the western rim of the Pacific Ocean, the northeastern edge of the Indian Ocean, and the western and southern edges of the Atlantic. A large area of the ocean floor is occupied by vast rolling abysses and flat abysses separated by isolated anticline-block seamounts and volcanic ridges. The peaks of some of these volcanoes rise above the surface of the water, forming islands.

The geological structure and evolution of the Earth can be described quite well within the framework of the new global plate tectonics (or lithospheric plate tectonics) theory, developed in the late 1960s. This theory has been used to derive convincing explanations for the idea of continental drift proposed by Wegener at the beginning of this century.

According to lithospheric plate tectonics theory, seismic belts, within which at least 95 percent of the earthquakes on Earth occur, divide the rigid stony shell of the Earth—the

Table 2   Major characteristics of the moons of the inner planets

Planet	Satellite	Mean radius, km	Mass (in planetary masses)	Density, g/cm^3	Albedo (integrated spherical)
Earth	Moon	1738	1.23×10^{-2}	3.34	0.07
Mars	Phobos	13.5	2.0×10^{-8}	2.2	0.05
	Deimos	7.5	2.8×10^{-9}	1.7	0.07

Planet	Satellite	Orbital radius (in planetary radii)	Orbital radius (in 10^{3}km)	Orbital period, d	Orbital eccentricity	Inclination to ecliptic, deg
Earth	Moon	60.27	384.4	27.32	0.055	5.15
Mars	Phobos	2.76	9.4	0.319	0.015	1.02
	Deimos	6.91	23.5	1.263	0.001	1.82

lithosphere—into individual large blocks or plates ranging in diameter from 2000 to 10,000 km and in thickness from 20 to 100 km under the oceans and from 200 km under the continents. These plates move on top of the asthenosphere, a softened layer of reduced strength between crust and mantle. The largest plates include the Eurasian, African, Indian (which includes Australia), Pacific Ocean, American, and Antarctic plates.

The plate boundaries and associated seismic belts can be divided into three distinct major groups. The first includes the mid-oceanic ridges, which are considered to be regions of convective upwelling in the Earth's interior and spreading centers. In these regions, the plates on each side move away from the axes of the mid-oceanic ridges under the action of the horizontal component of the convective flows, which originate in the interior of the Earth as a result of the density differentiation of the Earth into an iron-oxide core and silicate envelope—the mantle. Such rift zones are formed in regions where the plates are moving apart (i.e., spreading), and the resulting free space is filled with basalts—lavas that melt and rise up from the mantle. When these lavas cool and crystallize, they form new oceanic crust; thus, the oceanic lithosphere is constantly being renewed.

The second group of plate boundaries forms a global system of deep ocean trenches, which are especially prominent around the periphery of the Pacific Ocean. Here solid lithospheric plates are submerged in the mantle of the Earth, causing earthquake epicenters to descend obliquely under the continents to depths of approximately 700 km. These regions are dominated by pressure that has led to the formation of many geological structures. The lithospheric plates draw close together in the deep ocean trench, and one (the oceanic plate) is subducted under the other (the continental plate). Extensive volcanism occurs along the boundaries where the plates approach one another and submerge (the so-called Zavaritskii-Benhoff zones); the famous "ring of fire" around the Pacific Ocean passes through these regions. In these zones (subduction zones), the submerged material is melted, and the continental crust is formed.

Finally, the third group of plate boundaries and seismic belts includes the large faults that dissect the mid-oceanic ridges and ocean floors (and, in spots, the continents). These are the transform faults, along which the lithospheric plates slide parallel to each other and scrape against each other.

The maximum velocity at which the lithospheric plates move across the Earth's surface is 15 cm per year, which is the maximum characteristic spreading rate for spreading centers along the Pacific Ocean mid-oceanic ridge. The spreading rate for the mid-Atlantic ridge is lower, on the order of a few centimeters a year.

C. Moon and Mercury

The situation is different for those celestial bodies where the surface did not experience the substantial changes that took place on the Earth, since they did not have the efficient sources for the accumulation of sedimentary rocks created by the presence of a hydrosphere and atmosphere, and where geological activity terminated earlier. The best examples of this are the Moon and Mercury. Mercury is of the greatest interest, since there is good reason to believe that the formation and evolution of the Moon were strongly affected by the Earth. Therefore, along with the asteroids, Mercury can be viewed as the best-preserved relic of the formation of the inner planets.

Figure 4 shows a current map of the lunar surface, compiled from all available data. The traditional designations "mare" and "continent" are used to characterize the large, well-resolved topographic regions, visible from the Earth with a telescope. The lunar surface is most prominently characterized by an abundance of craters (primarily of impact origin) ranging from hundreds of kilometers to a fraction of a meter (crater pits) in size. There are fewer craters in the maria (indicating that the maria are younger), and the regional variations in crater density are larger than on the continents. The surface of the maria is covered by a layer of pulverized rock—the lunar regolith, which has an estimated thickness ranging from 1-6 m in relatively young regions and 5-10 m in older regions. The load-carrying capacity of the regolith increases from 0.2-0.3 N/cm^2 in the top layer to 10 N/cm^2 at a depth of 8-10 cm. Another characteristic morphological trait of the lunar surface is the asymmetric distribution of maria: there are many fewer maria on the far side of the Moon. This asymmetry is generally explained using the hypothesis that the basalt melt was mainly concentrated on the visible side of the Moon, whereas the light crust melt was mainly concentrated on the opposite side.

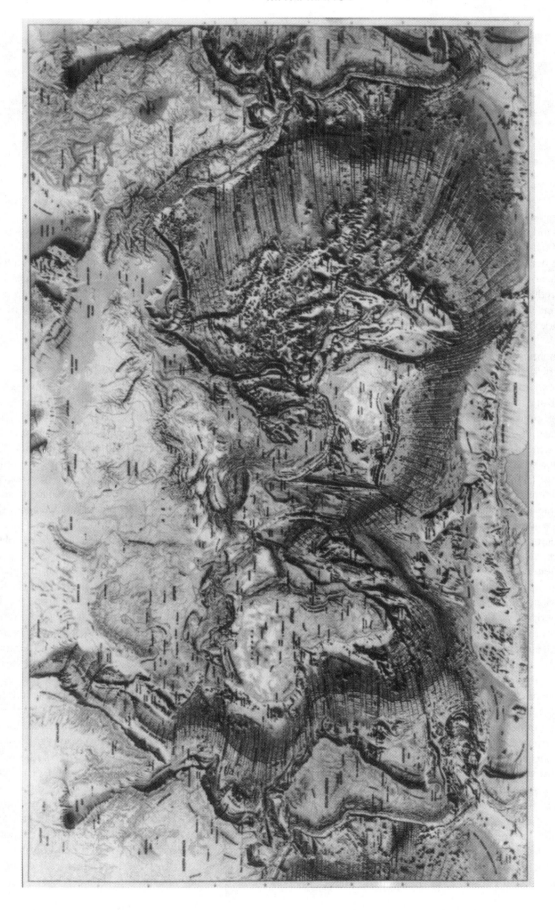

Fig. 3 The floor of the oceans. Topography of Earth's surface. Bathymetric map compiled by B. Heezen and M. Tharp, New York, 1964. Mercator Projection. (Based on Bathymetric studies by Bruce C. Heezen and Marie Tharp of the Lamont Doherty Geological Observatory, Columbia University Palisades, New York, 1963, reprinted courtesy of Marie Tharp.)

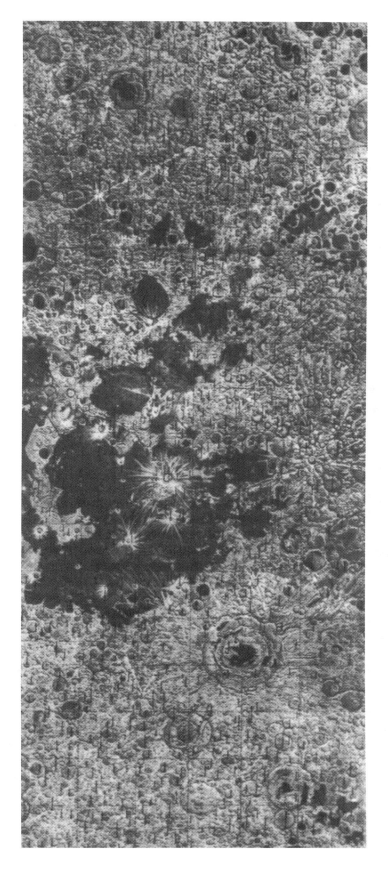

Fig. 4 Topography of the surface of the Moon. Map compiled from data of Luna 3, Zond 3, and Lunar Orbiter. Arbitrary cylindrical projection. (Courtesy of Shtenberg Astronomical Institute, Moscow, 1976.)

Table 3   Surface characteristics of the Moon and planets from radar data
(Source: Kotelnikov V.A., 1984. Personal communication.)

Planet	Reflection coefficient K, %	Dielectric permittivity ε	Density ρ, g/cm³	Microrelief (root-mean-square slope angle), θ, deg
Moon	5.7-6.3	2.6-2.8	1.2-1.3	6-7
Mercury	5.8-8.3	2.7-3.3	1.2-3.6	5-8
Venus	11-18	4-6	2-3	2.5-5
Mars	3-14	1.4-4.8	1-2.5	0.5-4

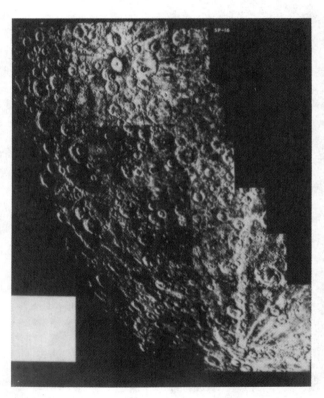

Fig. 5 Photomosaic of the surface of Mercury at middle and high altitudes of the southern hemisphere at the terminator. The radial texture resulting from meteor impacts associated with craters in the lower and upper portion of the picture can be seen clearly (Mariner 10). (Photograph courtesy of NASA.)

An important contribution to dating and interpreting the geological processes that occurred on the Moon (and, by association, on the Earth during the Precambrian era, over 570 million years ago) has come from the analysis of lunar soil. Analysis of the chemical and mineralogical composition of the surface soil led to the conclusion that the lunar maria largely consist of rock-forming minerals such as pyroxenes (which are rich in magnesium and iron), while the continents consist of lighter feldspathic rocks (anorthosites) in which aluminum and the alkali metals predominate. This pattern shows some analogy with the ocean floors and continents on Earth. It may be hypothesized that the anorthosites formed during the very early phases in the evolution of the Moon, during crystallizational differentiation of the basic gabbro-basalt magma, while the basalt-melt outcrops that filled the maria came much later. These ideas are supported by estimates of the absolute ages of various types of lunar material. The oldest continental crust on the Moon has an age approximately equal to that of the solar system (approximately 4.6 billion years), while "younger" rocks (less than 3.16 billion years) tend to dominate in the maria regions. This latter estimate apparently marks the end of the major active period in the evolution of the Moon. Current estimates indicate that the main activity on the lunar surface at the present time involves a continuous turning over of the soil by meteorite impacts; over the lifetime of the maria regions, the surfaces of the maria have probably been cycled in this fashion at least 100 times to a depth of approximately 40 cm.

It has been postulated that the mineral composition of rocks on Mercury is similar to that of rocks on the Moon, since Mercury reflects electromagnetic radiation almost as well as the Moon. Moreover, the intrinsic thermal emission shows similar characteristics to that of the Moon, while the thermal inertia values used to characterize the thermal and physical properties of the surface are also similar. However, Mercury turns out to have a slightly lower albedo in the visible spectrum than the Moon, and the reflection spectrum is brighter in the blue rather than the red. This suggests that the surface layer of Mercury is depleted of iron and titanium, so much so that the ferric oxide content is estimated to be only 3-6 percent—a fraction of that on Venus and Mars.

Radar results provide additional information. The intensity of the signal reflected by the planet is a function of the reflection coefficient K (in percent), which is directly related to the physical properties of the surface (primarily the density of the surface layer at a depth on the order of several wavelengths for the probe radiation) and the composition of the surface rocks. These properties determine the dielectric permittivity ε of the material reflecting the electromagnetic wave. We can also evaluate the scattering properties of the surface and the slopes of regions comparable to the wavelength in extent. The larger the scattering angles, the rougher the surface (or, in other words, the less homogeneous the microrelief).

The reflection coefficient of Mercury in the radio region, which proves to be almost identical to that of the Moon, was used to obtain the mean dielectric permittivity $\bar{\varepsilon} = 3$, which corresponds to a density of 1.4 g/cm^3 in the surface layer. This value is intermediate between the densities of surface rocks on the Moon and Earth and much smaller than the mean density of Mercury (see Table 1). This may have important consequences from the point of view of identifying the internal structure of Mercury. A summary of the results obtained in radar observations of the Moon and Mercury (and of Mars and Venus as well) is presented in Table 3.

Approximately 40 percent of the surface of Mercury was photographed in 1974 from the flyby trajectory of the Mariner 10 spacecraft at resolutions from 4 km to 100 m (in some areas). This enabled us to see Mercury approximately as well as the Moon can be seen using ground-based telescopes (see Fig. 5).

The most obvious characteristic of the surface of Mercury is the large number of craters. At first glance, this seems similar to the Moon. Indeed, the morphology of the craters is similar to that of the lunar craters, and there is no doubt that they are of impact origin. Most of the craters have a well-defined wall and traces of ejecta formed from materials fragmented during impact, accompanied in many cases by characteristic bright rays and a field of secondary craters. Many craters show a central peak and terrace structure on the inner slope of the crater wall. These properties occur not only in all large craters with diameters greater than 40-70 km (as on the Moon), but also in a much larger number of smaller craters.

The extent to which craters have been eroded and smoothed out is also different from the situation on the Moon. Clear ray structures indicate that the craters are only slightly eroded; however, some craters have rims that are barely discernible. Craters on Mercury are generally shallower than lunar craters, a fact that can be explained by assuming a larger kinetic energy for the infalling meteorites due to the greater acceleration of gravity on Mercury than on the Moon, so that impact craters fill with ejecta more rapidly. This is also why the secondary craters are closer to the central crater than on the Moon, and ejecta blankets mask the primordial topography to a lesser extent.

Just as on the Moon, on the basis of relief, we can identify generally rough "continental" areas and much smoother "maria" on Mercury. The maria are predominantly basins, although there are many fewer than on the Moon, and they are generally no larger than 400-600 km in size. Moreover, some of the basins are poorly defined against the background of the surrounding relief. One exception to this is the Caloris basin, which resembles the well-known Mare Imbrium on the Moon. In the predominantly continental portion of the surface of Mercury, we can identify regions with high crater density and a high degree of crater degradation as well as extensive regions occupied by old inter-crater highlands, indicating that volcanism was once widespread. These are the oldest relief forms on the planet. The flat areas in the maria and adjacent regions were formed at a later epoch, as indicated by the low density of relatively fresh (mostly small) craters in the plains. The flat surfaces in the basins are obviously covered by the thickest layers of pulverized rock—regolith. Definite evidence has been obtained concerning the volcanic origin of most of the basins; however, this volcanism occurred at a later time than the volcanism which formed the inter-crater highlands. These regions of Mercury seem to be roughly analogous to lunar maria (and the plains of Mars) in morphology and age. This period corresponds to the end of the most intense phase in the bombardment of the planets (after the accumulation phase) by large bodies, which in fact caused volcanism and led to the formation of the maria.

The unique steep rupes—scarps or escarpments—are characteristic indicators of tectonic activity on a global scale. These rupes range from 20-500 km in length and from a few hundred meters to 2 km in height. They differ in morphology and surface distribution from the usual tectonic rifts and faults observed on the Moon and Mars and were probably formed by overthrusting and stratification caused by stress in the surface layer associated with the shrinking of the planet. Some crater walls shifted and this shift was probably due to the decrease in the size of the craters, which occurred as the total crustal area of the planet shrank. Existing estimates are that there has been a total shrinkage of 100,000 km^2, equivalent to a decrease of 1-2 km in the radius of Mercury. This process had enormous consequences for the formation of the planet's topography. We can conclude from this that the crustal shrinkage occurred during the formation of the maria as Mercury cooled, some 4 billion years ago.

D. Venus

Radio methods are the most effective means of studying Venus, which is surrounded by a dense gaseous envelope and clouds that are opaque at visible wavelengths. The window of transparency for radiation emitted by the surface or for probe radiation of any kind is limited: radio waves with wavelengths between 10 cm and 10 m pass virtually unimpeded through the venusian atmosphere, while considerable absorption is observed at longer and shorter wavelengths. Unexpectedly, the first estimate of the radio brightness temperature of the surface of Venus (T_B), obtained in the 1950s, proved to be unusually high and provided the first evidence for a hot atmosphere.

At radio wavelengths, we can study both the reflective properties of the surface and altitude differentials, and such studies have been performed from the Pioneer spacecraft as well as from the surface of the Earth. However, the most effective technique is radar mapping, with the so-called "side-looking radar" method based on the Doppler effect, used on the Venera 15 and 16 and Magellan spacecraft.

It was found that, on the whole, Venus is a rather flat planet: almost 90 percent of the surface lies within ± 1 km of the mean level, which corresponds to a radius of 6051.5 km (Fig. 6). Extensive highlands, which may be compared to the continents on Earth, are concentrated in the equatorial region (Aphrodite Terra, Beta Regio) and in the northern hemisphere (Ishtar Terra).

There is no doubt that the surface of Venus was formed

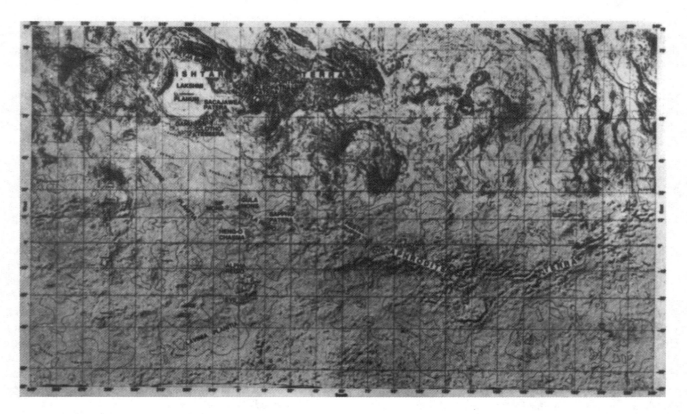

Fig. 6   Map of Venus at latitude 65 S-78 N, compiled from data from radar mapping (Venera 15, 16) and Pioneer Venus altimetry.   The largest plains are Aphrodite Terra and Ishtar Terra. (Saunders, R.S., Arvidson, R.E., Head III, J.W., Schaber, G.G., Stofan, E.R., Solomon, S.C., An overview of Venus geology. *Science,* **April 12, 1991, vol. 252, p. 250. Copyright 1991 by AAAS.)**

primarily as a result of extensive volcanic activity and tectonic deformation of the crust. Vast areas with approximately constant radio reflectivity are occupied by extensive volcanic plains, with low mountain ranges, hills, depressions, and ridges. These were probably formed by basaltic lava outflow. The morphologically more complex rolling plains are marked by thousands of volcanic cones several kilometers in diameter, many with summit pits. Impact craters are often present in these regions; however, there are no more than 150 of these, and the lower threshold of their diameters is ~3 km, which can be explained by the screening effect of the atmosphere for smaller meteoroids (projectiles). Due to fragmentation by the atmosphere, larger projectiles sometimes form chains of craters. Craters greater than 15-20 km in diameter show a clear central peak. The zones of rough ejecta on the flanks of the craters are also obviously associated with the effects of the atmosphere (Fig. 7).

The signs of powerful deformation of the surface resulting from tectonic and volcanic/tectonic activity reflect different types of disruptions (dislocations) of the primordial crustal strata. These deformations can be classified as linear fold fault forms; systems of chaotic disruptions in the form of extended ridges and grooves resembling a parquet (tesserae); and unique ring-shaped structures ranging from 150-600 km in diameter, which are composed of concentric ridges and troughs and are

called "coronae." A typical representative corona is the Nightingale Corona in Atalanta Planitia (Fig. 8). This feature consists of a massive ring-shaped wall (annulus), with a fragmented trough extending around its outside base. It is crossed by a series of short transverse fractures and covered in spots by shallow volcanos and lava, which obviously flowed from the crest of the wall onto the surrounding plain. There are smaller structures of this type, also with traces of lava flow, resembling gigantic spiders and called arachnoids.

The extensive area of linear folded structures in the form of a system of almost parallel ridges and valleys, from 5-10 km to 30-50 km wide, corresponding to folded mountain belts on Earth, form the mountain systems of Maxwell Montes, Freyja Montes, and Akna Montes in Ishtar Terra (Fig. 9). These systems surround the enormous Lakshmi Planum volcanic plateau, which is approximately equal to Tibet in size with two flat-bottomed craters approximately 150 km in size, resembling the calderas of the shield volcanos on Mars in its central region. The altitude of this mountainous region is no lower than 4-5 km, and the crests that surround it are several kilometers higher. It is separated from the surrounding plains by steep escarpments. One of the peaks toward the center of the Maxwell massif reaches an altitude of 11.5 km above the mean surface level, exceeding the highest peak on Earth, Mount Everest, by a factor of 1.5. The enormous Cleopatra

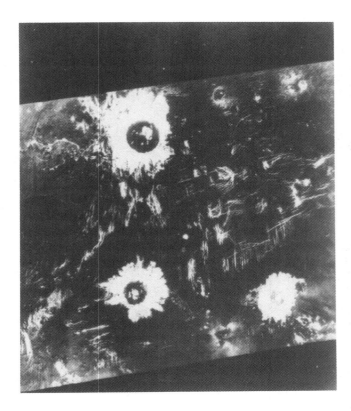

Fig. 7 Impact craters on the surface of Venus in the southern hemisphere with fragmented ejecta on the slopes (from results of Magellan radar mapping). (Photograph courtesy of NASA.)

impact crater, 95 km in diameter, with another crater 55 km in diameter inside it and almost a kilometer deeper, is located on the slopes of this mountain.

Areas of regional tectonic deformation—tesserae with systems of intersecting extensional ridges and grooves—are particularly widespread in a number of regions of Ishtar Terra, Tethus Regio, Tellus Regio, Leda Regio, and others. They are sometimes crossed by fractures (cracks) due to crustal spreading caused by internal stress. These structures are younger than the ancient plains and are hypothesized to have formed as a result of horizontal displacements of surface strata several kilometers thick with respect to local elevations. Characteristic traces of plastic deformations suggest an analogy with systems of transform faults in the vicinity of oceanic rift zones on Earth.

Structures resembling rift zones are also characteristic of the Beta Regio, the size of which is approximately 2000 × 2300 km, in which fault forms (Devan Kazma) are combined with large shield volcanoes (Theia and Rhea). This region was probably formed as a result of volcanic uplift and subsequent extension of the lithosphere. Here, as on Aphrodite Terra, there is a strong positive correlation between long-wavelength topography and gravitational anomalies, suggesting the high depth of isostatic compensation for the uplift.

This in turn attests to the close association between forma-

tion of topography and convective processes in the mantle. It has been hypothesized that the higher surface temperatures of Venus have led to hotter magma rising to the crust from the upper mantle. As a result, there is more intense melt of the substance of the crust, and it thickens more during the subsequent cooling in the areas of intrusion (zones of mantle upwelling). Depending on the size of the mantle "plumes," either large features like Beta Regio are formed, or comparatively small formations of coronae, without analogs on other planets. Thus, unlike the ringed basins on the Moon, Mercury, and Mars, resulting from the ebb and flow of magma at the site of impact craters, coronae most likely are magma structures originating later, during the formation of the tectono-volcanic complexes of the surrounding region.

The most fundamental question about the morphology and origin of the topographical features on the surface of Venus is whether it is possible to associate them with processes of global plate tectonics, such as those that occur on Earth. At present it is difficult to give an unambiguous answer. However, a number of intriguing features have been discovered on Aphrodite Terra; for example, the equatorial mountain massif 3.5-4.5 km in altitude, extending for 16,000 km (Fig. 10). In this region, especially its western portion, several features resemble those characteristic of divergent boundaries of lithospheric plates in the mid-oceanic ridges on Earth, which are centers of spreading. On Venus, however, these morphostructures are more complex, particularly the subparallel linear faults, which occur at an angle to the spreading axis. These and certain other differences may in principle be attributed to both the different pattern of convective movements in the mantle of Venus and the significantly greater flexibility of the lithospheric plates that respond to these movements and undergo substantially greater deformation.

On the basis of these ideas, one might conclude that the equatorial regions of Venus have the youngest crust, and that crust age increases with distance from the spreading axis in the direction of moderate and high latitudes. The plastic deformations associated with extension and deformation of the crust have a strong effect on relief, causing redistribution of tectonic stress. At the same time, processes of partial submersion occur, extending for almost 40,000 km in zones of linear deformation (ridge belts), resembling subduction zones on Earth.

Evidently, the geological activity of Venus continues, and the age of its crust may be estimated to be between 0.45 and 1 billion years. The lower limit corresponds to the mean age of the Earth's crust, whereas the upper is significantly below the age of the crust of the remaining smaller inner planets (≈ 3.5 billion years). Thus, Venus without a doubt resembles Earth more than Mars (not to mention the Moon and Mercury), since intensive tectonic activity on Mars was completed during the phases of formation of giant shield volcanos and canyons probably no less than 1.5 billion years ago.

Important information about the nature of Venus' surface was provided by photographic panoramas, transmitted first from the Venera 9 and 10 lander spacecraft, and then by

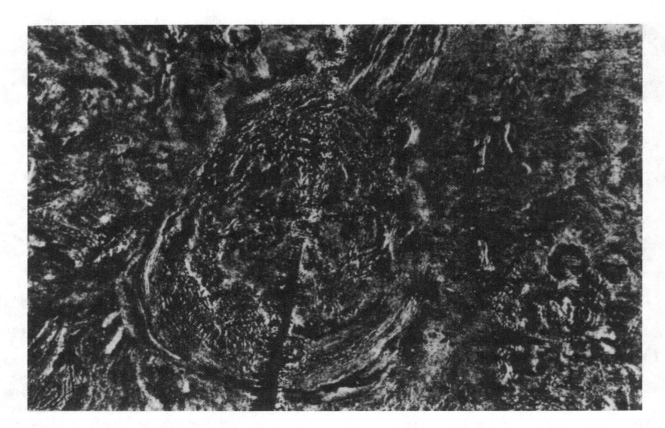

Fig. 8   An example of an annular structure—the Nightingale Corona—600 km in diameter on the Atalanta Planitia.   These and other similar topographic forms were formed by concentric grooves and ridges, providing additional evidence for powerful tectono-volcanic processes in the geological history of Venus (from Venera 15 and 16 data). (Photograph courtesy of the U.S.S.R. Academy of Sciences.)

Venera 13 and 14. These images of landing sites close to the Beta Regio clearly show the stratified horizontal layering of the rock, with the width of individual layers no greater than several centimeters and the number of layers reaching 10 and more (Fig. 11). This suggests cyclic deposition of layers (possibly with different chemical composition) on the surface of the material; in other words, processes of sedimentation. The sources of these processes may be volcanic eruption followed by deposition of the ejecta (ash) on the surface, or stratification of magma flows. It is not impossible that the products of sedimentation are tuffs, such as those well-known on Earth, corresponding in composition to igneous basalt rock.

Synthesized color images have indicated that the surface of Venus has a reddish-orange color when observed in visible light. This color is due to the diffuse incident solar radiation, which is reddish because of the much higher absorption and scattering of blue light by the dense atmosphere.

Information on the chemical composition and physical and mechanical properties of the surface rocks is extremely important for understanding the geology of Venus. The mean value obtained for the dielectric permittivity of the venusian surface from radar data, $\varepsilon = 4.5$ (see Table 3), implies an estimated density of 2.5 g/cm^3, much higher than that for the Moon or various regions of the martian surface. This value of

permittivity corresponds to dry silicate rocks such as basalt. The mean radio reflectivity of the venusian surface is in good agreement with a model involving reflection from a stony conductive surface having a thin coating of fine-grained material with low conductivity. However, in a number of the highland regions (Maxwell Montes, Sif, etc.), the reflectivity was considerably higher, $\varepsilon \geq 25$, suggesting that the surface layer has an unusually high level of electrical conductivity.

Direct measurements of the composition of the surface rocks by the Venera and Vega landers confirmed these ideas. The measurements were made with gamma-ray spectrometers, which determined the natural radioactivity of the rock by recording the intensity of hard gamma radiation in several characteristic lines of uranium (U), thorium (Th), and potassium (K) from the radioactive decay of these radionuclide elements, which are present in the crust of a planet. The intensity ratios derived make it possible to identify the rocks with respect to their petrochemical composition. Table 4 summarizes information about the composition and U and Th ratios of various rocks of the Earth, Moon, Venus, and Mars. The table also identifies various families of igneous rock, including analogs of terrestrial basalts.

This conclusion was confirmed by measurements of the elemental composition of venusian soil performed using X-

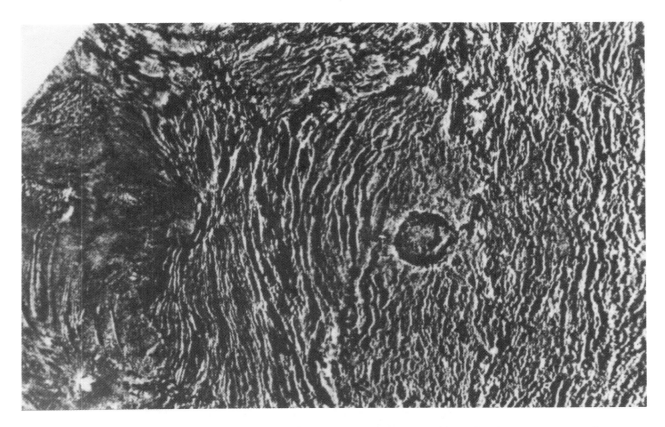

Fig. 9 A fragment of Ishtar Terra with the Maxwell Montes. The entire region is an enormous high-land, rising among the basalt plains. The mountain ranges that embay it, Freyja and Akna Montes (from the west), are examples of linear folded fault structures due to tectonic processes. The highest point in Maxwell Montes is 11.5 km, the Cleopatra crater on its slope has a diameter of 95 km (based on results of Venera 15 and 16 radar surveys). (Photograph courtesy of U.S.S.R. Academy of Sciences.)

ray radiometry on the Venera 13 and 14, and Vega 2 landers (Table 5). In the Beta Regio, rocks were discovered that were potassium-rich, high-magnesium alkaline basalts, as well less acid toellite basalts. The first type is an igneous rock consisting mainly of potassium feldspar and plagioclases. It is fairly rare on Earth, found mainly on islands and on the continental rifts of the Mediterranean Sea. The second type is a common component of the oceanic crust of the Earth and of ancient lava flows on the Moon. Rocks measured on Aphrodite Terra, in a typical area of gradual transition from rolling plains to highlands, also are of this type.

It is striking that samples of venusian rock have high sulfur content. Thermodynamic computations of mineral composition suggest that high sulfur level is consistent with current ideas concerning cyclical processes of surface-atmosphere interactions. Erosion of basic and acid rocks should lead to high accumulations of sulfur, which can reach a level of 10 percent by mass. A sulfur-calcium compound, anhydrite ($CaSO_4$), has been identified as the most likely candidate.

To summarize, the basalt rocks that make up a large part of the Earth's crust are also characteristic of Venus. This in turn suggests that the relationship between continental crust and widespread outflows is similar on all of the Earth-like bodies

in the solar system: the Moon, Mercury, Mars, and Venus. However, the surface of Venus is believed to be more uniform than that of the Earth with respect to structure and morphology as well as chemical composition. The point is that the basalt melts that make up the crust of water-poor Venus obviously did not undergo any significant metamorphosis; thus, there should be much less variety in the surface rocks on Venus than on Earth, where the situation was quite different.

Data on the basic physical and mechanical properties of the surface of Venus are presented in Table 6. The measured densities of the surface rocks in several regions of the planet, in general agreement with radar estimates, range from 1.2 to 2.7 g/cm^3.

E. Mars

The traditional interest in Mars has long been fed by illusions resulting from the inaccurate interpretation of ground-based optical observations with limited spatial resolution (on the order of 500 km). Such exotic phenomena as the "seasonal variation in plant cover," "canals," etc., were discussed, although the validity of these terms was questioned even before space missions had begun. Global mapping of Mars

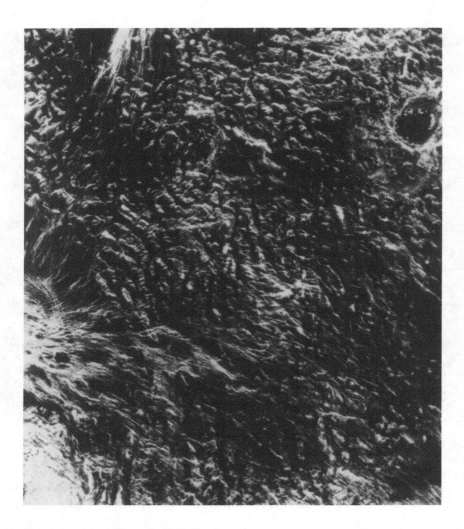

Fig. 10 A photomosaic of the Ovda region in the western portion of Aphrodite Terra, which extends for approximately 600 km. The predominant geological forms are alternating large- and small-scale systems of ridges with isolated rises. The grooves between these ridges are filled with dark material, probably outpourings of basalt lava. To the left is an impact crater. Photograph taken from Magellan. (Photograph courtesy of NASA.)

from spacecraft enabled us to obtain images of the surface to resolutions of a few hundred or even (in some rare areas) a few dozen meters. This finally allowed us to find out what the bright and dark features on the disk of Mars really were, to determine what caused the periodic changes in their outlines and contrast, to understand how real the boundaries between other barely observable spots were, and to get a good look at the polar caps.

The major regions and features of the martian topography are shown on the map in Fig. 12. The difference in the altitudes of the mean surface level due to the asymmetric nature of the figure, as noted above, is quite visible in the surface morphology: plains predominate in the northern hemisphere, whereas cratered regions predominate in the southern hemisphere. Large (over 2000 km in circumference) basins ("maria"), such as Hellas Planitia, Argyre Planitia, Amazonis Planitia, and Chryse Planitia, as well as elevated plateaus ("continents") such as Tharsis Montes, Elysium Mons,

Thaumasia, etc., are visible. The latter are similar in size to terrestrial continents and rise some 4-6 km above the mean surface level (R = 3394 km).

The maria and continents have different surface reflectivities due to the characteristics of the surface material, which largely consists of loose fines with different dominant particle sizes. Comparison of the albedo of the martian surface as a function of wavelength against laboratory reflection spectra of terrestrial rocks in the visible and near infrared indicates that the dark regions probably consist of basalt fines with grain sizes greater than 0.5 mm, while the grain sizes in the bright regions are less than 0.05 mm. Satellite measurements of the Th/U ratio and elemental composition of the soil at the Viking landing sites proved to correspond to igneous basalt rocks with a higher iron and lower silicon content (Tables 4 and 5). This indicates that the differentiation of substances in the interior of Mars was less complete than on Earth. The mean density of the surface layer of soil, determined from satellite-

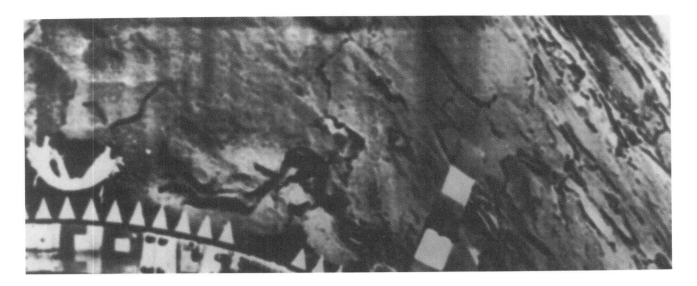

**Fig. 11 Fragments of a panorama of the surface of Venus, transmitted from
Venera 13 and 14 landers. (Photograph courtesy of U.S.S.R. Academy of Sciences.)**

based measurements using infrared radiometers (1.5-2 g/cm³),
was confirmed by the results of analyses of the depth to which
the legs of the landers penetrated the ground and of operations
with the surface sampling system (1.2-1.8 g/cm³). These
values are much higher than the rock density on the Moon, but
somewhat lower than those for Venus.

The temperature of the martian surface shows strong
seasonal and diurnal variations—as much as 100 K. However, the diurnal variations decrease quite rapidly in amplitude with depth—the amplitude decreases by nearly a factor
of 3 for every 5 cm increase in depth, which means that that
there is virtually no temperature variation at depths of a few
dozen centimeters. This shows that martian soil has very low
thermal conductivity, and this has a significant effect on the
meteorology of the planet.

The physiography of the martian surface shows a wide
variety of types of relief. In addition to large cratered regions,
there is direct evidence of tectonic and volcanic activity in the
form of characteristic volcanic cones and faults, the juxtapo-
sition of comparatively young structures and comparatively
old structures, and traces of various types of erosion and
deposition processes.

Impact craters, concentrated primarily in the southern
hemisphere, show varying degrees of obliteration. The degree
of obliteration (especially the breakdown of the crater walls)
can be used to determine the age of the crater and the rate of
the smoothing processes. The craters on Mars are generally
shallower than those on the Moon and Mercury, but considerably deeper than on Venus. The outer slopes of the crater walls
in typical craters generally have slopes of about 10° relative to
the horizontal, while the inner walls have slopes of 20-25°.
The crater floors are generally flat due to filling by eroded
material.

Associated with the dominant relief forms in the northern

hemisphere are active geologic processes. The most prominent features here are signs of volcanism—enormous shield
volcanos with well-defined craters at their peaks. Such
craters are formed when the top of a volcano is destroyed by
violent eruption.

The largest volcanic cones are in the Tharsis Plateau—
Arsia Mons (Fig. 13), Ascraeus Mons, Pavonis Mons, and
Olympus Mons. They reach 500-600 km across the base and
rise some 20-21 km above the surrounding plain. Relative to
the mean surface level on Mars, Arsia Mons, Ascraeus Mons,
and Pavonis Mons have altitudes of 24-26 km, while Olympus
Mons reaches 27 km. The diameters of the craters at the peaks
are approximately 100 km for Arsia Mons and 60 km for
Olympus Mons. No mountain on Earth is of comparable
dimensions.

The lack of impact craters in the regions of Mars where
volcanos are concentrated and the well-preserved traces of
lava flows on the slopes of the mountains suggest that the
volcanos were active until relatively recently (from a few
hundred million to a billion years ago). Evidence of widespread volcanism on the planet is also provided by the well-
preserved traces of lava flows captured in the Viking 2
panoramas. The landing site in Utopia Planitia, a large martian plain, was literally strewn with a multitude of stones with
the characteristic fragmentation and porous pumice-like surfaces. Similar rock fragments from the fragmentation of
pumice lavas occur in the form of friable lumps on Earth.

The numerous faults and rifts in the martian surface, which
form cliffs, grabens, and large canyons with a system of
smaller branching canyons, attest to intense tectonic activity.
They are as much as several kilometers deep, several dozen
kilometers wide, and hundreds or even thousands of kilometers long. The large rift that extends for over 4000 km along
the equator in an east-west direction (Valles Marineris) re-

**Table 4   Thorium and uranium content of various types of rocks
from Earth, Moon, Venus, and Mars**

(Basic data from Surkov, Yu. A. *Chemical Studies of the Planets and Their Satellites*. Moscow, Nauka, 1985, pp. 36 and 48.)

Planetary body	Type of rock	Th, g/metric ton	U, g/metric ton	Th/U
Earth	Ultrabasic	0.08	0.03	2.7
	Toellite oceanic basalts	0.18	0.1	1.8
	Alkali olivine basalts	3.9	1.0	3.9
	Platform plateau basalts	2.5	0.8	3.1
	Geosyncline basalts	2.4	0.7	3.4
	Granites, granodiorites, granite gneiss	15.6	3.9	4.0
Moon	Continental rocks	0.8	0.21	3.8
	KREEP[*]	9.3	2.8	3.3
	High-Ti, high-K maria basalts	3.98	0.68	5.9
	Low-Ti, low-K maria basalts	1.18	0.64	1.8
	High-Ti, moderate-K maria basalts	0.61	0.16	3.8
Venus	High-K basalt rocks (alkali)[‡]	6.5	2.2	3.0
	Low-K basalt rocks (toellite type)[3]	1.5	0.6	2.5
Mars	Volcanic	5.0 ±2.5	0.2±0.14	2.5
	Continental	0.7±0.35	0.2±0.14	3.5

[*]KREEP consists of basalts high in potassium, rare earth elements, and phosphorus.

[‡]Venera 8 measurements showed a high level of K (4.0 ± 1.2), while Veneras 9, 10 and Vegas 1, 2 measurements were approximately an order of magnitude lower (0.3 to 0.47)

sembles the rift zones along the mid-oceanic ridges on the floors of the oceans on Earth. Networks of large canyons are partially separated from one another by flat plateaus or flat-topped mountains with steep sides. These mountains are evidently composed of the strongest, most weathering-resistant rocks. These features and the chains of craters were evidently what created the illusion of the "canals" in ground-based observations from Earth—one of the most well-known and attractive hypotheses in late 19th-century and early 20th-century astronomy.

The enormous quantity of fine-grained, sand-like material that is characteristic of the surface of Mars attests to the high efficiency of erosion on Mars. Under water-free conditions, sand carried by the wind (both wind due to local meteorological processes and wind due to global planetary circulation processes) causes periodic variations in the outlines of the dark and light regions, and the dark regions systematically become a few degrees warmer than the light regions. During relatively quiet periods, these fines tend to collect in the depressions, but later are blown out of these regions during periods of strong wind, forming characteristic bright plumes around the edges of the craters oriented to the direction of the wind. This orientation may also be retained for a certain period of time inside the craters, where larger dust and sand particles dominate. Sand dunes resembling those in deserts on Earth have been observed on the floors of such craters. Traces of sand dunes are also clearly visible in the panoramas transmitted from Chryse Planitia (Fig. 14).

Dust transport due to seasonal alterations in circulation patterns and the dynamics of the polar cap explain the well-known "wave of darkening," which used to be attributed to plant growth cycles. When spring comes, this wave propagates from a latitude of approximately 70° toward the equator at a rate of approximately 1 m/s, and reaches it in less than 2

Table 5 Chemical composition of rocks from Venus and Mars, mass percent
(Source: Barsukov, V.L., Surkov Yu.A., et al. Geochemical studies of Venus on the Vega 1 and Vega 2 landers. *Geokhimiya*, 1986, no. 3, pp. 275-288; Clark, B.C., Baird, A.K., Rose, A.J., et al. The Viking x-ray fluorescence experiment: Analytical methods and results. *Journal of Geophysical Research*, 1977, vol. 82, pp. 4577-94; Baird, A.K., Toulmin, P., Clark, B.C., et al. Mineralogic and petrologic implications of Viking geochemical results from Mars: Interim results. *Science*, 1976, vol. 94, pp. 1288-1293.)

Venus

Element (oxide)	Venera 13	Venera 14	Vega
MgO	11.4±6.2	8.1±3.3	11.5±3.7
Al_2O_3	15.8±3.8	17.9±2.6	16.0±1.8
SiO_2	45.1±3.0	48.7±3.6	45.6±3.2
K_2O	4.0±0.63	0.2±0.07	0.1±0.08
CaO	7.1±0.96	10.3±1.2	7.5±0.7
TiO_2	1.59±0.45	1.25±0.41	0.2±0.1
MnO	0.2±0.1	0.16±0.08	0.14±0.12
FeO	9.3±2.2	8.8±1.8	7.74±1.08
SO_3	1.62±1.0	0.88±0.77	4.7±1.5
Cl	<0.3	<0.4	<0.3
Na_2O	2.8±0.5	2.5±0.4	0.2

Mars

Element (oxide)	Viking 1 Sample I	Viking 1 Sample II	Viking 1 Sample III	Viking II
MgO	8.3±4.2	-	8.6	-
Al_2O_3	5.7±1.7	-	5.5	-
SiO_2	44.7±5.3	44.5	43.9	42.8
K_2O	0.1±0.1	0.1	0.1	0.0
CaO	5.6±1.1	5.5	5.6	5.0
TiO_2	0.8±0.3	0.8	0.8	1.0
Fe_2O_3	18.2±2.9	18.1	18.7	20.3
SO_3	7.7±1.3	9.4	9.5	6.5
Cl	0.7±0.3	0.8	0.9	0.6

Table 6 Physical characteristics of Venus rocks and terrestrial analogs (Kemurdzhian, A.L., Brodskiy, P.N., et al. Preliminary results of measuring the physicomechanical properties of the venusian soil using the Soviet Venera 13 and 14 stations. *Kosmicheskiye Issledovaniya*, 1983, vol. 21, no. 3, pp. 323-330.)

Experiment	Venera 13	Venera 14
Measurement of the physical properties of rocks with a penetrometer	Load-bearing capacity 2.6-10 kgf/cm^2 (heavy clays, densely packed sand grains)	Load-bearing capacity 62-250 kgf/cm^2 (volcanic tuffs, fractured rocks)
Study of the dynamics of lander impact	Load-bearing capacity 4.5-5.0 kgf/cm^2 (foam concrete)	Load-bearing capacity of layer above 5 cm depth 2 kgf/cm^2, at greater depth 4.0-5.0 kgf/cm^2 (packed sand, foam concrete)
Analysis of the operation of the soil sample collector	Packed volcanic ashfall tuff	Packed volcanic ashfall tuff
Analysis of the TV panoramas	Laminated igneous rocks partially covered by loose soil	Laminated igneous rocks sedimentary in nature

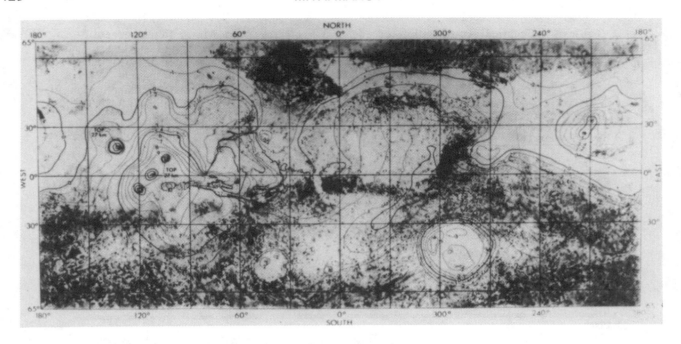

Fig. 12 Topographic map of the surface of Mars for the latitude band of ±65°. The isolines showing altitude differential are at 1 km intervals. The 0 point for altitude corresponds to a surface level with atmospheric pressure of 6.1 mbar. The heavily cratered, old, and generally higher surface of the southern hemisphere contrasts to the more level, younger surface of the northern hemisphere. The two highest regions with shield volcanoes are Tharsis (0°, 105°W) and Elysium (30°N, 210°W). (Reprinted from: Wu, S.S.C. Mars Synthetic Topographic Mapping. *Icarus*, 1978, vol. 33.)

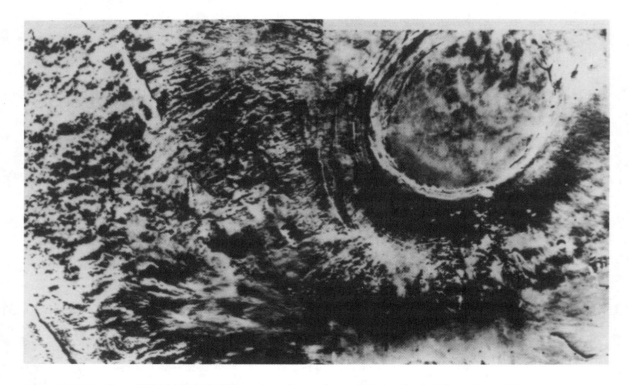

Fig. 13 One of the largest volcanoes on the surface of Mars, Arsia Mons, has a diameter greater than 500 km at the base, with caldera diameter of 120 km and height of 27 km. Radial texture formed by ancient lava outflows is faint. (NASA photograph 211-5170.)

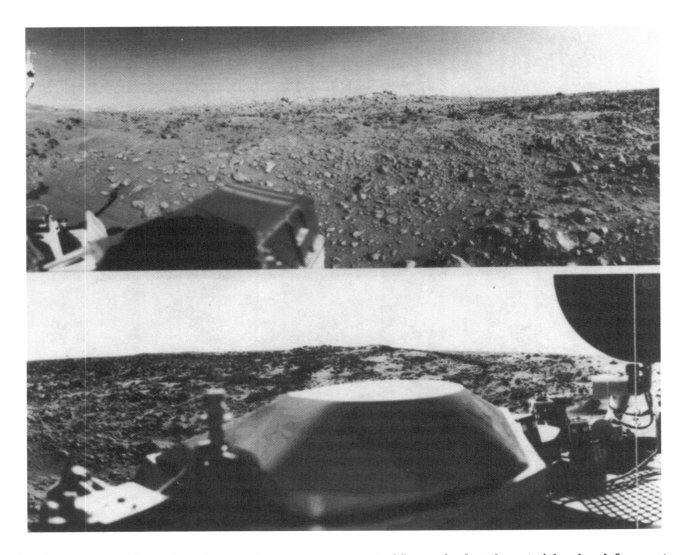

Fig. 14 Panorama of the surface of Mars. Among the abundance of fine-grained sandy material and rock fragments (top picture), there may be areas of bedrock, right foreground (Viking 1 photo). (NASA photograph 76-H-557.)

terrestrial months, covering a distance of more than 4000 km. By summer, when the polar cap has reached its minimum size, the dark band reaches 40° latitude in the opposite hemisphere; by fall, when the polar cap has begun to grow, the dark band rapidly shrinks, and the "maria" become brighter.

The abundance of dust and the intensive dust transport also explain albedo variations and the lack of any well-defined relationship between relief features and reflectivity on the surface of Mars, as well as the low soil density in a number of regions of the planet (as indicated by the large range of variation in ε—see Table 3). Intense local dust storms (called dust devils) sometimes occur. The situation becomes global in scope during the periodic planet-wide dust storms—a colossal natural phenomenon in which the dust is carried to an altitude of 10 km or more and the entire surface of the planet is shrouded in a featureless yellowish haze.

Long, branching valleys hundreds of kilometers in extent, which morphologically resemble dried-out riverbeds, and smooth ravines with traces of destruction of rock and scouring of the surface (exaration) have been observed on Mars. These characteristic configurations, present mainly on the ancient surface of the southern hemisphere, attest to the effectiveness of water and ice (fluvioglacial) erosion during an early period of martian history, more than 3.8 billion years ago. At the same time, the surface of the planet was furrowed by flowing water, which created riverbeds with meanders and a well-developed tributary system, as well as valles, along which glaciers moved (Figs. 15 and 16), although the nature of this drainage system is still not clear. In particular, we cannot yet answer the questions of: what mechanism was primarily responsible for the formation of valley systems (sapping or run-off); how far the channels flowed; (especially, if we assume climatic conditions were cold); and what volume of erosion is implied.

The decrease in altitude in the direction of flow for these ancient rivers from source to discharge also indicates that the

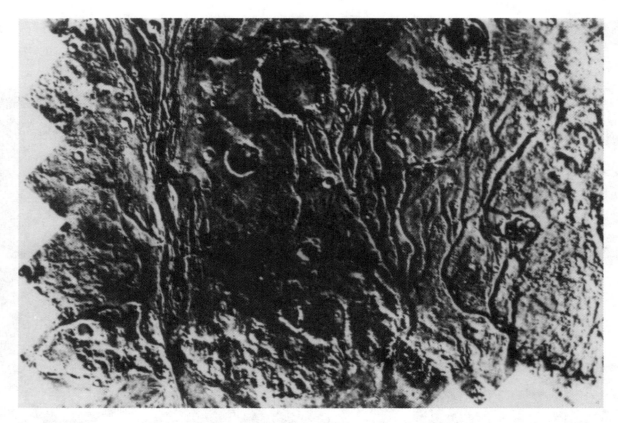

Fig. 15 Meandering dried river beds on the surface of Mars—the Vallis Maja and Vedra, crossing old, heavily cratered landscape (approximately 300 km shown in the photograph) between the regions Luna on the left and Chryse on the right (Viking photo). (NASA photograph 211-5190.)

numerous riverbeds present today (of which there are estimated to be tens of thousands) were originally carved by water flow. Some of these riverbeds extended between depressions in cratered regions of the surface, which apparently served as local water reservoirs. It is possible that predominant precipitation of carbonate due to binding of carbonic acid from the atmosphere in the carbonate-silicate cycle occurred in these paleolakes, possibly involving the participation of microorganisms (by analogy to the Earth). For this reason, such sediments are of high-priority interest to exobiologists. For example, the Gusev crater, located south of Apollinaris Patera (14.6S; 184.6W), which is probably filled with fluvial deposits from a river that flowed into it, and areas of transition from ancient topography, with traces of water-filled depressions, to young plains are likely to be promising from this standpoint. Such areas are naturally considered promising future landing sites.

The fundamental geochemical laws governing the exhalation of water from the interiors of planets during the course of thermal evolution long ago suggested that the bulk of the water on Mars (estimated as between ~1 and ~30 percent of the water on the Earth) would be concentrated in a layer of permafrost near the surface, especially in deposited layers and large basins such as Hellas Planitia. It is not impossible that, due to the geothermal temperature gradient within these

basins, temperatures under the ice layer could have been sufficient to maintain the water in liquid form, while it is not clear how large the geothermal heat flow was and what its current level is.

A number of pieces of evidence favor the existence of extensive regions of permafrost on Mars. In particular, these include certain valleys that have depressions on their flanks similar to those in karst areas on Earth (Fig. 17), which were most likely formed by the initial exposure and subsequent sublimation of layers of ice (ice lenses) and subsequent liquid water outflow. The regions of chaotic relief on Mars may be similar in nature. They were probably formed by settling of the exterior layers due to loss of subsurface material. It is not impossible that ground ice reservoirs could have been efficiently recharged on a cold planet such as Mars. Also relevant is the unique form of the ejecta blanket on the outer slopes of some craters, resembling a snowslide. Such features, which have no analogs on other planets, may be attributed to melting of subsurface ice on meteorite impact and mud flows down the outer slopes of the resulting crater.

Periodic deposition under permafrost conditions can also explain the morphological characteristics of the surface near the south pole, where several hundred quasiconcentric terrace-like layers formed by rock deposits ranging in thickness from several meters to several dozen meters are observed. It

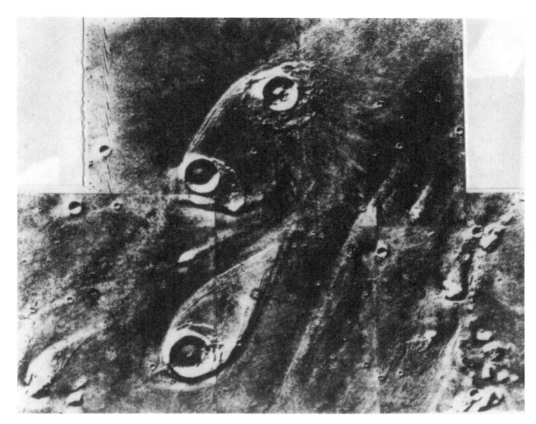

Fig. 16 "Teardrop" shaped islands in the southern Ares Valles, formed by flow of water and/or movement of glaciers around regions of increased density in impact craters (crater diameter ≈40 km). (Viking image, NASA photograph 4A50-54.)

is tempting to associate these structures with the cyclic activity of the ice caps, since the angle of inclination of the planet's axis (see Fig. 2), which strongly controls the intensity of melting in the ice caps, varies. It is possible that successive deposition and melting of the ice cap (accompanied by the formation of "water cushions," and of icebergs that partially smoothed out irregularities in the topography as they moved) occurred within a period of several hundred thousand years.

The iron-rich clays and hydrated metal oxides in the surface layer of Mars may (since they affect the exchange of water between the surface and atmosphere) give Mars its characteristic rusty-red color, similar to that of terrestrial deserts. Viking measurements confirmed that almost 80 percent of the soil probably consists of clay minerals (probably montmorillonite and nontronite) with a high concentration of iron oxides (see Table 5). This soil may have been formed by weathering of ultrabasic magmatic rocks (dunites and basalts) in the dry, nearly oxygen-free atmosphere of the planet.

Additional evidence for the existence of extensive permafrost regions on Mars is provided by the presence of igneous rocks of the palagonite type. Palagonite is a yellow-brown or dark brown glossy mineral that occurs on Earth in basalts,

diabases, and tuffs, especially in polar regions—the tundra of Bolshaya Zemlya, Iceland, Franz Josef Land, and Antarctica. Palagonites are formed when magma interacts with water or erupts through a layer of ice. They are rich in iron and poor in silicon, in precise agreement with the analysis of the elemental composition of martian surface rocks. Moreover, the lower atmospheric pressure means that martian palagonites may have a lower volatile content and weaker structure than terrestrial palagonites.

The white polar caps of Mars consist largely of normal water ice, with some solid carbon dioxide ("dry ice"). Carbon dioxide gas condenses out of the atmosphere at the temperature that occurs at the poles (-125 °C), forming a layer several centimeters thick. This layer vanishes rapidly with the onset of spring, leaving behind a residue (largely consisting of ordinary ice at -70 °C) that does not melt over the summer.

It is also not impossible that the polar caps contain extensive inclusions of clathrate-hydrates. These compounds are formed by the inclusion of molecules of carbon dioxide in interstices in the crystalline structure of water ice; they resemble packed snow. The deposits of condensate within depressions and craters observed in Viking photographs and provisionally called "white rock" may be similar in nature.

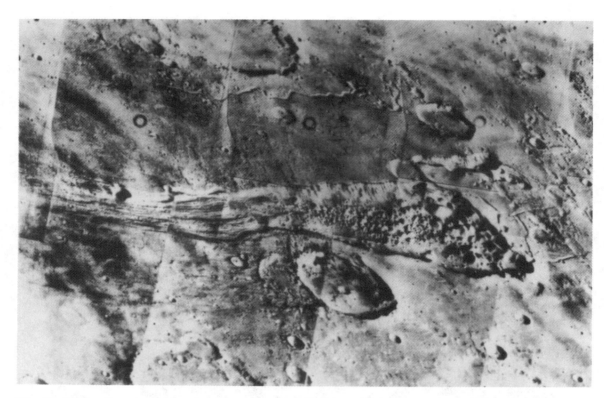

Fig. 17 "Chaos" structure in a martian valley (analogous to the karst type on Earth) probably associated with the exposure and melting of subsurface ice. (Viking photo, NASA photograph P-16983.)

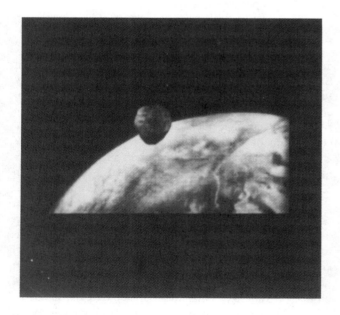

Fig. 18 Mars' moon Phobos seen against the planet. The difference in reflectances shows the extremely low albedo of the moon's material (image from Phobos 2). (Courtesy of the U.S.S.R. Academy of Sciences.)

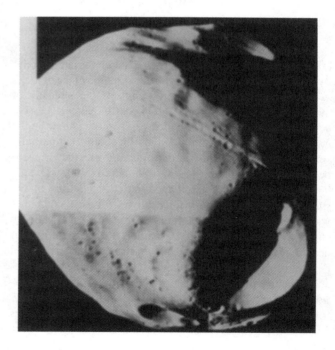

Fig. 19 The surface of Phobos with the largest crater (Stickney), 11 km in diameter with its characteristic linear grooves, possibly occurring when the satellite was formed. (Viking, NASA photograph P-20776.)

F. Phobos and Deimos

Mars's satellites—Phobos and Deimos—are most likely asteroids captured at a certain point in the evolution of the planet, but might also be relics of the last phase of its accretion.

The satellites of Mars have very low reflectivity (albedo less than 5 percent), meaning that they are among the darkest bodies in the solar system (Fig. 18). Carbonaceous chondrites (a small group among the ordinary chondrites, the most common type of stony meteorite) are the most likely low-albedo material; the carbonaceous chondrites characteristically have high volatile content and high porosity. However, measurements carried out by the Phobos 2 spacecraft placed this identification in doubt, since the spectral characteristics of the surface of Phobos between 0.3 and 3 μm turned out to be quite different from those of carbonaceous chondrites. Given the relatively low mean density of the martian satellites (approximately 2 g/cm^3), these data are consistent with the most probable model for the internal structure of the satellites, according to which only the outer layers surrounding a denser core consist of the porous material. In this case the idea of carbonaceous chondrites bulk composition would still hold

The crater densities on the surfaces of the satellites are higher than those on the planet itself. Due to intensive meteorite bombardment, their surfaces are probably covered by a layer of dust. This layer of dust resembles the lunar regolith, but is deeper and less dense than the Moon's, due to the very weak gravity on the two satellites. The low escape velocity (approximately 13 m/s for Phobos and roughly 8 m/s for Deimos) means that one might also expect a higher density of dust particles along the satellite orbits (in other words, dust rings of a kind around Mars).

The surface of Phobos is characterized by several remarkable linear grooves oriented perpendicular to the axis that points towards Mars (Fig. 19). Various hypotheses have been advanced to explain the origin of these structures. The most convincing of these ideas seems to be that they are associated with the formation of the large crater Stickney, which is approximately 10 km in diameter, while their complex morphology can be explained by interaction with the surface regolith. The impact of such a large body clearly would have been catastrophic for such a satellite, nearly leading to its disintegration. [1-3, 5-11, 26, 42,43]

III. Internal Structure and Thermal History

A. Initial Assumptions and Limitations of Models

There is a direct connection between the current appearance of the planets and their satellites and various processes that occurred in their interiors. Ultimately, the features of each planet were determined by a number of general laws and stages in the evolution of planetary material. Current experimental data and theoretical models based on these data have made it possible to advance several well-founded theories of the past and present geology of the planets, as well as to develop some understanding of their internal structural characteristics.

Mechanical properties—mass, size, figure, and rotation—place extremely important constraints on models of internal structure. The mass distribution within the interior of the planet determines its gravitational potential and moments of inertia. Deviations in the density distribution from spherical symmetry and hydrostatic equilibrium reflect features in the internal structure of the planet. Theoretical description of the thermodynamic state of the medium under the high pressures and temperatures occurring in planetary interiors is relevant to this problem. Information on the behavior of matter under extreme conditions can be derived from an equation of state and is based on principles of statistical physics and quantum mechanics used to solve problems in the hydrodynamics of planetary interiors.

The internal structure of the terrestrial planets has the following characteristics: rocks throughout the thickness of the planet, with a liquid core, a partially molten mantle and a solid crust whose surface is imprinted with traces of the geological history of the planet. However, the substantial differences in actual density of the planets (see Table 1) and results of modelling their interiors imply that the initial material in the protoplanetary nebula from which the planets were formed may not have had a uniform chemical composition. The equilibrium condensation model postulates that the decrease in temperature with distance from the proto-Sun led to fractionation into elements, even on a scale of 1-2 astronomical units (AU), due to differences in the temperature of condensation of the hot gas of which the Sun was composed. This is particularly relevant for metal-silicate fractionation, leading to differing concentrations of iron and silicon at different distances from the Sun, as well as fractionation of iron and sulfur (or, more precisely, fractionation of the so-called siderophilic and chalcophilic element groups).

The relatively small amount of material in the circumsolar protoplanetary nebula, from which the planets and asteroids formed, was similar in composition to meteorites, especially the most common of them—chondrites. Meteorites passing through various stages of evolution thus retained information about the "building blocks" of the solar system. The common source material of meteorites and asteroids suggests that the difference in their sizes was due to the fact that their parent bodies themselves were at different evolutionary stages. While the chondrites originated from relatively small, chemically undifferentiated bodies formed by condensation of primordial material at different distances from the Sun, iron meteorites and achondrites are fragments of larger asteroids that underwent a process of interior differentiation.

To facilitate understanding of condensation in the protoplanetary nebula, it is useful to consider the abundance of chemical elements in space. The most abundant and chemically active elements in space are hydrogen, carbon, oxygen, magnesium, silicon, sulfur, and iron (see Fig. 20). The relative iron content would have increased with increasing temperature, due to the loss of silicates (which condensed

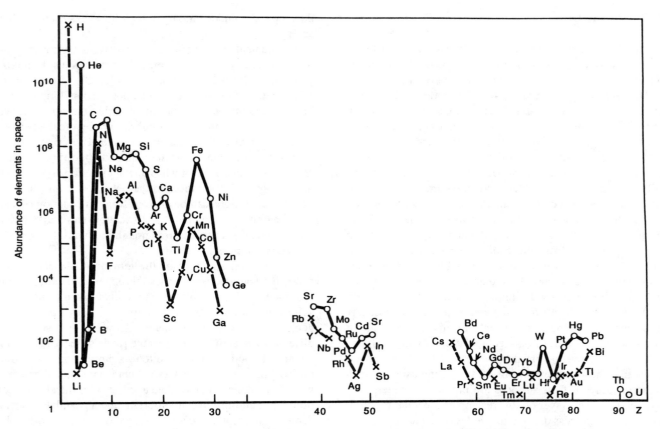

Fig. 20 Relative abundance of chemical elements in space. Solid curve identifies elements with even atomic numbers, Z, and the dashed curve, those with odd atomic numbers. (Reprinted from: Marov, M.Ya. *Planets of the Solar System,* **2nd edition, Moscow, Nauka, 1986, p. 184.)**

out mainly in the form of refractory compounds) and the fact that loss of volatiles causes reduction processes to dominate over oxidation processes. Ordinary iron-rich chondrites are classified as type H meteorites, while iron-poor chondrites are classified as type L meteorites. Enstatite chondrites, which consist mainly of minerals in the magnesium-silicate family-enstatite ($MgSiO_3$) and nickel-iron, are the most highly reduced, while carbonaceous chondrites (type C), where almost all of the iron is bound up in magnetite (Fe_3O_4), are the most highly oxidized. The latter thus are closest to the primordial chemical mixture from which the terrestrial planets and asteroids later formed. They also have the highest content of volatile (atmophilic) elements and are therefore of special interest from the cosmogonic point of view.

It can thus be concluded that iron meteorites and enstatite chondrites, which show the highest level of reduction, were formed primarily at high temperatures (i.e., very close to the Sun—roughly in the vicinity of the orbit of Mercury), while the most highly oxidized meteorites—carbonaceous chondrites—were formed at much lower temperatures (primarily beyond the orbit of Mars). The regions of space corresponding to the orbits of Venus and Earth were characterized by intermediate conditions. The overwhelming majority of the bodies in the asteroid belt (and probably the cores of the giant planets), which are presumed to consist of a mixture of metal

oxides and the hydrated silicates that occur in carbonaceous chondrites, were also formed from chondrites.

According to these ideas, condensation conditions were responsible for the differences in composition and mean density between the various terrestrial planets, and thus for the subsequent thermal evolution of each planet. Radioactive elements (both short-lived and long-lived radionuclides) were included in the high-temperature fraction of the condensed solid particles; these radioactive elements subsequently served as a heat source. This is why these planets experienced such dramatic changes, resulting in compositional differentiation and the formation of secondary gaseous envelopes, or atmospheres.

B. Composition and Internal Structure of Earth

Studying the internal structures of the terrestrial planets is made somewhat easier by using the Earth as a reference object. Earth's interior can be studied by the powerful method of measuring the propagation velocity of seismic waves. This method records variation in elasticity (density) with depth, revealing the basic internal structural characteristics of the body. These characteristics are determined by the chemical composition of the material and by its phase and thermodynamic parameters. This same method has also been effec-

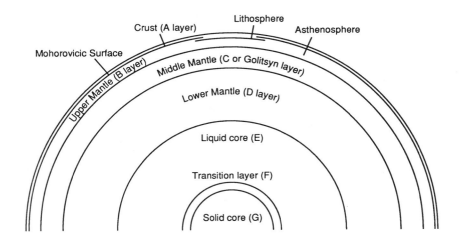

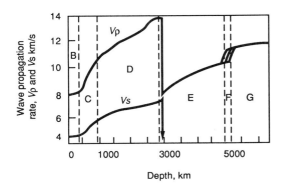

Fig. 21 A model of the interior structure of the Earth and the rate of propagation of longitudinal (V_p) and transverse (V_s) seismic waves. (Reprinted from: Marov, M.Ya. *Planets of the Solar System*, 2nd edition, Moscow, Nauka, 1986, p. 202.)

tively used to study the lunar interior.

Current ideas concerning Earth's internal structure are illustrated in Fig. 21, which identifies the major zones where the propagation velocities of the longitudinal (P) waves and transverse (S) waves change. These waves are called body waves, and originate with seismic energy released at earthquake epicenters as a result of tectonic processes. The velocities of these body waves vary as they move through the Earth's interior and are reflected and refracted at the interfaces between shells with different physical properties.

Each of the Earth's three major shells (crust, mantle, and core) has a number of additional peculiarities (zones) that affect the velocities of seismic waves. The outermost solid shell—the crust—is separated from the underlying mantle by an interface called the Mohorovicic Surface, or Moho. The depth of this interface varies with the thickness of the Earth's crust from 30-60 km under the continents to 5-10 km under the oceans, coming closest to the surface near the axial zones of the mid-oceanic ridges occupied by rift valleys.

The Earth's crust (A layer), formed through partial melting of material from the mantle, consists of typical lithophilic elements with the characteristics of silicate rocks. The most

abundant element (49.13 percent by mass) is oxygen (in metal oxides and silicon oxides), followed by silicon (26 percent), aluminum (7.45 percent), and iron (4.2 percent). These elements have the highest abundance by mass (or abundance ratio). Oxygen, silicon, and aluminum predominate because most of the minerals are silicates and aluminosilicates, i.e., salts of silicic and aluminic acids. Replacement of the hydrogen in the aluminosilicic acid by potassium, sodium, or calcium produces feldspars (the most common mineral), including the well-known sodium-calcium-aluminosilicates (plagioclases). Replacement of the hydrogen in silicic acids by magnesium, iron, and calcium produces olivines, pyroxenes, and amphiboles. The basic crust consists of igneous magmatic rocks—basalts and granites. These rocks can be subdivided on the basis of silicon dioxide (SiO_2) content into acidic rocks (over 65 percent), neutral rocks (52-65 percent), basic rocks (40-52 percent), and ultrabasic rocks (less than 40 percent).

Underlying the crust is the upper mantle (B layer). Its top layer, adjacent to the crust, is sometimes called the substratum. With the crust, it forms the lithosphere, the most rigid shell of the Earth. Below the lithosphere is a nearly molten layer with diminished strength—the asthenosphere. The lower boundary of the asthenosphere lies at a depth of 250-350 km, while the upper boundary comes closest to the surface under the axes of the mid-oceanic ridges. As Fig. 21 indicates, the velocities of longitudinal seismic waves increase at its boundary with C layer, which is called the middle mantle (or Golitsyn layer), and continue to increase all the way down to the boundary of the D layer (the lower mantle), 1000 km deep.

The increased seismic velocities in the C layer are due to phase transitions caused by the restructuring of minerals into modifications with more densely packed atoms. Unlike the crust's acidic and basic rocks, the mantle consists of ultrabasic rocks containing extremely small quantities of SiO_2 in the form of mineral quartz and large quantities of magnesium oxide in minerals of several types. The main rock-forming minerals occurring in the basic and ultrabasic rocks here (basalts, dunites, gabbros, peridotites, diabases, etc.) are iron- and magnesium-containing silicates—olivines and pyroxenes [$(Mg, Fe)_2SiO_4$ and $(Mg, Fe) SiO_3$, respectively]. The primordial mantle of the Earth before differentiation of the planetary material presumably consisted of olivine-pyroxene rocks (so-called pyrolites).

As pressure increases olivines are transformed into a denser crystal modification — the spinel form, starting at about 400 km. Another phase transition is presumed to exist between the spinel zones and perovskite zones (perovskite is a mineral with clear cubic cleavage, i.e., especially close cubic packing) in the middle mantle at a depth of approximately 700 km. Here, a corundum structure might change into an ilmenite structure with aluminum atoms replaced by iron and titanium atoms. Seismic wave velocity continues to increase through the homogeneous D layer (which apparently consists entirely of perovskite), but this is attributable only to its compression under the pressure of the overlying layers and increases in its density.

The pattern of propagation velocities of longitudinal and transverse waves implies that there is an E layer with a liquid outer core approximately 3460 km in radius and a G layer with an inner (or, rather, partially molten) core 1250 km in radius. The entire core has a mass equal to approximately 30 percent of the total mass of the Earth, while the inner core makes up approximately 1.2 percent. This mass distribution is fully consistent with theoretical models of the Earth's interior and the characteristics of the Earth's gravitational potential.

The composition of the Earth's core is apparently similar to that of iron meteorites, and is made up of an iron-nickel alloy (abbreviated NiFe), which is approximately 89 percent Fe, 7 percent Ni, and 4 percent FeS. It is currently believed that the temperature at the center of the Earth is approximately 6000 K with a pressure of 3.65 mbar, while temperature is 4300 K and pressure approximately 1.4 mbar at the boundary between the core and lower mantle.

Obvious physical considerations suggest that the temperature distribution in the Earth's interior should be roughly adiabatic; this result has been confirmed by theoretical model-based calculations in which the main mechanism for heat transfer is convection. At this point, there is essentially no doubt that the Earth's interior (including both the core and the mantle) is in a convective state. The geothermal gradient (directly related to the heat flux from the interior of the Earth) has only been experimentally determined for the topmost layer. The mean value of the geothermal gradient at the Earth's surface is 20 K/km, with substantial variations from one region to another. However, the increase in temperature slows down with depth. The true melting points of the mineral associations at large depths impose certain limitations here. The corresponding temperature variation along the melting curves thus corresponds to the boundaries describing the transition from one modification to another. The presence of well-developed convection in the core is also usually invoked to explain the large magnetic moment of the Earth as being due to electromagnetic induction in a moving medium. According to the hydromagnetic dynamo hypothesis, the motion of the conductive fluid leads to a self-excited magnetic field in much the same way as a current and magnetic field are generated in a dynamo machine with self-excitation.

C. Internal Structure of the Moon

Our model of the structure of the lunar interior also takes into account constraints placed on the interior structure by data on the figure of a celestial body and the propagation of P and S waves. The true figure of the Moon, determined by analyzing the orbits of manmade satellites around it, proved to be close to spherical equilibrium. Analysis of its gravitational potential indicates that the density of the Moon does not vary strongly with depth; i.e., unlike the Earth, the Moon has no large concentration of mass at the center.

The outermost layer of the Moon is the crust. Its thickness has been determined to be 60 km in the basin regions. The crust under the extensive continental areas on the far side of the Moon is probably roughly a factor of 1.5 thicker. The crust consists of crystallized igneous rocks—basalts. However, there are significant differences in composition between the basalts in the continental regions and those in the maria regions. While the oldest continental regions on the Moon consist primarily of light rocks—anorthosites (which consist almost entirely of neutral and basic plagioclase, with small amounts of pyroxene, olivine, magnetite, titanomagnetite, etc.), the crystalline rocks from the lunar maria consist mainly of plagioclases and monoclinic pyroxenes (augites). They were probably formed by cooling of the magmatic melt at or near the surface. Since the lunar basalts are less oxidized than terrestrial basalts, this means that they crystallize with a lower oxygen/metal ratio. Some volatile elements have lower abundances, while many refractory elements have higher abundances than in terrestrial rocks. Olivine and especially ilmenite impurities make the maria regions appear darker; these regions also contain higher density rocks than the continents.

Under the crust, there is a mantle that, like the Earth's, can be divided into an upper, middle, and lower mantle. The upper mantle has a thickness of approximately 250 km, the middle mantle has a thickness of approximately 500 km, and its boundary with the lower mantle lies at a depth of 800-1000 km. Transverse waves have virtually constant velocities above this level, and this means that the interior material is in the solid state, forming a thick, relatively cold lithosphere within which seismic vibrations extinguish relatively slowly. The upper mantle probably consists of olivine and pyroxene, with spinel and melilite, a mineral that occurs in ultrabasic alkaline rocks, at a greater depth. At the boundary with the lower mantle, the temperatures approach the melting points of the materials, which leads to intense absorption of seismic waves. This region is called the lunar asthenosphere. The very center of the Moon appears to have the form of a small liquid core, less than 350 km in radius, opaque to transverse waves. The core may consist of either iron sulfide or iron. In the latter case, the core would be smaller, which is in better agreement with estimates of the distribution of density with depth. The core makes up no more than 2 percent of the Moon by mass. The temperature of the core would depend on its composition, and appears to be between 1300 K and 1900 K. The lower temperature corresponds to the assumption that the heavy fraction of the lunar protomaterial was rich in sulfur, primarily in the form of sulfides, so that a core consisting of Fe-FeS eutectic (with a melting point of 1300 K, which depends only slightly on pressure) was formed. The higher temperature is more consistent with the hypothesis that the lunar protomaterial was rich in light metals (Mg, Ca, Na, Al), which were then included along with silicon and oxygen, in the most important component minerals in basic and ultrabasic rocks—pyroxenes and olivines. This latter hypothesis is also supported by the Moon's low iron and nickel content, as clearly indicated by its low mean density.

D. Models of Planetary Interiors and the Thermal Evolution of Planets

Differentiation of planetary material into a silicate envelope and a heavy, dense core is currently thought to begin as early as the accumulation stage or immediately after it, primarily as a result of gravitational energy of accretion and energy of radioactive decay. Tidal dissipation, heat released during adiabatic compression of the inner layers and in collisions of the bodies that formed the planet, electromagnetic and corpuscular radiation from the Sun, and Joule heating all played important roles as heat sources during the initial phase. However, evolutionary paths differed, primarily as a function of the size of the body (and thus the storage of radioactive isotopes), which determined the structure and thermal regime of the planetary interiors.

The course of evolution is determined by the balance between the intensity of thermal energy production and cooling due to convection and heat conduction. The most important energy source here is the radiogenic heat generated by the long-lived isotopes of uranium, thorium, and potassium (which are lithophilic elements): ^{238}U, ^{235}U, ^{232}Th, and ^{40}K. Short-lived radioisotopes, especially ^{26}Al (aluminum), ^{10}Be (beryllium), ^{129}I (iodine), ^{36}Cl (chlorine), and various transuranium elements such as ^{244}Pu (plutonium) and ^{247}Cm (curium) also could have played important roles in the early stages of the evolution of the primordial planetary material. Since ^{26}Al and most of the other isotopes have half-lives less than 1 million years, these isotopes have all disintegrated by now. However, they appear to have contributed to the rapid heating of large condensed meteoritic bodies and the protoplanets, thereby accelerating the process of chemical differentiation (this explains the fact that meteorites with different compositions are of similar ages). Unlike the heavy-element isotopes, the light isotopes (^{26}Al, ^{10}Be) appear to be supernova explosion products implanted in the protoplanetary nebula.

Formation of the core, mantle, asthenosphere, and lithosphere involves a multistage differentiation process that operates on the constituent material at practically all levels. Since the long-lived uranium, thorium, and potassium isotopes are lithophilic elements with an affinity for silicates, i.e., they can replace atoms in silicon dioxide (SiO_2) crystalline lattices, they will drift upward with the silicates under gravitational differentiation. They therefore accumulate mainly in basic crustal rocks, and their abundance falls off sharply in the less acidic ultrabasic rocks that make up the mantle. The heat generated by these radioactive isotopes is evidently released by radiation from the surface and makes up most of the observed heat flow. Very little of this heat is expended heating material at large depths. This implies that the greater the heat flow, the higher the differentiation in the interior of the body.

It can thus be asserted that when a long time had elapsed after the gravitational differentiation of the interior substance of planets was completed, and in the absence of substance exchange between the upper and lower mantles (as is believed to be the case for Earth), the major sources of internal heat on the planet had to be radioactive substances in the crust and mantle, primary heat, and heat flux from the core to the mantle. Here, radiogenic sources of heat entering the basaltic crust when it melted from the upper mantle were the major sources of heat generation.

The total heat released within the Earth over the past 4.6 billion years has been estimated at approximately 2.5×10^{38} erg, while the total loss due to heat flow at the current value of 61.5-80 erg/(cm$^2 \cdot$ s), or 1.8×10^{-4} cal/(cm$^2 \cdot$ s) would be no greater than 0.54×10^{38} erg. This means that approximately 1.8×10^{38} erg of accumulated heat went into heating and melting the interior of the Earth. Only the core became molten, since almost twice as much energy (approximately 3.2×10^{38} erg) would be required for complete melting at all levels, which means that the Earth did not pass through this stage. This can in turn be taken to imply that the maximum possible mass-averaged initial temperature of the Earth's interior was 1700 K, and that the actual temperature was probably 300-400 K lower.

Figure 22 shows curves calculated for the Moon and terrestrial planets describing the heat release E per unit mass

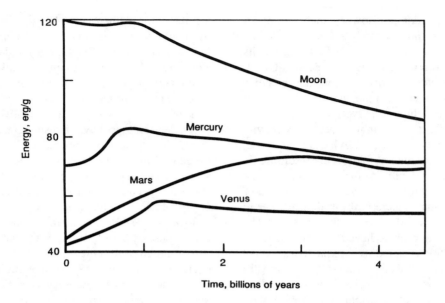

Fig. 22 Total thermal energy as a function of time over the course of thermal evolution for the Moon, Mars, Mercury and Venus. (Reprinted from: Toksoz, M.N., Hsui, A.T., Johnston, D.H. Thermal Evolution of the Planets. *The Moon and the Planets,* **1978, vol. 18, pg. 311.)**

of the planet as a function of time. The changes in the intensity of heat production are directly associated with the evolutionary stages through which a planet passes. On the Moon, this sequence of evolutionary changes, roughly corresponding to the early Precambrian on Earth, shows up most distinctly in the chronology of lunar rocks, thereby enabling us to develop a definite scenario for the formation of the other planets.

1. The Moon

The first stage that can be identified for the Moon is early widespread vulcanism, which brought the light fraction of the melt to the surface and formed the feldspar core beginning approximately 4.6 billion years ago. The remaining irregularities were smoothed after completion of accretion, which was followed by a phase of continuous magmatic activity between 4.0 and 4.4 billion years ago that resulted in the formation of aluminum- and calcium-rich rocks—anorthosites. During this stage, fragmental rocks—breccias—were formed and the magmatic rocks were either partially or completely remelted in meteorite falls and metamorphization of the primordial crust.

The most intense surface bombardment by large meteorites evidently dates back to the formation of the lunar maria approximately 3.9-4.0 billion years ago. The meteorites broke through the thin crust, exposing regions of basalt melt, leading to filling of the resulting cavities and, possibly, some subsequent settling, as well as the formation of local mass concentrations (mascons) associated with anomalies in the lunar gravitational field.

This appears to have been the most intense period in the evolution of the Moon, since it corresponds to the peak in the energy-release curve $E(t)$ in Fig. 22 and the largest scale of

magmatic activity. This was accompanied by a change in the distribution of heat sources with depth due to the fact that silicate magma, rich in lithophilic radioisotopes, was brought to the surface, while the heavier elements sank towards the center. This led to an increase in the temperature of the mantle and its melting. The filling of the lunar maria probably ended some 3 billion years ago. This is consistent with the age of the youngest crystalline rocks brought back to Earth, which were dated at 3.16 billion years. The period of melting was followed by rapid cooling and the formation of an extended solid lithosphere, which is currently estimated to have thickened at a rate of approximately 200-300 km/billion years. The molten region of the mantle was displaced toward the interior, so that the partially molten asthenosphere currently only occupies a region near the center.

2. Mercury

Mercury appears to have undergone a similar evolutionary process. This is suggested not only by the shape of the $E(t)$ curve in Fig. 22 but also by the many topographic features shared by the Moon and Mercury, each of which possess unique examples of extremely old structures little affected by subsequent processes. However, the initial composition of Mercury appears to have been somewhat different at condensation, largely consisting of the relatively high-condensation-temperature iron-meteorite fraction. The mean density of Mercury is indeed much higher than that of the Moon, and only slightly below that of the Earth. However, Earth's density can be explained by the fact that the material in its interior is at higher pressure because of the Earth's greater mass. Thus, in order to have nearly the same density, Mercury must contain a relatively greater fraction of heavy elements.

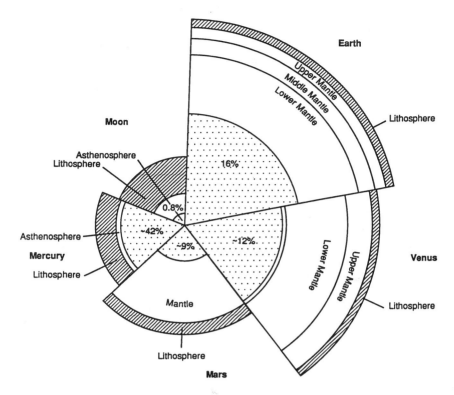

Fig. 23 Comparison of models of the interior structure of planets of the terrestrial group. The relative sizes of the cores are expressed as percentages of volume. (Reprinted from: Marov, M.Ya. *Planets of the Solar System,* **2nd edition, Moscow, Nauka, 1986, p. 223.)**

Considering their cosmic abundances, the most important of these should be iron. The Fe/Si ratio for Mercury is estimated to be three times as large as that for Earth and five times that for Mars.

As indicated by the traces of early volcanism on the surface of Mercury, differentiation probably occurred very early, soon after the end of the initial accumulation phase. The high conductivity of iron (which makes up approximately 70 percent of the planet by mass) may have strongly affected the subsequent thermal evolution of the planet. Current models (see Fig. 23) indicate that the iron-nickel core of Mercury, occupying approximately three-fourths of the planet's diameter (meaning that the core is approximately equal to the Moon in size), should have solidified almost completely some 2 billion years ago. The core is surrounded by a thin mantle, which probably consists of magnesium-silicate rocks of the olivine type. The mantle and upper crustal layer of Mercury form a solid lithosphere with a thickness of approximately 50 km. This thick lithosphere suggests that the tectonic activity of Mercury is currently quite low. However, its longer cooling time suggests that global tectonics and primordial volcanism covered a longer period in the history of Mercury than of the Moon. This then implies that the age of the youngest rocks in the lowland sections of the planet (crater floors and basins) filled with lava outflows should have a minimum age much below that determined for lunar rocks (i.e., less than 3.16 billion years).

3. Venus

The similarity between the geometric and mechanical properties of Earth and Venus at first glance suggests that the major features of their internal structure might also be extremely similar. However, the true situation on Venus is very likely to differ substantially from that on Earth. This difference is primarily due to the strong deviation of Venus's figure from that corresponding to hydrostatic equilibrium. In other words, it corresponds to a rotation rate several dozen times higher than the current actual value. This suggests that the rotation of Venus may have been slowed in the distant past by tidal friction, but was unable for a variety of reasons to reach an equilibrium form consistent with the new period of rotation. This situation suggests a two-layer model capable of supporting the nonhydrostatic loads, probably at the interface between the mantle and core, rather than a model that is homogeneous and elastic throughout the entire interior, as applies to the Earth.

The temperature distribution in the interior of Venus to a depth of ~200 km is associated with an estimated crust thickness that is a function of the amount of material exchange between the crust and the mantle. If the mechanism of plate tectonics exists on Venus, then the thickness of its crust should be approximately the same as that of the Earth's crust (10-30 km); if not, it may be significantly greater (70 km). The heat flux from the interior, which, evidently, is less than that on Earth, is a function of the thickness of the crust (lithosphere). Part of the heat may be released in areas of crustal spreading, although the effectiveness of this mechanism would be diminished by a factor of at least 4-5 compared to that on the Earth. Heat removal due to dispersed vulcanism (i.e., the large number of small volcanos on the surface) is also of low efficiency, and thus the major mechanism is likely to be heat conduction.

The distributions of temperature and pressure in the interior of Venus and the major mineralogical zones seem to generally correspond with those of Earth (Fig. 23). Olivines and pyroxenes dominate in the mantle, and the high-pressure modifications of these minerals dominate at larger depths. An *a priori* estimate of the temperature at the boundary between the lithosphere and mantle of $T \approx 1200$ K (for a lithosphere thickness of 70 km) corresponds to a temperature $T \approx 3500$ K at the boundary between the core and mantle. If the core is in adiabatic equilibrium (i.e., if heat transport in the interior is convective), the temperature at the center of the planet becomes ≈ 4670 K. However, the size of Venus's liquid core and the presence of an inner solid core remain open issues. These questions, in turn, are directly related to the explanation of why Venus currently has no intrinsic magnetic field, if we assume that a magnetic field is generated in the core of the planet by the hydromagnetic dynamo mechanism in the presence of thermal or chemical (crystallizational) convection.

4. Mars

Mars is larger than the Moon and Mercury, and smaller than the Earth and Venus. The characteristic traits of the geological structures on the surface provide good criteria for theoretical evolutionary models and indicate that Mars also underwent early differentiation of its interior material, as revealed by traces of ancient magmatic activity in some of the oldest regions of the surface and the chemical composition of the surface rocks. However, it turns out to be impossible to obtain the high initial temperatures required to heat the central regions to their melting point, if we consider only metal/silicate fractionation of the original material and the overall depletion of iron on Mars, which explain its low density. We evidently must also consider iron/sulfur fractionation and the fact that additional chalcophilic elements were retained at the relatively low condensation temperatures characteristic of the orbit of Mars. This implies that a liquid core consisting of an iron-iron sulfide mixture formed at a relatively low temperature (approximately 1300 K) and corresponding to the Fe-FeS eutectic. Assuming that potassium also went into the sulfide phase, the decay of ^{40}K would mean that radiogenic heat sources were still present.

The significant fraction of the iron bound to sulfur suggests that Mars's mantle is also rich in iron sulfide and that the silicates in the mantle contain more minerals with high iron content than minerals with high magnesium content. The surface rocks have also been clearly observed to be iron-rich. This implies that gravitational differentiation was not as deep and complete on Mars as on the other terrestrial planets. The insufficient free metallic iron gives rise to the high abundance of iron in martian rocks (see Table 5), even though the overall relative iron content of Mars is apparently no greater than ~25 percent, or much less than that of Earth, Venus, and, of course, Mercury. The characteristics of the gravitational potential of Mars also place strong constraints on the extent to which the planet could have been differentiated. These characteristics deviate relatively little from those expected for a homogeneous density distribution; this is consistent with the idea that there is a comparatively small iron sulfide core (Fig. 23). This core is estimated to be approximately 800-1500 km in radius, with a presumed mass equal to 9 percent of the total mass of the planet.

According to the scenario for the thermal evolution of Mars supported by model calculations, core formation began soon after accumulation was complete and lasted for ~1 billion years, which corresponds to the early volcanic period. Approximately another billion years later, a partially molten silicate zone formed in the mantle and slowly expanded inward. This phase was characterized by intense volcanic and tectonic activity and the formation of basalt plains and volcanic shields. At the end of this period (3 billion years ago), Mars reached the peak of its evolution before gradually beginning to cool (see Fig. 22). Over the next 1 billion years, thermal energy was maintained at an approximately constant level, global tectonic activity occurred on a very large scale, and enormous shield volcanos were formed.

Mars continues to cool. The thermal flux from the interior of Mars is currently estimated to be 40 erg/cm$^2 \times$ s, almost a factor of 2 smaller than the mean flux for the Earth. The lithosphere evidently has a thickness of several hundred kilometers, of which approximately 100 km makes up the martian crust. The relatively thick lithosphere suggests that the seismic activity on Mars is currently moderate. This conclusion is supported by Viking data.[1, 12-18, 26, 28, 44]

IV. Atmospheres of the Inner Planets

The atmosphere is the outer gaseous envelope of a planet and reflects various important characteristics of the planet's evolution. The chemical composition, structure, and dynamics of the atmosphere are strongly affected by the position of the planet in the solar system, its mass, and the parameters of its motion. This means that the properties of the planetary atmospheres vary widely, even within the relatively small region of the solar system occupied by the inner planets. The large differences in chemical composition reflect the laws governing the condensation and evolution of the primordial material released from the protoplanetary nebula and the subsequent evolution of the planet as a whole.

A. Chemical Composition

If we compare the solar abundance of the inert gases, which are the most characteristic representatives of the group of

Table 7 Properties of the atmospheres of the inner planets
(Source: Marov, M. Ya. *Planets of the Solar System. Second edition.* Moscow, Nauka, 1986.)

Planet	Mercury	Venus	Earth	Mars
Chemical composition (percent by volume)	$He \leq 20$ $H_2 \leq 18$ $Ne \leq 40\text{-}60$ $Ar \leq 2$ $CO_2 \leq 2$	$CO_2 = 95$ $N_2 = 3\text{-}5$ $Ar = 0.01$ $H_2O = 0.01\text{-}0.1$ $CO = 3 \times 10^{-3}$ $HCl = 4 \times 10^{-5}$ $HF = 10^{-6}$ $O_2 < 2 \times 10^{-4}$ $SO_2 = 10^{-5}$ $H_2S = 8 \times 10^{-3}$ $Kr = 4 \times 10^{-5}$ $Xe = 10^{-6}\text{-}10^{-5}$	$N_2 = 78$ $O_2 = 21$ $Ar = 0.93$ $H_2O = .01\text{-}3$ $CO_2 = 0.03$ $CO = 10^{-5}$ $CH_4 = 10^{-4}$ $H_2 = 5 \times 10^{-5}$ $Ne = 2 \times 10^{-3}$ $He = 5 \times 10^{-4}$ $Kr = 10^{-4}$ $Xe = 10^{-6}$	$CO_2 = 95$ $O_2 = 2\text{-}3$ $Ar = 1\text{-}2$ $H_2O = 10^{-3}\text{-}10^{-1}$ $CO = 4 \times 10^{-3}$ $O_2 = 0.1\text{-}0.4$ $Ne = < 10^{-3}$ $Kr = < 2 \times 10^{-3}$ $Xe = < 5 \times 10^{-3}$
Mean molecular mass		43.2	28.97	43.5
Surface temperature T_{max}, K T_{min}, K	700 110	735 735	310 240	270 148
Mean surface pressure P, atm	10^{-15}	90	1	6×10^{-3}
Mean surface density, g/cm^3	10^{-17}	61×10^{-3}	1.27×10^{-3}	1.2×10^{-5}

atmophilic elements and are not affected by chemical reactions (making them the most stable throughout the evolutionary process) with their abundances in the atmospheres of the terrestrial planets, we observe a large deficit in the planetary atmospheres. Similar depletion of atmophilic elements is also observed in chondritic meteorites. Taking the successive nature of the condensation process in the protoplanetary nebula (as discussed above) into account, this suggests a well-defined concept of the genesis of planetary atmospheres. This concept is based on the assumption that, unlike the atmospheres of the giant planets, the original reducing atmospheres of the terrestrial planets, which included free volatiles, were lost during or at the end of the accretion process. The present-day secondary oxidizing atmospheres were formed from condensed material (in which some of the volatiles were chemically bound or absorbed) during the thermal evolution of the planets by outgassing from the interior, mainly in volcanic eruptions.

Table 7 presents the basic data concerning the chemical composition, temperature, pressure, and density of the atmospheres of the terrestrial planets. The chemical compositions of the atmospheres of Venus and Mars (which are dominated by carbon dioxide) are easier to understand in terms of the outgassing concept than the nitrogen-oxygen atmosphere of

Earth. The latter is usually explained by assuming that photosynthesis upon exposure to solar radiation (which led to the presence of free oxygen in the atmosphere) played a dominant role in the evolution of the primitive reducing atmosphere of the Earth. This in turn led to oxidation of the ammonia and ammonia compounds in volcanic gases and the release of free nitrogen into the atmosphere, which, due to its weak chemical activity, does not interact directly with the surface rocks, and, furthermore, has a high threshold of dissociation.

A photosynthetic origin for oxygen can be ruled out for Venus and apparently Mars as well. Moreover, the composition of volcanic gases can be used to explain the presence of halogens in the form of compounds of fluorine and chlorine with hydrogen ("acid smoke," which is generally given off in copious quantities along with sulfur dioxide and hydrogen sulfide by volcanic craters and fumaroles on Earth). These gases are then washed out of the Earth's atmosphere by rain or dissolved in the oceans, where they combine chemically with solid material in the crust or form thermal springs for underground water. On Venus, these gases react much less effectively with the surface. As far as sulfur compounds are concerned, the chemical reactions involved in the formation and maintenance of equilibrium in the clouds of Venus (which

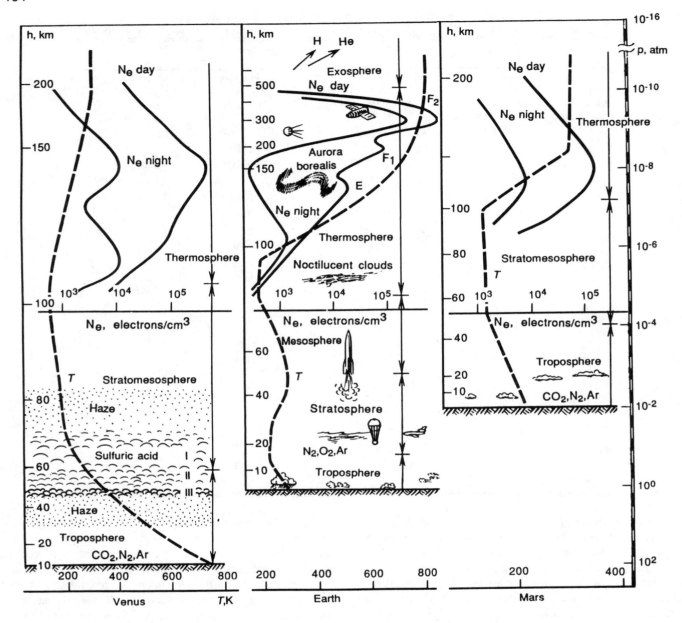

Fig. 24 Structure of the atmospheres of Venus, Earth, and Mars For each planet the figure shows profiles of temperature and electron density in the ionosphere and cloud structure as a function of altitude and pressure. (Reprinted from: Marov, M.Ya. *Planets of the Solar System.* 2nd edition, Moscow, Nauka, 1986, pp. 198-199.)

are primarily sulfuric acid) play the dominant role in removing them from the atmosphere.

The martian atmosphere and the atmosphere of Venus below the clouds are characterized by a low relative water vapor content—water vapor is present at the hundredths or thousandths of a percent level. However, on Venus there may be one or two orders of magnitude more water in the cloud deck. Approximately 80 percent of the H_2O in the martian atmosphere is concentrated in a surface layer a few kilometers thick, and (unlike Venus) the water vapor content varies by nearly two orders of magnitude, depending on season, latitude, and time of day. The atmosphere is driest during the winter at high latitudes and wettest above the polar regions in summer. Isolated regions of increased moisture content at middle latitudes have also been observed on Mars, along with an overall decrease in the water content during dust storms.

B. Temperature and Pressure

The atmospheric structures of Venus, Earth, and Mars are shown in Fig. 24. In this figure, the most characteristic regions have been identified by analogy with the Earth, from the troposphere at the surface (where meteorological processes occur) to the thermosphere and exosphere (where shortwave

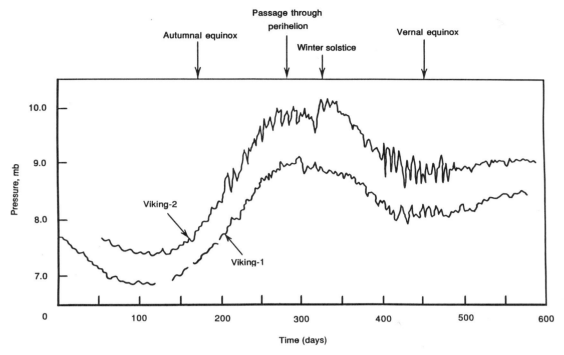

Fig. 25 Seasonal variations in atmospheric pressure of Mars due to CO_2 exchange between the atmosphere and the surface (condensation-evaporation) from measurements on Viking landers (Reprinted from Levy, C.B., Mars meteorology. Annual Review of Astronomy and Astrophysics, 1979, vol. 17, p.389, © 1979 by Annual Reviews, Inc.)

solar radiation is absorbed and aeronomic processes occur). The boundary between the troposphere and stratomesosphere is called the tropopause and that between the stratomesosphere and thermosphere is called the mesopause.

Direct measurements of the temperature and pressure in the atmosphere of Venus show that the temperature and pressure at the surface are 735 °C and 90 atm (at the mean level corresponding to a planetary radius of 6051.5 km). Venus's troposphere is several times thicker than the Earth's—approximately 70 km thick—and its temperature gradient is close to adiabatic. On the whole it is stably stratified, with a few regions of convective instability and turbulence between 30 and 50 km. Because of its enormous heat content, diurnal variations in temperature do not exceed 1 K. However, they become several times greater in the upper troposphere and stratomesosphere, in the region of clouds.

The association between temperature and latitude is much stronger: between 40 and 60 km altitude, the atmosphere becomes colder in the direction from the equator to the pole; the latitude variations are less than 10 K in the atmosphere below the clouds, but increase to 10-30 K at cloud level. As latitude increases, the boundary of the tropopause decreases by several kilometers.

The latitude variations are more complex in the stratomesosphere and include inversion layers—the deepest inversion layer occurs immediately above the upper boundary of the cloud layer at high latitudes. This is the coldest region—the "polar collar"—surrounding the pole and centered at an altitude of 65 km and a latitude of 65°. It divides the atmo-

sphere into two regions: below ~70 km, as latitude increases, temperatures drop; but between ~70 km and 90 km, on the contrary, they increase. On the dayside the temperature minimum (mesopause) lies at an altitude of approximately 100 km at a temperature of 160-180 K, above which in the thermosphere the temperature increases to $T \approx 400$ K. On the night side, on the other hand, temperatures continue to decrease at these altitudes, called the cryosphere, to $T \approx 100$ K.

In the rarefied martian atmosphere, the thermal differences at the surface are quite sharp (unlike those on Venus and Earth), and the temperature profile shows strong diurnal and seasonal variations of as much as 100-150 K. Because of the low thermal inertia of the soil and the low heat capacity of the atmosphere, as well as the lack of any surface water reservoirs to assist in smoothing out diurnal temperature contrasts, the surface temperature turns out to be close to its radiative-equilibrium value at each point on the planet's surface. In the northern hemisphere, the mean temperature of the mid-latitude atmosphere at the surface is 200-220 K by the end of summer, with the daytime temperature of the atmosphere being 10-15 K lower than that at the surface. The situation at night proves to be the reverse, because the surface cools more rapidly than the atmosphere. The maximum temperature recorded (during the summer afternoon) at the Viking lander sites was 244 K, and the surface temperature was above the freezing point of water, while the minimum temperature was 188 K. The temperature at high latitudes is still lower, dropping below the CO_2 phase transition (148 K at a pressure of 6.1×10^{-3} atm) during the winter at the poles, and atmo-

Table 8   Structure and microphysical properties of the clouds of Venus

[From data obtained in nephelometer measurements on Venera 9-14 (Marov, M.Ya. et al., Study of the structure of the clouds of Venus using nephelometers on Venera 13 and Venera 14. *Kosmicheskiye Issledovaniya*, vol. 21, no. 2, 1983, p. 277.)]

Layer	Altitude range, km	Effective particle radius, μm	Number of particles per cm^{-3}	Index of refraction	Optical depth τ	Mass density ρ_a, $mg \cdot m^{-3}$
Upper	65-58	1.0-1.4	200-350	1.46±0.01	3-20	1-3
Middle	57-53	1.7-2.5	250-350	1.35±0.02	10-26	5-11
Lower	52-49	1.7-0.9	50-150	1.41±0.01	5-12	~2
Haze beneath clouds	48-35	0.15	2	1.70	<3	—

spheric CO_2 freezes. The greatest temperature variations are those occurring in the boundary layer near the surface (which is from 4 to 6.5 km thick). This is the region where most of the convective activity is concentrated—during the daytime, the thermal mechanism for the excitation of convection is roughly an order of magnitude more efficient than in the Earth's atmosphere (per unit mass). In contrast, convection turns out to be completely blocked during the night (this is virtually never observed on Earth) by the formation of a surface inversion layer having a positive temperature gradient.

The amplitude of the variations decreases rapidly with altitude. A value of approximately 6.1×10^{-3} atm (or 6.1 mbar, which corresponds to the triple point in the phase diagram of water) is assumed for the mean level surface on Mars. The surface pressure varies from ~0.5×10^{-3} atm at the peaks of volcanic cones to ~10^{-2} atm in depressions. Condensation of CO_2 gas at the winter polar cap is an additional factor that leads to the well-defined pressure variation with season in the martian atmosphere (Fig. 25). This variation has an amplitude of 3 mbar, with the deeper minimum corresponding to CO_2 condensation at the southern polar cap (at the end of northern-hemisphere summer before the fall equinox) and the shallower minimum corresponding to condensation onto the northern ice cap (at the end of northern-hemisphere winter). This change in pressure is associated with restructuring of the circulation system, whereas the local fluctuations reflect changes in the overall wind regime, including the onset of dust storms.

The temperature profile as a function of altitude in the martian atmosphere shown in Fig. 24 corresponds to mean conditions (equatorial latitudes in the afternoon). The temperature gradient during the day is nearly adiabatic from the surface to altitudes of 20-30 km, and the atmosphere is approximately isothermal at higher altitudes (i.e., in the stratosphere), with isolated inversion layers. Carbon dioxide can condense here, just as at the poles. However, martian clouds have water ice crystals as their main constituent and lie at lower altitudes, in the troposphere. The position and temperature of the mesopause are approximately the same on Mars as on Venus; the dayside exospheric temperature is ~350 K, but shows much smaller diurnal variation.

The upper limit to the atmospheric pressure on Mercury is ~2×10^{-14} atm (density 10^{-17} g/cm³). This corresponds to conditions in the terrestrial atmosphere at approximately 800 km altitude and places Mercury in the same class as the Moon, which has an extremely rarefied gaseous envelope of similar density and composition. This implies that the exosphere (the region where the particle mean free path is much larger than the radius of the planet, leading to dissipation of atoms and molecules into space) is in direct contact with the surfaces of these bodies. The solar wind (which supplies protons and α-particles in addition to heavier elements such as Ne, C, O, etc.) obviously plays the dominant role in the creation and maintenance of the mercurian atmosphere. Continuing evolution of volatiles (primarily helium from the radioactive decay of uranium and thorium) from the planetary crust may also make some contribution. Because of the large difference between the dayside and nightside temperatures (see Table 7), the mercurian atmosphere is markedly asymmetric. The intrinsic magnetic field of the planet makes an additional contribution to the asymmetry. Most of the direct interaction between the solar wind plasma and the surface of Mercury (as well as atmospheric replenishment) occurs in the so-called polar cusps in the dayside polar regions. Charged particle streams due to acceleration in the magnetosphere also play an important role. (This is discussed in more detail in Section VI.C.)

C. Sulfur Cycle on Venus

The phase transitions of minor atmospheric species are responsible for the formation of clouds. The clouds of Venus are a unique phenomenon in the inner planets. Their main constituent is a concentrated sulfuric acid solution (75-80 percent) in the form of small droplets, also containing a small amount of polymerized crystalline sulfur. Three main cloud zones occupy a wide region from an altitude of 48-68 km. Including the haze above and below the clouds, this altitude range covers the region from 35-90 km. Despite the low density of the clouds, this creates a total optical depth of $\tau \approx 30$ in the visible region of the spectrum, and, together with the dense atmosphere, prevents the surface of the planet from being seen. This unbroken blanket of clouds (with no visible gaps) is made up of two particle fractions with mean diameters of 2 and 4 -5 μm (see Table 8).

The sulfur cycles in the atmosphere of Venus are controlled

by competing photochemical and thermochemical gas-phase reactions, with most of the sulfur existing in the form of SO_2 and SO_3 oxides (and probably the SO radical). The chemical processes involved in the formation of the H_2SO_4 aerosols are closely related to the reactions that lead to the photolysis of CO_2. These reactions are probably catalyzed by radicals containing hydrogen and chlorine. A fast atmospheric sulfur cycle (based on oxidized forms of sulfur) and a slow one (which also includes reduced forms) have been identified. The sulfur reaction chains are closed through a very slow geological sulfur cycle.

The fast atmospheric cycle includes all the photochemical reactions in the atmosphere above the clouds and within the cloud layer, and can be represented by either of two alternative reaction schemes. In the first scheme, most of the oxygen is produced by photolysis of CO_2, and the OH and HO_2 (hydroxyl and perehydroxyl) radicals act as catalysts for the oxidation of SO_2 to SO_3; these radicals are in turn produced in the photodissociation of HCl. In the second scheme, the oxygen required for oxidation of the sulfur-containing gases to SO_3 comes directly from SO_2, which undergoes photolysis in the atmosphere above the clouds. This process produces elemental sulfur as a by-product. Both of these reaction schemes (shown in Fig. 26) are consistent with the observational data; i.e., the much lower SO_2 and H_2O content of the stratosphere relative to the troposphere.

The concentrated sulfuric acid condensates formed within the cloud layer undergo thermal decomposition at altitudes of 47-49 km and temperatures of 365-380 K, and this determines the position of the lower boundary of the cloud layer. The fast cycle is probably closed in the atmosphere below the clouds, where SO_3 is reduced to SO_2 by reactions involving CO. The maximum residence time for SO_2 molecules in the fast cycle is estimated at several years.

The slow atmospheric cycle occurs in the lower atmosphere, and involves processes associated with the reduced forms of sulfur-containing gases (H_2S and COS), as well as elemental sulfur in the gas phase and in condensed form. The atmosphere above the clouds and the cloud layer itself are considered sources of H_2S and COS, either oxidized to SO_3 by molecular oxygen or undergoing photodissociation. Elemental sulfur is formed either by photolysis of H_2S and COS or by oxidation of H_2S in the presence of CO and S_2O and the HS and H radicals. Sulfur production has been associated with the intense absorption of ultraviolet radiation in the upper cloud layer. This cycle may be partially closed by thermochemical reactions in the troposphere below the clouds. The residence time for atomic sulfur in the slow atmospheric cycle is estimated to be at least 10 years, in view of the fact that the maximum lifetime for oxidized sulfur (H_2SO_4 aerosol) in the fast atmospheric cycle has also been calculated to be 10 years.

The full system of atmospheric reactions is closed by reactions with minerals in surface rocks. In this third (geological) cycle (Fig. 26), we start from the assumption that the surface rocks contain the mineral pyrite (FeS_2) and that the reduced sulfur-containing gases H_2S and COS were initially

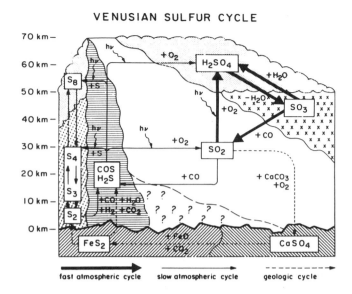

VENUSIAN SULFUR CYCLE

Fig. 26 Sulphur cycle on Venus. Zones of stability and relative concentration of the major sulphur-containing components are indicated by the position and size of the corresponding shaded areas, for each such component. The sequence of transformations in rapid atmospheric, slow atmospheric and geological cycles are indicated by heavy solid arrows, fine solid arrows, and dotted arrows, respectively. (From: Lewis, J.L., Prinn, R.G. *Planets and their Atmospheres. Origins and Evolution.* New York, Academic Press, 1984, p. 160; reprinted courtesy of R.G. Prinn.)

outgassed and then converted into SO_2, which is also formed through the decomposition of the sulfuric-acid aerosol in the clouds. However, as theoretical calculations show, if the surface and atmosphere of Venus are in chemical equilibrium, SO_2 cannot be the dominant sulfur-containing component. Thus, surface thermochemical reactions should lead either to the incorporation of SO_2 into anhydrite $CaSO_4$ and thus into the surface rocks, or to the reverse transformation of SO_2 into other reduced forms, such as H_2S and COS.

Thus, H_2SO_4 and elemental sulfur are probably formed in a common cyclical process. The dominant processes in the clouds involve the production of particles by photochemical oxidation of SO_2 and hydration of SO_3 at the upper boundary of the cloud layer, followed by condensation of H_2SO_4 all the way down to the base of the cloud layer. Below this level, the condensate decomposes and SO_2 is regenerated. The conversion of SO_2 into S and H_2SO_4 depends on the concentrations of water vapor and oxygen. The most likely mode for particle condensation on drops of H_2SO_4 involves gas-phase sulfur allotropes. These processes lead to the absorption of solar ultraviolet radiation and the formation of contrast features (so-called "ultraviolet clouds") on the disk of Venus. The most likely absorbent here (in addition to SO_2) is amorphous sulfur formed as a by-product of the sulfur cycle in the atmosphere and clouds.

D. Thermal Regime and Dynamics

The thermal regime and dynamics of the atmosphere form the basis for the meteorology and climate of a planet. Heat input to the atmosphere is the result of incident solar radiation, and is a constant nonadiabatic factor. The energy production and energy loss, which depend on the divergence of the heat flux, determine the nature of heat exchange in the medium. In a state of radiative equilibrium (e.g., in the stratosphere), the incoming flux of solar energy is approximately equal to the rate of atmospheric cooling due to infrared radiation. In a state of radiative/convective equilibrium (in the troposphere), on the other hand, the incoming solar energy flux at each level of the atmosphere is balanced by the total heat outflow due to thermal radiation and convective transport. These two states can serve as local approximations to the overall heat transport pattern on a planetary scale, where dynamic processes (especially circulation) play a key role.

The greenhouse effect, which leads to deviations from local equilibrium, plays an important role in heat exchange in the tropospheres of Earth, Venus, and Mars. This effect is due to the fact that the atmospheric transparency is different for incoming solar radiation and the outgoing thermal radiation reradiated by the surface and atmosphere, leading to heating of the lower troposphere, which then has a temperature greater than the equilibrium temperature of the layers at higher altitudes. In other words, the atmosphere (and clouds) prevent the outgoing radiation from leaving, and the excess heat is redistributed by various kinds of motions. The additional tropospheric heating at the surface is approximately 30 K for the Earth, insignificant in the current atmosphere on Mars, and nearly 500 K on Venus. This is due to the modification of the absorption band structure of carbon dioxide, water vapor, and sulfur dioxide by the high temperatures and pressures, so that the greenhouse effect plays a much more important role.

Planetary dynamics reflect the balance between the rate at which potential energy is generated by solar radiation and the rate at which kinetic energy is lost due to dissipation. From this point of view, the atmosphere of a planet is frequently compared to a heat engine in which the equatorial regions serve as heat sources and the poles serve as cold reservoirs. This engine has low efficiency—no more than a few percent. Thus, motion on various spatial scales is due to a lack of equilibrium between the incoming and outgoing energy in various regions of the planet (although overall thermal balance is strictly observed on a global scale). The wind system on a planet depends on whether the thermal effects have a period shorter or longer than the rotation period of the planet itself, as well as on the characteristic time scales for thermal relaxation. Substantial differences of this type are observed between the Earth, Venus, and Mars, and affect the characteristics of the mechanisms for thermal balance and dynamic exchange on the planetary, intermediate, and local levels.

The simplest way to think of the circulation pattern on the Earth is as follows. Thermal expansion causes air that has been more intensely heated and is thus less dense to rise, while cooler, heavy air moves downward. Differentials in solar heating lead to pressure differentials (pressure gradients) and heat transport associated with the flow of air masses. A giant closed convective cell (Hadley cell) is formed along the meridian, with hot air transported from the equator to the poles in the top half of the cell and cold air transported from the poles towards the equator along the surface.

In reality, this type of symmetric flow with respect to the equator does not exist on Earth or any other planet, because of the Coriolis force due to the planet's rotation. In atmospheric dynamics (and on Earth, also in the ocean) a key role is played by the horizontal component of this force, which causes air flows to deviate to the right in the Northern Hemisphere and to the left in the Southern Hemisphere. This severely limits the extent of the meridional circulation. In the Earth's atmosphere, the Hadley cells dominate only at the lowest latitudes (approximately 30° on each side of the equator). In the high- and mid-latitude atmosphere, on the other hand, the circulation becomes zonal in nature, with the motion occurring along parallels of latitude. Since these motions are primarily caused by temperature gradients, the winds themselves are called thermal. In the troposphere, we have west winds, which blow from west to east; in the stratosphere, the winds change direction, blowing from west to east in winter and from east to west in summer, with velocities of up to 50-100 m/s observed.

A convenient approximation (which holds for the atmosphere of any rapidly rotating planet) for determining the wind field on Earth is the concept of geostrophic wind (or geostrophic flow). This corresponds to the condition under which the horizontal pressure gradients are balanced by the Coriolis force. The strength of this wind is determined by the pressure gradient and is directed along lines of equal pressure—isobars.

The true circulation is a superposition of several types of motion, and the degree of disorder in these motions is a strong function of the angular rotation velocity of the planet. Wave motions, called Rossby waves, develop on a rotating planet. These waves become unstable as angular velocity increases, and eddies develop as the waves break up. In the Earth's atmosphere, these eddies vary widely in size from a few millimeters to several thousand kilometers in diameter. The small and medium-size eddies form turbulent elements in the atmosphere, while the largest form regions of high and low pressure—cyclones and anticyclones. Their lifetime in the atmosphere corresponds to the estimated rate of conversion for potential energy into kinetic energy (for the Earth, this is on the order of a week). Rossby-wave instability associated with large-scale weather systems is the most effective mechanism for atmospheric mixing in the meridional direction, heat transport from the equator to the poles, and smoothing of temperature differences on the Earth's surface.

On Venus, the Coriolis force has little effect because of the very slow rotation. We therefore have a different situation, governed by the "cyclostrophic-motion condition." This condition has the characteristic that although the temperature decrease from equator to pole does give rise to planetary circulation, the velocity of its zonal component increases with altitude. As a result, the atmosphere appears to be "unwinding" in the direction of the planet's rotation from 0.5-1 m/s at the surface to approximately 100 m/s at the level of the clouds. This type of motion, first observed by the Venera spacecraft, is called atmospheric superrotation, and the circulation pattern itself is sometimes called "carousel" circulation. The velocities in the meridional direction are approximately an order of magnitude smaller and resemble Hadley cells symmetrically distributed relative to the equator.

The superrotation of the atmosphere of Venus is readily apparent in the drift of the "ultraviolet clouds," whose structural features repeat approximately every 4 days (which is consistent with a zonal velocity in the atmosphere of approximately 100 m/s). The cloud configuration also indicates that the motions are ordered and become more and more spiral-like with increasing latitude, leading to the formation of an enormous (cyclonic) eddy around the poles. In this circulation pattern, the air must rise at the equator and descend at high latitudes, leading to the observed warming tendency in the polar regions. As in the Earth's atmosphere, eddy motions on various spatial and temporal scales and turbulence are important elements in the patterns of the atmospheric dynamics on Venus, which is associated with planetary circulation and convective processes.

Planetary circulation on Mars is very different from that in the atmospheres of Earth and Venus. A general circulational model based on the geostrophic balance condition predicts an identical wind distribution at the surface and in the overlying atmosphere in which the prevailing wind blows eastward at high latitudes during the winter, eastward in the subtropics during the summer, and westward elsewhere. The available information on the meridional component of the circulation is less definite. It is assumed that the driving mechanism for this component is associated with the seasonal exchange of carbon dioxide between the atmosphere and polar caps (Fig. 25). Hadley cell-like configurations probably occur at the equinox, with air flowing towards the summer pole at the surface, flowing upward in the summer subtropics, towards the winter pole along a high-altitude return path, and downward in the winter hemisphere mid-latitudes.

The surface topography has a strong effect on the winds. The topography introduces complications into the idealized picture of the dynamic processes in the general circulational model (GCM) description. Topography also induces wave processes that are superposed on the structure of flows on various spatial scales and are associated with the irregularities of the profiles of temperature with altitude in the stratomesosphere. The diurnal and semidiurnal thermal tides also give rise to a variety of dynamic phenomena in the martian atmosphere. One important characteristic of these thermal tides is that, in contrast to the atmospheres of the other planets, they lead to positive feedback between atmospheric heating and dust content, since atmospheric heating leads to stronger convection, increasing the amount of dust in the atmosphere. Dust is a good absorber of heat, and convection is damped. During major dust storms, when this absorption occurs at high altitudes, solar radiation is completely prevented from penetrating to the surface. This leads to tropospheric cooling by a mechanism that could be called the "reverse greenhouse effect." This was precisely the situation observed on Mars during the planet-wide dust storm of 1971. Analysis of this dust storm led to the concept of a "nuclear winter" on Earth.[1-2, 5, 18-19, 21-27]

V. Formation of the Atmosphere and the Problem of Climate

It is now generally accepted that the planets and their atmospheres were formed by the agglomeration of cold material from a protoplanetary gas and dust cloud. A number of models are based on common assumptions concerning particles of dust and gas from which bodies of larger and larger size (planetesimals) were formed as they combined through collisions into the protoplanets. The gas in the protoplanetary nebula may have played a variety of roles in the final phase of the formation process. The accretion of material may have occurred within the gas, or the protoplanetary gas may have been lost before the completion of the formation process, so that accretion proceeded in several stages, including one involving solar-wind particles. Cosmogonic models are invoked to explain not only the accretion process itself, but also the observed ratios between various volatiles, especially the noble gases and their primordial isotopes, which were incorporated in the initial material and then along with juvenile gases evolved into the atmospheres of the planets.

The bulk of the differentiation process on Earth (accompanied by large-scale emission of gas from the interior) appears to have occurred only a few hundred million years after its formation (which has been dated to a period 4.6 billion years ago). Large portions of the atmosphere and hydrosphere were formed during this process. The initial formation of the atmospheres of Mars and Venus probably dates to approximately this same period. However, we can assume that there might have been some differences between the outgassing mechanisms that operated on neighboring planets, since each planet had a somewhat different thermal history due to the different volatiles inventory of each one's mantle and the heterogeneous migration of solutions and melts during melting and formation of the crust. The different physical conditions and the processes through which the lithosphere and atmosphere interacted seem to have played a key role in determining the subsequent evolution of the planets.

A. Formation of the Atmosphere

If we assume that the initial albedo of the Earth was determined completely by the surface and was similar to the Moon's (~0.07), then at current solar luminosity its effective temperature would have been 275 K. At this temperature, beginning with a threshold value of pressure of approximately

5 mbar, the Earth could have retained its water, most of which went into the formation of the oceans. As far as carbon dioxide is concerned, at this relatively low temperature it would have accumulated in the Earth's hydrosphere and sedimentary carbonate rocks, both biogenically through deposition of lime sea organism skeletons and through being chemically bound to metal oxides in minerals from the oceanic crust in the upper mantle. Some of the carbon was deposited in sedimentary rocks in the form of fossil fuels—coal and petroleum. The main nonbiogenic process involves reactions between carbon dioxide dissolved in water and various well-known minerals such as olivines (orthosilicates containing iron and magnesium) and plagioclases/anorthites (aluminosilicates containing aluminum and calcium). These reactions lead to the formation of minerals containing hydroxyl (OH) groups (i.e., hydrated silicates)—serpentine and kaolin. The first of these reactions is thus called serpentinization, while the second is called kaolinization. [The role currently believed to have been played by hydration reactions and the low-temperature phase in the condensation of th eprotoplanetary material should be emphasized. When minerals in the olivine and pyroxene groups react with water vapor, this leads to the formation of the hydrated silicates—such as serpentine, talc, and tremolite—which are most common in carbonaceous chondrites. These silicates in fact serve as the main reservoirs of latent water, which is later outgassed from the planetary interior. This makes it obvious why we must treat the origin of the Earth's atmosphere and hydrosphere as a single unified evolutionary process. This also appears to hold on a qualitative level for the other inner planets, if we ignore any possible differences in the composition of the protoplanetary material during the stage when solar gas condensed into mineral particles of various size and composition. The latter may later have had an effect on the differentiation of the primordial mantle (in particular, on the extend to which low-melting-point, volatile-rich silicate fractions are fused), the formation of the basalt magma, and the accumulation of typical lithophilic and atmophilic elements, outgassed with the basalt magma, on the surface.]

The value given above for the temperature on the early Earth is actually too high, since it does not take into account the increase in the Sun's luminosity soon after its formation, when it moved onto the main sequence in the Hertzsprung-Russell diagram. Current estimates indicate that the increase in luminosity over the past 4.5 billion years has been 25 to 30 percent. The increase in the Earth's albedo as the atmosphere began to form must also be considered. But if the standard model of solar evolution is correct (as opposed to the non-standard mass-losing solar models that are currently also under consideration), then the temperature implied on the young Earth would be below the freezing point of water (even sea water). However, this is in conflict with recent geological and paleontological data indicating that primitive photogenic autotrophs appeared on Earth at least 2.5 billion years ago, and that the oceans were formed even earlier than this. The oldest stromatoliths—layered formations in limestone and

dolomite beds formed by blue-green algae colonies—also date to this same time period.

This contradiction may be resolved by assuming that the Earth's atmosphere during the early Precambrian era contained a relatively small quantity of ammonia (on the order of a few ten-thousandths of a percent) in addition to carbon dioxide and water, and probably also methane and hydrogen sulfide, or by assuming that it contained much more carbon dioxide than the present atmosphere, with an equivalent surface pressure on the order of 60 atm. The required increase in temperature is provided by the greenhouse effect.

If it had an initial albedo comparable to that of the early Earth, Venus would have an equilibrium temperature of at least 325 K, which is above the boiling point of water, up to a pressure of 0.2 atm. Thus, in order to have retained any water, Venus should have had an initial atmospheric density two orders of magnitude higher than that of the early Earth. This is highly unlikely given that the rates of outgassing and atmospheric dissipation for the two planets were virtually identical. A better assumption is that carbon dioxide gradually accumulated in the atmosphere, along with water vapor. This in turn would have led to a further increase in surface temperature and the transfer of more and more carbon dioxide and H_2O into the atmosphere until some equilibrium state was reached. This equilibrium state corresponds to a specific relationship between the mineral phases and volatiles on the surface. The most important of these relationships is that between carbonates and silicates in the upper layer of the planet's crust. In other words, what occurred was a typical characteristic of positive-feedback systems, where an initial perturbation is amplified rapidly rather than damped. For this reason, what occurred on Venus has come to be called the "runaway greenhouse effect.[1]"

Climatic evolution on Mars obviously took a different path. The equilibrium temperature of Mars is much less than zero (centigrade or 273 K), and any water expelled from the interior could have remained on the surface in the liquid state only if the atmosphere were dense enough due to the greenhouse effect and temperature increases. That such conditions existed is demonstrated by traces of early water in the form of numerous ancient river beds. These date to the first billion years of the history of Mars, soon after the major phase of meteorite bombardment. It is not impossible, however, that water basins on the surface could have disappeared completely after the sharp change in climate, which resulted from the sharp decrease in release of internal heat. The final phase of volcanic activity took place during this period. We do not know, however, with regard to the model of the evolution of solar luminosity, which greenhouse gases are likely to have been present in the ancient martian atmosphere and if the equatorial and middle latitude regions of the planet could have been warmer than the rest of the planet. Finally, the attractive idea that the martian climate continued to fluctuate, analogously to the great ice ages on the Earth, with a period on the order of a million years, cannot be totally rejected. Such fluctuations in climate could have resulted from periodic

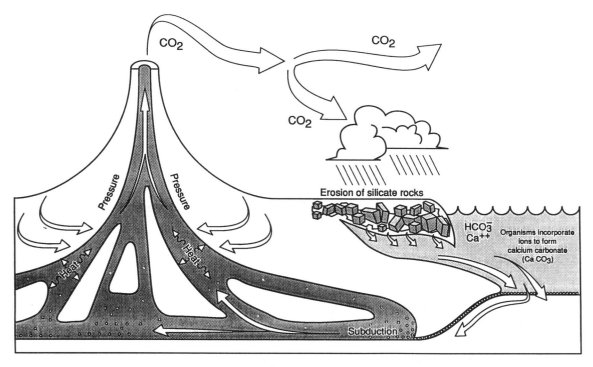

Fig. 27 The carbonate-silicate geochemical cycle. This figure represents CO_2 being removed from the atmosphere when it dissolves in rain and reacts chemically ascarbonic acid (H_2CO_3)with rocks containing calcium silicate minerals. The calcium and bicarbonate ions released by these reactions into the ground water eventually find their way into the ocean, where sea organisms incorporate them to form calcium carbonate shells. These shells are deposited as sediment on the ocean floor, which is carried underneath the continents through subduction. Under the influence of increased pressure and temperature, this sediment (calcium carbonate) reacts with silica (quartz) and releases CO_2, which may then enter the atmosphere through volcanic eruption and certain other processes. The time scale of this cycle exceeds 500,000 years.

variations in the obliquity of Mars, caused by tidal perturbations of the planets and the Sun, and thus changes in insolation at the poles (see Fig. 2). Computations show that a steady state of Mars's atmosphere with a density approximately equal to that of the Earth is possible in principle only when the rotation axis is inclined by at least 4-5° more than it is today.

Most of the carbon dioxide that outgassed during the geological history of Mars appears to be concentrated in carbonate deposits in areas of the ancient water basins, and is also bound in the surface regolith in deposits of finely dispersed dust near the poles, and in laminated plains near the polar caps. Especially large deposits of frozen soil would be expected in the northern polar regions because of the difference in insolation between the martian hemispheres (winter is longer in the northern hemisphere). Since the equilibrium between the amount of adsorbed carbon dioxide and its partial pressure in the atmosphere is temperature-dependent, it seems reasonable that atmospheric density would increase by a factor of approximately 100.

B. Carbon Dioxide and Water

The equilibrium between the carbon dioxide pressure in the atmosphere and the carbonate content of the crust is one of the most characteristic features of the chemical interaction between a planet's atmosphere and lithosphere. Upon reacting with silicic acid, carbonates, of which the most common on Earth are calcites and magnesites (dolomites), give off carbon dioxide gas and form calcium or magnesium silicates (i.e., the calcium and magnesium salts of silicic acid—pyroxenes and amphiboles called wollastonite and enstatite, respectively). On Earth, this cycle is quite rapid in the presence of water. Flowing water washes Ca and Mg cations out of silicate rocks on the surface, and these cations then react with carbonate anions in sea water (Fig. 27). Sea organisms play an important role in this process. Carbonates accumulate in sedimentary rocks, are remelted at great depths in metamorphic processes, and then return carbon dioxide to the atmosphere. One full cycle requires more than half a million years. The carbon dioxide ratio in the atmospheres of Venus and Mars is also controlled by these or similar reactions in most calcium- and magnesium-rich regions of each planet's surface. However, while the carbon dioxide on Earth and Mars is locked in sedimentary rocks, on Venus virtually all of it was evolved into the atmosphere. Indeed, the amount of carbon dioxide locked in the Earth's sedimentary mantle (estimated to be approximately 3.7×10^{23} g) turns out to be comparable to the carbon dioxide content of the venusian atmosphere

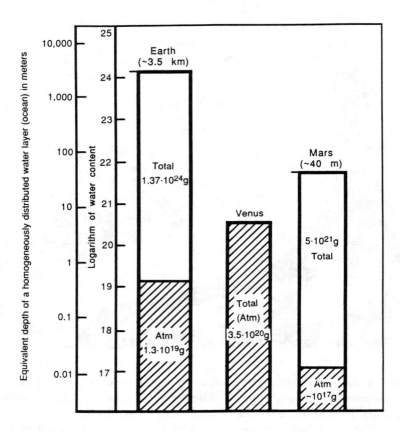

Fig. 28 Ratio of inventories of H_2O (overall and atmospheric) on Earth, Venus, and Mars. Estimates for Venus and Mars are based on analysis of the chemical composition and isotope ratios of atmospheric gases. (Reprinted from Marov, M.Ya. *Planets of the Solar System*, 2nd edition, Moscow, Nauka, 1986, p. 305.)

assuming a temperature of 750 K (4.8×10^{23} g). This temperature thus corresponds to the heating level at which carbonates became unstable mineral forms at the planet's surface and decomposed.

The true situation is somewhat more complex: the interaction processes include, in addition to the carbonate-silicate cycle, a large number of other minerals and mineral associations in equilibrium with the atmosphere and a large number of atmospheric gases, which affect carbonate stability. For Venus, for example, we should include thermochemical reactions with participation of sulfa-containing components, halogens and certain other volatiles, and also the pyrite-calcite-anhydrite buffer reaction, which prevents free oxygen from being present in the atmosphere and at the same time additionally facilitates release of carbon dioxide.

It is more difficult to explain the situation with water. The cosmogenic condensation theory implies that Mars must contain more volatiles than Earth and Venus. However, such ideas are not supported either by the data from chemical analyses of the isotopic composition of the martian atmosphere or soil, or by material from SNC (shergotites-nakhlites-chassignites) meteorites, which are believed to have originated on Mars. These data suggest that the total concentration of outgassed water (in the form of an equivalent layer uniformly distributed on the surface of Mars) would range from

approximately 10 to 100 m thick. At the same time, geomorphological analysis of the structure of troughs formed by streams of water on the surface of Mars suggest that the amount of water could be as much as 0.5-1 km. Thus, there is uncertainty of at least one order of magnitude associated with these estimates.

On Venus, assuming "geochemical congruence" between the processes of interior evolution and outgassing of volatiles on different planets, the amount of water outgassed should be equivalent to the volume of the Earth's hydrosphere (approximately 1370 million km^3, or over 1.37×10^{24} g, which corresponds to the mean depth of the World Ocean of 3.5 km). However, no water can be present on the surface of Venus despite the high atmospheric pressure, since the temperature is above the critical point (647 K). [This assertion also holds for aqueous solutions (brines) for which the critical temperature is somewhat higher than 675-700 K.] As far as the atmosphere is concerned, given a mean relative atmospheric water vapor content of 0.05 percent, the total water content does not exceed 3.5×10^{20} g. This is significantly more than in the Earth's atmosphere (1.3×10^{19} g), but almost four orders of magnitude below its total mass in the hydrosphere. A comparison of the water stores on the three planets is presented in Fig. 28.

It should be noted that, by analogy with the Earth, a certain amount of water may remain in the crust of Venus in the form of water chemically bound in minerals (water of crystallization and water of constitution). The amount of water in the Earth's crust, along with free (gravitational) water, is estimated at from 4-5 percent to 30-50 percent of the mass of the hydrosphere, with approximately 25 percent of the crustal water being in the form of bound water. For Venus this value is probably substantially lower. Analysis of soil from Aphrodite Terra indicates that the rocks of Venus may have been formed from a melt containing water (with 1-1.5 percent H_2O in the original material).

Did Venus have a "primordial" ocean that was lost in the subsequent climatic evolution, or did it form initially as a "dry" planet?

Various arguments in favor of the idea that Venus once had a relatively large hydrosphere can be derived from analysis of the concentration of hydrogen and its heavy isotope deuterium (D) (whose mass is twice that of H) in the atmosphere. The D/H ratio on Venus $[(1.6 \pm 0.2) \times 10^{-2}]$ turned out to be two orders of magnitude larger than in the Earth's atmosphere (on Mars the D/H ratio is only six times higher). This high abundance of deuterium in the atmosphere of Venus can be explained in terms of the isotope separation associated with thermal loss of hydrogen from the atmosphere, where it could have accumulated as water outgassed from the interior (the "primordial ocean"), evaporated, and then been dissociated by ultraviolet radiation. The D/H ratio suggests that the mass of this ocean was a few percent of Earth's. However, the idea that the thermal escape mechanism only operated during the final phase of the process, when the relative concentration of hydrogen in the atmosphere had decreased below a value of roughly 2 percent, implies it may even have been comparable to Earth's. Up to this point, the situation could have been controlled by a different hydrodynamic loss mechanism, in which hydrogen/deuterium fractionation does not occur; furthermore, when the dissipation rate for H atoms is high, they may take other heavier elements with them (blowoff-assisted escape). (This process enables us to explain the fact that the atmosphere of Venus is rich in deuterium, as well as other similar phenomena, such as the loss of sulfur atoms on Io, a satellite of Jupiter, where they may be carried off by a flow of atmospheric oxygen.)

However, other effective nonthermal loss mechanisms based on aeronomic rather than hydrodynamic principles could also explain the D/H ratio on Venus. An example is the 40-percent enrichment of the martian atmosphere with the heavy nitrogen isotope ^{15}N. In this case a process of recharging of hydrogen atoms with hot solar wind protons could have played the predominant role in the separation of D and H. This process is most likely still effective in the current atmosphere of Venus. This concept is consistent with the idea that Venus evolved under conditions of negligible amounts of water, a circumstance that was virtually unaltered throughout the geological history of the planet. This "waterless" model postulates that the source of hydrogen enriched with deuterium could be cometary matter. This is one version of the hypothesis of accretion heterogeneity—the idea that material from various regions of the solar system successively fell onto the planets during their formation.

If, nonetheless, Venus at one time had an ocean comparable to those on Earth, how could such an enormous mass of water have been lost? Several alternative mechanisms have been proposed, including dissociation of water molecules by solar ultraviolet rays; decomposition of outgassed water in a reaction with ferric oxide (FeO); a reduction reaction of water vapor with concurrently evaporated gasses, especially CO-forming carbon dioxide; and cyclic conversion of water in the interior of Venus, with partial thermal dissociation. Each of these mechanisms, however, must confront another difficult problem: how to evacuate from the atmosphere the enormous quantity of hydrogen that would form, the flow rate of which would reach $7 \times 10^{10}/(cm^2 s^1)$, which is three or four orders of magnitude faster than the rate of the current dissipation of hydrogen from the atmosphere of the Earth and Venus.

C. Noble Gases

Data on the abundances of minor atmospheric constituents, especially the noble gases (see Table 7), and the major isotopic ratios are extremely important for determining the evolutionary paths of a planet and its ancient climate, including the issue of the primordial ocean. It is especially important to compare the abundances of these gases in the atmospheres of Earth, Venus, Mars, and in the gaseous fraction of meteorites, since this will enable us to estimate the primordial fractionation during the accumulation phase as well as the amount of outgassing and dissipation of volatiles on the planet over geological time scales.

Unexpectedly, the ratio of the radiogenic isotope ^{40}Ar to the primordial isotopes ^{36}Ar and ^{38}Ar turns out to be approximately equal to unity on Venus, although this ratio is approximately 300 times larger on Earth and 3000 times larger on Mars. Moreover, Venus and Earth have approximately the same absolute abundance of ^{40}Ar, with Mars being roughly an order of magnitude lower. In other words, the atmosphere of Venus has more primordial argon than the atmosphere of Earth and especially of Mars. Although Venus has approximately one-third as much ^{40}Ar as Earth, it has nearly 100 times the ^{36}Ar. The atmosphere of Venus also contains an order of magnitude more neon, although there is little difference between the isotope ratios for the two planets. A similar tendency can also be followed for krypton and possibly xenon, although here the data are not as clear.

Comparison of these abundances for each of the three planets with primordial meteoritic matter—C1 carbonaceous chondrites (Fig. 29)—indicates that all three planets are extremely poor in noble gases. The deficit is especially large for Mars, smaller for Earth, and still smaller for Venus. The lighter the element, the greater the deficit compared to the heavier elements. Venus is closest to the carbonaceous chondrites (especially with respect to Ne and Ar). Moreover, the noble gas abundances on Venus are quite different from

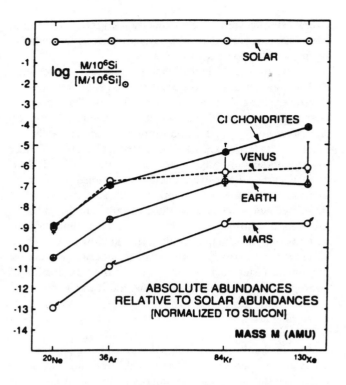

Fig. 29 Depletion of absolute noble-gas abundances in terrestrial planet atmospheres (atoms per 10^6 Si atoms on the planet) and C1 carbonaceous chondrites with respect to solar noble gas/Si ratios. (Hunten, D.M., et al. Planetary atmospheres. In: J.F. Kerridge and M.S. Matthews (Eds.). *Meteorites and the Early Solar System.* Tucson AZ, University of Arizona Press, 1988, © University of Arizona Press.)

the so-called planetary ratio observed on Earth and Mars. While the $^{36}Ar/^{20}Ne$ ratio is approximately the same for Earth and Venus, the $^{36}Ar/^{84}Kr$ ratio for Venus is much closer to the solar value than the planetary value.

An explanation of these facts apparently can be found in the previously discussed sequential nature of the condensation process in that the material in the planets and meteorites was formed at various distances from the Sun, as well as the accompanying mechanisms during the accumulation and subsequent evolutionary phases. We can assume that three basic mechanisms—heterogeneous accretion, nonidentical outgassing rates, and fractionation of the primordial protoplanetary cloud—were operating at different efficiencies. Analysis of the abundances of volatiles in the material making up the terrestrial planets and meteorites favors the model that postulates heterogeneous accretion during the last stage over the one that postulates significant fractionation within a radius of less than 1 AU. The fall of meteorites, consisting of the latest low temperature condensates, and comets, consisting of more than half water ice, could have been the source of most volatiles. However, since the number of impacts in the inner solar system has remained approximately constant throughout geological time, differences in planetary position could

not have played any significant role in the accumulation of volatiles. The amount of subsequent outgassing from the planet, including the surface layer (veneer) of primitive material that had fallen on the planet, may have played a more important role.

These late condensates primarily include the carbonaceous chondrites, which are rich in hydrated silicates, gases, and even organic materials. The hypothesis of intense bombardment by comets and meteorites in the inner solar system, which was especially intense during the early phases of the solar system's evolution, but has undoubtedly continued into the present, is generally favored by the ratios of outgassed volatiles for the Earth, Venus, and Mars. The history of water on these planets was also probably associated with these processes, while early stages of formation would also influence the accumulation of water at the end of planetary formation.

D. Carbonate-Silicate Cycle and Climatic Evolution

We have seen that, in addition to a planet's mass and distance from the Sun, the nature of the atmosphere-lithosphere interaction (which is determined by the carbonate-silicate cycle) plays a decisive role in the formation of climatic conditions on that planet. In this case, a scenario is possible in which the positive-feedback effect usually postulated, i.e., amplification of the greenhouse effect (for example, in response to an increase in the carbon dioxide content of the Earth's atmosphere) is replaced by a negative feedback mechanism that leads to stabilization of an equilibrium state. On Earth, for example, an increase in atmospheric temperature will not only increase evaporation of the oceans, but also rainfall and the elution of cations from silicate rocks ("weathering"). As a result, more atmospheric carbon dioxide will be bound in carbonate rocks, thereby attenuating the greenhouse effect. Conversely, if the temperature decreases, for example, to the point where the oceans freeze, there will be less moisture in the atmosphere, and silicate weathering will decrease. At the same time, the continuing process of carbonate metamorphosis will lead to the gradual accumulation of carbon dioxide in the atmosphere, amplification of the greenhouse effect, and an increase in temperature, i.e., a return to the original temperature. If this cyclical mechanism is postulated, it follows that the Earth's climate has always been relatively temperate.

The situation was different on Mars, which has probably had a temperate climate for only the first billion years. Thus it was most likely the small size of the planet, and not the fact that it is 1.5 times farther from the Sun, that played the determining role in the further climatic evolution of Mars. The smaller inventory of radiogenic elements (which serve as internal heat sources) in this relatively low-mass planet disrupts the process of carbonate metamorphosis (which puts free CO_2 into the atmosphere), and this is what ultimately led to the current state of Mars. This also implies that carbonate deposits in the martian crust are larger than on Earth.

As for Venus, it might have had a temperate climate for a certain period of time (advanced and considered in detail by Kasting et al., 1988) if a much gentler negative-feedback mechanism, called the "moist" greenhouse effect, had operated instead of the "classic" runaway greenhouse effect. Such a situation could have arisen on Venus, given a solar radiation flux approximately 1.1 times that of the Earth (considering planetary position and the change in solar luminosity) and atmospheric water vapor content of, at most, 20 percent. In this scenario, weathering of the silicate rocks and rainfall would have led the carbon dioxide to be efficiently bound in carbonates, preventing its accumulation in the atmosphere and blocking any increase in the greenhouse effect. In other words, this would have been the case had the situation resembled that discussed above for the Earth, with increased surface atmospheric temperature (a 20-percent water vapor content in an atmosphere with 1 atm pressure corresponds to a temperature of 70 °C). However, these conditions could only have existed on Venus until the point where further increases in solar luminosity caused the H_2O content of the atmosphere to exceed the threshold value of ~20 percent, leading to an increase in the heat of condensation and an increase in the altitude of the temperature minimum in the atmosphere (the so-called "cold trap"). From this point on, the scenario is virtually identical to that for the runaway greenhouse effect, and Venus would have lost its hydrosphere due to hydrogen escape over the course of a few hundred million years. Thus, until a certain point, distance from the Sun would not have precluded quite temperate climatic conditions from existing on Venus, and the loss of the carbonate-silicate cycle feedback mechanism (due to the decrease in atmospheric water precipitation, followed by a complete cessation of precipitation, followed by carbonate decomposition, CO_2 accumulation in the atmosphere, and increased temperature) played a critical role in the radical change in these conditions.

Since Venus currently receives even less energy from the Sun than the Earth due to reflection by the clouds, it is easy to imagine a planet completely different from our present neighbor. The transition from the moist to the runaway greenhouse effect might not even have occurred if the planet's albedo had increased earlier and compensated for the increase in incident solar energy. In that case, Venus probably would have had a moist carbon-dioxide atmosphere with a surface pressure of a few bars and temperature on the order of tens of degrees Celsius. Such a planet would in principle be suitable for organic life.

It should be noted that the scenario described also places quite serious restrictions on the initial position of an inner planet relative to the Sun from the point of view of the formation and evolution of the climate. Estimates indicate that the Earth would only have to be 0.01 AU (1.5 million km) closer to the Sun in order for the runaway greenhouse effect to occur; i.e., the Earth proves to be at the very inner edge of the zone of habitability. However, the outer edge of the zone of habitability extends 0.5 AU beyond the orbit of

Mars, implying that an Earth- or Venus-sized planet in Mars orbit could also have conditions entirely suitable for life. [1, 13, 17, 20-21, 28-34]

VI. Neutral Upper Atmosphere, Ionosphere, and Magnetosphere of Earth

A. Structure and Chemical Composition of the Middle Atmosphere, Thermosphere, and Exosphere

The structure of the Earth's atmosphere and the names of its major regions are shown in Fig. 24. The middle atmosphere includes the regions lying above the troposphere. The thermosphere lies above the mesopause, which is the coldest region of the atmosphere. Most of the energy exchange due to direct absorption of short-wave solar radiation in the far-ultraviolet and soft X-ray regions (from approximately 2000 Å to 10 Å) and solar corpuscular radiation occurs in the thermosphere. The longer-wave ultraviolet radiation (3200-2000 Å) largely responsible for the formation of the ozonosphere is absorbed lower in the middle atmosphere along with the high-energy (up to 30 MeV) solar protons generated in flares and galactic cosmic rays.

The structure of the upper atmosphere—its temperature, density, and chemical composition—is determined by absorption of solar, electromagnetic, and corpuscular radiation, mass, energy, and momentum transport from underlying regions in the lower atmosphere and processes involving magnetosphere-ionosphere interactions. The latter interactions include the high-latitude precipitation of energetic particles, the excitation of current systems, leading to intense heating, and the formation of large local density gradients.

Variations in structure and composition of the upper and middle atmosphere are determined by perturbations of various kinds as well as by atmospheric dynamics. The altitude profiles for minor gaseous components in the middle atmosphere are shown in Fig. 30. A complex set of physical, chemical, and biological processes associated with interactions between the atmosphere and the lithosphere, hydrosphere, and biosphere plays an important role in the formation and destruction of these components (which have relative concentrations equal to 10^{-13}-10^{-5} of the major constituents N_2, O_2, and Ar) in addition to a variety of photochemical and chemical reactions, phase transformations, and dynamic exchange processes.

The entire chemistry of the middle atmosphere (and, to a certain extent, the thermosphere) depends in some way on the formation of chemically active atomic oxygen. Its formation begins in the stratosphere through photodissociation of O_2. The fast reaction between O_2 and O leads to the formation of ozone (O_3), which itself is an effective absorber of ultraviolet radiation (at $\lambda < 3200$ Å). Ozone is rapidly destroyed in this photochemical reaction and the reaction between O_3 and O, and the oxygen atoms recombine. This sequence of processes is what makes up the well-known Chapman cycle.

Chemical radicals such as NO, NO_2, OH, HO_2, Cl, and ClO

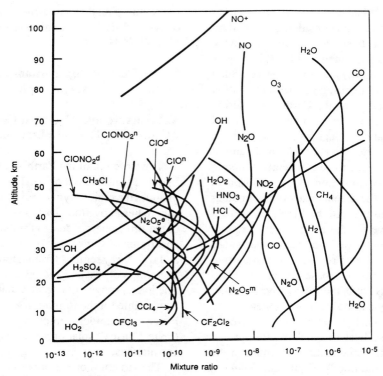

Fig. 30 Altitude profiles of concentrations of minor components in the middle atmosphere of Earth. Concentrations are shown as ratios to a unit volume composed of $N_2 + O_2 + Ar$. Superscripts d, n, m, and e stand for concentrations of the components during the day (afternoon), night, morning, and evening. (Reprinted from: Report of the Science Definition Working Group, Upper Atmosphere Research Satellite, courtesy of the Jet Propulsion Laboratory, California Institute of Technology.)

also have a substantial effect on the ozone concentration. The flow of these radicals from the troposphere into the ozonosphere is largely controlled by photochemical reactions involving halogen compounds, methane, nitrous oxides, and water. This leads to additional catalytic paths for the destruction of ozone. The anthropogenic factor is coming to play an increasing role in the observed increase in the concentration of the parent molecules for these radicals [primarily dichlorodifluoromethane (CCl_2F_2) and trichlorofluoromethane (CCl_3F)—freon—and the carbonated halogens ($C_2H_3Cl_3$, C_2Cl_4, etc.), as well as N_2O and CH_4].

Radical-radical reactions in the stratosphere lead to the formation of a number of intermediate compounds that have relatively low catalytic activity but readily decompose into the original radicals photochemically. These include radicals such as HNO_3, $ClONO_2$, H_2O_2, $HOCl$, HO_2NO_2, etc. The formation of hydrocarbonates (H_2CO, etc.) and CO is also important from the point of view of stratospheric chemistry. Other chemical reaction products serve as initial products for the formation of aerosols. These are primarily SO_2 and COS, which serve as a basis for the formation of droplets of sulfuric acid (with concentrations ranging from $0.5/cm^3$ to $10/cm^3$) concentrated in a stratospheric layer at approximately 20 km altitude, as well as NH_3. Although the concentrations of all these minor gaseous constituents typically do not exceed millionths of a percent, they have a substantial effect not only

on atmospheric chemistry but also on energy exchange processes in the middle atmosphere.

The upper atmosphere generally has a simpler chemistry. The chemistry of the mesosphere and lower thermosphere is largely driven by atomic oxygen formed through the photodissociation of O_2. The concentration of atomic oxygen begins to exceed that of molecular oxygen above an altitude of approximately 120-140 km. Another important component in this region is nitric oxide (NO), whose concentration depends on the concentration of atomic nitrogen. NO is most efficiently produced by collisions with O_2, and the main loss channels include photodissociation, photoionization, and vertical transport. Atomic nitrogen (like atomic hydrogen) is formed via ionization processes in the middle atmosphere accompanying the dissociation of molecular nitrogen and water vapor. N and H initiate a chain of catalyzed chemical reactions involving oxygen and ozone. The catalytic action of odd nitrogen and hydrogen compounds (in the form of NO_x and HO_x) significantly accelerates the destruction of ozone in reactions between O_3 and O.

On the average, N_2 (the major component of the atmosphere at the Earth's surface) remains the dominant component to 180 km altitude, because the efficiency of its dissociation is low. O becomes the dominant component higher in the thermosphere; at even higher altitudes, H and He begin to dominate (Fig. 31). He and O concentrations are approxi-

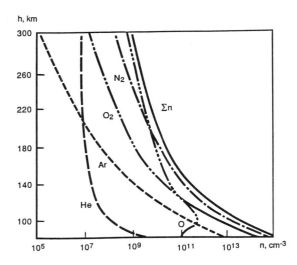

Fig. 31 Altitude profiles of neutral components of the thermosphere for the mean conditions of solar activity. (Reprinted from: Keldysh, M.V. and Marov, M.Ya. *Space Research*, Moscow, Nauka, 1981, pp. 35.)

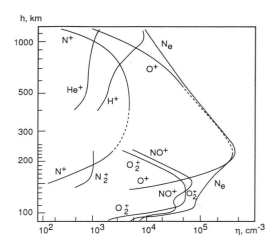

Fig. 32 Ion composition of the Earth's atmosphere (N_e is the profile of electronic concentration) (Reprinted from: Reprinted from: Keldysh, M.V. and Marov, M.Ya. *Space Research*, Moscow, Nauka, 1981, pp. 37.)

mately equal between 500 and 700 km, and those of H and He between 900 and 1800 km, depending on the phase of the solar cycle, which affects the temperature of the upper atmosphere. Concentrations of N_2, O_2, and O in the thermosphere increase with increasing temperature, while the concentration of H_2 decreases (due to the increase in its rate of dissipation). The variations in He concentration are more complex. The concentration of He is highest at solar minimum (especially in the winter hemisphere—the so-called "winter helium bulge"). Note that, although the hydrogen and hydrogen compounds (such as CH_4, H_2O, and OH) are minor constituents of the thermosphere, they may still play a significant role in chemical transformation and radiative heat exchange mechanisms.

B. Ionosphere

Photoionization and impact ionization by energetic electrons of major and minor components (which are responsible for the formation of the ionosphere) play important roles in the energy balance of the upper atmosphere, as well as in atmospheric chemistry, and lead to various important chains of aeronomic reactions that affect the structure and dynamics of individual regions in the atmosphere. However, the ionosphere itself exerts a strong influence over the macroscopic properties of the medium, even at levels of the atmosphere where the electron density is relatively low (no greater than ~$10-9$ at $z = 100$ km). The density of the ionosphere increases with altitude, and plays an extremely important role in electrodynamic interactions and in the dynamics of the atmosphere as a whole. In dynamic terms, the Earth's atmosphere can generally be treated as a neutral medium below ≈150 km; at higher altitudes, it must be treated as a thermal plasma that is primarily controlled by the geomagnetic field.

Electron density profiles and the D, E, and F regions generally distinguished in the ionosphere are shown in Fig. 24. The ionic composition of the mid-latitude ionosphere under conditions of mean solar activity is shown in Fig. 32. The maximum electron density (up to $10^6/cm^3$) is observed during the daytime at approximately 280 km altitude (the F_2 layer). Less well-defined maxima occur at altitudes of 150-200 km (F_1 layer), approximately 110 km (E layer), and 80 km (D layer), with electron densities ranging from $10^5/cm^3$ in the F_1 layer to $10^3/cm^3$ in the D layer. The density of each of these layers is substantially lower at night.

The lower layers of the ionosphere (D and E layers), from approximately 60 km to approximately 150 km, consist primarily of NO^+ ions, although the ratio of neutral NO molecules to N_2 molecules is no more than 10^{-8}. O_2^+ ions are also present in comparable quantities. The ionosphere from the F_1 layer (160-180 km) up to 600-800 km at solar minimum and 800-1000 km at solar maximum consists mainly of O^+ ions. Above 1000 km at mid-latitudes and low latitudes, the ionosphere is dominated by atomic hydrogen ions H^+; at latitudes corresponding to the outer plasmasphere, the O^+ ion begins to predominate up to altitudes of several thousand kilometers. It should be noted that ions of the metals Mg, Fe, Ca, and Si, apparently meteoritic in origin, have been observed at altitudes of 100-110 km. The drift of these long-lived ions in the large wind gradients at these altitudes leads to the appearance of the sporadic E_s layer.

We have given a rather simplified description of the ion component distribution that corresponds to a temporal and spatial average for undisturbed conditions. This structure undergoes major deviations as a result of variations of the initial neutral composition, and the rate of ion generation and recombination. These variations are due to changes in the flux intensity of ionizing radiation and the efficiency of dynamic exchange processes. At mesospheric altitudes, an important role is also played by cyclic variations in water vapor concentration, which is subject to photodissociations associated with changes in production of atomic oxygen. The concentration of NO and other minor components depends on this effect as well as the rate of vertical transport.

The increased downward flux of NO molecules out of the thermosphere and the decreased photolytic destruction rate during the winter in turn lead to an increase in the concentration of NO^+ ions. This increase, together with the seasonal restructuring of the wind system in the middle atmosphere, is associated with the anomalous winter increase in electron density in the D layer. Meteorological control over the lower ionosphere is one of the notable factors affecting variation in NO^+ concentration as well as of more complex formations, cluster ions. In the night ionosphere NO^+ ions may predominate throughout the F_1 region, up to 250-300 km near the equator. Under such conditions, density of electrons and ions is almost invariant with altitude, which is conducive to the development of ionospheric irregularities and instabilities.

The situation in the F layer of the ionosphere is more complex, especially at high latitudes. Thus, the region of anomalously low electron density at the altitude of the F layer (the main ionospheric trough) on the nightside shows significant variations. This trough serves as a kind of boundary between the mid-latitude ionosphere and polar ionosphere. The position of the trough is highly dependent on solar and geomagnetic activity as well as time of day and season. The entire structure of the ionosphere undergoes dramatic changes during geomagnetic disturbances, largely due to dynamic processes in the atmosphere.

C. Energy Balance and Variations in the Parameters of the Upper Atmosphere

The various atmospheric constituents are involved in a wide variety of complex chemical transformations. Products of these reactions have come to play a determining role both in the composition of the atmosphere and ionosphere and in heat exchange. The energy balance of the middle atmosphere is largely governed by the heating of the ozonosphere, while absorption of solar extreme ultraviolet radiation (EUV) and the action of particles and fields from the magnetosphere play decisive roles in the energy balance of the thermosphere. The energy input to the atmosphere above 100 km from EUV radiation is approximately 10^{12} W (or 2 erg/cm²s). The mean energy input from the magnetosphere due to solar-wind particles and the resulting current systems is 5×10^{10} W [or approximately 0.1 erg/(cm²s)]. However, during geomagnetic storms associated with solar flares, the energy input from this source may become comparable to, or even several times larger than, the energy input due to electromagnetic radiation, reaching tens of erg/cm² × s. A significant fraction of the energy from the charged particles injected into the magnetosphere is released in the auroral zones, while even more of the energy is trapped in the so-called ring current that encircles the planet at middle and low latitudes. Energy of ~0.1 erg/(cm²s)

is released when the ring current decays.

Various dynamic processes, including wave processes, also make a significant contribution to the energy balance of the middle atmosphere and thermosphere. Dynamic processes are primarily responsible for energy redistribution on a global scale. However, tides, acoustic and internal gravity waves, and turbulence also play an important role in the thermal balance of various individual regions and in observed spatial and temporal variations of structural parameters. For example, the bulk heat release rate due to the dissipation of internal gravity wave energy in the lower thermosphere is comparable to that of the other energy sources.

The chemical composition and related energy input determine the global structure of the upper atmosphere—primarily the vertical profiles of macroscopic parameters such as the temperature T and the density ρ. These parameters undergo substantial changes at high altitudes.

Temperature variations in the stratosphere and mesosphere are (like the temperature variations at the surface of the Earth) generally no greater than 50-60 K. Annual and semiannual components with altitude-dependent phase and amplitude are clearly present in the temperature and pressure variations. Semiannual variations in the atmospheric parameters are especially characteristic of the upper stratosphere at tropical latitudes, while quasibiennial variations are observed in the lower stratosphere near the equator.

Temperature variations in the thermosphere and exosphere reach 500-600 K in amplitude, which means that the variations in the density ρ are just as large. The basic variations in temperature and density may be divided into two major groups. The first group includes those due to changes in the influx of solar electromagnetic radiation, which depend on solar activity and time of day. This group includes the 27-day cycle frequently observed in density variations, which is associated with the rotational period of the Sun and the existence of long-lived local active regions on its surface. These variations are generally well-correlated with the decimetric radio flux of the Sun ($F_{10.7}$) and Wolf numbers (W), which are proportional to the number of sunspot groups on the Sun. These two characteristics (regularly recorded by ground-based observatories) serve as a measure of the effectiveness with which the upper atmosphere is heated by EUV radiation. The second group of variations is generally subdivided into geomagnetic disturbances and a semiannual effect comparable in magnitude to the diurnal effect. This group may be considered the overall response of the neutral atmosphere to magnetospheric-ionospheric interactions. These variations show the best correlation with the planetary geomagnetic disturbance indices (K_p or A_p), which are also regularly recorded by ground-based geophysical observatories and serve as a measure of the effect of the solar plasma on the Earth's geomagnetic field. In addition to the variations mentioned above, relatively small variations in T and ρ as a function of latitude and season have been observed, along with variations in ρ as large as 25 percent in amplitude and periods ranging from several minutes to several hours (with

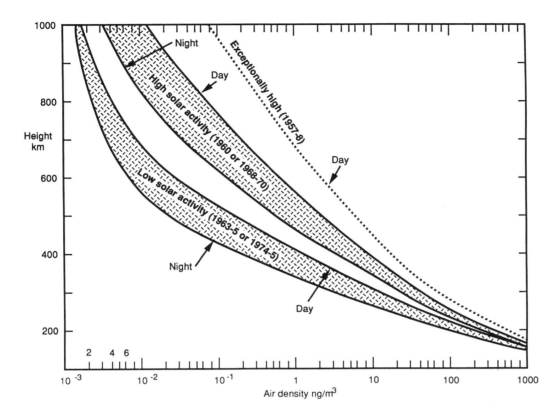

Fig. 33 Variation in density of the upper atmosphere at altitudes of the thermosphere and exosphere as a function of level of solar activity and time of day. (Reprinted from: King-Hele, D.G., Earth's Neutral Upper Atmosphere, *Space Physics*, 1978, vol. 16, no. 4. p. 735.)

24-, 12-, and 18-hour periods—multiples of the solar and lunar days—being especially prominent).

The largest variations in the neutral upper atmosphere are those involving the 11-year solar cycle. One characteristic indicator of this variation is the temperature of the upper thermosphere, which is nearly isothermal. This temperature is virtually identical to the exospheric temperature (T_∞). Including the diurnal variations, the latter temperature varies from 500-700 K at solar minimum ($F_{10.7} \approx$ 70-80) to 800-1300 K at solar maximum ($F_{10.7} \approx$ 200). As far as density is concerned, the expansion and contraction of the upper atmosphere due to these temperature variations (i.e., the diurnal and semiannual variations) cause the mean density to vary severalfold near 300 km altitude and by over two orders of magnitude at 500-600 km altitude (Fig. 33).

The diurnal variations in T and ρ are the most regular: the minima occur at approximately 0400-0500 LT (local time), while temperature reaches its maximum value at 1600 LT and density at 1400 LT. This is due to various special characteristics of the diurnal atmospheric expansion as well as the dynamics of the atmosphere. The largest diurnal variations in the thermosphere occur at 400-500 km altitude. The maximum of the diurnal variations shifts to lower altitude as solar activity decreases.

The variations associated with geomagnetic activity are particularly complex in nature. Even relatively weak mag-

netic disturbances cause global changes in T and ρ, with the relative effect of these variations being more apparent at solar minimum. During strong disturbances, temperatures of up to 3000 K have been recorded in auroral regions, whereas the density variations in the mid-latitude atmosphere (at 500 km altitude) have been as large as a factor of 8. The semiannual density variation has two peaks, in June-July and December-January, with the second peak having a slightly larger amplitude. This variation includes a larger range of altitudes than the diurnal density variations, from 90 to 1200 km. The largest variations (up to a factor of 3) are observed near 500 km, with virtually no dependence on phase of solar cycle. No direct source for the semiannual variations has as yet been identified; it has been suggested that they might be due to periodic variations in the heliographic latitude of sunspot activity centers.

These variations provide convincing evidence of the fact that the parameters of the upper atmosphere can only be adequately interpreted and utilized if accompanied by specification of the time of day, latitude, level of solar activity, level of geomagnetic activity, etc. Appropriate empirical models describing the structure of the atmosphere and the variations in its structure as a function of a limited number of parameters have been derived through the generalization and systematization of experimental results. This approach makes it possible to characterize the state of the upper atmosphere in a given region of space under certain geophysical conditions to high accuracy.

D. Dynamics of the Middle and Upper Atmosphere and Thermosphere

The fact that the variations in temperature and density are global is a reflection of the extremely dynamic nature of the middle and particularly upper atmosphere and their reaction to the external disturbances that affect energy and mass exchange. These variations lead to motions on various spatial scales all the way from planetary-scale circulation to local flows and wave processes.

The most important characteristic of middle atmosphere dynamics is the global circulation system. Its distinguishing feature is stable zonal flow, which periodically shifts direction over the course of the year from west to east during the winter to east to west in the summer. This flow is most prominent at altitudes of 60-70 km, and is due to the variation in insolation with latitude, which leads to a change in the amount of ultraviolet radiation absorbed by ozone and the subsequent reradiation of energy in bands of O_3, CO_2, and H_2O. The corresponding wind system, sometimes called the monsoon, is characterized by the stratospheric circulation index (SCI), which is the mean wind velocity in a layer 10 km thick at the level of the stratopause (~50 km). The SCI may reach values as high as 50-60 m/s.

Wave processes have a significant effect on the distribution of temperature, pressure, and density, as well as on wind velocity, degree of ionization, and atmospheric emissions. The wave field in the middle atmosphere reflects the close connection between the troposphere and the dynamics of overlying regions. The planetary waves, which have horizontal dimensions comparable to the radius of the Earth and periods on the order of a day or more, have an especially strong effect on mean zonal flow. The so-called sudden high-latitude stratospheric warmings in particular are due to these waves. Deviations from the regular restructuring of the mid-latitude circulation system (especially in the mesosphere) and the observed asymmetry in the middle-atmosphere circulation pattern relative to the poles during winter (in contrast to the symmetric pattern that occurs during summer) are also associated with these planetary waves.

Winds due to tidal oscillations are superposed on this wind system. Short-period variations—acoustic waves and internal gravity waves (caused by perturbations associated with the restructuring of meteorological processes, instabilities of various types, such as wind shear, heating in the auroral regions, etc.)—are also active in these same regions of the middle atmosphere. These waves have both vertical and horizontal (zonal and meridional) components. The periods of these acoustic-gravity waves range from several milliseconds to several hours, with wavelengths ranging from a few to hundreds of kilometers. Energy dissipation due to internal gravity wave modes makes a significant contribution to the thermal balance of the upper mesosphere and lower thermo-sphere.

Like the middle atmosphere, the thermosphere is characterized by a broad dynamic spectrum of motions, from large-scale wind systems to wave processes. The motions in the equatorial and mid-latitude thermosphere are largely determined by variations in the flux of EUV radiation, but are also strongly affected by the high-latitude regions most influenced by the magnetosphere-ionosphere interaction. The high-latitude neutral-gas circulation can also be stimulated by ions undergoing ionospheric convection, the effectiveness of which depends to a great extent on the amount of heating that occurs as energetic charged particles penetrate the auroral zones. The release of thermal energy in these more-or-less regularly occurring processes does make some contribution to the overall thermospheric circulation system. And since the redistribution of energy in these local heating processes is global in nature, the thermosphere, which as a whole has a stable structure and an effective energy dissipation mechanism in the form of viscosity and thermal conductivity, is essentially in a state of constant dynamic restructuring.

The system of zonal and meridional winds in the thermosphere at altitudes above approximately 100 km is comparatively stable. These winds, caused by density gradients due to diurnal and seasonal variations in solar energy flux, lead to meridional flow of air masses from the summer to the winter hemisphere. The stable nature of this circulation is strongly affected by increases in geomagnetic activity, leading to the formation of an additional system of large-scale eddies that may reach the equator after their formation in the winter auroral zone. One distinguishing feature of the zonal wind is that the "evening" winds (from west to east) and "morning" winds (from east to west) have different velocities. The terms "morning" and "evening" winds refer to the time periods 1800-2400 LT and 0400-1200 LT, respectively. As a result, the atmosphere at an altitude range of 200-400 km at latitudes of 30°-40° rotates with velocity $v \approx 100$ m/s, which on the average is above the Earth's intrinsic rotation.

The wind system at high latitudes, on the other hand, is primarily directed poleward and to the west during the night, switching to equatorward and to the east in the morning. This wind system depends strongly on the level of geomagnetic disturbance. The morphology of the wind systems and waves excited during disturbances initiated by the full set of electrodynamic interactions is unusually complex. The global "response" of the thermosphere to heating in the auroral regions largely involves changes in the dynamic regime of the atmosphere.

The dynamics of the thermosphere, under the influence of the ionospheric plasma, has a strong effect on the behavior of the ionosphere, which is the determining factor below ~150 km; above this level, the motion of the electrons and ions is largely controlled by the electrical and magnetic fields. At middle and low latitudes, the electrical fields are generated by winds associated with thermal tides, while the electrical fields in the high-latitude atmosphere are largely generated by interactions between the magnetosphere and ionosphere.

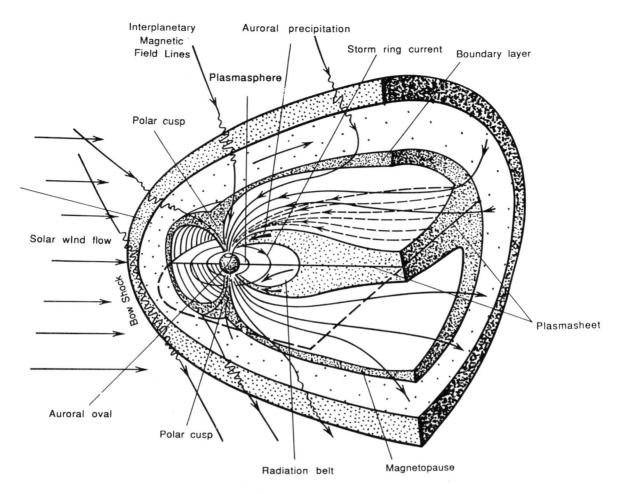

Fig. 34 A schematic diagram of the structures and various regions of the Earth's magnetosphere. (Courtesy of J.G. Roederer, Geophysical Institute, University of Alaska, reprinted from Exploration of the Polar Upper Atmosphere-1981. In: Biennial Report of the Geophysical Institute, 1983-84, p. 29.)

E. Magnetosphere

A model of the flow of the solar wind around the Earth and the structure of the magnetosphere is provided in Fig. 34. The pattern of relationships between the Earth's magnetosphere, ionosphere, and neutral upper atmosphere is complex. The solar wind deforms the geomagnetic field at distances on the order of 10 Earth radii (R_E) and brings lines of force originating in the polar regions over to the nightside. These lines of force and associated plasma form a magnetotail or plume behind the Earth consisting of two branches, a northern branch and a southern branch, separated by a neutral sheet with a maximum field strength of 1 gamma (1 gamma=10^{-5} TM). The magnetotail extends outward over a distance of at least 1000 R_E. A shock wave is formed as the supersonic solar plasma flows into the magnetosphere, the characteristics of the flow changing radically with flow passage. The region between the shock wave and the boundary of the magnetosphere contains a turbulent plasma layer with a highly fluctuating magnetic field. The thickness of this layer—the magnetosheath—increases with distance from the frontal point, but is almost

independent of the level of geomagnetic disturbance. Near the frontal point, the thickness of the transition zone averages 2-4 R_E. Immediately behind this region is the magnetopause (which is characterized by diffusion and large pressure gradients) and the polar cusp regions, which are constantly occupied by high-velocity plasmoids and very strong electric fields. This leads to constant replenishment of the magnetosphere with solar-wind particles. The neutral sheet, a plasma sheet containing plasma as hot as the solar wind, plays an important role in this process.

The topology of the magnetosphere and the position of its outer boundary on the side facing the Sun (the dayside magnetopause) are determined by the dynamic pressure of the solar wind flow and the orientation of the interplanetary magnetic field. When the flow of solar plasma is decelerated, the magnetosphere is compressed, the magnetopause moves closer to the Earth, and the strength of the magnetic field increases, marking the initial phase of a magnetic storm. The electric current systems formed at the boundary of the magnetosphere cause the lines of force to deform. The deformation of the outer magnetosphere and the fact that some of the lines of force are swept back to the nightside cause the magnetosphere to be asymmetric. The magnetopause can be likened to a pulsating membrane through which some of the kinetic energy of the solar wind is transferred to the magnetosphere. Instabilities in the magnetopause and shock wave zone convert some fraction of this energy into energy of plasma oscillations and electromagnetic radiation radiated from the magnetosphere into interplanetary space with a broad wave spectrum.

The magnetosphere is divided into two main regions filled with plasma having different properties—the inner magnetosphere and the outer magnetosphere. The inner magnetosphere (out to radius ~R_E in the equatorial plane)—the plasmasphere—contains a low-temperature plasma at relatively high density. The plasmasphere is structurally and morphologically related to the ionosphere, and in fact appears to be a continuation of it. The outer magnetosphere is filled with both high-temperature and relatively low-temperature plasma formed by particles trapped by the geomagnetic field. These two plasma states are determined by the initial nature of the charged particles. The hot plasma is injected through the dayside magnetopause and from the magnetotail, whereas the thermal plasma comes from the ionosphere via hydrodynamic light-ion acceleration at high latitudes (the so-called polar wind) and acceleration due to longitudinal electric currents in the auroral regions. The polar wind, a relatively thin supersonic flow of low-energy protons and helium ions directed upward, is subject to strong spatial and temporal variations. The motion of the thermal plasma in the plasmasphere, as well as energetic protons and electrons in the outer magnetosphere associated with the radiation belts, is largely controlled by large-scale electric fields resulting from magnetospheric convection, which leads to systems of electric currents directed parallel to the magnetic lines of force, with the return current flowing through the polar ionosphere. The boundary of the plasmasphere, where the thermal plasma accumulates for long periods of time, is called the plasmapause. The thermal ions experience a sharp "cutoff" near this boundary.

Particles in the magnetosphere move along complex trajectories determined by their rotation about the magnetic line of force, their oscillation between the Northern and Southern Hemispheres, and their drift in longitude. If the angle formed by the velocity vector of the particle and the magnetic field strength (pitch angle) decreases below the critical value and the point at which the particle is reflected (mirror point) descends into the ionosphere, the particle will lose all its energy in collisions with atoms and molecules in the upper atmosphere.

The mean density of charged particles in the magnetosphere is controlled by the balance between sources and losses. Ionospheric particles are an important source in addition to the solar-wind particles (electrons, protons, and α particles) transported into the magnetosphere from its boundary by fluctuating electric and magnetic fields. Ionized hydrogen, helium, nitrogen, and oxygen formed in photochemical processes (as well as electrons) enter the magnetosphere from the ionosphere. The plasmasphere (which is trapped by mid-latitude lines of force and lies relatively close to the Earth) is mainly filled with protons formed in the ionosphere by charge-exchange reactions between oxygen ions and atomic hydrogen, as well as He^+ and O^+ ions. During magnetic storms, the relative fraction and energy of thermal O^+ ions increase, reaching several tenths of a percent. Another source of particles for the magnetosphere includes protons, helium and hydrogen ions heated in the auroral regions of the ionospheric plasma, where they are accelerated and flows are formed along magnetic field lines.

Magnetospheric loss mechanisms include, first, exchange with the solar plasma through the magnetopause and the ejection of magnetospheric plasma into the magnetotail, and second, scattering of high-velocity particles due to so-called cyclotron instability. Characteristic manifestations of the cyclotron instability mechanism accompanying particle precipitation into the upper atmosphere include pulsating aurorae, various types of low-frequency electromagnetic radiation of magnetospheric origin covering a wide frequency range, and the excitation of geomagnetic field pulsations. All of these phenomena are in some way associated with the development of electric fields and current systems in the magnetosphere and ionosphere, leading to energy and mass exchange.

Aurorae are a prominent manifestation of the powerful energy and mass exchange processes and the interaction between current systems in the high-latitude upper atmosphere at high levels of geomagnetic disturbance. Aurorae are among the most well-known phenomena in the entire chain of effects linking the Sun and Earth. They occur in some form almost continuously within the so-called polar ovals located asymmetrically about the geomagnetic poles in the Northern and Southern Hemispheres at the edges of the polar caps. The closest approach of the polar ovals to the geomagnetic poles occurs on the dayside, while the largest separation occurs on the nightside. Strong diffuse auroral emission is almost always present along the band of the oval, along with discrete aurorae of various form and intensity. Under quiet geomagnetic conditions, the auroral boundaries lie at 78° and 68° geomagnetic latitude. Intense aurorae generally occur on the nightside, but sometimes also occur on the dayside. During intense magnetic storms, bright discrete auroral forms encompass the entire polar oval for 360° around the magnetic pole. When particles of magnetospheric origin (mainly electrons and protons) precipitate into the atmosphere, this leads to collisional excitation of atmospheric atoms and molecules and the emission of photons in several characteristic lines and bands—especially prominent are various molecular band systems and characteristic lines from oxygen and nitrogen, which give rise to the observed range of colors. The types and intensity of the aurorae depend on the energy spectrum of the electrons and/or protons and the spatial and temporal characteristics of the acceleration process. The complex morphology of this phenomenon is also determined by the structure and evolution of the current systems along the magnetic lines of force, the microstructure of the electric and magnetic fields within individual auroral arcs, and the overall dynamics of the polar atmosphere during the magnetic storm. Dissipation of energy from current systems provides the basic energy input to the high-latitude thermosphere.[1, 19, 35-41]

VII. Upper Atmospheres and Ionospheres of the Inner Planets / Circumplanetary Space

A. Neutral Upper Atmospheres

Unlike the Earth's upper atmosphere, where oxygen plays a dominant role, processes in the upper atmospheres of Venus and Mars are largely controlled by the photochemistry of carbon dioxide, which, with its dissociation products CO and O, remains the dominant component to altitudes of approximately 200-250 km. Above this altitude, helium and hydrogen gradually become the dominant components in the atmospheres of these planets, as in the Earth's atmosphere.

The processes of CO_2 dissociation and ionization are accompanied by the inverse processes of association and recombination under conditions of intense dynamic exchange (turbulent diffusion and circulation). Minor atmospheric constituents, primarily H_2O—and on Venus sulfur compounds—also play an important role in atmospheric chemistry, affecting the altitude distribution of various components and the thermal regime. Photochemistry and atmospheric dynamics explain the predominance of CO_2 to high altitudes in the thermospheres of both planets.

The bulk of the energy of EUV radiation is converted to heat in photolysis reactions, as well as in the thermalization of newly created photoelectrons. However, the association reactions involving CO and O have low efficiency at high altitudes, and only play an important role in the mesosphere and lower thermosphere, where photolysis products are removed most actively. The remainder of the EUV energy is scattered and reradiated by the atmosphere, providing important information on its properties.

An analysis of the dayglow in the martian atmosphere has provided an estimate of the temperature of the exosphere $T_\infty = 350$, and emission line data have been used to calculate the profiles of CO_2, CO, and O with altitude, which are in good agreement with mass-spectrometer data. Approximately the same value was obtained for the exospheric temperature from measurements of the characteristics of the upper-atmosphere dayglow on Venus: $T_\infty = 375 \pm 100$ K. This value of $T_\infty \approx 400$ on the dayside was confirmed by measurements of the drag on the Pioneer-Venus probe. The temperature on the nightside proved to be 100 K—much lower even than the temperature of the mesopause in the Earth's atmosphere.

The fact that the mean exospheric temperatures of Venus and Mars are much lower than that of the Earth can be explained primarily by the large amount of energy radiated in the infrared bands of CO_2. This also explains why the base of the exosphere is approximately 200 km lower for these planets than for the Earth's atmosphere. As for the unusually low temperature of the nightside upper atmosphere (cryosphere)

of Venus, it can probably be explained by turbulent heat conduction, in addition to the radiation.

B. Ionospheres

Venus and Mars have ionospheres, but they are less dense and closer to the surface than the Earth's.

One substantial difference between the ionospheres of Mars and Earth is that the former does not have the F_2 maximum formed in the Earth's ionosphere due to O^+ ions as a result of the relationships between the processes of ionization, recombination, and diffusion. This difference is apparently due to the fact that the charge-exchange reaction between O^+ and CO_2 is faster than that between O^+ and N_2, which continues to be the dominant atmospheric constituent in the Earth's atmosphere to relatively high altitudes. This prevents the accumulation of O^+ ions on Mars at altitudes less than approximately 200 km. The maximum electron density N_e in the dayside martian ionosphere occurs at altitudes $z = 135$-140 km and is $\leq 2 \times 10^5/cm^3$, i.e., an order of magnitude lower than the density in the F_2 layer of the Earth's ionosphere. Another, less well-defined maximum (small inflection point) in the N_e (z) profile occurs at an altitude of approximately 110 km, with an electron density of $\approx 7 \times 10^4/cm^3$. On the nightside, the peak N_e moves down to an altitude of 100-110 km, with a maximum density of $5 \times 10^3/cm^3$.

The main constituent of the martian ionosphere is O_2^+, which is mainly formed in the charge-exchange reaction between CO_2^+ and O. A model of the photochemical equilibrium based on this reaction and several associated reactions is consistent, to the first approximation, with the measured distributions of various components up to an altitude of ~2000 km. Above this level, the relative concentration of the lighter ions increases.

The lower ionosphere of Venus also consists mainly of O_2^+, but with a significant quantity of O^+ as a secondary constituent. CO^+ and CO_2^+ ions are also present in significant quantities. O^+ ions dominate above 160 km on the nightside and 200 km on the dayside, except for during the predawn hours, when concentration of H^+ ions is approximately the same as that of O^+ ions. The dayside maximum [with density $(2$-$5) \times 10^5/cm^3$] occurs at 140 km, while a sharp decrease in electron density is observed at the 250-300 km level. The ionopause—the boundary between the thermal ions in the ionosphere and streams of energetic particles from the solar wind—is located at approximately this same level (with an altitude ranging from 290 km on the nightside to 1000 km at the terminator). On the nightside, an extended region of moderate electron density ~$10^3/cm^3$ (up to over 3000 km in altitude) forms. This region contains several local maxima, which have density 5-10 times higher, near 150 km altitude. The ion density and composition in the lower ionosphere are subject to substantial variations.

The dayside ionosphere of Venus generally satisfies the condition of photochemical equilibrium, i.e., is largely controlled by local processes involving the formation and destruction of ions, like the ionosphere of Mars and the E layer in the Earth's ionosphere. The situation on the nightside is more complex. The narrow maximum in N_e that forms at the same (or perhaps slightly higher) altitude as the maximum in the dayside ionosphere is probably due to processes involving the transport of ions from the dayside and bears a closer resemblance to the F_2 layer of the Earth's ionosphere in morphology and nature. This horizontal transport of ions to the nightside hemisphere is presumably due to the diurnal pressure gradient of the ionospheric plasma, which does not undergo any appreciable drag because the planet has no intrinsic magnetic field. Precipitation of energetic electrons due to electromagnetic interactions also contributes to the ionization of the nightside thermosphere, and is probably responsible for the secondary peak in N_e below the main peak.

One of the interesting characteristics of Venus's ionosphere is the extremely high electron ($T_e \approx 5000$ K) and ion ($T_i \approx 1000$ K) temperatures, which are both much higher than the temperature of the neutrals. This is indicative of the low efficiency of thermal relaxation processes (in contrast to Earth, where there are no substantial differences between temperatures of electrons and ions and of neutrals up to an altitude of ≈ 500 km). We should also note that these high values of T_e and T_i are maintained on the nightside, against the background of a neutral cryospheric temperature of ≈ 100 K, which confirms the high efficiency of horizontal transport and ionization processes on the nightside.

C. Characteristics of Circumplanetary Space

The problems treated in planetary aeronomy are closely linked with the interactions between the celestial body and the solar wind.

Mercury's magnetosphere is small compared to that of the Earth. One of its distinguishing features is that the solar plasma approaches quite close to the planet's surface because of the rather weak magnetic field (350 gammas) and the lack of an atmosphere. The shock front (detected from the sharp increase in the magnetic field) is ≤ 1.5 R_M from the center of the planet. The boundary of the magnetosphere (i.e., the magnetopause, which carries the electrical currents responsible for sudden changes in the direction of the magnetic field) lies at approximately the same distance. This means that the planet itself occupies a significant fraction of the magnetosphere, so that there is no room for a magnetic trap. Thus, Mercury does not have a region where energetic charged particles are trapped within a regular magnetic field; there are essentially no radiation belts. Second, there are no longitudinal currents in Mercury's magnetosphere due to the lack of an atmosphere, since they cannot be closed by transverse conduction in the ionosphere. Solar-wind plasma is mainly present in the outer magnetosphere and subject to strong boundary fluctuations in the regions where the field is disturbed.

The solar wind flow around Mars does not form anything analogous to the magnetospheres of Earth or Mercury. The configuration of circumplanetary space around Mars is most similar to that observed for Venus, which implies that Mars has no intrinsic magnetic field (except for remnant magnetism in the crust). A number of features actually do support a gas-dynamic model for the solar plasma flow around the magnetosphere and direct exchange of mass between the solar plasma and the upper atmosphere in which the intrinsic magnetic field does not play a critical role. These features are as follows: the properties of the detached shock wave, whose position does not show any significant deviation from a mean altitude of ~1500 km, even when there are variations in solar-wind pressure (in contrast to the model magnetosphere); formation of a boundary layer (where a decrease in flow velocity and drops in electron and ion temperature are observed) on the dayside and nightside of the planet; and evidence suggesting the presence of streams of O^+ ions in the boundary region, moving away from the planet. Nevertheless, further research is needed on the origin of the structure of circumplanetary space around Mars, because the patterns observed are not completely congruent with solar plasma interaction with a non-magnetized body.

The topology of space in the neighborhood of Venus is completely determined by the direct interaction of the solar plasma and the ionosphere. The most characteristic feature of this interaction is the formation of a transitional region—the ionopause—which forms on the dayside of the planet in a region behind the shock wave, at altitudes above ~300-500 km. Here the pressure of the solar wind is in approximate equilibrium with the kinetic pressure of atmospheric gases and the pressure of the magnetic field induced by the currents in the ionosphere. In addition to the formation of the transitional zone identified with the ionopause, the processes in the solar plasma flow area around Venus also include successive heating and thermalization of ions; the formation of a region of reduced density behind the shock wave (i.e., the ionosheath, roughly analogous to the magnetosheath in Earth's magnetosphere); the important role played by the dynamics of the ionosphere and the electric fields within the ionosphere; and the formation of a zone of reduced density behind the planet.

This model for the solar plasma flow around Venus is consistent with ideas concerning the important role played by ionospheric convection and the interaction between the ionospheric and interplanetary magnetic fields. In this model, the pressure in the dayside ionosphere is much lower than the thermal plasma pressure, and can be comparable to it only near the terminator, where it presumably has the greatest effect on the morphology of movement. The strongest magnetic fields are expected in the nightside ionosphere, primarily in the vicinity of the large-scale holes reflecting the interaction between the zone of reduced density (magnetotail) and the ionosphere. All of these processes taken together reflect the special nature of the interaction between Venus and the solar wind, which is fundamentally different from that observed in the interaction between Earth (or any other planet with a magnetic field) and the solar wind.[1, 19, 44-48]

VIII. Conclusion

We have attempted to acquaint the reader with the most important characteristics of the inner planets using a comparative planetological approach, which in our opinion is the best way to reveal the properties shared by the planets and how they differ. This sort of approach was made possible by the enormous progress that has been made during the last two decades, especially in space exploration. The large amount of empirical data that have been obtained and the interpretational models based on these data have laid the foundation for an in-depth understanding of the evolutionary mechanisms responsible for current conditions on the celestial bodies closest to the Sun. And this, in turn, casts a new light on the origin of life, promising a better understanding of the interrelationship between physicochemical and biological processes and the uniqueness of the Earth within the family of solar system planets.

It can be asserted that, now, on the threshold of the next millennium, we have completed the reconnaissance phase in the study of this entire family of planets. It is understandable that the largest body of information has been obtained about the Earth's nearest neighbors—Venus and Mars. Obviously, the focus of attention will continue to be on them in the future, as is required by the need for a comprehensive approach to understanding the Earth itself, as well as the unquestionable desirability of an incremental approach to the next phase in the development of manned space flight—the era of interplanetary flight. We may thus expect further stimulation of virtually all the branches of the planetary sciences (planetary geology and geophysics, space chemistry and physics of the atmosphere, meteorology and climatology, etc.) and the close association between these sciences and space biology and medicine.

In conclusion, we suggest that even a brief survey of contemporary knowledge of the inner planets requires reference to an enormous number of primary sources. For this reason, because of space limitations on this chapter, and also the difficulty of objective citation of works of historic or scientific interest, we have preferred not to use this approach, but to limit ourselves generally to a number of references to monographs and outstanding reviews. In these, the demanding reader interested in a deeper understanding of one or another issue can find a more complete bibliography.

References

[1] Marov, M.Ya. *Planets of the Solar System.* 2nd edition. Moscow, Nauka, 1986 (in Russian).

[2] Kuzmin, A.D. and Marov, M.Ya. *The Physics of the Planet Venus.* Moscow, Nauka, 1974 (in Russian).

[3] Murray, B.C., Belton, M.J.S., Danielson, G.E., Davies, M.E., Gault, D., Hapke, B., O'Leary.B., Strom, R.G., Suomi, V., and Trask, N. Venus atmospheric motion and structure from Mariner 10 pictures. *Science,* 1974, vol. 85, pp. 1307-1315.

[4] Keldysh, M.V. and Marov, M.Ya. *Space Research.* Moscow, Nauka, 1981 (in Russian).

[5] Marov, M.Ya. and Davydov, V.D. Earth-type planets (Mercury, Venus, Mars). In: M. Calvin and O.G. Gazenko (Eds.) *Foundations of Space Biology and Medicine.* Washington, D.C., NASA, 1975, pp. 133-197.

[6] Kotelnikov, V.A. (Ed.) *Atlas of Venus.* Moscow, Glavnoye Upravleniye Geodesy i Kartografii, 1990 (in Russian.)

[7] Basilevsky, A.T. and Head, J.W. The geology of Venus. *Annual Review of Earth and Planetary Sciences,* 1988, vol. 16, pp. 295-317.

[8] Keldysh, M.V. *First Panoramas of the Surface of Venus.* Moscow, Nauka, 1979 (in Russian).

[9] Carr, M. N. *The Surface of Mars.* New Haven, Connecticut, Yale University Press, 1981, p. 232.

[10] Chapman, C.R. and Jones, K.L. Cratering and obliteration history of Mars. *Annual Review of Earth and Planetary Sciences,* 1977, vol. 5, pp. 515-540.

[11] Carr, M.N. The morphology of the martian surface. *Space Sciences Review,* 1980, vol. 25, pp. 231-284.

[12] Zharkov, V.N. and Trubitsyn, V.P. *Physics of Planetary Interiors.* Moscow, Nauka, 1980, p. 448 (in Russian).

[13] Monin, A.S. *History of the Earth.* Moscow, Nauka, 1977 (in Russian).

[14] Zharkov, V.N. *Interior Structure of the Earth and Planets.* Moscow, Nauka, 1983 (in Russian).

[15] Wasserburg, G. and Papanastassiou, D.A. *Nuclear Physics.* Mir, Moscow, 1986, p. 85 (translated into Russian).

[16] Vinogradov, A.P. (Ed.) *Cosmochemistry of the Moon and Planets.* Moscow, Nauka, 1975 (in Russian).

[17] Urey, H.C. *The Planets, Their Origin and Development.* New Haven, Yale University Press, 1952, p. 345.

[18] Ksanfomaliti, L.V. *The Planet Venus.* Moscow, Nauka, 1985 (in Russian).

[19] Marov, M.Ya., and Kolesnichenko, A.V. *Introduction to Planetary Aeronomy.* Moscow, Nauka, 1987 (in Russian).

[20] Vinogradov, A.P. *Introduction to the Geochemistry of the Ocean.* Moscow, Nauka, 1967 (in Russian).

[21] Prinn, R. and Lewis, J. *Origin and Evolution of the Planetary Atmospheres.* New York, Academic Press, 1984.

[22] Marov, M.Ya., Lystsev, V.Ye., et al. Structure and microphysical properties of the Venus clouds: Venera .9, 10, and 11 data. *Icarus,* 1980, vol. 44, pg. 608.

[23] Moroz, V.I. *The Physics of the Planet Mars.* Moscow, Nauka, 1978 (in Russian).

[24] Kliore, A.J., et al. (Eds.) The Venus International Reference Atmosphere. *Advances in Space Research,* 1985, vol. 5, no.11.

[25] Hunten, D.M., et al. (Eds.) *Venus.* Tucson, Arizona, University of Arizona Press, 1983.

[26] Barsukov, V.L. and Volkov, V.P. (Eds.) *The Planet Venus.* Moscow, Nauka, 1989 (in Russian).

[27] Volkov, V.P. *Chemistry of the Atmosphere and Surface of Venus.* Moscow, Nauka, 1983, p. 208 (in Russian).

[28] Safronov, V.S. and Vityazev, A.V. The origin of the solar system. *Itogi Nauki i Tekhniki. Ser. Astron.,* 1983, vol.

24 (in Russian).

[29] Voytsevich, G.V. *Fundamentals of the Theory of the Origin of the Earth*. Moscow, Nedra, 1988 (in Russian).

[30] Holland, H.D. *The Chemistry of the Atmosphere and Oceans*. New York, Wiley, 1978.

[31] Pollack, J.B. and Yung, Y.L. Origin and evolution of planetary atmospheres. *Annual Review of Earth and Planetary Sciences,* 1980, vol. 8, pp. 425-487.

[32] Chamberlain, J.W. and Hunten, D.M. *Theory of Planetary Atmospheres*. New York, Academic Press, 1987.

[33] Hunten, D.M. et al. Planetary atmospheres. In: Kerridge, J.F. and Matthews, M.S. (Eds.) *Meteorites, the Earth, and the Solar System*. Tucson, Arizona, University of Arizona Press, 1988.

[34] Kasting, J.F. et al. How climate evolved on the terrestrial planets. *Scientific American*, 1988, vol. 256, no. 2, 90-97.

[35] Roble, R.G. Dynamics of the Earth's thermosphere. *Review of Geophysics and Space Physics,* vol. 21, no. 2, 1983, pp. 217-233.

[36] Nicolet, M. *Aeronomy*. Moscow, Mir, 1964 (translated into Russian).

[37] McEwan, M.J. and Phillips, L. *Chemistry of the Atmosphere*. Moscow, Mir, 1978 (translated into Russian).

[38] Bertelier, A. et al. In: Dier, C. and Holtet, J. (Eds.) *The Polar Upper Atmosphere*. Moscow, Mir, 1983 (translated into Russian).

[39] Bauer, S.J. *Physics of Planetary Ionospheres*. Berlin, New York, Springer, 1973.

[40] Koshelev, V.V. et al. *Aeronomy of the Mesosphere and Lower Thermosphere*. Moscow, Nauka, 1983 (in Russian).

[41] Akasofu, S.I. and Chapman, S. *Solar-Terrestrial Physics*. Oxford, Clarendon Press, 1972, 920 pages.

[42] Saunders R.S., Pettengill, G.H., Arvidson, R.E., Head, J.W., et. al. Magellan: Mission Summary; and other papers. *Science,* 1991, vol. 252, p. 247-312.

[43] Head, J.W. and Crumpler, L.S. Venus geology and tectonism: Hotspot and crustal spreading models and questions for the Magellan mission. *Nature,* 1990, vol. 346, no. 6284, p. 525.

[44] Tokosz M.N. and Solomon, S.C.. Thermal history and evolution of the Moon. *The Moon,* 1973, vol. 7, p. 251.

[45] Krasnopolskiy, V.A. *The Physics of Luminescence of Planet and Comet Atmospheres*. Moscow, Nauka, 1987 (in Russian).

[46] NASA. *Solar Wind Interactions with the Planets Mercury, Venus, and Mars*. NASA SP-397, 1975.

[47] Russell, C.T. Solar wind interactions. *Advances in Space Research*, 1986, vol. 6, no. 1.

[48] Russell, C.T. (Ed.) Venus Aeronomy. *Space Science Review*, vol. 55, 1991, pp. 1-4.

Chapter 4

The Outer Planets of the Solar System

Tobias Owen

I. Introduction

The distinction between the outer and inner planets can be traced back to the location in the primitive solar nebula where water could condense to form ice. If we examine a table of the cosmic abundances of the elements (Table 1), we see that oxygen is the most abundant chemically reactive element after hydrogen, which dominates everything else. It follows that H_2O should be the most abundant compound in the universe, and ice the most abundant solid. We will therefore suddenly have a huge supply of building material available for making planets in the solar nebula at the distance from the forming sun where the temperature dropped below 0°C. The best current calculations suggest that this must have occurred near the present location of Jupiter, largest of all the planets.

Closer to the Sun, only silicates were forming solid compounds. The planets we find there today—Mercury, Venus, Earth, Mars—are relatively small and dense. They are rocky bodies whose thin atmospheres—if they have atmospheres—contain gases like carbon dioxide and nitrogen. Hydrogen and helium, despite their overwhelming abundances in the cosmos (Table 1), have long since escaped into space. These planets do not have enough gravitational fields to overcome the kinetic energies produced by thermal motions of these light species. The combination of small gravitational fields, not much planet-forming material, and proximity to the extremely massive sun has denied the inner planets the systems of rings and grand retinues of satellites that are common in the outer solar system.

Except for Pluto, the outer planets are large, mostly gaseous bodies, with immensely deep atmospheres dominated by hydrogen and helium. Carbon is predominantly in the form of methane, and nitrogen is tied up in ammonia, etc. This means that their densities are low—so low that Saturn would float in champagne, if one just had a large enough glass in which to prepare this stunning cocktail! These giant worlds all have ring systems and are richly endowed with satellites (Table 2). Except for Uranus, all of these bodies are radiating more energy than they receive from the Sun.

Pluto doesn't fit into either of these categories. It is about two-thirds the size of our own Moon, but it appears to be at least half-composed of water ice mixed with other frozen gases. In these respects—size and composition—Pluto resembles Triton, the mysterious icy moon of Neptune. Pluto has at least one satellite of its own, called Charon, which is in a synchronous orbit. Both Pluto and Triton are so cold that methane is frozen on their surfaces.

We can characterize these two sets of planets, inner and outer, as evolved and primitive, respectively. The inner planets are like cosmic cinders, on which the light elements that are so abundant in stars and interstellar material are drastically depleted. In contrast, the composition of Jupiter is quite similar to that of the Sun and other stars. Somewhat enriched in heavy elements, it has preserved, almost intact, the cosmic composition of the cloud of gas and dust that collapsed to form the solar system 4.5 billion years ago. We find Saturn somewhat more enriched in heavy elements, while Uranus and Neptune seem to have 20 and 30 times the Sun's complement of carbon (and presumably other species) respectively. The increase in the relative abundances of heavy elements parallels an increase in the relative sizes of the cores of these bodies. These cores are the dense central regions whose existence and size can be deduced from models that match the mass, density, figure, rotation rate, composition, gravitational moments, etc. Yet in all four cases, hydrogen and helium dominate the atmospheres, since even the least massive of these bodies (Uranus) has a strong enough gravitational field to prevent these gases from escaping.

For our present purposes, we are especially interested in the fact that we can find chemical reactions taking place in the atmospheres of these planets today that must resemble, if not duplicate, the chemistry that occurred in the earliest history of our solar system. There may be lessons to be learned here about the first steps in chemical evolution that ultimately led to life on Earth. This is particularly true in the case of Saturn's large satellite, Titan, which is small enough that hydrogen can escape, yet cold enough to keep H_2O frozen on its surface with a very low vapor pressure. This combination means that the atmosphere remains in a reducing condition as it evolves with hydrogen escape, since there is no readily available source of oxygen or other oxidizing agent. Here we can expect to find low-temperature analogs for the reactions commonly invoked in the pre-biological Miller-Urey synthesis of organic compounds on the primitive Earth.

157

Table 1   Relative cosmic abundances

H	27,900
He	2,720
O	23.8
C	10.1
Ne	3.4
N	3.1
Mg	1.1
Si	1.00
Fe	0.90
S	0.51
Ar	0.10

A. Exploration by Spacecraft

Just how rich in phenomena these distant systems are became clear only in the last two decades, as spacecraft passed the planets and their moons, penetrating the magnetospheres in which they are immersed. This direct exploration began with Pioneers 11 and 12, two small, spinning spacecraft that reached Jupiter in 1974 and 1975, respectively. Before these pathfinder missions, it was not clear that spacecraft could safely be sent to the outer solar system. No one knew the extent of the possible hazard posed by the asteroid belt, or what would happen when the electronics on the Pioneers was bombarded by the protons and electrons trapped in Jupiter's magnetosphere. In fact, the missions were very successful. Pioneer 11 passed close enough to Jupiter to use the planet's gravitational field to deflect the spacecraft across the solar system for the first close fly-by of Saturn in 1979.

The Pioneers were followed by Voyagers 1 and 2, which reached Jupiter in March and July of 1979 (Fig. 1, color). (For this figure and all other color figures, please see the color section in this chapter.) Jupiter's gravity was then used to boost both spacecraft on to Saturn, where Voyager 1 arrived in November 1980 followed by Voyager 2 in August 1981. Voyager 1 (Fig. 2) was targeted to make a close encounter with Saturn's remarkable satellite Titan. This decision meant that the spacecraft could not pass close enough to the planet itself to be boosted on to Uranus and Neptune. However, the trajectory of Voyager 2 was chosen with this latter objective in mind, and this spacecraft flew through the Uranus system in January 1986. Uranus proved to be relatively bland itself, but its small inner moon, Miranda, revealed a surprising amount of geological activity to the Voyager cameras. The next stop was Neptune, encountered in August 1989. Voyager found, in addition to the striking cloud features on the planet, active vulcanism on the 37 K surface of Triton, Neptune's largest satellite.

Almost everything we know about the outer planets has come to us from the epic 12-year journey of the two Voyager spacecraft. This article will review the results from those missions that are particularly relevant to exobiology, adding the insights obtained from ground-based observations as appropriate. It is important to recognize that not only are new ground-based observations continuously bringing new insights, but even the Voyager observations themselves have not yet been completely analyzed. Thus we may expect new information about these distant planets before the Galileo spacecraft gives us our next big leap forward in 1995. It will go into orbit around Jupiter after deploying an instrumented probe into this giant planet's atmosphere.

Pluto, alas, was out of reach of both Voyager spacecraft. In one of nature's kinder coincidences, however, Pluto and its satellite Charon produced a series of eclipses and occultations during the 1980s that will not be repeated for 120 years, allowing some detailed inferences to be drawn about this system from ground-based observations.

II. Jupiter

A. System Overview

Aptly named for the king of the gods in the Greco-Roman pantheon, Jupiter is larger than all the other planets combined, with 318 times the mass of the Earth. Its magnetosphere is bigger than the Sun. If we could see the magnetosphere with our eyes, it would appear to cover an area in the sky equal to that of the full moon.

Jupiter possesses a thin, narrow ring, discovered by Voyager 1. The ring is surrounded by a diffuse cloud of particles that tapers away into a still thinner, gossamer ring that extends to the orbit of the satellite Thebe. This ring is apparently composed primarily of silicate dust generated by impacts on the tiny inner moons—Adrastea and Metis—with contributions from other satellites, especially Io.

The satellites themselves exhibit a wide range of characteristics (Table 2). The four largest can easily be seen with a small telescope, as Galileo found out when he discovered them in 1610. This discovery was one of the important observations that argued against the Church-supported view that the Earth was the center of the universe and all celestial bodies must therefore orbit around it. Galileo had found a miniature solar system, more similar to the actual one than he imagined.

Io is the most remarkable of the four Galilean satellites. As it moves around its orbit, this satellite is acted upon by massive tides from Jupiter that are countered by the attractions of the neighboring satellites. The result is a huge dissipation of tidal energy within Io, causing the interior to melt and producing the most volcanically active body in the solar system. This was one of Voyager's most spectacular discoveries.

In sharp contrast, Europa is covered by a thin layer of ice, making it the smoothest satellite we know. This coating must have occurred relatively recently (100 million to a billion years ago) since we see only a few impact craters on Europa. The icy surfaces of Ganymede and Callisto reveal a record of early bombardment similar to that found on the surfaces of Mercury and our Moon in the inner solar system. Evidently

VOYAGER FLIGHT PATHS

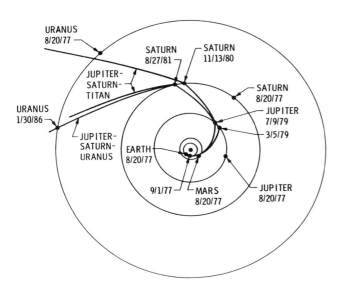

Fig. 2 The trajectory of the Voyager 1 spacecraft. The decision to make a close approach of Titan with Voyager 1 prevented the spacecraft from going on to Uranus and Neptune. (Owen, T., Morrison, D. Escaping from Earth, *The Planetary System.* Addison-Wesley, New York, 1988, Figure 2.15.)

we are looking at very ancient surfaces here, more than 3.5 billion years old.

The small outer satellites of Jupiter fall into two groups according to the direction of their orbital motions about the planet: four are in direct, and four are in retrograde orbits. Opinion is divided about the origin of these small bodies, but most scientists agree they must have been captured some time during the planet's formation. Neither of the Voyagers got close enough to any of them to provide direct observations.

The huge magnetosphere that surrounds the planet, its rings, and all of the satellites gets its energy and structure from Jupiter's magnetic field. As in the case of the Earth, Jupiter's field is generated deep within the planet by motions within a fluid, conducting core. On Earth, that fluid is molten iron and nickel. On Jupiter, it is liquid hydrogen, compressed so greatly by the overlying burden of gas that electrons have been stripped from their atoms and move freely, giving the hydrogen the properties of a conducting metal. The magnetic field strength at Jupiter's cloud deck is 12 times the value we experience on Earth. It is also oriented in the opposite direction with respect to the planet's spin axis, so a terrestrial compass taken to Jupiter would point south instead of north. There is nothing profound in this difference, however, since our planet's field has reversed its direction many times during the past millions of years, and the same may be true for Jupiter. The Sun, for example, reverses the direction of its field every 11 years.

B. The Atmosphere

Jupiter's hydrogen and helium dominated atmosphere contains a variety of additional gases (Table 3). As expected, other elements form compounds with hydrogen; carbon produces methane, nitrogen produces ammonia, oxygen produces water, etc. But there are also some surprises. Acetylene would not be anticipated from simple chemical equilibrium, nor would carbon monoxide or hydrogen cyanide. These substances are produced by chemical reactions within the atmosphere, driven by non-thermal (or at least nonlocal) sources of energy. These include solar ultraviolet light, lightning discharges, electrons and protons raining down in the polar regions from the magnetosphere, and the heat escaping from the planet's deep interior (Fig. 3). All four of these sources of energy have been observed in action on Jupiter. The polar auroras caused by particle precipitation are even visible from Earth (Fig. 4). Their effects on atmosphere chemistry are evident in Voyager ultraviolet images that show a darkening at the poles. Table 3 includes an attribution of the energy source considered to be primarily responsible for each of these non-equilibrium compounds.

This is still a somewhat controversial subject, since we do not yet have all the information that is necessary to make a clean choice in some cases. Thus, for C_2H_2 and HCN, both photochemistry and lightning discharges have been invoked as the key energy sources. It seems possible that in the case of HCN in particular, both sources may contribute. Ground-based observations seem likely to be able to determine soon which of these various energy sources is most important for which compounds.

It is somewhat disappointing that more complex compounds have not yet been identified spectroscopically. We can be rather certain that such compounds exist, however, because of the presence of subtle shades of color in the jovian clouds (Fig. 5, color). Simple condensation of the gases and vapors in Jupiter's atmosphere would produce white clouds, like the ones we are familiar with in our own skies. Color is one of the defining characteristics of discrete cloud systems on Jupiter. It is especially remarkable that on a planet with such a turbulent atmosphere, not only do these discrete colored cloud systems with well-defined boundaries exist, some of them occur only at very specific latitudes and altitudes. Perhaps the most striking examples of this specificity are the dark brown clouds at +18° and the Great Red Spot at 35°. The association with latitude is determined by simple inspection of photographs such as Fig. 5. The determination of altitude is more subtle, requiring the use of thermometers and/or barometers.

Thermal radiation from the planet itself offers a good thermometer. It can be observed directly at 5 μm, where reflected sunlight is negligible. Here one finds discrete hot spots showing up against a rather bland (cold) background, with the hottest regions appearing near the planet's equator (Fig. 6). Evidently we are "looking" more deeply into the planet's interior in these hot spots than we do in the adjacent

Table 2 Satellites of the outer planets

Satellites of Jupiter

Name	Discoverer(s)	Year of discovery	Magni-tude (V_o)[1]	Mean distance from Jupiter (km)	Sidereal period (days)	Orbital inclination (degrees)	Orbital eccentricity	Radius (km)	Mass (g)	Mean density (g/cm^3)
Metis	S. Synnott	1979	17.5	127,960	0.295	(0)[2]	0.00	(20)	?	?
Adrastea	D. Jewitt, E. Danielson	1979	18.7	128,980	0.298	(0)	(0)	12 x 8	?	?
Amalthea	E. Barnard	1892	14.1	181,300	0.498	0.4	0.00	135 x 75	?	?
Thebe	S. Synnott	1979	16.0	221,900	0.675	(0.8)	0.01	(50)	?	?
Io	S. Marius, Galileo	1610	5.0	421,600	1.769	0.04	0.00	1,815	8.94×10^{25}	3.57
Europa	S. Marius, Galileo	1610	5.3	670,900	3.551	0.47	0.01	1,569	4.80×10^{25}	2.97
Ganymede	S. Marius, Galileo	1610	4.6	1,070,000	7.155	0.19	0.00	2,631	1.48×10^{26}	1.94
Callisto	S. Marius, Galileo	1610	5.6	1,883,000	16.689	0.28	0.01	2,400	1.08×10^{26}	1.86
Leda	C. Kowal	1974	20.2	11,094,000	238.72	27	0.15	(8)	?	?
Himalia	C. Perrine	1904	15.0	11,480,000	250.57	28	0.16	(90)	?	?
Lysithea	S. Nicholson	1938	18.2	11,720,000	259.22	29	0.11	(20)	?	?
Elara	C. Perrine	1905	16.6	11,737,000	259.65	28	0.21	(40)	?	?
Ananke	S. Nicholson	1951	18.9	21,200,000	631	147	0.17	(15)	?	?
Carme	S. Nicholson	1938	17.9	22,600,000	692	163	0.21	(22)	?	?
Pasiphae	P. Melotte	1908	16.9	23,500,000	735	147	0.38	(35)	?	?
Sinope	S. Nicholson	1914	18.0	23,700,000	758	153	0.28	(20)	?	?

Satellites of Saturn

Name	Discoverer(s)	Year of discovery	Magni-tude (V_o)	Mean distance from Saturn (km)	Sidereal period (days)	Orbital inclination (degrees)	Orbital eccentricity	Radius (km)	Mass (g)	Mean density (g/cm^3)
Atlas	R. Terrile	1980	18.0	137,640	0.602	(0)	(0)	20 x 15	?	?
Prometheus	S. Collins and others	1980	15.8	139,350	0.613	(0)	0.00	70 x 40	?	?
Pandora	S. Collins and others	1980	16.5	141,700	0.629	(0)	0.00	55 x 35	?	?
Epimetheus	R. Walker	1966	15.7	151,422	0.694	0.34	0.01	70 x 50	?	?
Janus	A. Dollfus	1966	14.5	151,472	0.695	0.14	0.01	110 x 80	?	?
Mimas	W. Herschel	1789	12.9	185,520	0.942	1.53	0.02	195	3.8×10^{22}	1.17
Enceladus	W. Herschel	1789	11.7	238,020	1.370	0.02	0.00	250	8.4×10^{25}	1.24
Tethys	G. Cassini	1684	10.2	294,660	1.888	1.09	0.00	525	7.55×10^{23}	1.26
Telesto	B. Smith and others	1980	18.7	294,660	1.888	(0)	(0)	(12)	?	?
Calypso	B. Smith and others	1980	19.0	294,660	1.888	(0)	(0)	15 x 10	?	?
Dione	G. Cassini	1684	10.4	377,400	2.737	0.02	0.00	560	1.05×10^{24}	1.44
Helene	P. Laques, J. Lecacheux	1980	18.4	377,400	2.737	0.2	0.01	18 x 15	?	?
Rhea	G. Cassini	1672	9.7	527,040	4.518	0.35	0.00	765	2.49×10^{24}	1.33
Titan	C. Huygens	1655	8.3	1,221,850	15.945	0.33	0.03	2,575	1.35×10^{26}	1.88
Hyperion	W. Bond	1848	14.2	1,481,000	21.277	0.43	0.10	175 x 100	?	?
Iapetus	G. Cassini	1671	10.2-11.9	3,561,300	79.331	14.72	0.03	720	1.88×10^{24}	1.21
Phoebe	W. Pickering	1898	16.5	12,952,000	550.48	175.3	0.16	110	?	?

Satellites of Uranus

Name	Discoverer(s)	Year of discovery	Magnitude (V_O)	Mean distance from Uranus (km)	Sidereal period (days)	Orbital inclination (degrees)	Orbital eccentricity	Radius (km)	Mass (g)	Mean density (g/cm^3)
Cordelia	Voyager 2	1986	24	49,750	0.335	(0.14)	(0)	(15)	?	?
Ophelia	Voyager 2	1986	24	53,760	0.376	(0.09)	(0.01)	(15)	?	?
Bianca	Voyager 2	1986	23	59,160	0.435	(0.16)	(0)	(20)	?	?
Cressida	Voyager 2	1986	22	61,770	0.464	(0.04)	(0)	(35)	?	?
Desdemona	Voyager 2	1986	22	62,660	0.474	(0.16)	(0)	(30)	?	?
Juliet	Voyager 2	1986	22	64,360	0.493	(0.06)	(0)	(40)	?	?
Portia	Voyager 2	1986	21	66,100	0.513	(0.09)	(0)	(55)	?	?
Rosalind	Voyager 2	1986	22	69,930	0.558	(0.28)	(0)	(30)	?	?
Belinda	Voyager 2	1986	22	75,260	0.624	(0.03)	(0)	(35)	?	?
Puck	Voyager 2	1985	20	86,010	0.762	(0.31)	(0)	75	?	?
Miranda	G. Kuiper	1948	16.5	129,780	1.414	3.40	0.00	235	6.89×10^{22}	1.35
Ariel	W. Lassell	1851	14.4	191,240	2.520	0.00	0.00	580	1.26×10^{24}	1.66
Umbriel	W. Lassell	1851	15.3	265,970	4.144	0.00	0.00	585	1.33×10^{24}	1.51
Titania	W. Herschel	1787	14.0	435,840	8.706	0.00	0.00	790	3.48×10^{24}	1.68
Oberon	W. Herschel	1787	14.2	582,600	13.463	0.00	0.00	760	3.03×10^{24}	1.58

Satellites of Neptune

Name	Discoverer(s)	Year of discovery	Magnitude (V_o)	Mean distance from Neptune (km)	Sidereal period (days)	Orbital inclination (degrees)	Orbital eccentricity	Radius (km)	Mass (g)	Mean density (g/cm^3)
Naiad	Voyager 2	1989	25	48,000	0.296	(0)	(0)	(25)	?	?
Thalassa	Voyager 2	1989	24	50,000	0.312	(4.5)	(0)	(40)	?	?
Galatea	Voyager 2	1989	23	52,500	0.333	(0)	(0)	(90)	?	?
Despina	Voyager 2	1989	23	62,000	0.429	(0)	(0)	(75)	?	?
Larissa	Voyager 2	1989	21	73,600	0.554	(0)	(0)	(95)	?	?
Proteus	Voyager 2	1989	20	117,600	1.121	(0)	(0)	(200)	?	?
Triton	W. Lassell	1846	13.6	354,800	5.877	157	0.00	1,350	2.14×10^{25}	2.07
Nereid	G. Kuiper	1949	18.7	5,513,400	360.16	29	0.75	(170)	?	?

Satellite of Pluto

Name	Discoverer(s)	Year of discovery	Magnitude (V_o)	Mean distance from Pluto (km)	Sidereal period (days)	Orbital inclination (degrees)	Orbital eccentricity	Radius (km)	Mass (g)	Mean density (g/cm^3)
Charon	J. Christy	1978	16.8	19,640	6.387	98.8	0.00	595	(1.77×10^{24})	(2.0)

NOTES AND EXPLANATIONS

[1]V_0 is an object's magnitude in visible light at opposition. [2]Values in parentheses are uncertain by more than 10 percent. [3]Probably detected by H. Reitsema and others during an occultation in 1981. (Table information from *The New Solar System*, J. Kelly Beatty and Andrew Chaikin, eds., 1990.)

Table 3   Compositions of the atmospheres of Jupiter and Saturn

Main Constituents (percent)

Gas	Formula	Jupiter	Saturn
Hydrogen	H_2	86.1	92.4
Helium	He	13.8	7.4
Methane	CH_4	0.09	0.2
Ammonia	NH_3	0.02	0.02
Water vapor	H_2O	0.008(?)	—

Trace Constituents
(parts per billion)

				Energy Sources
Acetylene	C_2H_2	800	100	UV, Lightning (?)
Ethane	C_2H_6	40000	8000	UV
Carbon monoxide	CO	3	2	Internal Heat
Hydrogen cyanide	HCN	2	7	UV, Lightning (?)
Germane	GeH_4	0.6	0.4	Internal Heat
Phosphine	PH_3	400	3000	Internal Heat
Methyl acetylene	C_3H_4	?	trace	UV
Propane	C_3H_8	trace	trace	UV, Charged Particles (?)

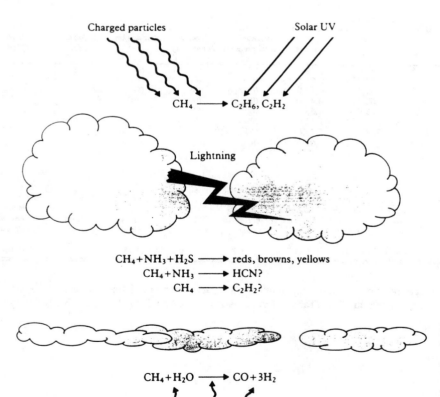

Fig. 3 This schematic diagram shows the various energy sources available on Jupiter to drive chemical reactions. (Owen, T., Morrison, D. Escaping from Earth, *The Planetary System*. Addison-Wesley, New York, 1988, Figure 11.8.)

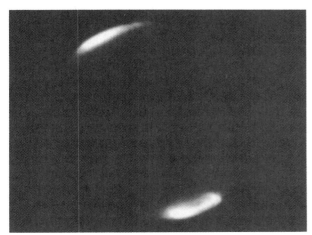

Fig. 4 This image of Jupiter was recorded with a special infrared camera at a wavelength of 3.4 μm. The planet itself is barely visible because we are looking into a strong methane band at this wavelength, so the incident sunlight is efficiently absorbed. But bright auroras are evident high in the atmosphere, above the methane, at each pole, as H_3+ is excited by charged particles precipitating into the atmosphere from Jupiter's radiation belts.

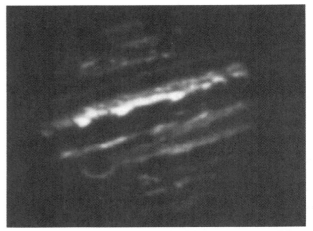

Fig. 6 The same camera used in Fig. 4 recorded this image of Jupiter at a wavelength of 4.9 μm. In this part of the spectrum, thermal radiation escaping from the interior of the planet dominates over reflected sunlight. Hence the bright areas on this picture are breaks in the clouds where heat from the interior can emerge.

regions, the opacity being provided by the clouds themselves. This means that one can make the best search for trace constituents in this part of the spectrum, since the optical path through the atmosphere is longest here.

Barometric measures can come from other deductions of optical path. Thus a region on the planet exhibiting strong absorption in a methane band, for instance, signals a deeper level than an adjacent feature that exhibits less overlying absorption. Another example is offered by photographs of the planet in ultraviolet light, since here one is dealing with Rayleigh scattering and the imaging is therefore constrained to the upper atmosphere. On all three counts—lack of 5 μm thermal radiation brightness in methane band photography, and its appearance in ultraviolet maps of the planet—the top of the Great Red Spot is one of the highest cloud features on the planet.

We have demonstrated that the dark brown clouds at +18° appear to be holes in a widespread layer of clouds characterized by a tawny color.[1] The proof consists of ground-based 5 μm observations showing that these features are warmer than the surrounding cloud layer (Fig. 6). Evidently, at this latitude a lower cloud layer of brown material exists which is absent in the planet's equatorial region, since the even hotter holes in the clouds observed here have a purplish coloration. One small brown hole was detected at -33° in Voyager 1 imagery, but was absent during the Voyager 2 encounter. It is possible that the brownish material defining small circular "storm systems" that tend to occur generally at high latitudes is made of the same material, as these features also appear to be warm at 5 μm. The oval-shaped dark brown clouds near 18° have been observed for over 100 years from Earth.[2]

This association of specific atmospheric chemistry with specific regions of the atmosphere is even more dramatic in the case of the Great Red Spot. Little red spots have been observed at +30°, but unfortunately none was available for inspection during the two Voyagers' encounters. Their absence proved the basic point: none of these small disturbances has exhibited lifetimes anywhere near that of the Great Red Spot. This feature has been well-observed for the past 150 years, and is probably the same object that was recorded by Robert Hook over 300 years ago.[2]

At the time of the Voyager flyby, the Great Red Spot could be characterized as an ellipse with axes of 21,000 km and 10,400 km (compared with Earth's diameter of 12,750 km). Voyager observations indicated that velocities around the periphery were about 100 km/sec in a counterclockwise direction, appropriate for an anticyclonic or high pressure system in the planet's southern hemisphere. Within 4000 km of the center of the Great Red Spot, the velocities appeared to be random, in keeping with the general appearance at Voyager's high resolution that resembled the surface of a choppy lake. The center was very quiescent, with velocities less than 10 m/sec.[3]

These descriptions tell us how the various clouds appear, but they have not yet helped us identify the chromophores responsible for their appearance. Today, the leading contenders seem to be organic polymers composed of $C_xN_yH_z$ sulfur compounds of some type, perhaps including carbon, and red phosphorus. Despite searches in various wavelength intervals by many investigators, no absorption features specific to any of the discrete, colored cloud systems have been discovered. Thus the chemical identification(s) depend(s) on indirect arguments tied to colors and altitudes, which are very poor discriminants.

Of the three hypotheses mentioned above, the Voyager

investigations and recent laboratory work appear to argue against the last one—red phosphorus. This idea was originally proposed[4] on the basis of laboratory experiments showing the production of red phosphorus from phosphine (PH_3). However, these experiments were carried out in the absence of other gases known to exist in the jovian atmosphere, and therefore it is not obvious they are applicable to Jupiter. Furthermore, there is some doubt that the phosphorus produced by the photodestruction of PH_3 is red, it may be yellow. The original argument[4] proposing this hypothesis cited the altitude of the Great Red Spot as one of the key points. The idea was that upwelling of gases over this region of Jupiter brought PH_3 higher in the atmosphere above the Great Red Spot than over adjacent cloud features. The data available to date do not support this prediction, but more work is needed to provide a definitive test.

If P_4 is not the answer, what are the alternatives? What is so special about this region of Jupiter? One suggestion is that the great height of the Great Red Spot also implies that the disturbance extends to great depth. Thus there is the potential for the upwelling of compounds that do not reach visible levels in the atmosphere at other locations on the planet, or at least do not appear in the same concentrations. This is also a testable hypothesis, in that one could look for anomalous concentrations of compounds like AsH_3, GeH_4, HCN, etc., within the Great Red Spot. No such anomalies have yet been uncovered.

The proposal that sulfur compounds could be responsible for most of the colors we see on Jupiter received a serious setback a few years ago, when a very sensitive search failed to turn up any evidence of H_2S. A limit of S/H $<10^{-3}$ of the solar abundance in the column of jovian atmosphere above a pressure level of 1.2 bars was set.[5] This is consistent with the presence of an NH_4SH cloud deck at 2.0 bars, since the vapor pressure of H_2S above these clouds would be too low to be detectable. The existence of such clouds was first postulated on thermochemical grounds[6] and their reality is generally accepted, although there is not yet any direct observational proof. The important point for our discussion is that if infrared photons penetrating to 1.2 bars cannot find any evidence of the dominant sulfur compound expected in the atmosphere, then ultraviolet photons won't find it either. In other words, production of chromophores by ultraviolet irradiation of H_2S isn't going to work. The remaining possibility, then, is lightning discharges in the clouds themselves.

We are thus left in a very unsatisfactory position. The jovian clouds are undeniably colored, and those colors bespeak the presence of molecules more complex than (or at least profoundly different from) any of the substances discovered in the atmosphere to date. Some of these compounds may be very relevant to our concerns about prebiological chemical evolution. Unfortunately, at this stage we simply don't know what they are!

Additional progress on this subject can be expected from ground-based spectroscopy with high spatial resolution during the next few years. The Hubble Space Telescope may also be able to help, but only with the Great Red Spot since this is the only colored region that reaches high enough in the atmosphere to be accessible in the ultraviolet. Finally, we have the Galileo mission, which will send a probe into Jupiter's atmosphere in December 1995. It is unlikely that the mass spectrometer on this probe will be able to identify chromophores directly, because they must be present in such tiny traces. Nevertheless, the detailed information that will be obtained about atmospheric composition, its variation with altitude and with the existence of clouds at different levels, all seems certain to advance our knowledge.

C. The Volcanoes of Io

Because of its unusual volcanic activity and sulfur chemistry, Jupiter's remarkable satellite Io deserves some additional attention. The first observational clue that something must be different about Io came from ground-based observations that showed it had a unique reddish color, yet was highly reflective in the near infrared. The early Voyager pictures revealed a surface with no impact craters, indicating very young terrain. Some process had to be continually resurfacing this satellite, and that process was soon identified as tidally driven volcanism. The reddish color, in turn, appears to be the result of various forms of sulfur and sulfur compounds that have been distributed over Io's surface by the volcanic activity.

This activity had been predicted by Stan Peale and his colleagues before the Voyager encounter. They had noticed that the gravitational attraction exerted on Io by the satellites Europa and Ganymede through orbital resonances would force Io to have an eccentric orbit. This means that the distance of Io to Jupiter varies around the orbit and the speed of Io in its orbit changes with time although its rate of spin remains constant. Taken together, these two effects occurring deep within Jupiter's powerful gravitational field lead to the dissipation of a huge amount of tidal energy inside the satellite, enough to cause extensive melting and—so these authors correctly surmised—widespread volcanic activity.

The volcanoes of Io are not like those of Earth or Mars in appearance. Apparently because of the lower viscosity of the satellite's "lavas"—which may be the result of their high sulfur content—Io's volcanoes do not form the large cones or shields typically associated with terrestrial volcanic activity. Instead one finds vents with very little surface relief producing flows that are sometimes hundreds of kilometers in intensity. There is no doubt about the extent of the activity. The Voyager spacecraft found nine eruptions in progress during their encounters in 1979.

These eruptions take the form of plumes rising vertically from the satellite's surface to altitudes near 300 km, where they spread out into a mushroom shape as the material rains down around the vent (Fig. 7). Two types of vulcanism have been postulated, one in which SO_2 is the working fluid, the other, of shorter duration, relying on sulfur itself. The entire interior of the satellite should be partially molten as a result of

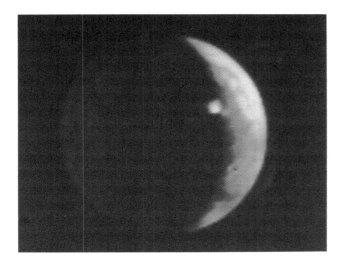

Fig. 7 This image of Io led to the discovery of the famous volcanoes by Linda Morabito, who noticed the mushroom shape of the plume on the satellite's limb. Another plume is evident as a bright blotch on the terminator (line between day and night). NASA photograph P-21306.

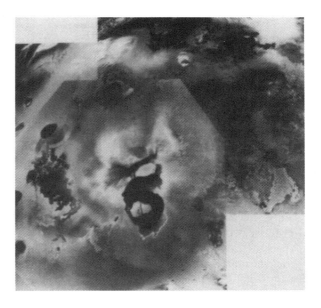

Fig. 8a A close-up view of the feature known as Loki on Jupiter's volcanically active satellite Io. The diagonal vent at the top is the source of a vertical plume, while the dark, semicircular feature may be lake of molten sulfur. NASA photograph 260-642B.

the dissipation of tidal energy. The surface layers must contain relatively large amounts of sulfur and SO_2, including lakes of liquid sulfur such as the one located near the Loki vent (Fig. 8). (See also color plate Fig. 8b, a color view of Io.) All of the water that was originally present on the satellite must have disappeared long ago, boiled out to the surface where it would rapidly evaporate and dissociate.

Io is also remarkable because of its interaction with the jovian magnetosphere. The planet, with its magnetic field, rotates in a little less than 10 hours, whereas the period of revolution of Io about Jupiter is nearly 2 days. Thus the planetary magnetic field is sweeping over this satellite with a velocity approaching 60 km/sec, which could lead to the generation of an electric potential difference of 600,000 volts across Io's diameter.

Charged particles from the jovian magnetosphere are continually impacting Io's surface. The first measurements by J. Van Allen with the Pioneer spacecraft showed that the flux encountered by the satellite amounts to $2 \times 10^5/cm^2s^{-1}$ for electrons with energies greater than 21 MeV. The cumulative exposure for each spacecraft during its passage amounted to 400,000 rads, which may be compared with the lethal dose of 400 rads for a human being. The Voyager spacecraft added information on the proton flux, found to be more than $10^4/cm^2s^{-1}$ for protons with energies greater than 2.5 MeV. The surface of Io is therefore an extremely hostile environment!

This flux of high energy electrons and protons does produce an interesting side effect, however. The bombarding particles can dislodge atoms from surface materials on Io through a process known as sputtering. The result is that a torus of atoms surrounds the satellite's orbit, with sodium, potassium, oxygen, and sulfur present in the neutral state,

together with ions of sulfur and oxygen. This torus had been detected from Earth before the arrival of any spacecraft through observations of the glowing of cloud of sodium atoms.

Io is obviously an extremely interesting satellite for geologists and geochemists, offering a spectacular natural laboratory for testing ideas about volcanism, mantle plumes, sulfur chemistry, etc. While that chemistry may also seem alluring to exobiologists, we must recognize that the hostile radiation environment will necessarily limit the development and survival of the kind of complex, information-containing molecular structures with only moderately strong bonds that are generally assumed to be prerequisites for any type of life. A possible exception to this conclusion may be afforded by special environments in subsurface layers that are protected from the lethal fluxes of electrons and protons. But an even friendlier subterranean environment may be waiting on Europa.

D. An Ocean on Europa?

This completes our discussion of the Jupiter system except for one more object that may hold some interest for exobiology. This is the satellite Europa, smallest of the four discovered by Galileo, with the smoothest surface of any body we have seen so far. The density of this object is below that of its sister satellite Io, whose rocky surface is wracked by intense volcanism. If these two moons are made of the same material, the lower density of Europa is most easily accounted for by assuming that its smooth icy surface is the top of a layer of ice

Table 4   Relative abundances on Jupiter and Saturn

Element	Jupiter/Sun	Saturn/Sun
O	~2	~10 (?)
C	2.3 ± 0.2	4 ± 2
N	~2	$\sim 3 \pm 1$
S	$<10^{-3}$	?
P	0.9 ± 0.2	9 ± 2
As	0.5 ± 0.2	7 ± 2
Ge	~0.05	~0.05

some 10 to 100 km thick.

Living on a planet whose oceans are equivalent to a global layer only 3 km thick, we may regard this as a great deal of ice. However, recall that Jupiter is on the far side of the ice line in the solar system, where ice is more abundant than rock. Thus we should be more surprised that the ice layer on Europa isn't at least a factor of 5 thicker, as it is on the Ganymede and Callisto, whose mean densities are only 1.9 gm/cc. Current thinking suggests that this layered composition is probably connected to the smoothness of Europa's surface. Like Io, Europa is subject to tidal heating that was apparently much more intense in the past than it is today, although still not as intense as that suffered by Io. As a result, the ice and water that was in the mix of material that formed the satellite were brought to its surface in a warm enough state to allow rapid evaporation into space. This process must have continued well past the end of the initial heavy bombardment, some 3.8 billion years ago; hence the absence of the widespread impact craters that characterize the icy surfaces of Ganymede and Callisto. The freezing of this global ocean has left Europa in the state we find it today. The question is, to what depth is the ocean frozen?

Given that tidal energy is still being dissipated inside Europa, one may legitimately ask whether sufficient heat from the interior reaches the surface of the rocky core to melt the ice to some height above this level. If so, perhaps the icy surface we see is in fact a relatively thin crust overlying a deep ocean. This model could explain the pattern of dark cracks with bright central ridges that appear to run over the satellite's surface (Fig. 9, color). Subsurface seawater could be extruded out onto the surface. If this water contains a rich enough mixture of dissolved material (e.g., organic compounds), photochemical and/or cosmic ray-induced reactions on the surface could act to darken it with time.

This model has been developed in considerable detail.[7] These authors carry the argument further to suggest two interesting extremes. At the surface of the ocean, thermal energy appearing at local "hot spots" might be available to colonies of organisms similar to those found around the famous "black smokers," hydrothermal vents occurring at places along the sea floor associated with plate boundaries on Earth. At the other extreme on Europa, enough sunlight may penetrate the ice sheet at the top of the ocean to permit photosynthesis by marine flora.

These ideas are certainly intriguing, but confront several difficulties. Perhaps the first of these is the issue of whether or not life could *begin* under these ultra-aqueous conditions. Could a freeze-thaw cycle near the upper ice boundary substitute for the drying and wetting of the more traditional tide pool? If they can, we must still ask if there is some way to concentrate the important precursor chemicals.

Even more fundamental than these arguments is the basic question of whether there is an ocean of liquid water beneath Europa's icy surface. Perhaps the satellite is simply covered by a thick sheet of ice. Under certain circumstances—for example, detection of Io-like eruptions of liquid water—the Galileo spacecraft may be able to help us here. If not, we must await a much more elaborate, specific mission to this intriguing moon. Meanwhile, we should at least be aware of this unusual possibility for a habitable environment, much farther from the Sun than conventional wisdom would allow. It might be well to keep such possibilities in mind when solving the Drake equation, with which one tries to estimate the number of "Earth-like planets" around nearby stars.

III. Saturn

A. System Overview

This giant planet is a beautiful sight in a telescope of modest size, with its magnificent system of rings and its extensive family of satellites (Fig. 10, color). Galileo could not see the rings clearly (he first thought the planet was three distinct bodies), but Christian Huygens deduced their true nature some 45 years later, discovering the satellite Titan as well.

The appearance of Saturn's globe is more subdued than that of Jupiter's. It does not show the same intricate cloud systems, although the banded structure of the overall cloud cover is similar. Voyager did discover a small reddish feature in one of the buff-colored cloud layers, but like other less colorful clouds on Saturn, this was a relatively short-lived phenomenon. A huge storm was observed by ground-based observers and by the Hubble Space Telescope in the fall of 1990, but it was white, and therefore probably ammonia cirrus. In fact, the basic cloud deck that we observe on Saturn is probably composed primarily of solid ammonia. The lower gravity on Saturn could make this layer much thicker than the ammonia cirrus found on Jupiter, so perhaps the saturnian clouds are more colorful at lower, inaccessible altitudes. The

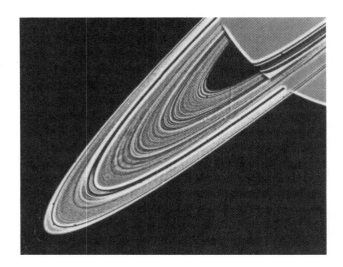

Fig. 11 The Voyagers found that Saturn is actually surrounded by thousands of rings, as the three main rings seen for 300 years from Earth were discovered to be full of structure. NASA photograph P-23068.

yellowish cast of the upper cloud deck may again be caused by sulfur compounds, but just as in the case of its giant neighbor, no surlfur-containing gases have yet been found in Saturn's atmosphere.

The list of gases that are known to exist there is very similar to the list for Jupiter (Table 3). The one major difference is the smaller relative abundance of helium on Saturn. This gas is evidently condensing and raining out of the atmosphere deep within Saturn's interior, mixing with the liquid hydrogen. The heat released by this process contributes to the excess energy the planet is observed to radiate.

There are some other interesting differences in the atmospheric compositions of the two planets, as illustrated in Table 4. Some elements, such as carbon, phosphorus and oxygen, are significantly enhanced on Saturn compared with Jupiter, while others, like germanium, are essentially identical in the two cases. As in the case of helium, these differences probably result from processes occurring deep in the planetary interiors. We might reasonably expect that the chemistry in the upper atmospheres of these planets is quite similar.

Unfortunately, there is no probe scheduled for deployment into Saturn's atmosphere that could produce results comparable to those to be obtained by Galileo on Jupiter. However, the Cassini spacecraft that will deliver such a probe to Titan, Saturn's intriguing satellite, will be equipped with a powerful infrared spectrometer that can be expected to improve our present understanding of the composition of Saturn's atmosphere.

The wind patterns on Saturn are also somewhat different from those of Jupiter, featuring a broad equatorial jet that reaches a speed of 1000 miles per hour. The alternating pattern so prominent on Jupiter doesn't begin on Saturn until latitudes approaching 40° from the equator. The reasons for this major difference between the two planets are not yet understood.

Saturn's extraordinary system of rings consists of a sheet of thousands of millions of icy particles ranging in size from dust grains to large boulders. There is a bewildering amount of structure in the rings that the Voyager spacecraft were able to record in detail (Fig. 11).

Saturn's magnetosphere is smaller than Jupiter's, but still much larger than Earth's. Again we have a rich array of phenomena as the whirling charged particles interact with the satellites and the planet. But no aurora was seen on Saturn by Voyager cameras, because the dark side of that planet is never truly dark. Light from the rings provides an illumination great enough to obliterate any auroral glow. An aurora was detected by the Voyager ultraviolet spectrometers, however. The presence of dark polar caps in visible and near infrared reflected sunlight suggests that chemical reactions are taking place at the poles of this planet, just as they are on Jupiter, producing compounds that are not found at other latitudes.

B. Satellites

Unlike Jupiter, Saturn has only one large satellite, Titan. But this satellite is so remarkable and so interesting for exobiology that it merits a separate section. Here we shall just mention three other moons that have some relevance to our topic: Enceladus, Iapetus, and Phoebe. (See Table 2 for a complete list of Saturn's satellites.)

Enceladus is remarkable for its astonishingly bright surface and its association with Saturn's E-ring (Fig. 12, color). It is a small (D = 500 km), icy satellite whose surface reveals a variety of impact craters and some smooth regions that look as if they had melted. The reflectivity of Enceladus is close to 100 percent, making it the best reflector in the solar system. This requires a continuous renewal of the icy surface material, which would otherwise darken with time. Other evidence for such activity comes from the fact that the orbit of the satellite is located in the densest part of the E-ring, a tenuous band of fine particles that would dissipate in just a few million years. Some process must be episodically repopulating this ring. Perhaps it is the same process that refreshes the satellite's surface. After our experience with Io, we might expect icy volcanism. But no volcanoes or active vents have been observed, and no one has yet been able to find a suitable energy source to power this activity. Is this another case like Europa, of possible ice covered ocean? We just don't know.

Iapetus is another mysterious moon. The leading side of this satellite is roughly 10 times darker than the trailing hemisphere, for reasons that still aren't clear. The rotation of Iapetus is locked in resonance with its period of revolution, so the dark side always leads as the satellite orbits the planet. This hemisphere is so dark it appears to be coated with a carbon-containing substance similar, perhaps, to the equally dark material covering the nucleus of Halley's Comet. But how did it get there? Why is it only on one side of one satellite in the entire solar system? The distant views afforded by Voyager 2 could not resolve the problem (Fig. 13, color).

It was once thought that this material might be coming from Phoebe, Saturn's outermost satellite. Phoebe is itself a very interesting body, with a diameter of only 200 km and a very dark surface. Because it is in a retrograde orbit, Phoebe is almost certainly a captured object, and may be a large comet nucleus. Whatever its origin, however, Phoebe is not the source of the dark material on the leading hemisphere of Iapetus, as spectra of these two dark surfaces are distinctly different. Some scientists think that the dark material on Iapetus originated on this satellite itself. They support this view by pointing out that on the border between the light and dark hemispheres, the dark matter is found preferentially in the bottoms of craters. On the other hand, Hyperion, orbiting Saturn between Iapetus and Phoebe, exhibits the same spectrum as the dark side of Iapetus, simply with a higher albedo. This would suggest an external origin, which could coat Hyperion uniformly since this satellite exhibits chaotic rotation.

Again we need help from a spacecraft to resolve these questions. Cassini, equipped with a near infrared spectrometer, will make the same measurements on Phoebe, Hyperion, and Iapetus. The close encounters of Cassini with Iapetus will permit a hundredfold increase in the resolution of images obtained by the cameras, further improving our chances of understanding the processes responsible for coating Iapetus in such a unique way.

IV. Titan

A. Introduction

Titan was first glimpsed as a tiny "star" accompanying Saturn by the Dutch astronomer Christian Huygens in March 1655. In the 1940s, Gerard P. Kuiper discovered that Titan's spectrum exhibited the same absorption bands of methane that were well known in the spectra of Jupiter and Saturn. Evidently this satellite has an atmosphere. This initially surprising result is simply a consequence of Titan's relatively large mass and low temperature. Methane, having a high vapor pressure at low temperatures and a relatively high molecular weight is a reasonable candidate for the atmosphere of this distant satellite.

Obviously a number of other gases satisfy these criteria as well, but most of them are difficult to detect from Earth. Unlike Jupiter and Saturn, Titan was certainly not expected to retain large amounts of hydrogen and helium, as these gases can easily escape from the satellite's relatively weak gravitational field. Nitrogen, argon, and carbon monoxide are all good possibilities. Even determining the abundance of methane on Titan proved difficult, however, since measurements made at different wavelengths gave different results. This suggested the presence of clouds, but just what these clouds were made of and how widespread they were remained obscure. Earth-based observers struggled with these and other questions for many years, finding various, often contradictory answers. Titan appears as a barely resolvable disk even in our best telescopes, a serious handicap for any efforts to unravel its mysteries at this distance.

The Voyager 1 spacecraft flew past Titan in November 1980. The trajectory of this spacecraft had been optimized for a close encounter, at a distance of only 4000 km. The full array of instruments on board was brought into play, and we learned more about Titan in those few days than in all the preceding 325 years since its discovery. The high resolution pictures turned out to be very disappointing (Fig. 14, color), but the other experiments produced a rich harvest of results.

B. Origin

Titan must be seen as a member of a class of large, icy objects in the outer solar system. Other members of this class include Ganymede and Callisto at Jupiter, Triton at Neptune, and the Pluto-Charon system (Table 2). The similarities and differences among these objects and their relationship to the smaller icy satellites, the giant comet Chiron, and other comet nuclei are not yet completely clear. What we do know is that all of these larger objects are made of a mixture of water ice and rock, with the ice apparently containing increasing amounts of frozen, trapped, and adsorbed gases the farther the body is from the Sun.

It is not just distance from the Sun that determines the final composition of these bodies. The specific location in which the object formed is also extremely important. Each giant planet had a major influence on the gas and dust in the solar nebula in the region of its formation. We can thus speak of planetary sub-nebulae, in which conditions varied as a function of distance from the primary planet in an analogous way to the variations found within the solar nebula with varying distance from the Sun.

In both cases, temperature was a key variable. The formation of the giant planets produced large amounts of heat as gravitational potential energy was turned into kinetic energy when the dispersed matter in the solar nebula "condensed" into the much smaller volume of a planet. Calculations show that in the early phases of its history, Jupiter was radiating so much thermal energy it must have glowed. Some of this primordial heat is still escaping from that giant planet today.

For the Saturn system, the effect is more subtle, since Saturn is more than three times less massive than Jupiter and therefore the heat generated during its formation was correspondingly less. Instead of a distinction between rocky inner satellites (Io and Europa) and icy outer ones (Ganymede and Callisto), we find icy bodies throughout the Saturn system, from the ring particles to Phoebe. But the proportion of other volatiles in the ices contained in these bodies may follow the early thermal gradient set up by the presence of the hot, forming planet at the system's center. Thus we expect substances such as methane, ammonia, nitrogen, carbon monoxide, and argon to have been more prevalent in the materials that formed the more distant satellites.

Similarly, the generally lower temperatures in the Saturn system compared with Jupiter may explain why Titan has an atmosphere while Ganymede and Callisto do not, although the

Table 5   Composition of the atmosphere of Titan

Gas		Formula	Amount
A.	Main Constituents (percent)		
Nitrogen		N_2	82-99%
Argon		Ar	0-12[a]
Methane		CH_4	1-6[a]
B.	Trace Constituents (parts per million)		
Hydrogen		H_2	2000
Hydrocarbons			
Ethane		C_2H_6	20
Propane		C_3H_8	20
Ethylene		C_2H_4	0.4
Diacetylene		C_4H_2	0.1-0.01
Methylacetylene		C_3H_4	0.03
Nitrogen compounds			
Hydrogen cyanide		HCN	0.2
Cyanogen		C_2N_2	0.1-0.01
Cyanoacetylene		HC_3N	0.1-0.01
Oxygen compounds			
Carbon monoxide		CO	50-150
Carbon dioxide		CO_2	0.015

[a]The presence of argon can only be deduced indirectly. There may be none at all, in which case the abundance of nitrogen would increase. The amount of methane varies with altitude and is still poorly determined.

similar densities of all three satellites suggest similar bulk compositions. Laboratory studies of the ability of water ice to trap and retain gases as it forms have demonstrated that this ability rapidly diminishes with increasing temperature. In particular, at temperatures above 135 K (-138 °C), gases that have either been trapped in the crystal structure of ice or merely absorbed on icy surfaces leave the ice with ease. In other words, even if the ice that now composes Ganymede and Callisto was formed at lower temperatures, once it had been heated above this temperature, its gas content would have been markedly depleted. This is apparently what happened to the materials that formed these satellites before their incorporation: they were in effect "baked out." In the cooler environment at Titan's distance from Saturn, however, temperatures evidently remained well below 135 K and the gases were not released until the satellite formed.

Heat liberated during the accretion of Titan would have been more than sufficient to liberate gases from the infalling ices. It could also have driven reactions among them, forming new species. These gases then became the satellite's earliest atmosphere. Additional heat was generated by the energy released from the decay of short-lived radioactive elements in the rocky component of Titan. Just as the inner rocky planets melted and differentiated, this distant satellite must have formed a core of dense (rocky) material that became surrounded by a mantle of ice. Thus the formation of a secondary, outgassed atmosphere on Titan followed the same general pathway that produced the early atmospheres on Mars, Venus,

and Earth.

In this discussion of Titan's origin, we have not considered where the material that formed the satellite came from and how it got organized in such a way that one large satellite was formed instead of several smaller ones. These are problems whose solutions are still unknown. As stated above, the current consensus is that the giant planets and their satellites formed from "sub-nebulae" in a similar manner to the formation of the Sun and the planets form the primordial solar nebula. But a significant difference was afforded by the fact that it is commonly assumed that no material came from outside the solar nebula to affect the forming sun and planets. In contrast, material from outside the planetary sub-nebulae was able to contribute to the formation of individual planets and satellites. Hence the composition of these sub-nebulae may have been closer to that of the main nebula that one might otherwise expect. This relationship is one of the many unresolved problems that require a new mission to the Saturn system for their resolution.

C. The Atmosphere: Composition and Evolution

As Voyager 1 approached Titan in the fall of 1980, it quickly became apparent that there are layers of airborne material in the satellite's atmosphere that completely hide the surface. Yet the reflectivity of Titan showed a sharp demarcation, with the northern hemisphere noticeably darker than the southern. Just how the airborne particles on Titan know where the satellite's equator is remains an unresolved problem of Titanian meteorology. Layering of the aerosols could also be observed at the limb, and there was a dark northern cap (Fig. 15, color).

The dominant gas in the atmosphere is molecular nitrogen, just as on the Earth. There is about 10 times as much nitrogen on Titan as on our planet, giving a value for the surface pressure of 1.5 times the sea-level pressure on Earth. Methane, the one gas identified with certainty before Voyager, turned out to be a minor constituent, with an abundance of a few percent. Present uncertainties in the determination of the mean molecular weight of the atmosphere allow as much as 10 to 15 percent of primordial argon (^{36}Ar + ^{38}Ar), but this gas may also be present only in tiny quantities. The infrared spectrometer revealed a rich variety of other compounds, principally hydrocarbons such as ethane (C_2H_6) and acetylene (C_2H_2) and nitriles such as hydrogen cyanide (HCN). A list of all the compounds detected so far is given in Table 5. Nitrogen and methane molecules are being broken apart by cosmic rays, high energy ultraviolet photons from incident sunlight, and electrons bombarding the atmosphere from Saturn's magnetosphere, and the fragments are recombining to make the minor constituents shown in Table 5. In this process, some hydrogen is produced; the amount of H_2 we see in Table 5 represents a steady state between production and escape.

In other words, Titan has an atmosphere that is still in the process of evolution from a primitive hydrogen-rich state. This is not too surprising, given the extremely low temperature at the satellite's surface. Voyager measured a value of 94 K, only a few degrees warmer than the temperature that would be assumed for a body with Titan's reflectivity and no atmosphere at all at this distance from the Sun. At this low temperature, the vapor pressure of water is vanishingly small. If we could magically move Titan closer to the Sun, say to the orbit of Mars, we would find that the character of the atmosphere would immediately change. The warmer surface temperatures would allow plenty of water vapor to enter the atmosphere, and the resulting supply of oxygen would rapidly convert methane and its byproducts to carbon dioxide, exactly the dominant carbon-carrier we find on Mars.

Meanwhile, back on the real Titan as we find it today, Table 5 indicates that a tiny amount of carbon dioxide is present, as is carbon monoxide. There are at least two solutions to this apparent paradox. First, the carbon monoxide may be primordial—it may have been one of the gases trapped in the ices that formed the satellite, that was then released into the atmosphere as Titan formed. Electrons from Saturn's magnetosphere that are continually bombarding Titan's atmosphere can break carbon monoxide apart, leaving the oxygen in an excited state. If one of these oxygen atoms encounters a methane molecule, it forms a molecule of OH that can then combine with another CO molecule to make CO_2, while the hydrogen escapes. In other words, given the presence of CO from the beginning, the formation of a small amount of CO_2 is understandable without the presence of water vapor.

Alternatively, water vapor could be supplied to this low temperature atmosphere from the outside, as showers of ice particles formed by meteoritic and cometary impacts with icy satellite surfaces, or directly, when this debris gravitationally captured by the Saturn system is swept up by Titan as it orbits the planet. In this case, the small amounts of CO and CO_2 observed could be produced from photochemical reactions between the resulting water vapor and the already present methane.

Which of these two alternatives is correct? Perhaps some of each. Today we cannot be certain, but recent evidence suggests that at least some primordial CO may be present. This evidence is in the form of microwave observations of CO in Titan's stratosphere that indicate a much lower abundance of this gas than that reported from the infrared observations that discovered it in the satellite's troposphere. In other words, it appears that this gas is more abundant at lower altitudes on Titan, which is consistent with its formation there (by outgassing) and destruction at high altitudes (by photochemistry). Since both sets of CO observations were made from Earth, there are hopes of improving the data during the next few years and finding an answer to this basic question.

The ultimate test of this hypothesis is a search for solid CO_2 on the surface of Titan. If the CO we now find in the atmosphere is a relic from a large primordial abundance, then a correspondingly large amount of CO_2 should have been produced and deposited in Titan's surface during the ensuing 4.5 billion years. This could be equivalent to a layer 10-100 meters thick. A properly instrumented probe that reaches the surface—an experiment planned for the year 2002—would be able to make this measurement.

Meanwhile, there is one more piece of evidence we can bring to bear on the problem of the origin of Titan's atmosphere, the relative abundance of deuterium. On Titan, most of the hydrogen is in the methane, and it has proved possible to detect the deuterated form of this molecule—CH_3D—in addition to CH_4. It turns out that the ratio of deuterium to hydrogen in the methane molecules on Titan is eight times higher than the ratio we find in the methane in the atmospheres of Jupiter and Saturn. About one-fourth of this enrichment, a factor of 2, has apparently been caused by processes acting on the satellite's atmosphere since it formed. For example, the escape of hydrogen from Titan's upper atmosphere produced an increased concentration of deuterium owing to its larger mass. Yet the other factor of 4 in the observed enrichment must be caused by something else. One possibility is that the high value of D/H on Titan is original, an indication that an interstellar ratio of deuterium to hydrogen has been preserved in Titan's ices.[8] Even higher ratios than this have been observed in hydrogen-containing molecules in dark interstellar clouds. These high values of D/H are produced by ion-molecule reactions that can occur in these cold, low density environments. In other words, the ices that formed the satellite and the gases that these ices contained were never subjected to high enough temperatures to allow them to reach equilibrium with either the gas in the proto-saturnian nebula or the hydrogen in the solar nebula itself. Since CO is at least

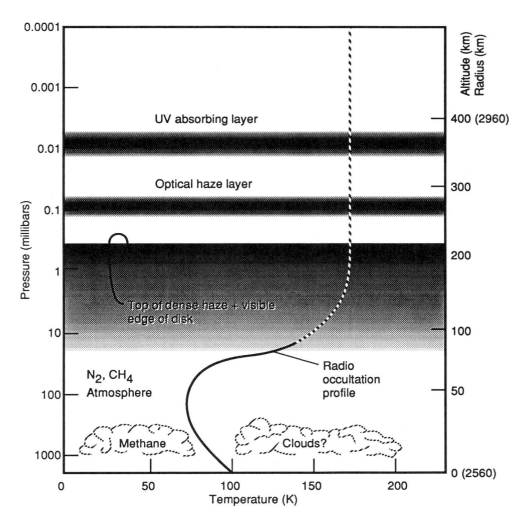

Fig. 16 The temperature profile in Titan's atmosphere reveals that this satellite has an extensive stratosphere that is warmer than the surface. The haze is formed continuously in this warmer region. (Owen, T., Morrison, D. In *Deep Freeze: Planets We Cannot See*, *The Planetary System*. Addison-Wesley, New York, 1988, Figure 13.24.)

100 times as abundant as methane in the interstellar medium, this apparent preservation of interstellar deuterium abundances also lends support to the idea that at least some fraction of the CO we find on Titan today is primordial in origin.

D. Aerosols

Figure 16 shows that temperature initially decreases with altitude from Titan's surface until the tropopause is reached at an elevation of about 60 km. At this point, there is a turnaround, and temperature begins to increase with height, eventually reaching a value of 175 K, some 80° *higher* than the surface temperature. This unusual structure is caused primarily by the absorption of ultraviolet light in Titan's upper atmosphere. Absorption occurs not only in the photochemical processes described in the previous section, but also in nondestructive excitation of the resulting molecules, and in the dark material making up the aerosol.

We can now see that some of this aerosol material is simply

condensed forms of the gases shown in Table 5. With the exception of hydrogen and carbon monoxide, everything in the table will condense at the tropopause temperature. The aerosol layers we see (Fig. 15) are not just simple condensation products, for in that case, they would be white or gray. The dirty-orange color suggests that some additional chemistry is occurring, transforming the simple molecules of Table 5 into more complex substances. Some of these are probably polymers. Both hydrogen cyanide and acetylene are known to form dark polymers that could certainly contribute to the observed effects. Laboratory experiments starting with the principal ingredients of Titan's atmosphere and using a variety of energy sources to drive the reactions have little difficulty in producing dark organic material that may well offer a good analog to Titan's aerosols. A long list of compounds has been identified in this laboratory material, but it has not yet proved possible to demonstrate a close match between laboratory and Titan observations.[9]

This aerosol cannot remain suspended in the atmosphere.

As the particles grow, they will precipitate out, and fall through the cold trap formed by the tropopause, ending up on Titan's surface. Inspection of Table 5 indicates that ethane is the most abundant photochemical product. As the condensed ethane falls through the lower atmosphere, it may form clouds or hazes, but when it reaches the surface, it will accumulate as a liquid. In principle, methane could also condense at the low temperature on Titan's surface, but careful analysis of the decrease of temperature with altitude just above the surface indicates that this is not the case. Clouds of methane may form in the lower atmosphere, but significant condensation of this species on the surface is unlikely. In contrast, Titan may be covered by a global ocean of methane with an average depth of 1 km.[10] This ocean would contain nitrogen and methane dissolved within it, along with all of the other products shown in Table 5.[11] The bottom could be lined with a mixture of nonsoluble aerosols (unless they are very "fluffy," they won't float) and solid CO_2. Projecting surface topography would also be coated by this mixture.

In the absence of oceans, one might expect a landscape similar to those found on Ganymede and Callisto, such as some mixture of impact craters and their debris plus the effects of a primitive kind of plate tectonics (present on Ganymede but not on Callisto). On the other hand, Enceladus and Io have taught us that it is very risky to extrapolate the geological history of one body to another. There may have been internal sources of energy on Titan such as resonance-induced tides from earlier configurations of the saturnian satellites. Giant impacts may have left huge basins. Yet whatever is present, it should be covered with a coating of precipitated smog particles if not by the global ocean.

Today, we cannot discriminate between these two possibilities. Ethane may undergo further reactions that produce more complex substances so efficiently that there is not enough of this compound left to form a global ocean. Yet ponds or seas seem likely, and the ability of a large ocean to serve as a reservoir for methane that can resupply the atmosphere as this gas is broken down makes the idea especially attractive. What we are lacking are definitive observations that tell us how much liquid is present, what its composition is, and how it is distributed over Titan's surface. Improvements in ground-based radars over the next few years may answer some of these questions even before we actually visit this fascinating satellite.

E. The Next Step: Cassini-Huygens

This account of Titan and its atmosphere should indicate just how much this satellite can tell us, if only we can learn more about it. Titan is a member of a class of volatile-rich icy planetesimals whose influence extends from the cores of the giant planets, through icy satellites to comet nuclei. Comets are capable of delivering these volatiles to the atmospheres of the inner planets, so studies of Titan may be closer to home than we might think. In Titan, we can examine a secondary atmosphere produced by the degassing of the volatiles trapped in such a planetesimal. The similarities and differences between these gases and those found in other representatives of this class of body—e.g., the comets—will tell us something about the conditions in which these objects formed and the processes involved in their formation. As we have seen, there appear to be opportunities to reach back in time through the process of solar system formation to study the chemistry in the natal cloud of gas and dust in the Interstellar Medium. Finally, this time travel also allows us to investigate an evolving, oxygen-poor atmosphere in which complex chemical reactions are occurring today that may resemble some of the reactions responsible for the first steps along the path from chemistry to biology on the early Earth.

This is a rich harvest indeed, so how do we go about reaping it? The most likely answer is a mission called Cassini-Huygens that has been initiated as a joint project by the European Space Agency (ESA) and the National Aeronautics and Space Administration. This mission will consist of a Saturn orbiter (Cassini) built by NASA and a Titan probe (Huygens) built by ESA. It is currently scheduled for launch in 1997, with arrival scheduled for 2004.

The orbiter is designed to carry a radar experiment that will allow it to map the surface of Titan right through the smog layers, much as the Magellan radar is mapping the surface of Venus. The orbiter would also carry cameras and infrared and ultraviolet spectrometers that will be much more capable than the equipment (launched 19 years earlier) on Voyager.

But the big news about Titan will surely come from the probe. Descending slowly through the atmosphere on a trajectory that allows it nearly 3 hours of measurements, the probe will take direct samples of the atmosphere with a gas chromatograph-mass spectrometer (GCMS) to determine composition and isotopic ratios. A special device will trap and volatilize the aerosols. Pictures of the scene below will be recorded by a sensitive camera while the ambient pressure and temperature are continuously monitored.

The descent is sufficiently slow that the probe could even survive its landing, be it a splash or a thud, and make additional measurements at the surface. In particular, the GCMS will have a heated inlet that will allow it to sample the material on which the probe will land. It will therefore be able to distinguish easily among an ethane ocean, deep deposits of aerosols, or an exposed icy surface consisting of CO_2, H_2O and other frozen volatiles.

V. Uranus

A. Overview

Uranus was the first of the planets to be discovered. All the rest were known to the ancients. William Herschel found this planet during a systematic survey of the stars in March 1781. He initially thought he had discovered a comet, but the true nature of the object soon became apparent. Two hundred and five years later, Voyager 2 passed through the Uranus system, discovering new satellites, rings, and features on the satellites

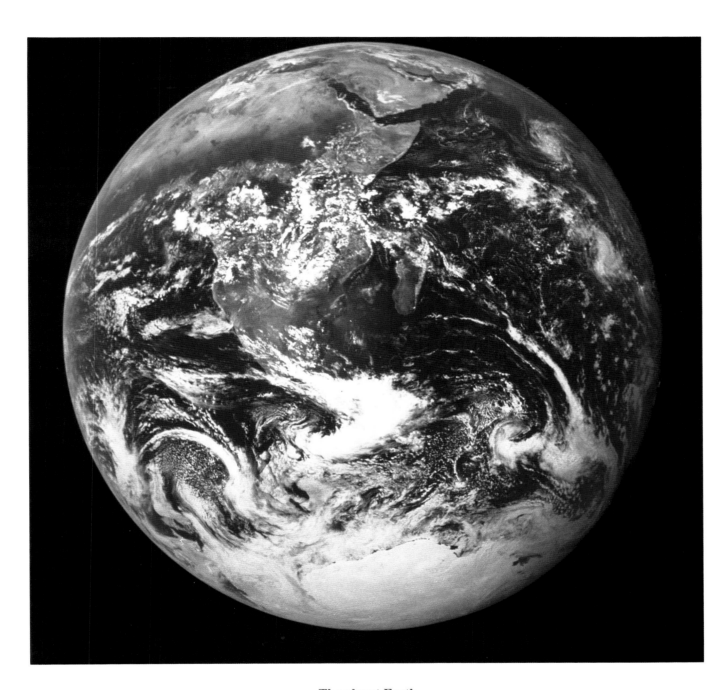

The planet Earth

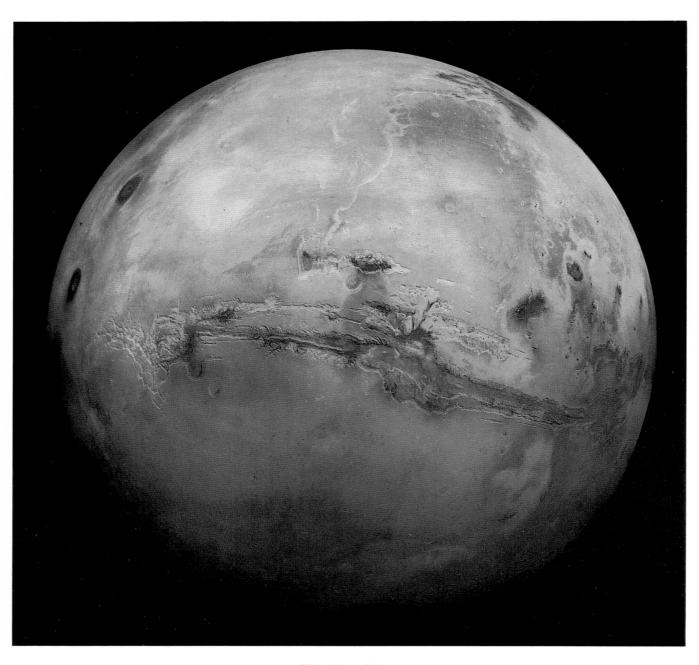

The planet Mars

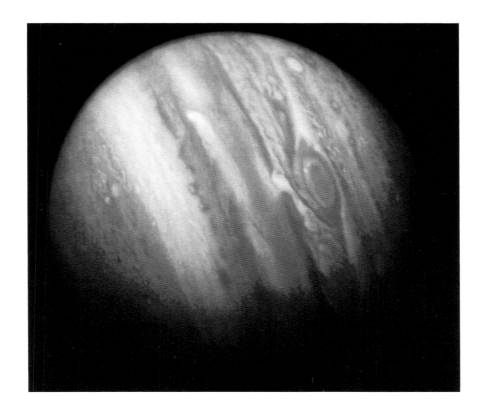

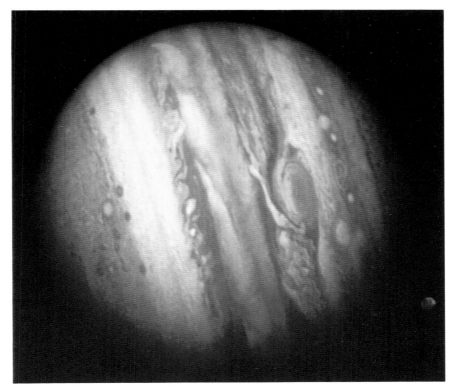

Chapter 4, Fig. 1   These two images of Jupiter were obtained by Voyager 1 (top) in March 1979 and Voyager 2 (bottom) in July 1979. Note the changes in appearance of the visible clouds resulting from the different velocities of wind currents at differing latitudes. (NASA photograph P-21599).

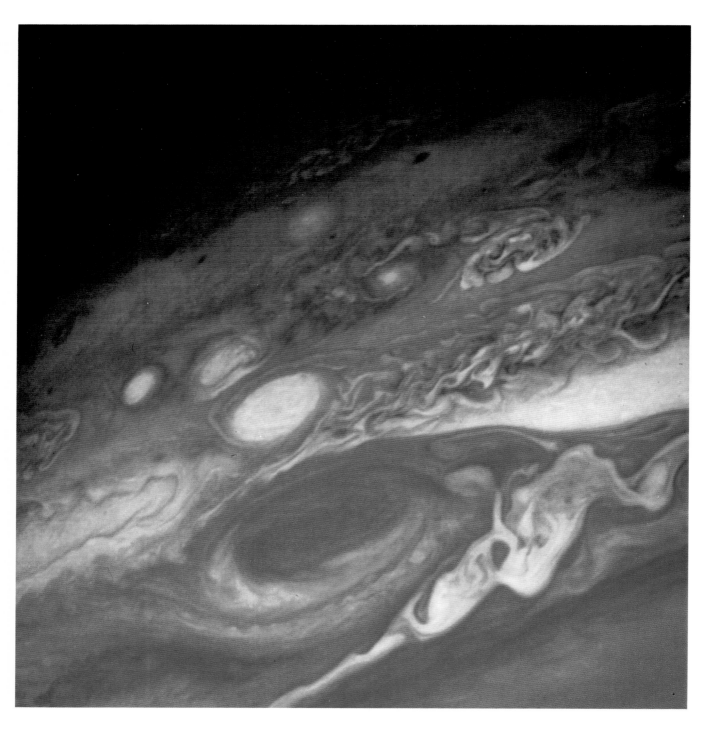

Chapter 4, Fig. 5   This close-up view of Jupiter by Voyager 1 shows the color (exaggerated for reproduction) associated with the Great Red Spot and the surrounding clouds. (NASA photograph 79-HC-280).

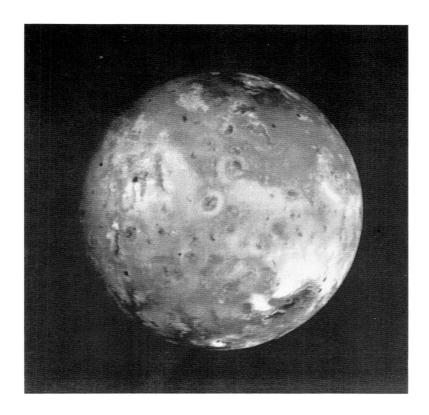

Chapter 4, Fig. 8b   Color plate of Io.

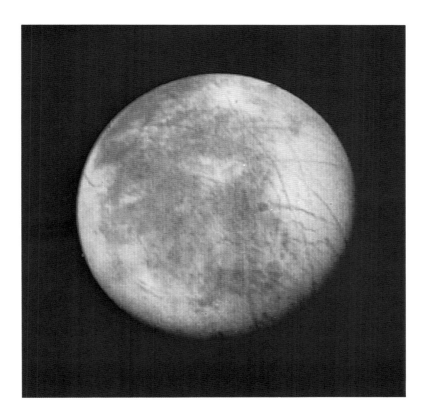

Chapter 4, Fig. 9   Europa is the smoothest satellite we know. Like Io, it has no impact craters; however, instead of volcanoes, we find a smooth, icy sphere decorated with a random pattern of dark streaks. (NASA photograph 82-HC-84).

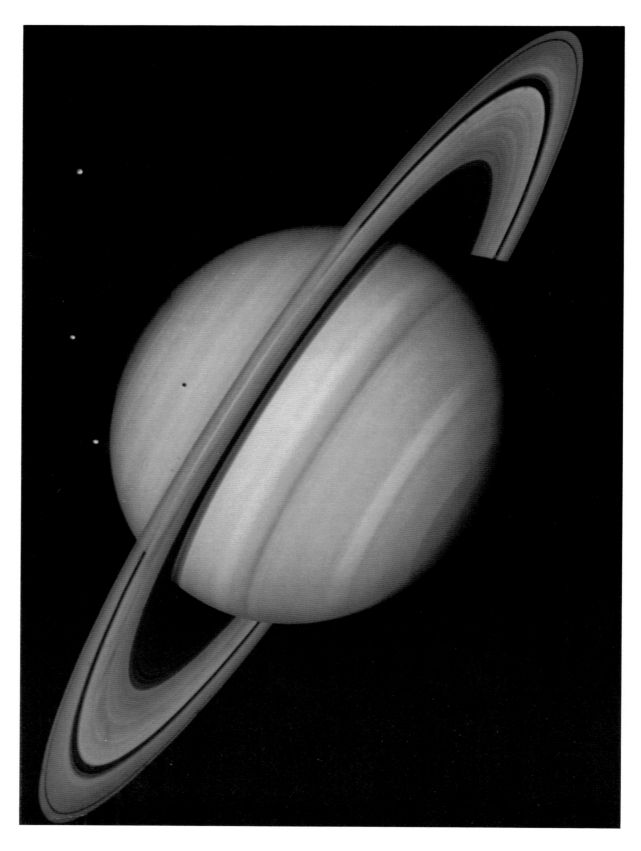

Chapter 4, Fig. 10   Saturn has a much more uniform cloud cover than Jupiter, as a comparison of this Voyager image with Fig. 1 demonstrates. (NASA photograph P-23887C/BW).

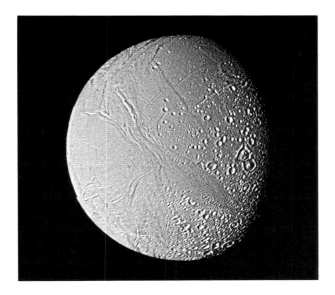

Chapter 4, Fig. 12   Parts of the surface of Enceladus appear to have melted, but no one has yet identified the source of energy required to do this, or to produce the particles populating the E-ring. (NASA photograph 82-HC-76).

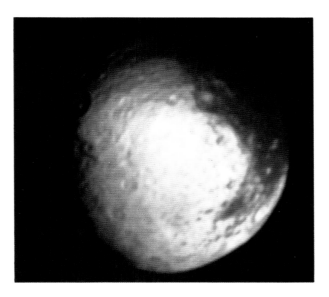

Chapter 4, Fig. 13   In this view of Iapetus, we should see the entire disk illuminated. The fact that we do not is caused by the very low reflectivity (3-5 percent) of the satellite's dark hemisphere, at the left-hand side of this image. (NASA photograph 81-HC-540).

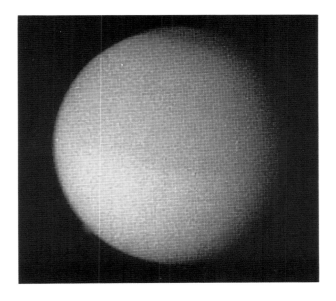

Chapter 4, Fig. 14   Titan was a disappointment to the Voyager 1 cameras, showing only a smog-filled atmosphere with an intriguing difference in reflectivity between northern and southern hemispheres. (NASA photograph P-23076).

Chapter 4, Fig. 15   The ubiquitous haze in Titan's atmosphere is not uniformly distributed with altitude. Discrete layers can be seen in this picture of the satellite's limb. (NASA photograph P-23107).

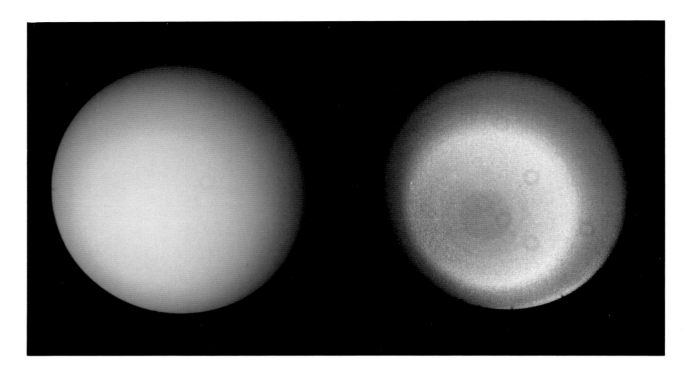

Chapter 4, Fig. 18   Uranus from Voyager 2. The image on the left shows the planet as it would appear to human eyes. On the right we see a false-color image that reveals an ultraviolet absorbing haze forming a cap centered on the south rotational pole of the planet. (NASA photograph P-29478C).

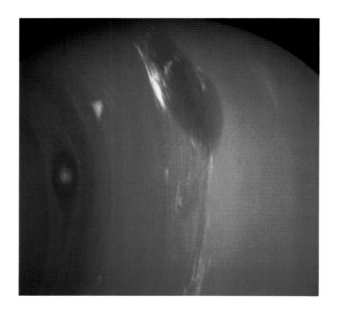

Chapter 4, Fig. 19   As Voyager 2 approached Neptune, the bright clouds suspected from ground-based observations became clearly apparent, along with a large dark oval and a dark collar of haze. Seen close up, the Great Dark Spot of Neptune shows certain resemblances to Jupiter's Great Red Spot (Figs. 1 and 4). (NASA photograph 89-HC-488).

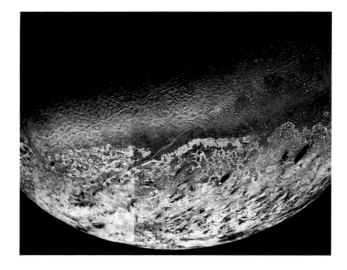

Chapter 4, Fig. 20   Neptune's satellite Triton has a tenuous atmosphere with a surface pressure of only 16 millionths of the sea-level pressure on Earth. Nevertheless, that atmosphere is evidently capable of producing winds that can move material around on Triton's surface, judging by the presence of these aligned, fan-shaped dark streaks. (NASA photograph 89-HC-461).

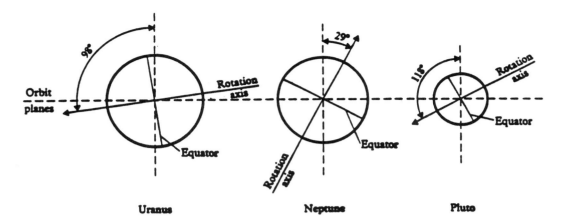

Fig. 17 Of the three outermost planets, only Neptune has a moderately inclined rotational axis. (Owen, T., Morrison, D. In Deep Freeze: Planets We Cannot See, *The Planetary System.* Addison-Wesley, New York, 1988, Figure 12.14.)

that could never be found from Earth.

Uranus is both smaller and denser than Jupiter or Saturn, indicating that it is enriched in elements heavier than hydrogen and helium. These two elements still dominate its composition, however. Perhaps the most striking characteristic of this planet is the orientation of its rotational axis, which is nearly in the plane of its orbit (Fig. 17). Only Pluto shares this peculiar configuration, commonly attributed to a glancing impact by a large planetesimal during the formation of the planet.

In appearance, Uranus is extremely bland (Fig. 18, color). The low temperature of the visible atmosphere (-218 °C) ensures that ammonia clouds will form below the levels to which we can see. Methane is condensing in this part of the atmosphere, but only a thin haze is readily apparent. A few clouds could be seen at low latitudes in the Voyager pictures. The beautiful aquamarine color of Uranus is caused by the absorption of red light by the methane gas in the planet's atmosphere. Sunlight reflected by the planet is thus deficient in red rays, but the short wavelengths are scattered strongly, just as in our own blue skies. The result is that when we view Uranus from a distance, we see a greenish disk.

Uranus has a system of 11 dark, narrow rings, quite different from the ring systems of either Jupiter or Saturn. Some of these rings are just 1 kilometer in width, while the widest has a variable width, ranging from 22 to 93 km. This ring is apparently held in place by two small satellites, one on either side.

Uranus has 15 known satellites, of which 10 were discovered by Voyager 2 (Table 3). The new ones are all tiny objects, less than 150 km in diameter, and very dark. Of the five discovered before the spacecraft encounter, the most remarkable is surely Miranda. Although this object is only 500 km in diameter, its surface reveals a variety of geological processes that indicate the dissipation of large amounts of energy. Some geologists have speculated that the entire satellite might

have been disrupted by a collision and then reformed. Another possibility is that the initial process of differentiation was somehow arrested prior to completion.

The magnetic field of Uranus is also unusual. In general, one expects a planet's magnetic axis to be oriented within a few degrees of the rotational axis. On Uranus this is not the case. The angle between the two axes is an astonishing 55°! This has the potential effect of causing the planet's auroral zone to occur near its equator, rather than at the pole.

B. Chemistry

Of special interest for our purposes is the dark haze in the upper atmosphere, covering the sunward pole (Fig. 17). This is not condensed methane, since it absorbs strongly in the ultraviolet, and occurs at a high altitude. Acetylene has been identified in the upper atmosphere of Uranus, so once again we have the case of an outer planet atmosphere in which methane is being photodissociated and producing other compounds. Evidently the end result is some ultraviolet absorbing components, perhaps similar to those found in the upper atmospheres of Saturn, Jupiter, and Titan.

It is also interesting that the icy satellites and the rings are so dark. These dark coatings are not like those on either Phoebe or Iapetus. So we seem to have yet another example of carbon chemistry producing solid components that coat the surfaces of icy bodies. In this case, if the starting material were CO and/or CO_2 instead of CH_4 we could account for the singular neutral color of these objects. They are almost uniformly dark at all wavelengths, unlike Iapetus and Phoebe, which are especially dark in the ultraviolet. What are the compounds? Since we find dark, carbon-rich material on so many icy bodies, we may also ask why any satellites of Saturn are bright. We cannot answer either of these questions at the present time.

VI. Neptune

A. Survey of the System

Neptune was discovered by means of mathematical calculations that were made to try to explain deviations in the apparent motion of Uranus. These deviations were thought to be caused by the gravitational attraction of a new, as yet unseen planet. John Couch Adams in England and Urbain Jean Joseph Leverrier in France independently solved the problem. Leverrier was able to persuade Johann Gottfried Galle in Berlin to look for the planet. Galle found Neptune the day after he received Leverrier's letter (September 23, 1846) within a few degrees of the positions predicted by Adams and by Leverrier.

Like Uranus, Neptune exhibits a depletion in hydrogen and helium compared with Jupiter and Saturn. It also exhibits an aquamarine color resulting from methane absorption in its atmosphere. But its rotational axis is oriented at a more rational 29.5°.

Voyager 2 reached Neptune in August 1989. Unlike the bland appearance of Uranus, Neptune exhibited bright, discrete clouds of condensed methane as well as dark clouds contrasting with the general blue-green background (Fig. 19, color). The planet is encircled by a system of three rings, the outermost of which includes three sausage-like condensations of material. Six small, dark satellites were discovered close in to the planet, occupying nearly circular orbits in Neptune's equatorial plane. The spacecraft made a close flyby of Triton, Neptune's largest satellite, which turned out to be an extremely interesting object from the standpoint of the chemical reactions that are taking place there.

B. Chemistry

As on Uranus, Voyager 2 found that the visible pole of Neptune was also surrounded by a haze of material that was dark in the ultraviolet. In fact, this material is thick enough and dark enough that it shows up as a dusky collar around the pole even in visible light (Fig. 19). In the case of Uranus, we attributed the formation of the polar haze to the continuous flux of ultraviolet irradiation received by the atmosphere. The same mechanism may be responsible for the haze on Neptune, although the distribution of the haze—as a collar rather than a cap—is distinctly different. For both planets, these circumpolar hazes cannot be the simple result of charged particle precipitation along magnetic field lines, since the magnetic field orientation of Neptune, like that of Uranus, is inclined at an angle of nearly 60° to the rotational axis.

Neptune also offers a possible example of internally driven chemistry, perhaps analogous to Jupiter's Great Red Spot. This is the huge oval storm system that is often referred to as the Great Dark Spot (Fig. 19). Here too, we seem to have dark material that is different in composition from the white condensation clouds we see nearby. At this writing, we still do not have a good value for the color of this feature, since the blue-green tint of the overlying atmosphere has to be substracted once the altitude of the top of the spot is known.

Nevertheless, this giant storm is clearly an example of chemical reactions taking place on this distant world. Observations of the energy emitted by Neptune show that, like Jupiter, it radiates more than it receives, so Neptune also has an internal source of heat. Thus chemistry can occur at great depths with the products convected up to levels where we can see them, just as in the case of CO and GeH_4 on Jupiter.

Unfortunately, Neptune is too faint and too cold at the levels we can probe to permit the kind of high resolution spectroscopy that revealed the rich variety of trace gases found on Jupiter and Saturn. The fact that methane is highly enriched suggests that other, heavier elements should also be enhanced in the lower atmosphere. Both ethane and acetylene have been found in Neptune's upper atmosphere, however, indicating that the first steps in a process of haze-producing photochemistry do indeed occur.

On Triton, the situation is even more revealing. Despite the extremely tenuous nitrogen atmosphere (16×10^{-6} of the sea-level pressure on Earth) and the low surface temperature (37 K!), we again find dark and colored compounds on the satellites' surface. Voyager 2 could not obtain spectra of Triton, but ground-based observations show a number of as-yet-unidentified absorption features that must be caused by solid forms of various photochemical reaction products.

The surface in general is very bright, indicating that it is continually renewed. Sublimation and deposition of nitrogen seem the likely processes. But it is not quite so simple, since the dark northern hemisphere appears distinctly reddish, compared with the sunlit south. This implies a difference in composition, but what is it? Isolated patches of dark material show clear evidence of being blown by local winds (Fig. 20, color). Some of these patches are the end points of vertical columns that are carrying this dark material up into the atmosphere. Are these columns dust devils? Low-temperature volcanism? Thermal chimneys punching through an inversion layer? We just don't know. But they provide a useful illustration of energetic reactions at very low temperatures. Clearly, we have much to learn about the chemistry that can occur under these conditions and what it can tell us about the compounds we find in comets and meteorites (see Chapter 5).

VII. Pluto

A. Survey of the System

Pluto was discovered by Clyde Tombaugh in February 1930, 6 months after the initiation of a systematic search for a trans-Neptunian planet. It moves in an inclined, eccentric orbit that allows it at times to be closer to the Sun than is Neptune, as is the case just now (1979-1999).

Pluto's satellite, Charon, was discovered by James Christy in 1978. Until this discovery, neither Pluto's mass nor the orientation of its rotational axis could be accurately defined. We now know that the inclination of the axis takes it below the

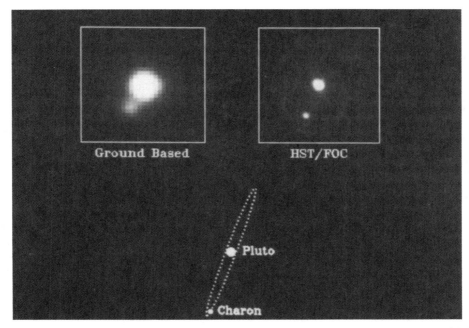

Fig. 21 The most distant known planet in our solar system is Pluto, shown here with its satellite, Charon, in a picture taken by the Hubble Space Telescope. NASA HQL-277.

orbital plane and that the mass is only 3/1000 the mass of the Earth. The respective diameters of Pluto and Charon are 3000 and 1300 km, making them closer in size than any other planet-satellite pair (Fig. 21).

Unfortunately, neither Voyager spacecraft could reach Pluto in the course of their epic journeys through the outer solar system. But through one of nature's kinder coincidences, we have just passed through one of the two periods in Pluto's orbital journey around the Sun (separated by 120 years!) when mutual occultations and eclipses of Pluto and Charon are visible to Earth-based observers. Much of what we know about this distant system has been gleaned from meticulous observations of these phenomena by Earth-based astronomers.

Charon is in a synchronous orbit about Pluto, i.e., its period of revolution is exactly equal to the period of the planet's rotation, the only such case in the solar system. This is an unusually long rotation period, 6.4 days compared with the less than 20 hour periods of the four giant planets. The synchronicity of the two periods means that for one hemisphere of Pluto, Charon always stays in the same place in the sky, day and night, whereas it is never visible from the planet's other hemisphere.

It appears that Titan, Triton, and Pluto are all closely related objects, much like the family of inner planets. But in this case we are speaking of bodies that are half ice and half rock, rather than rocky planets like our own. Frozen methane has been detected on Pluto's surface, and a small amount must also be present in its atmosphere, reminding us of conditions on Titan and Triton.

This tenuous atmosphere was first suspected on the basis of spectroscopic observations showing the presence of methane

absorptions. But the recent occultation of a star by Pluto, coupled with infrared determinations of Pluto's surface temperature, indicates that the atmosphere, like that of Triton, must be very tenuous. Some CO should be present on both of these objects, in addition to the N_2 that has been specifically found on Triton. Interestingly, spectra of Charon suggest that this satellite has no methane on its surface, although it does show absorption bands of water ice. There may be an important clue here about how these icy bodies form atmospheres. If the main source of volatiles for these atmospheres is in the form of compounds of carbon, nitrogen, and hydrogen that are devolatilized during accretion (see Titan discussion, Section IV) then it may be that the mass of Charon was simply too small to allow it to retain the resulting gases.

Although repeated attempts have been made to find more distant planets (most recently, in 1984 with the Infrared Astronomy Satellite), Pluto remains the planet whose average position is farthest from the Sun.

B. Chemistry

Because of their many similarities one might well expect Pluto and Triton to have similar chemistries. But this doesn't quite seem to be true. Pluto is darker on average than Triton, and its reflectivity is nonuniform at the large scales mapped by the occultation technique Fig. 22).[12] Furthermore, there is no indication of the putative N_2 absorption that is present at 2.15 μm in the spectrum of Triton. (The data for Pluto are not quite as good, however, so one must await better spectra to be certain this difference is real.)

These two observations are in fact consistent, since it is generally assumed that the reason Triton is so bright is that the

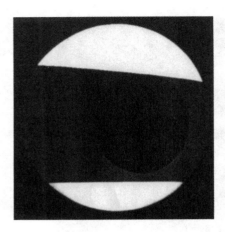

Fig. 22 As Pluto and Charon went through a series of eclipses and occultations, it became evident that Pluto must have dark and light markings on its surface. This model by March Buie gives an impression of what these markings may be like. (Owen, T., Morrison, D. In Deep Freeze: Planets We Cannot See, *The Planetary System.* **Addison-Wesley, New York, 1988, Figure 12.15.)**

seasonal transport of N_2 by the atmosphere continuously refreshes the surface. In the absence of a large deposit of N_2, this mechanism will not work on Pluto. If, instead, CO and methane are the dominant gases, we would expect the accumulation of dark material that was different in composition from that found on Triton, where nitrogen should be one of the important constituents of at least some of the dark solids. Detailed ground-based spectroscopy over the next few years may clarify this distinction between these two small, distant worlds.

VIII. Conclusion

This brief survey of the outer solar system has demonstrated that there are records on satellite surfaces of chemical reactions that took place early in the solar system's history. There is chemistry taking place in the atmospheres of planets and satellites today that is continually building more complex substances from simple ones. If our goal is to find a path from the naturally occurring reactions that took place in the primitive solar nebula to the origin of life on Earth, the outer solar system appears to be an excellent place to look.

We can expect steady progress in this endeavor during the next few years as our remote investigations achieve even better signal-to-noise and higher spectral resolution, thanks to the new giant telescopes that are becoming available. The first of these will be the Keck 10-meter reflector atop Mauna Kea in Hawaii, which should begin making observations in 1992. The resulting huge gain in light-gathering power will permit much more sensitive searches for trace constituents in the atmospheres of both planets and satellites, better spatial resolution on planetary disks, and spectrophotometry of more dark satellites. The greatest gains in our knowledge of the distant worlds will undoubtedly come from the planetary missions already described in the text: Galileo reaching Jupiter with an atmospheric probe and an orbiter in December 1995 and Cassini, with a probe into Titan's atmosphere and a Saturn orbiter, arriving in 2004. The data obtained can then be compared with the results of the reactions taking place today in the atmosphere of Titan.

Will we find detailed similarities in the compounds produced in these different environments? Will this knowledge lead to new insights into the origin of life on Earth? The 2005 edition of this book may have the answers!

References

[1] Owen, T., Terrile, R. "Colors on Jupiter," *Journal of Geophysical Research*, 1981, vol. 86, no. A10, p. 8797.

[2] Peek, B.M. *The Planet Jupiter*, London, Faber & Faber, 1958.

[3] Mitchell, J.L., Beebe, R.F., Ingersoll, A. P., Garnean, G.W. *Journal of Geophyisical Research*, 1981, vol. 86, p. 8751.

[4] Prinn, R.G., Lewis, J.S. *Science*, 1975, vol. 190, p. 274.

[5] Larson, H.P., Davis, D.S., Hoffman, R., Bjoraker, G.L. *Icarus*, 1984, vol. 60, p. 621.

[6] Lewis, J.S. *Icarus*, 1969, vol. 10, p. 365.

[7] Reynolds, R.T., McKay, C.P., Kasting, J.F. *Advances in Space Research*, 1987, vol. 7, p. 125. (See also Reynolds et al. *Icarus*, 1983, vol. 56, p. 246.)

[8] Owen, T., Lutz, B.L., de Bergh, C. *Nature*, 1986, vol. 320, p. 244.

[9] Thompson, W.R., Henry, T.J., Schwartz, J.M., Khare, B.N., Sagan, C. *Icarus*, 1991, vol. 90, p. 57.

[10] Lunine, J.I., Stevenson, D.J., Yung, Y.L. *Science*, 1983, vol. 222, p. 1229.

[11] Raulin, F., Toupance, R. *Advances in Space Research*, 1987, vol. 7, p. 120.

[12] Tholen, D., Buie, M. *Icarus,* 1990, vol. 88, p. 326.

Chapter 5

Asteroids, Comets, and Other Small Bodies

David Morrison

I. Remnants of Creation

A. Introduction

Where did we come from? The origin of the planetary system and of life on Earth are among the most basic questions asked by astronomers (or anyone else). Many clues to the origin of the solar system are to be found in the configurations of the planets and their satellites. Other clues come from an understanding of the process of star formation, including observations of the disks of dust that accompany many young stellar objects, which are presumably analogs of our own solar nebula 4.5 Gyr ago. But some of our most important information on solar system origins is derived from the study of primitive material in the solar system today.

The comets, asteroids, and meteors are surviving remnants of this primitive material—all objects that preserve vital information about conditions in the solar nebula at the time of the birth of the planetary system. They are either remnant planetesimals from the solar nebula—objects that did not accrete into larger planets or satellites—or fragments of planetesimals subsequently broken up by collisions.

The asteroids and comets differ from each other primarily in their volatile content, with the asteroids greatly depleted in volatiles relative to the solar nebula. In practice, astronomers distinguish comets from asteroids in terms of an observational criterion: the presence or absence of an atmosphere of gas or dust. A comet is defined as a small object that possesses a visible transient atmosphere near the perihelion of its orbit. If there is no atmosphere, a small body is called an asteroid. According to this definition, an object originally classed as an asteroid could become a comet if it later outgassed an atmosphere as a result of solar heating, which is just what happened to the object Chiron in 1988.

B. Meteors and Their Parent Bodies

The interpretation of astronomical studies of comets and asteroids is greatly assisted by comparisons with the meteors, which can be studied in the laboratory. By themselves, meteors provide essential information on the nature of the solar nebula. This information is of still greater value if the meteors can be associated with their source regions, or even with specific parent bodies.

A fragment of interplanetary debris in space is called a meteor. Occasionally, a meteor survives its flight through the atmosphere and lands on the ground as a meteorite. This happens with extreme rarity in any one locality, but over the entire Earth hundreds of meteorites fall each year.

One way to investigate the source of meteors is to determine the orbit of the meteor while it is still in space, before it encounters the Earth's atmosphere. Successful orbits have been calculated from photographs of the meteoric fireball for the Pribram meteor (Czechoslovakia, 1959), Lost City (U.S., 1979), and Innisfree (Canada, 1977). All three of these meteoroids were on eccentric orbits that carried them from the main asteroid belt to the Earth, similar to the orbits of many Apollo asteroids. Although not conclusive, these results suggest the asteroids as the source for at least some of the meteors.

The meteors in our collections include a wide range of compositions and histories, but traditionally they have been placed into three broad classes. First, there are the irons, which are composed of nearly pure metallic nickel-iron. Second, there are the stones, which is the term used for any silicate or rocky meteor. Third, there are the much rarer stony-irons, which are (as the name implies) made of mixtures of stony and metallic materials.

Stones are much more common than the irons, but harder to recognize. Often a laboratory analysis is required to demonstrate that a particular sample is really of extraterrestrial origin, especially if it has lain on the ground for some time and has been subject to weathering. The most scientifically valuable stones are those that are collected immediately after they fall, or the Antarctic samples that have been preserved in a nearly pristine state by the ice. Most stones are primitive, are called chondrites (Fig. 1), and are named for the chondrules they typically contain. Chondrules are small, spherical fragments that solidified from a liquid or vapor state. The other class, called the achondrites, are derived from differentiated parent bodies.

Meteorites are fragments of larger parent bodies. We know this because microscopic examination reveals the tracks of energetic ions that struck the meteor while it was in space. In most cases the relatively small number of such atomic tracks indicates that the meteor was exposed to the rigors of space for

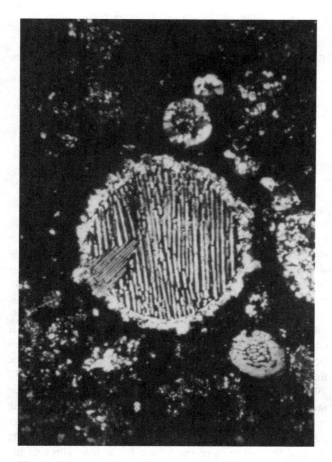

Fig. 1 Cross-section of a stony chondrite meteorite, showing a barred, olivine chondrule. (Smithsonian Institution, Museum of Natural History)

no more than a few tens of millions of years. Before that time it must have been part of a larger parent object, which shielded it from most such particles.

What were the parent bodies of the meteorites like? They cannot have had permanent atmospheres, as we can tell by the composition of the meteors themselves, which have not been exposed to great chemical weathering. They must have been subject to heavy cratering, as we can determine from the large numbers of meteor breccias, which are made up of the recemented bits and pieces from a hierarchy of impact fragmentation. Estimates of the sizes of meteor parent bodies are possible from the fact that most high-pressure minerals are absent, with the exception of a few forms (such as tiny diamonds) that are the result of high-speed impacts. Their mineralogy limits the pressures in the meteor source regions to less than about 1000 bars. Therefore, the meteors either all come from shallow sources in the crusts of large parent bodies, or (more likely) their sources are distributed within smaller parent bodies, not more than a few hundred kilometers in radius—typical of the larger asteroids in the main belt.

We can also ask how many different parent bodies are needed to account for the meteors in our collections. Detailed chemical and isotopic analyses of the meteors reveal that they cannot all have come from the same source. At least 20 different parents are required, and the number is probably greater than 50. We therefore conclude that the parent bodies of the meteors were a large number of relatively small bodies, similar to the asteroids we see today. In addition, detailed comparisons of the spectra of meteors with those of asteroids reveal that the minerals present on asteroidal surfaces are the same as those typically found in meteors.

C. Message of the Meteors

The true significance of meteors as remnants of solar system formation was not appreciated until their ages were measured and techniques were developed for the detailed analysis of their chemistry and isotopic compositions. Almost all of the meteors have radiometric ages near 4.53 Gyr. The few exceptions are igneous rocks that are thought to have originated on the surfaces of the Moon or Mars. This age of 4.53 Gyr is taken to represent the age of the solar system—the time since the first solids condensed from the solar nebula and began to accrete into larger bodies.

The iron meteors all have approximately the same composition, primarily metallic iron with from 5 to 15 weight-percent nickel and trace quantities of other metals. They are divided into three groups on the basis of their nickel content, which shows up in crystal patterns (called Widmannstatten patterns) that can be observed when the meteor is polished and etched. Most iron meteors are called octahedrites. Those with more than 13-percent nickel are the ataxites, and those with less than 6 percent are the hexahedrites.

There are two main groups of stony-iron meteors. The pallasites are the most beautiful of all of the meteors, consisting of crystals in all meteors, as well as crystals of the transparent green mineral olivine embedded within a metallic nickel-iron matrix. They are thought to be samples from the core-mantle interface of their parent body. The second main type of stony-irons is the mesosiderites, which are breccias with mixed iron/silicate composition.

The differentiated stony meteors are called achondrites. One group of achondrites consists primarily of the mineral enstatite; these are called enstatite achondrites, or aubrites. They are presumably fragments from the mantles of their differentiated parent bodies. The second major group of achondrites is the basaltic achondrites, which are lavas from the crusts of their parents. The basaltic achondrites include the eucrites, which appear to be fragments from asteroid Vesta, and the SNC meteors (shergottites, nakhlites, and chassignites), which appear to come from Mars.

The great majority of meteors are primitive chondrites. In spite of their name, the chondrites are defined by their general chemical nature and not by the presence (or absence) of chondrules.

One small group of chondrites is composed primarily of the mineral enstatite and is known as enstatite chondrites; these may be condensates from a hot, oxygen-depleted region of the solar nebula. Most primitive meteors, however, fall into the

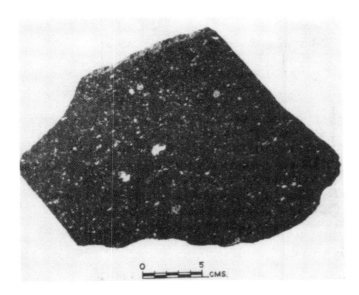

Fig. 2 Allende carbonaceous meteorite that fell in Mexico in 1969. (NASA/Johnson Space Center)

category of ordinary chondrites, characterized by the presence of silicates formed in a moderately oxidizing environment together with some tens of percent metallic iron. They are classified primarily on the basis of their iron content, which in turn reflects their degree of oxidation. These classes are called high-iron (H chondrites), low-iron (L chondrites), and very-low-iron (LL chondrites).

Of great interest to a student of the origin of the solar system are the carbonaceous chondrites (Fig. 2), which contain significant quantities of carbon and water but relatively little iron. They are also more highly oxidized than the ordinary chondrites. All of these distinctions refer to the basic chemical composition of the chondrites, and presumably they reflect conditions in the solar nebula where they formed.

An additional classification of the ordinary and carbonaceous chondrites can be made on the basis of their degree of thermal or chemical alteration since formation—in other words, their degree of metamorphism. The most common system uses a number from 1 to 6 to express the degree of metamorphic alteration. Thus, for example, an L5 chondrite is a rather highly modified low-iron meteor. In the case of the carbonaceous chondrites, the least modified types (equivalent to class 1 for the ordinary chondrites) are usually called CI chondrites, whereas more modified types are called CM, CO, and CV chondrites. Generally, the degree of thermal alteration is less for carbonaceous chondrites than for other chondrites, but their aqueous modification may be significant.

The asteroids are the most likely parent bodies for most meteors. Laboratory studies of meteors provide us with critical information that cannot be derived from remote sensing of the asteroids. However, to make full use of that information we need to identify at least the general classes of asteroids that are the most likely sources for the various types of meteors.

II. Asteroids

A. Discovery and Orbits

Asteroids (also called minor planets) are faint objects, named for their unresolved (starlike) images when seen through the telescope. Even the brightest are only marginally visible to the unaided eye. Most of the asteroids are located between the orbits of Mars and Jupiter, and it was here that the first asteroid, Ceres, was discovered in 1801, by the Sicilian observer Guiseppe Piazzi. Shortly thereafter came the discoveries of three more large asteroids also with orbital radii near 2.5 AU: Pallas in 1802, Juno in 1804, and Vesta in 1807. It was 1845 before the fifth asteroid was discovered, but visual discoveries continued throughout the 19th century, greatly supplemented after 1890 by photographic searches (begun by Max Wolf at Heidelberg). Today more than 4000 asteroids have well-determined orbits. By tradition, an asteroid is specified by both a number and a name; for example, 1 Ceres or 4 Vesta. (See Fig. 3 and Table 1.)

It would be a formidable task to discover, determine orbits, and catalog all of the asteroids bright enough to be observed with modern telescopes. Nevertheless, the total number of such objects can be estimated by systematically sampling regions of the sky. The number of asteroids bright enough to leave trails on photographs taken with the 50-cm Palomar Schmidt telescope are estimated to be about 100,000. Except in the outer part of the belt, this number includes essentially all objects down to a diameter of 1 km. In 1983 the Infrared Astronomical Satellite (IRAS) carried out from orbit an all-sky survey that was particularly sensitive to asteroids, which are strong emitters of thermal radiation. More than 10,000 individual observations were made, corresponding to perhaps 5000 separate objects.

The largest asteroid is Ceres, with a diameter of just under 1000 km. Two asteroids have diameters near 500 km, and about 30 are larger than 200 km. The number of asteroids increases rapidly with decreasing size following approximately a power law distribution: for each drop in size by a factor of 10, the number of asteroids increases by nearly a factor of 200. This size distribution is characteristic of a population of objects subject to collision and fragmentation. Most asteroids observed today are probably fragments, and initially there may have been many more asteroids than are observed today. Repeated collisions have shattered many asteroids and dispersed the fragments throughout the solar system.

It is estimated that our census of asteroids is 99-percent complete for objects down to 100 km diameter, and at least 50-percent complete down to 10 km. The total mass of the asteroids is about 1/20 the mass of the Moon, with Ceres alone accounting for nearly half of this total mass.

The asteroids all revolve about the Sun in the same direction as the planets (from west to east), and most of them have orbits that lie near the plane of the Earth's orbit, with a mean inclination of 10°. A few, however, have orbits inclined more

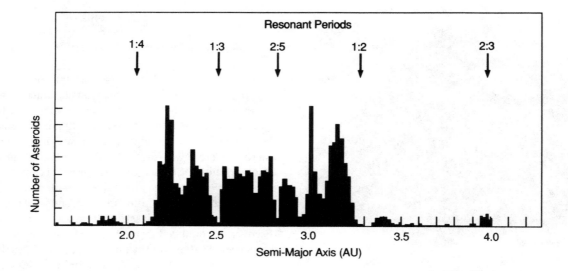

**Fig. 3 Distribution of the number of asteroids at various distances from the Sun (AU). Some of the reso-
nances are indicated at gaps (Kirkwood gaps) where the period of an asteroid would be a simple fraction of
the period of Jupiter. For example, an asteroid at 2.5 AU from the Sun would have a period one-third of
Jupiter's. (Figure from** *Realm of the Universe,* **Fifth Edition, by George Abell, David Morrison, and Sidney
C. Wolff, copyright © 1991 by Saunders College Publishing, reprinted by permission of the publisher.)**

Table 1 The 20 largest asteroids

Name	Discovery	Semimajor Axis (AU)	Diameter (km)	Class
1 Ceres	1801	2.77	940	C
2 Pallas	1802	2.77	540	C
4 Vesta	1807	2.36	510	*
10 Hygeia	1849	3.14	410	C
704 Interamnia	1910	3.06	310	C
511 Davida	1903	3.18	310	C
65 Cybele	1861	3.43	280	C
52 Europa	1868	3.10	280	C
87 Sylvia	1866	3.48	275	C
3 Juno	1804	2.67	265	S
16 Psyche	1852	2.92	265	M
451 Patientia	1899	3.07	260	C
31 Euphrosyne	1854	3.15	250	C
15 Eunomia	1851	2.64	245	S
324 Bamberga	1892	2.68	235	C
107 Camilla	1868	3.49	230	C
532 Herculina	1904	2.77	230	S
48 Doris	1857	3.11	225	C
29 Amphitrite	1854	2.55	225	S
19 Fortuna	1852	2.44	220	C
*Vesta has a very unusual (once thought unique) basaltic surface.				

than 25°; the orbit of 2102 Tantalus is the most inclined (64°)
to the ecliptic. The main asteroid belt contains minor planets
with semimajor axes in the range 2.2 to 3.3 AU, with corresponding periods of orbital revolution about the Sun from 3.3
to 6 years. The mean value of the eccentricities of the main
belt asteroid orbits is 0.15, not much greater than the average
for the orbits of the planets.

Some asteroids have orbits rather far outside the main
asteroid belt. A few with semimajor axes around 1.9 AU are
called the Hungarias (for the prototype 434 Hungaria), and a
few with larger orbits, near 4 AU, are called the Hildas (for 153
Hilda). There are asteroids with even more extreme orbits,
some of which cross the orbit of the Earth, and a few that cross
the orbit of Jupiter. We shall return to these objects later.

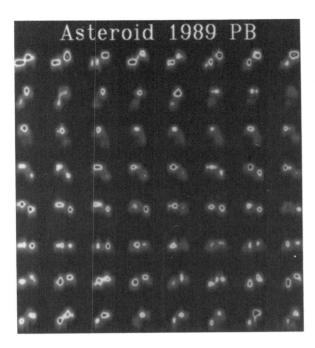

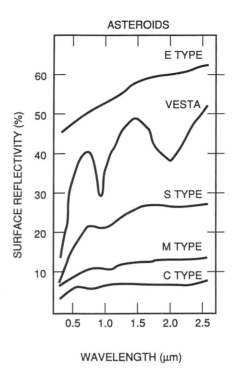

ASTEROIDS

WAVELENGTH (μm)

Fig. 4 Radar images of asteroid 1989 PB over a period of 3 hours, showing the elongated or "dumbbell" shape of the asteroid and its rotation. The resolution of these images is about 50 meters. (Courtesy of Arecibo Observatory, Steve Ostro, NASA/Jet Propulsion Laboratory)

Fig. 5 Examples of visible-infrared spectra of several asteroids of diverse compositional types. (Clark R. Chapman, Arizona University/ Planetary Science Institute)

B. Size, Composition, and Classification

Before 1970, no asteroid diameters had been measured, but today there are several methods of determining the sizes of asteroids. The most accurate technique is to measure the amount of time required for the asteroid to pass in front of (or occult) a star. From different places on Earth, different parts of an asteroid will appear to pass in front of the same remote star because the various observers see the asteroid from slightly different directions compared to the direction to the star. In effect, the asteroid casts its own moving shadow on the Earth. The combination of many observations of an occultation permits an accurate determination of the size and shape of the asteroid (in one orientation). About a dozen asteroid diameters measured by this technique are accurate to within a few percent.

Another approach that can yield accurate sizes and shapes of asteroids is radar imaging. This technique can be applied only to asteroids that come very close to the Earth. A series of images of asteroid 1989PB obtained by Stephen Ostro at Arecibo in 1989 (Fig. 4) shows this little object, only 400 m in average diameter, to be dumbbell shaped, as if two objects of similar size collided and stuck to each other.

The method that works best to estimate the sizes of large numbers of asteroids is to compare the asteroids' brightness in visible light (reflected sunlight) with the light the asteroids emit in the infrared—energy they have previously absorbed

from the Sun (Fig. 5). For a particular asteroid, we know its distance from the Sun and therefore how much sunlight falls on each area of its surface. The total sunlight it intercepts is equal to its cross-sectional area times the incident flux. Of that intercepted light, the asteroid reflects part, a fraction A (the albedo), and therefore absorbs the rest, the fraction 1-A. The asteroid re-emits the energy it absorbs at infrared wavelengths. When we measure the infrared radiation coming from the object, we are recording how much energy it must have absorbed from the sunlight falling upon it. If we compare this measure with that of the light reflected from the object, we find what its reflectivity is. Then we can calculate what its size must be to account for the amount of light it reflects to us, that is, its observed brightness.

The first clue to the composition of an asteroid is obtained from its derived albedo or reflectivity. The majority are very dark, with reflectivities of only 3-5 percent, about as dark as a lump of coal. However, there is another large group with typical reflectivities of about 15 percent, a little brighter than the Moon, and still others with reflectivities as high as 60 percent.

Further compositional information is contained in the visible and near-infrared spectrum, from about 0.3 to 3 micrometers. Ideally, we measure the reflectivity over this interval with high photometric precision at a spectral resolution sufficient to resolve spectral features due to ices or minerals. Considerable useful work has also been done with lower-resolution spectra, including eight-color photometry

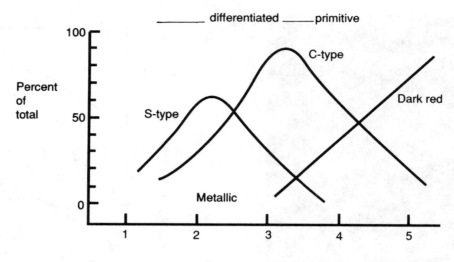

Fig. 6 Distribution of asteroid compositional types with the distance from the Sun. (Adapted from work carried out by D. Tholen and J. Gradie, University of Hawaii, and E. Tedesco, NASA/Jet Propulsion Laboratory. Figure from *Realm of the Universe*, Fifth Edition, by George Abell, David Morrison, and Sidney C. Wolff, copyright © 1991 by Saunders College Publishing, reprinted by permission of the publisher.)

Table 2 Asteroid masses and densities

Name	Mass (Moon = 1)	Density (g/cm^3)
1 Ceres	1.4×10^{-2}	2.4
2 Pallas	2.9×10^{-3}	2.6
4 Vesta	3.7×10^{-3}	3.8
10 Hygiea	1.3×10^{-3}	2.6
Phobos	1.5×10^{-6}	2.0

by David Tholen and others in a specially designed photometric system for determining asteroid colors (Fig. 6).

The majority of the asteroids are primitive bodies, composed of silicates mixed with dark organic carbon compounds. The presence of these dark materials reduces the asteroids' reflectivities to the 3 to 5 percent level observed. Many of these objects also include some water chemically bonded to the silicates. Two of the three largest asteroids, 1 Ceres and 2 Pallas, are primitive, as are almost all of the objects in the outer third of the belt. Most of the primitive asteroids are classed as C asteroids, where the C stands for "carbonaceous." The C asteroids are similar to the carbonaceous meteors. Beyond 3 AU, the C asteroids thin out and are replaced by other primitive forms with different spectra (classed as D, F, etc.), apparently not represented in our meteor collections.

The second most populous asteroid group is the S asteroids, where S stands for "silicaceous"; 3 Juno is an example. In these asteroids the dark carbon compounds are missing, resulting in higher reflectivities and clearer spectral signatures of silicate minerals. The minerals present are similar to those that make up many meteors, but the exact compositions of the S asteroids remain in dispute. In particular, we are

unable to answer the basic question of whether these asteroids are primitive bodies or whether they are differentiated.

Spectral observations have identified a few asteroids, not more than 5 percent of the total, that are clearly differentiated objects. These include the M class asteroids, which are thought to be made largely of metal (presumably the cores of differentiated parent bodies that were shattered in collisions). This supposition has been proven in the case of the largest M asteroid, 16 Psyche, which has a higher radar reflectivity than would a rocky object of the same size and distance.

Other differentiated asteroids have basaltic surfaces like the volcanic plains of the Moon and Mars. The large asteroid 4 Vesta is in the latter category. Apparently some of the asteroids were heated early in the history of the solar system, but why these, and why only a small percentage of the total number, we do not know.

Measurements of reflected sunlight provide compositional information on asteroid *surfaces* only. If densities were also known, we could draw some conclusions concerning their internal properties. Only for the largest have the masses been measured from the gravitational perturbations they produce on the orbits of other asteroids. Table 2 lists the best values now available, with the martian satellite Phobos included for

Table 3 Some near-Earth asteroids

(data in part from L.A. McFadden in **Asteroids II**, University of Arizona Press, 1989)

Name	Orbit Class	Discovery	Semimajor axis (AU)	Eccentricity	Diameter (km)	Type
433 Eros	Amor	1898	1.46	0.22	22	S
1036 Ganymede [1]	Amor	1924	2.66	0.54	37	S
1221 Amor	Amor	1932	1.92	0.44	-	-
1566 Icarus [2]	Apollo	1949	1.08	0.83	0.9	-
1620 Geographos	Apollo	1951	1.24	0.34	2.0	S
1862 Apollo	Apollo	1932	1.47	0.56	1.5	*
1866 Sisyphus [3]	Apollo	1972	1.89	0.54	8.2	-
2062 Aten	Aten	1976	0.97	0.18	0.9	S
2100 Ra-Shalom	Aten	1978	0.97	0.18	2.4	C
3200 Phaethon [2]	Apollo	1983	1.27	0.89	6.9	*
1989FC [4]	Apollo	1989	1.02	0.36	0.2	-
1989PB [5]	Apollo	1989	1.06	0.48	0.6	-

1. Largest Earth-approaching asteroid.
2. High eccentricity; possibly a dead comet.
3. Largest currently Earth-crossing asteroid.
4. Passed within 700,000 km of Earth on March 22, 1989.
5. Dumbbell shaped (see Fig. 4).

comparison. The densities of 1 Ceres, 2 Pallas, and 10 Hygiea are about what one would expect for primitive bodies, consistent with their surface spectra. Vesta apparently has a higher density, presumably the result of loss of volatiles when it differentiated.

C. Main Asteroid Belt

The main asteroid belt stretches from 2.2 to 3.3 AU. Probably more than 75 percent of the asteroid mass is in the main belt. Although there are 10^5 belt asteroids larger than 1 km diameter, the typical spacing between objects is several million kilometers.

For the most part, the more primitive objects are in the outer part of the belt, whereas the rarer differentiated objects are closer to the Sun. We may think of the belt as made up of overlapping rings of similar kinds of objects, with each ring having a width of about half an AU. The presence of this structure tells us that the asteroids must still be in approximately the positions where they formed; the belt has not been totally mixed and homogenized. By sampling the compositions of the different kinds of primitive asteroids, we can map out in some detail the nature of the solar nebula out of which they formed.

An interesting characteristic in the distribution of asteroid orbits is the existence of several clear areas or gaps in histograms of observed periods or semimajor axes. These Kirkwood gaps, which correspond to resonant periods, are the consequence of gravitational perturbations from Jupiter. If plots are made combining semimajor orbit axis with orbit eccentricity and inclination, the distribution does not seem random, as first pointed out in 1917 by Hirayama. Groups of asteroids with statistically correlated elements are called families. There are several dozen such families, and observations of the larger families (the Eos and Themis families in particular) show that their individual members are physically similar, as if they were fragments of a common parent.

D. Near-Earth Asteroids

The near-Earth or Earth-approaching asteroids have orbits that either come close to or cross the orbit of the Earth. Some of these are the nearest approaching celestial objects, except, of course, the Moon and meteors.

The near-Earth asteroids are divided into three groups on the basis of their orbits. The innermost are the Atens, named for 2062 Aten, which have orbits with semimajor axes less than 1.0 AU. The best-known group are the Apollos (for 1862 Apollo, discovered in 1948), which cross the orbit of the Earth (or nearly do so) but have semimajor axes greater than 1.0 AU. The Apollos include 1566 Icarus, which has its perihelion inside the orbit of Mercury. The outer group are the Amors (for 1221 Amor), which are Mars-orbit-crossing asteroids with perihelion distances between 1.017 and 1.400 AU.

About 100 near-Earth asteroids have been located (Table 3). The largest are similar in size to the satellites of Mars, although most are only a few kilometers in diameter. Chemically, they seem similar to the main belt asteroids, with several different compositional classes identified. Current searches for additional Earth-approaching asteroids lead to the discovery of several new objects each year. Eugene Shoemaker has carried out extensive calculations of the dynamics of the entire population; he estimates that there are between 1000 and 2000 Earth-approaching asteroids down to a diameter of 500 m. About half of these are Apollos and half Amors, with only a few Atens.

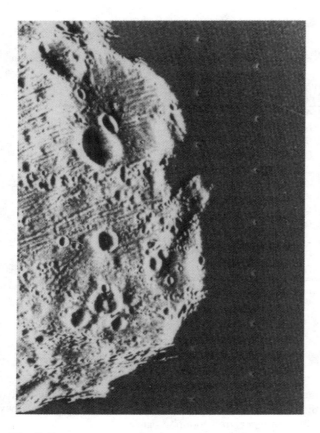

Fig. 7 Long "grooves" in the surface of Phobos, presumably features related to the ancient impact that produced the large crater Stickney. The frame is 9 km by 18 km. (NASA/Jet Propulsion Laboratory, courtesy of Peter Thomas, Cornell University)

As Shoemaker and others have shown, the orbits of near-Earth asteroids are unstable. These objects will meet one of two fates: either they will impact one of the terrestrial planets, or they will be ejected from the inner solar system as the result of a near encounter with a planet. The time scale for impact or ejection is only about 10^8 years, very short in comparison with the age of the solar system.

If the current population of Earth-approaching asteroids will be removed by impact or ejection in 10^8 years, there must be a continuing source of new objects. Some come from the main asteroid belt, where collisions can eject fragments into Earth-crossing orbits. Others may be dead comets that have exhausted their volatiles. Possibly as many as half of the Earth-approachers are the solid remnants of former comets. We will discuss the fate of old comets in Section III.E.

E. Phobos and Deimos

The two satellites of Mars are probably captured asteroids. However, there is no guarantee that Phobos and Deimos resemble other asteroids in detail. If they were captured, it must have been very early in solar system history. For more than 4 billion years they have been in orbit about Mars, and not

out among the other asteroids.

Phobos and Deimos were first studied at close range by the Viking orbiters in 1977. In 1989, Phobos was the target of the Soviet spacecraft named "Phobos." Unfortunately, the Phobos spacecraft failed before it could land experiments on the surface, but this mission did add to our knowledge of this little world.

Both Phobos and Deimos are rather irregular, somewhat elongated, and heavily cratered. The largest diameters of Phobos and Deimos are about 25 km and 13 km, respectively. Each is a dark brownish gray in color, and spectral analysis suggests that each is composed of dark materials similar to those out of which most asteroids are made. Apparently these two satellites are chemically primitive.

Some additional clues to the compositions of Phobos and Deimos can be derived from their densities, which have been calculated from the masses and volumes measured by the Viking and Phobos spacecraft. Each has a density of only 2.0 g cm^{-3}, remarkably low for a rocky object—substantially lower than the densities of Ceres or Pallas, for example. In fact, this is about the same density as Pluto or Triton, which are thought to be made in part of water ice. It therefore seems probable that these satellites contain substantial quantities of ice, although their surface layers have been determined to be dehydrated.

In addition to numerous impact craters, Phobos is laced by long groves or troughs associated with the large crater Stickney (Fig. 7). Apparently the impact that produced Stickney very nearly ruptured the satellite. If we want to imagine what a more "normal" asteroid might look like imaged up close, Fig. 8 is a better representation. Note the dark, rough surface, frequent small impact craters, and irregular contours—all probably typical of the appearance of small asteroids.

F. Primitive Bodies in the Outer Solar System

The largest populations of asteroids beyond the main belt are the Trojans, orbiting the Sun at 5.2 AU, in the L4 and L5 Lagrangian points of the jovian orbit. Between 1906 and 1908, four such asteroids were found, the number has now increased to several hundred. These asteroids are named for the Homeric heroes from *The Iliad* and are collectively called the Trojans.

To a first approximation, the Trojan asteroids circle the Sun with Jupiter's period of 12 years, one-sixth of a cycle ahead of or behind the planet. Their detailed motion, however, is very complicated; they slowly oscillate around the points of stability found by Lagrange, with some of their oscillations taking as long as 140 years.

Measurements of the reflectivities and spectra of the Trojans show that they are very dark, primitive objects like those in the outer part of the asteroid belt. They appear faint because they are so dark and far away, but actually the larger Trojans are quite sizable. Four of them have diameters between 150 and 200 km. The largest, 624 Hektor, is about twice as long as it is wide, leading to the suggestion that it is a double

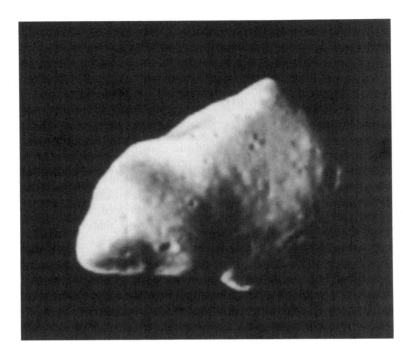

Fig. 8 This view of the asteroid Gaspra was taken aboard the Galileo spacecraft on October 29, 1991, from a distance of about 16,000 km. Illuminated portions of this photograph are approximately 16 × 12 km. (Produced by the U.S. Geological Survey and NASA/Jet Propulsion Laboratory)

asteroid, with two similar objects orbiting in contact with each other. Current estimates are that there must be more than 1000 Trojan asteroids in the region preceding Jupiter that are at least 15 km in diameter and about 250 in the region following Jupiter.

There are two asteroids known with orbits that carry them far beyond Jupiter. Asteroid 944 Hidalgo, with its semimajor axis of 5.9 AU and a very large eccentricity of 0.66, has an aphelion outside the orbit of Saturn. Still more distant is 2060 Chiron, which has a semimajor axis of 13.7 AU and a diameter estimated at 200 km. Its orbit (eccentricity 0.38) carries it from just inside the orbit of Saturn at perihelion out almost to the orbit of Uranus.

Ever since the discovery of Hidalgo and Chiron, astronomers have wondered about the relationship between such distant asteroids and the comets. If these two objects are composed of volatiles (like H_2O or CO ice), they would probably develop atmospheres if they were heated by the Sun. In that case we would call them comets, not asteroids.
In 1988 this speculation was confirmed for Chiron, when astronomers found that it had brightened by a factor of 2. Presumably the additional light was being reflected from gas or dust ejected from the surface. One year later, this new atmosphere was photographed. Chiron has been slowly approaching its perihelion for several years, and apparently the gradual increase in its temperature was sufficient by 1988 to initiate cometary activity.

There are many small satellites in the outer solar system that are also composed at least in part of dark, primitive materials. These include the eight outer satellites of Jupiter, which may be captured asteroids. In the Saturn system, both the outermost satellite, Phoebe, and the leading hemisphere of Iapetus are primitive. The 10 small inner satellites of Uranus discovered by Voyager are also dark and presumably primitive, as are all of the satellites of Neptune except Triton. Some of these satellites may be captured planetesimals that formed separately in the solar nebula, whereas others probably accreted within nebular disks associated with the formation of the giant planets. Because they are small, these satellites have not been subject to global melting or loss of volatiles, and they therefore retain their primitive chemical composition to the present.

G. Impacts and Earth History

Let us now comment briefly on the history of cosmic collisions with our own planet, the Earth. There is increasing evidence that the impacts of comets and near-Earth asteroids have had important effects, particularly in the field of biological evolution.

Twice in the 20th century large objects have collided with the Earth. The first such event took place on June 30, 1908, near the Tunguska River in Siberia, when a 10-megaton explosion about 8 km above the surface flattened more than 1000 square kilometers of forest. The blast wave spread around the world, recorded by instruments designed to measure changes in atmospheric pressure. Yet in spite of this violence, no craters were formed by the explosion. Although we do not know exactly what caused the Tunguska event, it certainly represented the disintegration of an impacting body weighing approximately 10^5 tons. The projectile, perhaps of cometary origin, did not have the strength to survive its plunge to the surface but dissipated its kinetic energy in the atmosphere.

The second impact event also took place in Siberia, near Vladivostok. On February 12, 1947, observers saw a fireball "as bright as the Sun." The impact produced 106 craters and pits ranging in size up to 28 m across. More than 23 tons of iron meteor fragments have subsequently been recovered from the area, demonstrating that the impacting bodies here were a swarm of iron meteors.

Both the Tunguska and the Vladivostok impacts were much too small to create large craters of the sort seen on the Moon. Meteor Crater in Arizona (about 1 km diameter) is the best example of a substantial young crater that has been identified on the land areas of the Earth; it is 50,000 years old. Even the Meteor Crater projectile, however, was no more than 100 m across. Impacts of objects the size of the smallest known Earth-approaching asteroids (about 400 m diameter) are much rarer yet.

More than 100 major impact scars have been identified on the Earth, mostly in the very old rocks of the continental shields. Rarely do they resemble the craters on other planets, however. Erosion and sedimentation have generally removed such characteristic features as the rim and the ejecta blanket. Often the only remaining indication of the impact is a circular region of shocked and shattered rock below the original location of the crater.

An interesting and relatively recent such impact feature is the Ries structure near the German town of Nordlingen. This crater, originally 27 km in diameter and 5 km deep, was formed about 15 million years ago. The impacting object was of rocky composition and had a mass of at least 10^9 tons. Presumably it was an Earth-approaching asteroid with a diameter of 2 to 3 km. An impact of this magnitude must have devastated much of central Europe and may have had significant global effects.

Still larger impacts can certainly disturb the whole planet and have a major influence on the course of evolution. The best-documented such impact took place 65 million years ago, at the end of the Cretaceous period of geological history. This break in the Earth's history is marked by a mass extinction of marine biota. Although there are a dozen or more mass extinctions in the geological record, the Cretaceous event has always intrigued paleontologists because it is coincident with the end of the age of the dinosaurs.

The body that impacted the Earth at the end of the Cretaceous period was an asteroid with a mass of more than 10^{12} tons and a diameter of at least 10 km. The size was inferred from the worldwide layer of sediment deposited from the dust cloud that enveloped the planet after the impact. First identi-

fied in 1980, this sediment layer is enriched in the rare metal iridium and other elements that are relatively abundant in an undifferentiated asteroid but are very rare in the crust of the Earth. Even diluted by the terrestrial material excavated from the crater, this asteroidal component is easily identified.

The Cretaceous impact released energy equivalent to more than a billion Hiroshima-size nuclear bombs, excavating a crater at least 100 km across and deep enough to penetrate through the Earth's crust. It can be compared with the lunar crater Tycho, the youngest major crater on the Moon (formed about 250 million years ago). The Cretaceous explosion lifted about 100 trillion tons of dust into the atmosphere, as can be determined by measuring the thickness of the sediment layer formed when this dust settled to the surface. Such a quantity of material would have blocked sunlight completely from reaching the surface, plunging the Earth into a period of cold and darkness that lasted at least several weeks, and more likely several months. The impact is also calculated to have produced vast quantities of nitric acid, and there is evidence of widespread fires that must have consumed much of the terrestrial biomass. Presumably these environmental disasters were responsible for mass extinctions, including the death of the dinosaurs.

Several other mass extinctions in the geological record have been tentatively identified with large impacts, although none is so dramatic as the Cretaceous event. But even without such specific documentation, it is clear that impacts of this size do occur and that their effects can be catastrophic for life. What is a catastrophe for one group of living things, however, may create opportunities for another group. Following each mass extinction, there is a sudden evolutionary burst as new species develop to fill the ecological niches opened by the event.

Impacts by comets and asteroids represent the only mechanisms we know of that could cause global catastrophes and seriously influence the evolution of life all over the planet. According to some estimates, the *majority* of all extinctions of species may be due to such impacts. Such a perspective fundamentally changes our view of biological evolution. A criterion for the survival of a species is not just its success in competing with other species and adapting to slowly changing environments, as envisioned by Darwinian natural selection. Of at least equal importance is its ability to survive random global ecological catastrophes due to impacts. The Earth is a target in a cosmic shooting gallery, subject to random violent events that were unsuspected a few decades ago.

III. Comets

A. Discovery and Orbits

Comets have been observed from the earliest times, and accounts of spectacular comets are found in the histories of many ancient civilizations. Yet early observers did not generally regard comets as celestial objects. The first investigation of a comet based on careful observation was Tycho

Table 4   Some well-known comets

Name	Period	Special interest
Great Comet of 1577	long	Found by Tycho to be beyond Moon
Great Comet of 1811	long	Largest head (>2 million km)
Great Comet of 1843	long	Brightest ever; visible in daylight
Donati's Comet of 1858	long	Multiple tails; very beautiful
Daylight Comet of 1910	long	Brightest comet of 20th century
Kohoutek (1973)	long	Widespread public interest
West (1976)	long	Best recent comet; nucleus broke up
Halley	76 yrs	First periodic; detailed spacecraft studies in 1986
Schwassmann-Wachmann 1	16 yrs	Outbursts at >5 AU from Sun
Biela	6.7 yrs	Broke up in 1846; disappeared
Kopff	6.5 yrs	Possible mission target
Giacobini-Zinner	6.5 yrs	First spacecraft encounter, 1985
Tempel 2	5.3 yrs	Probable mission target
Encke	3.3 yrs	Shortest period, nongravitational forces modelled by Whipple

Brahe's study of the comet of 1577. Had the comet been inside the Earth's atmosphere, as was then generally supposed, changes in its apparent direction would easily have been detectable to an observer who changed position by several kilometers. From the absence of such parallax, Tycho concluded that the comet was a celestial object, and he demonstrated that it was substantially more distant than the Moon.

Newton suggested that comets might be gravitationally bound to the Sun, like the planets. Edmund Halley, Newton's contemporary, calculated 24 cometary orbits. He noted that the orbits of the bright comets of 1531, 1607, and 1682 were so similar that the three could well be the same object, returning to perihelion at average intervals of 76 years. Halley successfully predicted that the object (now called Comet Halley) should return about 1758. Subsequent investigation has shown that Comet Halley has been observed and recorded on every passage near the Sun at intervals from 74 to 79 years since 239 B.C. The period varies somewhat because of perturbations upon its orbit produced by the jovian planets.

Observational records exist for about a thousand comets, with about 10 new comets discovered every year, many by amateur astronomers. Because the orbits of most comets appear to be nearly parabolic and therefore weakly bound to the Sun, the question arises whether all comets are members of the solar system or whether some might be coming from interstellar space. The evidence is conclusive, however, that comets are permanent members of the solar system. If comets were intruders from interstellar space, their orbits should nearly all be markedly hyperbolic, and this is not observed. Moreover, the orbits of long-period comets, unlike those of planets, are oriented at random in space. If comets were interstellar objects, there should be a preponderance of them approaching from the direction toward which the Sun is moving. It is generally accepted, therefore, that comets are members of the solar system following elliptical orbits of high eccentricity. The aphelia of new comets are usually at 50,000 AU from the Sun.

All comets approach the Sun on periodic orbits, but their periods may be very long (millions of years). Some of these very long-period comets are perturbed by Jupiter into orbits of smaller eccentricity and shorter periods. If the period is less than 200 years, it is classed as a short-period comet. The comet of the shortest known period is Comet Encke (3.3 years).

There are about 50 known comets whose orbits are inclined at less than 45° to the ecliptic, which travel from west to east (like planets), and whose aphelion distances are near Jupiter's mean distance from the Sun. They compose the Jupiter family of comets, with periods that range from 5 to 10 years. The Jupiter-family comets are objects that were strongly perturbed by Jupiter during one of their passes through the inner solar system.

Table 4 lists some well-known comets, including both bright recent comets and some of the fainter Jupiter-family comets that have been considered as possible targets for space probes.

B. Physical Nature of Comets

No two comets are alike, but they all have (by definition) an extended atmosphere that forms the comet's head, appearing as a round, diffuse, nebulous glow. Many comets also develop long tails that stream away from the head.

When we look at a comet we see its transient atmosphere of gas and dust, illuminated by sunlight. Since the escape velocity from such small bodies is very low, the atmosphere we see is rapidly escaping; therefore, it must be coming from somewhere. The source is in the heart of the comet's head, usually hidden in the glow of its atmosphere. The small, solid nucleus is found there. The nucleus is the *real* comet, the fragment of primitive material preserved since the beginning of the solar system.

The modern theory of the physical and chemical nature of comets was first proposed by Fred L. Whipple in a 1950 paper

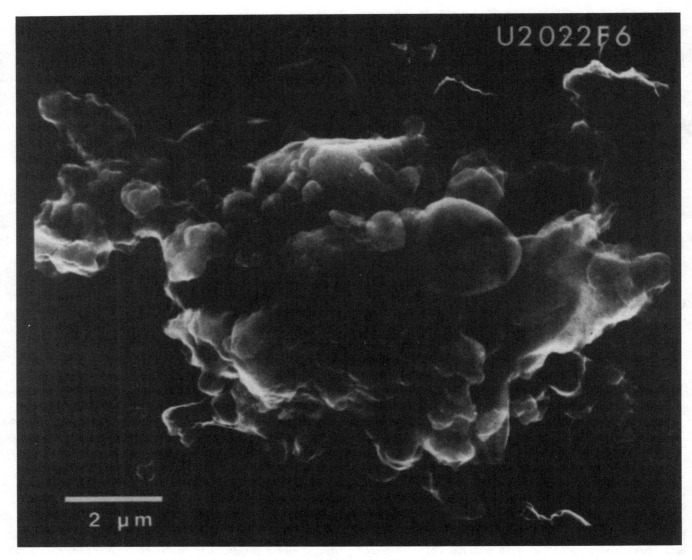

Fig. 9 Particle believed to be a tiny fragment of cometary dust, collected in the upper atmosphere of Earth. (NASA/Johnson Space Center U2022F6)

on Comet Encke. Before Whipple's work many thought that the nucleus of a comet might be a loose agglomeration of solids of meteoritic nature—a sort of orbiting "gravel bank." Whipple proposed instead that the nucleus was a solid object a few kilometers across composed in substantial part of water ice, mixed with silicate grains and dust. This proposal became known as the "dirty snowball" or "icy conglomerate" model for the nucleus of a comet.

Later observations detected large quantities of water vapor and its dissociation products in cometary atmospheres, confirming the importance of this material. Other ices may also be present, including CO_2, CO, NH_3, and CH_4. These are the same molecules that are expected to have condensed in low-temperature regions of the solar nebula.

We are somewhat less certain of the non-icy component of the nucleus. No large fragments of solid matter from a comet have ever survived passage through the Earth's atmosphere to be studied as meteors. Some very fine, microscopic grains have been collected in the Earth's upper atmosphere (Fig. 9), however, and collectors for interplanetary dust have also flown in Earth orbit on the NASA Long-Duration Exposure Facility. The Soviet and European spacecraft that encountered Comet Halley in March 1986 also carried instruments to analyze cometary dust.

From these various investigations it seems that much of the "dirt" in the dirty snowball consists of dark, primitive hydrocarbons and silicates similar to the material thought to be present on the distant asteroids and dark satellite surfaces, such as the leading hemisphere of Saturn's Iapetus. The presence of this dark carbon-rich material gives the comet nucleus a low reflectivity, particularly when the evaporation of ice concentrates the nonvolatile material at the surface. The darkness of the nucleus makes it faint and contributes to the problem of studying it telescopically.

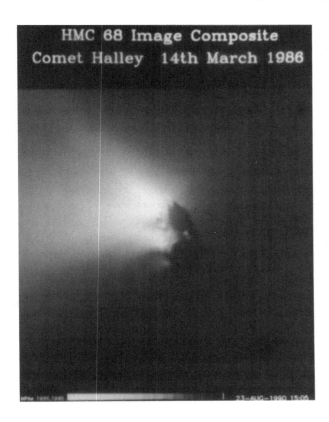

Fig. 10 Composite photographic image taken by the Halley Multicolour Camera on board the European Space Agency's Giotto spacecraft of the nucleus of Halley's Comet. The photograph is composed of 68 images of the nucleus taken during the approach from distances between about 25,000 km and 2500 km. (Max-Planck-Institut Fur Aeronomie, Lindau/Harz, Germany, courtesy of Dr. H. U. Keller)

A recent innovation in the study of the nucleus is to use radar to probe through the surrounding gas and dust. The typical diameter derived by radar for the nucleus of several faint comets seems to be 2 to 5 km. The more active Comet Halley, as measured in 1986, has dimensions of about 13 by 8 km, very similar to the martian satellite Deimos. The largest historic comets probably had diameters of the order of 100 km.

The mass of the nucleus of Comet Halley can be approximated from its observed volume, obtained from spacecraft photos, of about 600 km^3. If its primary constituent is water ice (density near 1.0 g cm^{-3}), the corresponding mass is then 6×10^{14} kg, or about 10^{-10} Earth masses. Comet masses have also been estimated from the evolution of their orbits, but these estimates are unreliable and may be in error by a factor of 3 or more; consequently, there are no direct measures of cometary densities.

C. Cometary Activity

The spectacular activity of comets that gives rise to their

atmospheres and tails results from the evaporation of the cometary ices when they are heated by sunlight. Beyond the asteroid belt, where even short-period comets spend most of their time, the ices are tightly frozen. But as a comet approaches the Sun, its temperature increases. If water is the dominant ice, significant quantities will outgas as temperatures rise toward 200 K, somewhat beyond the orbit of Mars. The evaporating water in turn releases the dust that was mixed with the ice. Since the comet nucleus is so small, its gravity offers no resistance to either the gas or the dust, both of which flow away into space at speeds of about 1 km/s.

The comet continues to absorb energy from the Sun as it approaches perihelion. Much of the solar energy goes into vaporization and evaporation of the ices. Observations of many comets indicate that the evaporation is not uniform, and that most of the gas is released in jets confined to a few areas of the surface. Such jets were observed directly on the surface of Comet Halley by the Soviet Vega and European Giotto spacecraft in 1986, where they resembled volcanic plumes or geysers (Fig. 10). Most of the surface was apparently inactive, with the ice buried under a layer of black silicates and carbon compounds.

On Comet Halley, the same two major plumes were photographed by each of the three spacecraft, indicating that these centers of activity persisted with little change over a period of a week. However, we do not know if they represented deep-seated eruptive centers, or if perhaps the plume regions migrate from one part of the surface to another on time scales of several weeks or more. To answer such questions, it will be necessary to send a spacecraft to orbit with a comet and observe it for longer periods of time.

The escaping jets of gas from an active comet can have an effect on its orbit. It was the problem of accounting for observed changes in cometary orbits that originally led Whipple to develop the dirty snowball model for the nucleus. His 1950 paper was primarily concerned with interpreting orbital variations seen in Comet Encke. As the gas streams away from the nucleus of an active comet, it exerts a reaction force on the nucleus. If the nucleus was very large, or if the gases were escaping from all directions equally, the resulting accelerations would not be observable. However, Whipple hypothesized that Comet Encke had a small nucleus rotating in a period of a few hours. The side of the nucleus facing the Sun would be the warmest, with the highest temperatures on the "afternoon" quadrant of the nucleus. The strongest forces would therefore be concentrated in one direction, and acting continuously over weeks they could measurably influence the comet's orbit. Such reaction effects of cometary activity are called nongravitational forces.

D. Cometary Atmospheres

When it is far from the Sun, the comet's spectrum is simply that of sunlight reflected from the nucleus. The spectrum changes, however, when the comet comes within about 3 AU and its atmosphere begins to develop. Bright emission bands

Table 5   Composition of the volatile fraction of Comet Halley
(from A. Delsemme, U. Toledo)

Parent	Percent	Parent	Percent
H_2O	80	N_2H_4	0.8
H_2CO_2	4.5	HCN	1.0
H_2CO	4.0	N_2	0.5
CO_2	3.5	$H_4C_5N_4$	0.5
CO	1.5	NH_3	1.0
CH_4	2.0	S_2	0.2
C_2H_2	1.5	H_2S	0.2
C_3H_2	0.2	CS_2	0.2

of the molecules and radicals carbon (C_2), cyanogen (CN), and hydroxyl (OH) are generally present. Ultraviolet light from the Sun dissociates the molecules in the head of a comet to produce these radicals or molecular fragments. Often NH, NH_2, and other molecules are detected as well. The parent molecules—the original molecules that were dissociated to form the radicals we measure—are presumed to be water (H_2O), carbon dioxide (CO_2), carbon monoxide (CO), methane (CH_4), and ammonia (NH_3). Direct spacecraft measurements of the inner atmosphere of Comet Halley revealed many other gases, including hydrocarbons. Table 5 lists the main volatile constituents of Comet Halley as identified or inferred from observations in 1985-86.

Many comets develop tails as they approach the Sun. The tail of a comet is an extension of its atmosphere, consisting of the same gas and dust that make up the head. As early as the 16th century, observers realized that comet tails point away from the Sun, not back along the comet's orbit. Newton attempted to account for comet tails by a repulsive force of sunlight driving particles away from the comet's head, an idea that is close to our modern view.

Actually the primary repulsive force that causes the tails of comets to point away from the Sun is the solar wind. This outward-streaming plasma interacts with the plasma in the comet tail and carries it along at a speed of about 400 km/s. Decades before the solar wind was detected directly by spacecraft its existence was inferred from the behavior of comet tails. The solar wind interacts strongly only with ionized gas, however; other forces, primarily radiation pressure, are important in repelling dust grains, as Newton had suggested. Tails generally grow in size as comets approach the Sun and have been known to reach lengths of more than 150 million km.

Most comets have two tails that are very different from each other. The most prominent is the plasma tail; it is usually nearly straight, and its spectrum shows emission by ions such as CO^+, N_2^+, and H_2O^+. The other tail is a dust tail, broad and generally curved, displaying the spectrum of reflected sunlight.

The nearly straight plasma tails sometimes have recognizable features or knots that can be tracked as they move away from the comet. Measures of such structures show that the streaming ions have speeds that increase from several km/s near the head of the comet to hundreds of km/s toward the end of the tail. From time to time, sudden solar outbursts (flares) result in a greater than average flow of plasma from the Sun. These changes in the solar wind intensity, and variations in the ejection of material from the comet's nucleus, probably account for the irregular features in its plasma tail.

The dust tails of comets are often broad or multiple because the particles of different sizes are accelerated by different amounts. Radiation pressure generally imparts smaller speeds to particles of greater mass, so that they trail farther behind the comet. Sometimes the dust tails are distinctly fan-shaped, the trailing edge of the fan consisting of the largest particles and curving back the most.

E. Origin and Evolution

The observed aphelia of new comets typically have values near 50,000 AU. This clustering of aphelion distances was first noted by Jan Oort, who in 1950 proposed a scheme for the origin of the comets that is still accepted today.

The gravitational sphere of influence of a star—the distance within which it can exert sufficient gravitation to hold onto orbiting objects—is about one-third of the distance to the nearest other stars. For the Sun, the radius of this sphere of influence is about 1 light year, or somewhat more than 50,000 AU. Oort suggested that the new comets were objects orbiting the Sun with aphelia near the edge of its sphere of influence. Furthermore, the perturbing effects of other nearby stars modified their orbits to bring them close to the Sun where we can see them.

The region of space from which the new comets are derived is called the Oort comet cloud. Oort calculated that if comets have been entering the inner solar system at their current rate for its entire history of 4.5 Gyr, then the source region must have originally held at least 10^{11} comets.

Just because most new comets have aphelia near 50,000 AU, we should be careful not to conclude that the Oort cloud consists of billions of comets in roughly circular orbits at this distance, like a shell around the Sun. There may be some comets in nearly circular orbits, but if so, we have no evidence of them. What we see are comets that are perturbed into the inner solar system from orbits that must have been already of very large eccentricity. A passing star can cause only a slight change in eccentricity, and so if a comet has an orbit with a perihelion of, say, 1 AU when we discover it, it must have had a perihelion of no more than a few AU on its previous unobserved passage near the Sun. For every comet that comes close enough to be seen, there must be many more skimming invisibly through the orbits of the outer planets, and still more with perihelia beyond Pluto.

Direct observations of comets beyond Pluto are lacking, but there is indirect evidence of a substantial reservoir of comets inside the traditional Oort cloud. The orbital statistics of the short-period comets suggest that most of them originated in a flattened, disk-shaped region rather than in the more nearly spherical Oort cloud. This additional reservoir of cometary objects is called the Kuiper belt. It may contain as many as 10^{13} comets, an order of magnitude more than the traditional Oort cloud.

What is the mass represented by 10^{13} comets? We can make an estimate if we assume that the nucleus of Comet Halley is typical with its mass of 10^{-10} Earth masses. The corresponding mass for all of the comets is about 10^3 Earth masses—greater than the mass of all of the planets put together. Cometary material may be the most important constituent of the solar system after the Sun itself.

There are two theories for the formation of the Oort cloud. The first hypothesizes that the comets are condensates from the outer fringes of the solar nebula. However, models suggest that the solar nebula thinned out rapidly with increasing distance from the Sun. It is difficult to understand how any substantial amount of material could have condensed at such huge distances, or how small grains might have accumulated into bodies several kilometers across.

A more likely hypothesis is that the comets were ejected into the Oort cloud from initial orbits near the present orbits of Uranus and Neptune. Calculations indicate that if many icy planetesimals were still present after the giant planets formed, a substantial fraction of them would have been ejected by gravitational encounters with these bodies. If this is correct, then the comets are leftovers from the building blocks of the outer planets, preserved for 4.5 Gyr years in the deep freeze of space.

Once a comet enters the inner solar system, its previously uneventful life history begins to accelerate. It may, of course, survive its initial passage near the Sun and return to the cold reaches of space. At the other extreme, it may impact the Sun or pass so close that it is destroyed on its first perihelion passage. Observations from space indicate that at least one comet collides with the Sun every year. Frequently, however, the new comet does not come this close to the Sun, but instead interacts with one or more of the planets.

A comet coming within the gravitational influence of a planet has three possible fates: 1) It can impact that planet, ending the story at once; 2) it can be ejected on a hyperbolic trajectory, leaving the solar system forever; or 3) it can be perturbed into a shorter period. In the last case, its fate is sealed. Each time it approaches the Sun, it will lose part of its material, and it still has a significant chance of collision with a planet. Once in a short-period orbit, the comet's lifetime is measured in thousands, not billions, of years.

Measurements of the amount of gas and dust in the atmosphere of a comet suggest that typical loss rates are up to a million tons (10^9 kg) per day from an active comet near the Sun, adding up to some tens of millions of tons per orbit. This is equivalent to stripping off the top several meters from the nucleus. Comparing these loss rates with the total mass of the comet, we see that they amount to about 0.1 percent per orbit. At that rate, the comet will be gone after a thousand orbits.

Whether the comet evaporates completely is not known. If the gas and dust are well mixed, we would expect the nucleus to shrink each time around the Sun until it has entirely disappeared. However, there remains the suggestion that many of the near-Earth asteroids are extinct comets. If there is a silicate core in the comet, or if the dirty snowball includes large blocks of nonvolatile material that are held gravitationally to the surface, then there could be a substantial solid residue after the ices are gone.

Some comets end catastrophically. Even if they avoid impacting a planet or being perturbed into an orbit that collides with the Sun, they can break apart for reasons that are not well understood. In 1846, for example, the nucleus of Comet Biela split into two parts, and on its next return in 1852 it appeared as two comets, separated by 2 million km. In 1866, the next perihelion year, nothing appeared; Comet Biela had disappeared. A more recent example of breakup is provided by Comet West. Shortly after its 1976 perihelion passage its nucleus split into four components, which drifted apart at a rate of several hundred kilometers per day. The smallest fragment survived only a few days, but the other three retained their identities until the comet became invisible with increasing distance from the Sun.

F. Meteors and Comet Dust

Whatever the fate of the remnants of a cometary nucleus after the volatiles are exhausted, we do know what happens to the dust that is carried away from a comet by the evaporation of the nucleus. This dust fills the inner part of the solar system. The Earth is surrounded by it, and each of the larger dust particles that reaches the Earth creates a meteor or "shooting star."

On a dark, moonless night an alert observer can see half a dozen meteors per hour. Over the entire Earth, the total number of meteors bright enough to be visible must total about 25 million per day. Meteors become visible at an average height of 95 km, and their luminous paths generally end by the time they reach altitudes of 80 km.

The typical bright meteor is produced by a particle with a mass less than 1 gram, although an object as large as 1 kilogram has a fair chance of surviving its fiery entry to become a meteor, if its approach speed is not too high. The total mass of meteoritic material entering the Earth's atmosphere is estimated to be about 100 tons per day.

Many—perhaps most—of the meteors that strike the Earth can be associated with specific comets. These interplanetary dust particles retain approximately the orbit of their parent comet, and the particles travel together through space. When the Earth crosses such a dust stream, we see a sudden burst of meteor activity, usually lasting several hours. These events are called meteor showers.

No shower meteor is known to have survived its flight through the atmosphere and been recovered for laboratory analysis. However, there are other ways to investigate the nature of these particles and thereby to gain additional insight into the comets from which they are derived. Analysis of the photographic tracks of meteors shows that most of them have densities less than 1.0 g cm^{-3}. Apparently a fist-sized lump, if you placed it on a table, would fall apart under its own weight. Such particles disintegrate in the atmosphere, accounting for the failure of even relatively large showers of meteors to produce meteorites.

Comet dust can be seen directly in the zodiacal light, which is a faint glow of sunlight reflected from this dust. The total mass of the material responsible for the zodiacal light is estimated at 10^{16} kg. These dust particles are gradually spiralling into the Sun, but they are replaced from the comets and from collisional fragmentation of objects in the asteroid belt, in the amount of about 10 tons (10^4 kg) per second. Spacecraft that have explored beyond the asteroid belt confirm that most of the interplanetary dust is located within a few AU of the Sun.

The zodiacal dust has also been detected in the infrared. In 1983 the IRAS carried out an all-sky survey at wavelengths from 10 to 100 micrometers, in which the presence of this material is obvious. IRAS also detected previously unrecognized structure in the emission, indicating the presence of three distinct dust bands. These bands apparently represent the debris from asteroid collisions, and they have been identified with two of the largest asteroid families, the Eos and Themis families. IRAS also located dust bands along the orbits of comets, and it led to the discovery of an asteroid (3200 Phaethon) that seems to have the same orbit as the Geminid meteor stream. This is the first association of an asteroid, rather than a comet, with a meteor shower.

G. Comets and the Earth

Statistical studies of their orbits indicate that comets collide with the Earth and other terrestrial planets with approximately the same frequency as do near-Earth asteroids. In the case of an airless target like the Moon, cometary impacts produce craters that are indistinguishable from those generated by asteroidal impacts. However, the effects on the Earth of cometary impacts may be different. As a consequence of both their weaker physical structure and their higher average impact velocities, comets may not survive passage through the atmosphere. However, the kinetic energy of the projectile is equally great even if its material is loose and fluffy, and so

the environmental effects of collisions with large comets may be similar to those from asteroids. The fact is that we do not know, for example, if the impact that terminated the Cretaceous was cometary or asteroidal. We measure the iridium and tend to assume that it came from an asteroid, but there is probably also iridium in the nonvolatile fraction of comets.

Early in solar system history, the rate of impacts by both comets and asteroids was much higher than today. The lunar cratering history tells us that as recently as 4.0 Gyr ago impact fluxes were several orders of magnitude higher than those observed today. If comets—that is, planetesimals containing large quantities of volatiles—were major contributors to this impact flux, this deposition must have been important for the early Earth.

During the late period of planetary accretion we can imagine that numerous cometary impacts transported significant quantities of water and organic material to the inner planets from the colder regions of the outer solar system. The oceans of the Earth, which amount to less than 0.1 percent of the terrestrial mass, probably originated in this cometary flux. The organic building blocks for life may have reached the Earth in the same way. However, we must also recognize that the largest impacts were capable of boiling the early oceans and stripping the Earth of much of its atmosphere. Detailed calculations are required to determine the balance between accretion and loss, which depended on the size distribution of the infalling materials and its variation with time.

IV. Future Studies

A. Spacecraft Missions to Asteroids

Asteroids are the last major component of the solar system to be investigated by spacecraft (unless the Mars missions that have studied Phobos and Deimos are counted). The first flyby of an asteroid took place on October 21, 1991, when the Galileo spacecraft encountered 951 Gaspra (spectral class S, longest dimension 20 km) at a range of 1600 km. A variety of remote sensing observations were made using cameras, spectrometers, and other instruments targeted for the later Galileo observations of the jovian satellites. The measurements reveal Gaspra to be an elongated, irregular, cratered fragment of an asteroid collision that took place no more than a few hundred million years ago. In 1993, a second Galileo encounter is planned with 243 Ida (spectral class C, diameter about 30 km).

NASA has established a policy to include asteroid flybys in missions that cross the asteroid belt en route to the outer solar system. Thus additional encounters are planned for the Cassini mission to Saturn. These flybys will take place late in the decade of the 1990s.

The U.S., European Space Agency, and the U.S.S.R. have all studied missions to the near-Earth asteroids. These are among the most accessible objects in the solar system, and they can be reached with relatively short flight times and modest launch capabilities. It is hoped that one or more missions to these objects can be undertaken before the end of the century.

B. Spacecraft Missions to Comets

In 1985 the first spacecraft encounter with the tail of a comet took place. The U.S. International Sun-Earth Explorer (ISEE) was diverted in a complicated set of maneuvers so that it left our planet and intercepted Comet Giacobini-Zinner. This spacecraft, renamed the International Comet Explorer (ICE), passed 7800 km behind the comet nucleus on September 11, 1985. Among the results was the discovery of an unexpectedly large and energetic region of interaction between the plasma tail and the solar wind, and a lower than anticipated density of dust (only about 50 hits measured). This spacecraft was not instrumented, however, to measure the nucleus; that was left to the flotilla of spacecraft that encountered Comet Halley the following March.

Six spacecraft made measurements of Comet Halley in March 1986, as the comet crossed the plane of the Earth's orbit a month after perihelion. Two of these—the U.S. ICE spacecraft mentioned above and a small Japanese craft named Sakagaki—served primarily to monitor the comet and the interplanetary medium from a distance of several million kilometers, while a second Japanese spacecraft—Suisei— passed about 1 million km from the comet. The primary exploration tasks, however, were undertaken by three craft targeted for the nucleus itself.

The Soviet Vega 1 and Vega 2 were the first craft to arrive, on March 6 and 9, 1986. Each plunged deeply into the inner atmosphere and dust cloud of the comet, passing within about 8000 km of the nucleus. In addition to making many direct measurements of the gas and dust, they photographed the dust-shrouded nucleus, but they were able to see little beyond the bright plumes of material jetting out from the two most active regions on its surface. The trajectory data for the Vega craft were provided to the ESA to allow them to target their Giotto spacecraft for an even closer encounter on March 14, 1986, just 605 km from the comet's nucleus. Giotto photographed the nucleus and carried out many measurements of the near environment of the nucleus, confirming and extending the Soviet results. Among the most exciting discoveries was the fact that much of the dust is in the form of very small particles consisting largely of carbon and hydrocarbon compounds, rather than silicates.

Halley is the only bright comet with a predictable orbit that can be targeted for spacecraft investigation. To take the next step, from a flyby to a rendezvous or lander mission, we must turn our attention to the smaller Jupiter-family comets, several of which have orbits of low inclination. A number of possible missions to these comets have been studied, most notably the NASA Comet Rendezvous Asteroid Flyby mission: CRAF. CRAF received funding in fiscal year 1990 for a planned launch in 1996 to comet Tempel 2, but it now appears that this mission is to be cancelled.

The CRAF spacecraft was designed to match orbit with the comet far from the Sun, more than 800 days before perihelion so that its initial characterization of the nucleus could be carried out with minimal interference from the comet's atmosphere. As the comet approached the Sun, the spacecraft was to observe the onset of activity and the development of the atmosphere. As the density of gas and dust increased near the nucleus, the spacecraft could back off to observe from a safe distance. The mission profile also included an excursion of more than 10,000 km along the tail near the comet's perihelion. Even if the CRAF mission is not implemented, a rendezvous mission of this type clearly represents the highest priority for comet exploration.

C. Other Studies

Spacecraft observations of asteroids and comets will greatly expand our understanding of these remnants from the formation of the solar system. However, it is difficult to imagine that more than a very small fraction of these objects can be investigated in this way. Therefore, it will be essential to continue remote astronomical observations from the ground and from Earth orbit. Only in this way can we begin to understand the diversity of the populations of small bodies and thus to place spacecraft studies in a broader context.

An important scientific objective in the exploration of members of the planetary system is the return of samples to the Earth for detailed laboratory investigation. In this respect, scientists who study comets and asteroids are fortunate. In the meteors, we have in hand samples of several dozen separate asteroids or asteroid-related bodies. Interplanetary dust particles of cometary origin are also beginning to receive detailed laboratory attention. These investigations will be critical for developing an understanding of these objects and of their role in solar system history.

Thus we can project a continuing scientific assault on the small bodies and their record of solar system history that has at least four essential components. Spacecraft observations will provide detailed information on a few bodies. Astronomical studies will place these detailed studies in context and will allow the characterization of the broad populations of comets and asteroids. Analysis of meteors and interplanetary dust will yield the type of precise mineralogical, chemical, and isotopic data that can be obtained only in the laboratory. And all of these studies will be further strengthened by astronomical observations of disks of gas and dust around other stars that are the present-day analogs of the solar nebula that gave birth to our solar system 4.5 Gyr ago.

References

[1] A'Hearn, M.J. Observations of Cometary Nuclei. *Annual Reviews of Earth and Planetary Sciences,* 1988, Vol. 16, pp. 273-293.

[2] Bell, J.F., Davis, D.R., Hartmann, W.K., Gaffey, M.J. Asteroids: The Big Picture. In: Binzel, R.P., Gehrels, T.,

Matthews, M.S. (Eds.), *Asteroids II,* University of Arizona Press, Tucson, 1989, pp. 921-948.

[3] Binzel, R.P. An Overview of the Asteroids. In: Binzel, R.P., Gehrels, T., Matthews, M.S. (Eds.), *Asteroids II,* University of Arizona Press, Tucson, 1985, pp. 3-20.

[4] Brownlee, D.E. Cosmic Dust: Collection and Research. *Annual Reviews of Earth and Planetary Sciences*, Vol. 13, pp. 147-174.

[5] Gradie, J.C., Chapman, C.R., Tedesco, E.F. Distribution of Taxonomic Classes and the Compositional Structure of the Asteroid Belt. In: Binzel, R.P., Gehrels, T., Matthews, M.S. (Eds.), *Asteroids II,* University of Arizona Press, Tucson, 1989, pp. 316-335.

[6] Keller, H.U., et al. Comet P/Halley's Nucleus and Its Activity. In: Grewing, M., Praderie, F., Reinhard, R. (Eds.), *Exploration of Halley's Comet*, Springer-Verlag, Berlin, 1988, pp. 807-823.

[7] Kerridge, J.F., Anders, E. Boundary Conditions for the Origin of the Solar System. In: Kerridge, J.F., Matthews, M.S. (Eds.), *Meteorites and the Early Solar System,* University of Arizona Press, Tucson, 1988, pp. 1149-1154.

[8] Langevin, Y., Kissel, J., Bertaux, J.L., Chassefiere, E. First Statistical Analysis of 5000 Mass Spectra of Cometary Grains Obtained by PUMA 1 (VEGA 1) and PIA (Giotto) Impact Ionization Mass Spectrometers in the Compressed Modes. In: Grewing, M., Praderie, F., Reinhard, R. (Eds.), *Exploration of Halley's Comet*, Springer-Verlag, Berlin, 1988, pp. 761-766.

[9] Tholen, D.J., Barucci, M.A. Asteroid Taxonomy. In: Binzel, R.P., Gehrels, T., Matthews, M.S. (Eds.), *Asteroids II*, University of Arizona Press, Tucson, 1989, pp. 298-315.

[10] Weissman, P.R. Dynamical History of the Oort Cloud. In: Wilkening, L. (Ed.), *Comets*, University of Arizona Press, Tucson, 1982, pp. 637-658.

[11] Wetherill, G.W. Origin of the Asteroid Belt. In: Binzel, R.P., Gehrels, T., Matthews, M.S. (Eds.), *Asteroids II*, University of Arizona Press, Tucson, 1989, pp. 661-680.

[12] Wetherill, G.W., Chapman, C.R. Asteroids and Meteorites. In: Kerridge, J.F., Matthews, M.S. (Eds.), *Meteorites and the Early Solar System*, University of Arizona Press, Tucson, 1988, pp. 35-70.

[13] Wyckoff, S. Overview of Comet Observations. In: Wilkening, L. (Ed.), *Comets*, University of Arizona Press, Tucson, 1982, pp. 3-55.

[14] Moroz, V.I. Halley's Comet (Part II): Space Studies. *Highlights of Astronomy*, 1989, No. 8, pp. 17-31.

[15] Shulman, L.M. *Nuclei of Comets*, Moscow, Nauka, 1987 (in Russian).

[16] Dobrovolsky, O.V. *Comets,* Moscow, Nauka, 1966 (in Russian).

[17] Simonenko, A.N. *Meteorites: Fragments of Asteroids,* Moscow, Nauka, 1979 (in Russian).

Bibliography

A'Hearn, M.J. Observations of Cometary Nuclei. *Annual Reviews of Earth and Planetary Sciences,* 1988, Vol. 16, pp. 273-293.

Bell, J.F., Davis, D.R., Hartmann, W.K., Gaffey, M.J. Asteroids: The Big Picture. In: Binzel, R.P., Gehrels, T., Matthews, M.S. (Eds.), *Asteroids II,* University of Arizona Press, Tucson, 1989, pp. 921-948.

Binzel, R.P. An Overview of the Asteroids. In: Binzel, R.P., Gehrels, T., Matthews, M.S. (Eds.), *Asteroids II,* University of Arizona Press, Tucson, 1985, pp. 3-20.

Brownlee, D.E. Cosmic Dust: Collection and Research. *Annual Reviews of Earth and Planetary Sciences*, Vol. 13, pp. 147-174.

Dobrovolsky, O.V. *Comets,* Moscow, Nauka, 1966 (in Russian).

Gradie, J.C., Chapman, C.R., Tedesco, E.F. Distribution of Taxonomic Classes and the Compositional Structure of the Asteroid Belt. In: Binzel, R.P., Gehrels, T., Matthews, M.S. (Eds.), *Asteroids II,* University of Arizona Press, Tucson, 1989, pp. 316-335.

Keller, H.U., et al. Comet P/Halley's Nucleus and Its Activity. In: Grewing, M., Praderie, F., Reinhard, R. (Eds.), *Exploration of Halley's Comet*, Springer-Verlag, Berlin, 1988, pp. 807-823.

Kerridge, J.F., Anders, E. Boundary Conditions for the Origin of the Solar System. In: Kerridge, J.F., Matthews, M.S. (Eds.), *Meteorites and the Early Solar System,* University of Arizona Press, Tucson, 1988, pp. 1149-1154.

Langevin, Y., Kissel, J., Bertaux, J.L., Chassefiere, E. First Statistical Analysis of 5000 Mass Spectra of Cometary Grains Obtained by PUMA 1 (VEGA 1) and PIA (Giotto) Impact Ionization Mass Spectrometers in the Compressed Modes. In: Grewing, M., Praderie, F., Reinhard, R. (Eds.), *Exploration of Halley's Comet*, Springer-Verlag, Berlin, 1988, pp. 761-766.

Moroz, V.I. Halley's Comet (Part II): Space Studies. *Highlights of Astronomy*, 1989, No. 8, pp. 17-31.

Shulman, L.M. *Nuclei of Comets*, Moscow, Nauka, 1987 (in Russian).

Simonenko, A.N. *Meteorites: Fragments of Asteroids*, Moscow, Nauka, 1979 (in Russian).

Tholen, D.J., Barucci, M.A. Asteroid Taxonomy. In: Binzel, R.P., Gehrels, T., Matthews, M.S. (Eds.), *Asteroids II*, University of Arizona Press, Tucson, 1989, pp. 298-315.

Weissman, P.R. Dynamical History of the Oort Cloud. In: Wilkening, L. (Ed.), *Comets*, University of Arizona Press, Tucson, 1982, pp. 637-658.

Wetherill, G.W. Origin of the Asteroid Belt. In: Binzel, R.P., Gehrels, T., Matthews, M.S. (Eds.), *Asteroids II*, University of Arizona Press, Tucson, 1989, pp. 661-680.

Wetherill, G.W., Chapman, C.R. Asteroids and Meteorites. In: Kerridge, J.F., Matthews, M.S. (Eds.), *Meteorites and the Early Solar System*, University of Arizona Press, Tucson, 1988, pp. 35-70.

Wyckoff, S. Overview of Comet Observations. In: Wilkening, L. (Ed.), *Comets*, University of Arizona Press, Tucson, 1982, pp. 3-55.

Part III:

Life in the Universe

Chapter 6

Exobiology

John D. Rummel

I. What is Exobiology?

Exobiology is the study of the origin, evolution, and distribution of life in the universe. The term itself was coined by Nobel prize-winner Joshua Lederberg in 1960,[1] at the beginning of the space age, but the nature of the science it connotes has grown throughout the last 32 years. Through the science of exobiology, answers are sought to interrelated questions such as how the development of the universe and the process of star and solar system development led to the existence of our own solar system, and how that development subsequently led to a planet suitable for life, how life originated on Earth, and what factors influenced the course of biological evolution? Working from this basis, exobiologists then ask where else life may be found in the universe, and how best to establish its existence.

These questions have broad scientific and cultural significance, addressing the possibility that life is unique to Earth while investigating prospects for its existence and detection elsewhere. A general theory for the natural origin and evolution of living systems within the context of the origin of the universe, may eventually arise from knowledge gained in the systematic search for answers to these age-old questions.

For the purposes of this discussion, we can define life as a property of self-replicating, mutating, metabolizing systems. Other definitions are possible, but in anticipating the potential variety of extraterrestrial life it is perhaps unwise to over-specify our expectations. Similarly, it is possible to conceive of life forms that do not rely heavily on carbon, hydrogen, nitrogen, oxygen, phosphorus, and sulfur (C, H, N, O, P, S), the "biogenic" elements that compose the bulk of biomass on Earth. Nonetheless, because these elements are among the most abundant in the universe (phosphorus being the exception), it is likely that they should be equally involved with living systems elsewhere. The chemistry of carbon, in particular, is unique. Its ability to form four stable covalent bonds allows it to form the three-dimensional molecules of large size and complexity that are essential to life. Such molecules are capable of performing an amazing variety of chemical activities when given an aqueous medium in which to react. Thus, the biogenic compounds of major interest are those normally associated with water and with organic chemistry, in which carbon is bonded to itself or to other biogenic elements.

Our present understanding of biological evolution and the natural history of life on Earth indicates that biology has been strongly influenced by planetary and solar system evolution, both in its origins and in its subsequent development. At the core of the science of exobiology are issues concerning the natural history of life in the universe, all of which can be addressed most fruitfully in the context of evolution. In the cosmic, galactic, solar system, planetary or environmental sense, "evolution" refers to the course of change over time as a consequence of the changing thermodynamic state of the universe. It is within this milieu that life arose from inanimate matter and evolved in concert with the physicochemical universe. Life, then, may be viewed as a unique product of countless changes in the form of primordial matter.

The exploration of space has provided a vast array of data on these cosmic influences, but despite a few initial (negative) attempts, we have yet to conduct a comprehensive search for life on the few other bodies of this solar system that we think could harbor carbon-based life. Nonetheless, evidence about life on Earth suggests that there is no reason to believe that life should be limited to this planet alone. It could (and probably should) arise and evolve on a multitude of other planets in this galaxy. For these reasons, unparalleled opportunities to contribute to the state of the biological sciences are embodied within the missions and projects associated with space exploration. In the U.S., such opportunities are integral to NASA's charter to promote "the expansion of human knowledge of phenomena in ... space" (National Aeronautics and Space Act of 1958). The rationale for conducting the science of exobiology in concert with our exploration of space is ultimately derived from the demands of the science itself.

Although the term "exobiology" is comparatively recent, the history of the subject dates back to ancient times, and the subject undoubtedly had a prehistory. A desire to understand the origin of life on Earth and the potential for life elsewhere are features of most of the world's religions, and those subjects have long been reflected in the literary world. In Greek mythology the universe came into being in the persons of Chaos, representing the emptiness of the universe, and Gaea, representing the mother Earth. The ancient Babylonians espoused a similar beginning with the deities Apsu and Tiamat. In the Hebrew tradition, "heaven and earth" are also the first products of creation, whereas in the Hindu Vedas the

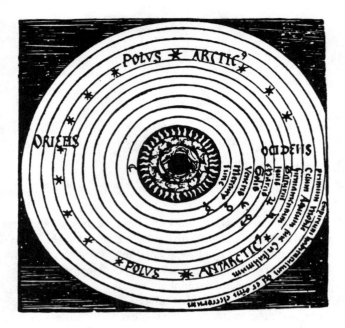

Fig. 1 The Aristotelian scheme of the universe. From inside to outside: spheres of the Earth, water, air, and fire composing the terrestrial region; planetary spheres carrying Moon, Mercury, Venus, Sun, Mars, Jupiter, Saturn; then to fixed stars.

oceans are postulated as the cradle of life that was derived from the primary elements.

There is also evidence that ancient thought on these matters went beyond a simple acceptance of mythology or religious tenets. The idea of life arising from non-life on a regular basis can be traced to Aristotle (322 B.C.), and was commonplace until the 17th century. This concept was supported by (flawed) experimental evidence: worms appeared in mud, maggots seemed to form in decaying meat, etc. Only with Pasteur's experiments in the early 1860s was this particular concept of the spontaneous generation of life put to rest.

Other ancient ideas about life in the universe were more general and more compatible with present thinking. Motivated by astronomical observations that suggested a vast universe and by the atomic theory of matter, philosophers of the ancient world had clearly conceived of a physical basis for the origin of the universe and of life. As a result, they were able to consider a non-Earth-centered cosmology and the possibility of other worlds, and therefore other living worlds. For example, the Greek philosopher Metrodorus of Chios, who applied himself to explaining astronomical phenomena, wrote in the 4th century B.C., "To consider the Earth as the only populated world in infinite space is as absurd as to assert that in an entire field of millet, only one grain will grow."[2]

Ancient tradition, however, contained both heliocentric and Earth-centered views of the solar system (and the universe). Between the 2nd and 16th centuries A.D. the prevailing concept in the Western World was the Ptolemaic view of a geocentric universe (cf., Fig. 1). Only when this view of the universe was overthrown by the ideas of Copernicus and Kepler, and when the concept of spontaneous generation was abandoned, did the concept of an "origin of life" make sense as a unique event in the context of the origin and evolution of the universe. Only in the early 20th century did the concept of an unchanging "clockwork" universe give way to concepts of the "Big Bang" and a truly evolving stage on which the drama of life could unfold.

In the middle of the 19th century, Charles Darwin and Alfred Russell Wallace each put forward the idea that evolution of life through natural selection provided a mechanism by which life could have been gradually altered from its beginnings in the distant past by the "Origin of Species" that has led to life in the present. Perhaps the most difficult aspect of their hypothesis resulted from the contemporary biological world's lack of knowledge of the mechanisms of heredity—a lack that persisted until results of the sort initially gained by Gregor Mendel in the mid-1800s became better known at the turn of the century. The concept of natural selection, however, opened up the possibility that the evolution of living systems was a continuous process, one that was shaped by the common forces of the physical world. Henceforth, the process of biological evolution could be no more mysterious than physics or chemistry (although working within an enormously complex milieu). What, then, of the origin of life itself?

Darwin himself retraced in his mind the process of natural selection to the time of life's origins. Rather than the "spontaneous generation" of evolved forms that had been fully laid to rest by 1871, Darwin envisioned, in a letter to Hooker, the formation of the simplest possible form of life from the buildup of complex components under much different conditions than now exist.

> It is often said that all the conditions for the first production of living organisms are now present, which could ever have been present. Assuming we could conceive in some warm little pond in the presence of all sorts of ammonia and phosphoric salts, light, heat, electricity, etc., a chemically formed protein compound prepared to undergo still more complex changes. Then, at the present day such matter would be instantly devoured or absorbed, which would not have been the case before living creatures were formed.[3]

Clearly conditions for the origin of life would require, at a minimum, the proper conditions, a source of components, and sufficient time in which to combine them.

Such thinking formed the basis for the hypothesis on the origin of life that was first published by Oparin in 1924,[4] and independently by Haldane in 1928.[5] In this hypothesis, the buildup of the starting materials for life on Earth was a direct consequence of the physical and chemical formation and evolution of the planet, and presumed a much different set of conditions on the early Earth than is found today. These ideas

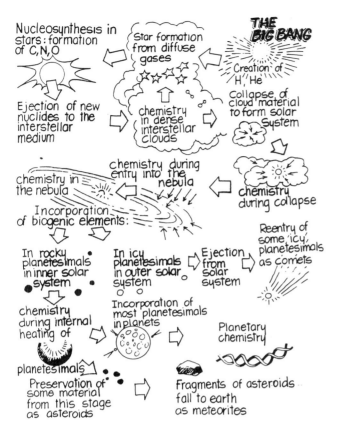

Fig. 2 The cosmic evolution of the biogenic elements and compounds from the "Big Bang," the birth of the heavier elements in stars, and the formation of the solar system, until their incorporation into the forming Earth.[6]

form the basis for the ideas of the origin of life espoused by exobiologists today, though the specific hypothesis has been substantially modified by the insights and data provided by a greater understanding of the Earth and through the exploration of space.

It is precisely these insights and data that have provided exobiologists with an understanding of the relationship between the origin of life on Earth and the formation of the entire universe. As our understanding of the universe has grown, it has become more apparent that life is a consequence of the evolution of the cosmos, and that widely separated events in time and space have all contributed to life on Earth. Two considerations directly follow from our present evidence: 1) that life is a direct result of the physical and chemical conditions that formed the universe in the first place; and 2) that if those conditions were common throughout the universe, then life, too, is likely to be widespread. The nature of that evidence is reviewed below.

II. Life in the Universe

Recognition of the evolutionary interplay between the universe and life has led to extensive scientific research on the natural history of that interplay. The study of exobiology can be divided conceptually into subject areas that correspond to the four major epochs in the evolution of living systems: 1) The Cosmic Evolution of the Biogenic Compounds, 2) Prebiotic Evolution, 3) The Origin and Early Evolution of Life, and 4) The Evolution of Advanced Life.

Through the study of these subject areas, exobiology traces the pathways leading from the origin of the universe through the major epochs in the story of life. Additional facets of the science of exobiology address the study of life-related compounds, and the search for life elsewhere in the universe. Exobiology advances through the study of life on Earth, its origin and evolution, the direct study of other planets and small bodies in the solar system, and by studying the universe from ground-based and Earth-orbital observatories.

A. The Cosmic Origin of the Biogenic Elements and Compounds

An understanding of life in the universe cannot be reached solely through an understanding of the living organisms that presently exist, or have existed, on the planet Earth. If the subject of exobiology is to have any generality, then Earth life must be understood in the context of the physical and chemical universe in which all life must originate. In particular, exobiologists focus on the origin and evolution of the elements and compounds associated with the origin and evolution of life on Earth—the biogenic elements and compounds. There is reason to think that these materials are truly universal in their distribution. The mechanisms that provided them to our own solar system appear to be taking place throughout this galaxy and elsewhere in the universe.

Although other conceptions of life might be possible, because of their abundance in the cosmos the elements that are biogenic on Earth are likely to be important to life elsewhere in the universe. Essential elements usually associated with inorganic rather than organic chemistry—e.g., iron, magnesium, calcium, sodium, potassium, and chlorine—are also important, but they are given secondary emphasis. The physical and chemical pathways taken by the biogenic elements and compounds can be traced from their origin in stars, through their residence in interstellar clouds, cloud fragmentation and protostellar collapse, into the evolution of the solar nebula, and to their incorporation and transformations in the pre-planetary bodies by which they were distributed throughout the solar system (Fig. 2).

In addition to their importance to living systems, measurements made in the galaxy and solar system using the biogenic elements and compounds as observational probes can help to develop models of the formation of the solar system and the chemistry that occurred in it. The physical and chemical properties of the biogenic elements and compounds have influenced the course of events during the formation of the solar system as a whole. Because water plays such a central role in the development of life and, therefore, in the environments in which prebiotic evolution could have occurred, the

Table 1　Identified interstellar molecules[7]

Simple Hydrides, Oxides, Sulfides, Halides, and Related Molecules

H_2	CO	NH_3	CS	$NaCl^x$
HCl	SiO	$SiH4$	SiS	$AlCl^x$
H_2O	SO_2	CC	H_2S	KCl^x
	OCS	CC_4x	PN	AlF^x
	HNO (?)	SiC^x		

Nitriles, Acetylene Derivatives, and Related Molecules

HCN	$HC{\equiv}C{-}CN$	$H_3C{-}C{\equiv}C{-}CN$	$H_3C{-}CH_2{-}CN$	$H_2C{=}CH_2{}^x$
H_3CCN	$H(C{\equiv}C)_2{-}CN$	$H_3C{-}{-}C{\equiv}CH$	$H_2C{=}CH{-}CN$	$HC{\equiv}CH^x$
CCO(?)	$H(C{\equiv}C)_3{-}CN$	$H_3C{-}{-}(C{\equiv}C)_2{-}H$	HNC	
$CCCO$	$H(C{\equiv}C)_4{-}CN$	$H_3C{-}(C{\equiv}C)_2{-}CN$ (?)	$HN{=}C{=}O$	
$CCCS$	$H(C{\equiv}C)_5{-}CN$	$HN{=}C{=}S$		
$HC{\equiv}CCHO$				
H_3CNC				

Aldehydes, Alcohols, Esthers, Ketones, Amides, and Related Molecules

$H_2C{=}O$	H_3COH	$HO{-}CH{=}O$	H_2CNH
$H_2C{=}S$	$H_3C{-}CH_2{-}OH$	$H_3C{-}O{-}CH{=}O$	H_3CNH_2
$H_3C{-}CH{=}O$	H_3CSH	$H_3C{-}O{-}CH_3$	H_2NCN
$NH_2{-}CH{=}O$	$NH_2{-}CH{=}O$	$(CH_3)_2CO$ (?)	$H_2C{=}C{=}O$

Cyclic

C_3H_2	SiC_2	C_3H

Ions

CH^+	HCO^+	H_3O^+ (?)
H_2D^+ (?)	$HOCO^+$	$HCNH^+$
$HN_2{+}$	HCS^+	SO^+
HOC^+ (?)		

Radicals

CH	C_3H	CN	HCO	C_2S
OH	C_4H	C_3N	NO	SO
C_2H	C_5H	H_2CCN	NS	
	C_6H			

NOTE:　The superscript x indicates detection only in the enveloped around evolved stars. A question mark (?) indicates molecules claimed but not yet confirmed.

cosmic history of water is especially important, particularly with respect to evidence of its interaction with other biogenic compounds, be they organic or inorganic.

It is useful at this point to identify six stages in the cosmic history of the biogenic elements and compounds: 1) nucleosynthesis and ejection to the interstellar medium, 2) chemical evolution in the interstellar medium, 3) protostellar collapse, 4) chemical evolution in the solar nebula, 5) growth of planetesimals from dust, and 6) accumulation and thermal processing of planetoids. Each of these stages has intrinsic scientific interest, and is related to the question of life in the universe. In general, those stages closer in time and space to the formation of our solar system and its planets have a stronger bearing on the specific events connected with the origin of life than do the more distant stages.

1. Nucleosynthesis and Ejection to the Interstellar Medium

Since the time of initial star formation after the universe began, the biogenic elements have been produced by the nuclear reactions within stars. During their life and upon the death of those stars, those elements have been ejected into the interstellar medium by stellar winds and cataclysmic explosions. The abundance of heavier elements in the interstellar medium results from the repeated addition of heavy elements produced by stars through multiple cycles of star formation and nucleosynthesis. This process has determined the elemental and isotopic abundances that are characteristic of the materials found in the interstellar medium. Supernovae, novae, and late-type giant stars are all potentially important sources of the biogenic elements. Organic compounds and

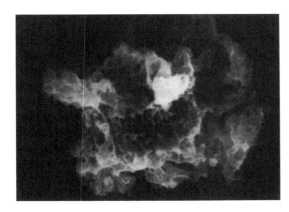

Fig. 3 Cosmic dust particles such as this one contain important clues to the formation of the solar system and the fate of the pre-solar organic compounds.

dust grains in planetary nebulae and circumstellar shells are indicators of the condensation of carbon and growth of grains from the gas phase production of these materials.

2. Chemical Evolution in the Interstellar Medium

Atoms of the biogenic elements combine in the interstellar medium to form organic compounds of interest to exobiologists (Table 1). Although a large number of organic and inorganic compounds containing the biogenic elements have been detected in the interstellar medium, the mechanisms of formation are poorly understood except in the cases of the simplest species containing three to four atoms. The full complexity of the ion-molecule and surface catalyzed reactions that are important for interstellar chemistry has not been determined. Nonetheless, the chemistry of gas-grain interactions in the interstellar medium, under the variable ultraviolet flux characteristic of dense molecular clouds, has prompted researchers to speculate that organic compounds such as glycine and adenine might even be found. The dust grains found in these clouds are thought to be particularly important to the chemistry of the complex organic compounds that are formed in them.

The chemistry of interstellar clouds is important to our understanding of life because these clouds form the materials and sites for star (and planet) formation of the sort that once led to our own solar system. Isotopic evidence from meteorites suggests that some of the complex organic materials manufactured in the clouds survive essentially unaltered through the process of star and planet formation, and therefore may make their way to the surface of a forming or formed planet. The origin of some of these materials, methane and carbon dioxide, for example, remains unclear. But if samples of those materials can be obtained, an understanding of the presolar processes that produced the interstellar grains, the carbonaceous chondrites, and the comets may become possible.

3. Protostellar Collapse

The star-formation process itself begins with the transition of matter from a low-density, cloudy structure to the higher-density nebulae of gas and dust surrounding the forming protostar. In this energetic process, chemical and isotopic fractionations develop between the gas phase and dust as a result of ion-molecule reactions and dust-gas interactions during the collapse of the interstellar cloud fragment. The state of the biogenic elements found in dust clouds can be altered in this process, and biogenic compounds can be formed, destroyed, or modified. These processes are poorly understood today, but can severely affect the distributional heterogeneity of biogenic compounds in the solar nebula that follows.

4. Chemical Evolution in the Solar Nebula

As observations and theoretical understanding of protostellar systems develop, more tightly constrained physical models of the solar nebula are emerging. These models provide better knowledge of the processes that contribute to the chemistry and govern the distribution of biogenic elements and compounds within the nebula over time. In our own solar system, photochemistry due to starlight and the early Sun, electric discharges, ion-molecule reactions in plasmas, and strictly thermochemical processes could all have yielded organic compounds and carbonaceous grains. Emerging evidence about the nature of cometary and meteoric materials that formed during this stage suggests that this period is particularly important in the provision of the organic materials that are later delivered to planets through the infall and impacts of comets, meteorites, and interplanetary cosmic dust particles (Fig. 3).

5. Growth of Planetesimals from Dust

In this stage of cosmic evolution, aggregation and accretion of dust and gas occur as particles settle to the mid-plane of the nebula, where they further agglomerate into kilometer-sized bodies. Indirect evidence exists that dust grains formed in interstellar space and their mantles of complex organic material survive through to this stage, and are instrumental in promoting the growth of planetesimals through collisions with other grains. At this stage, the surface chemistry of those grains is particularly important to the ability of the grains to bind to each other, and sticky carbon compounds may play a major role in initiating planetesimal formation. One outcome of the accretion process is a segregation of dust from gas, as the dust settles into the equatorial plane of the solar nebula.

6. Accumulation and Thermal Processing of Planetoids

In this stage, materials of stellar, interstellar or nebular origins initially accreted in comets, asteroids, and the parent bodies of meteorites would be altered to varying degrees. The degree of alteration would depend on the subsequent thermal

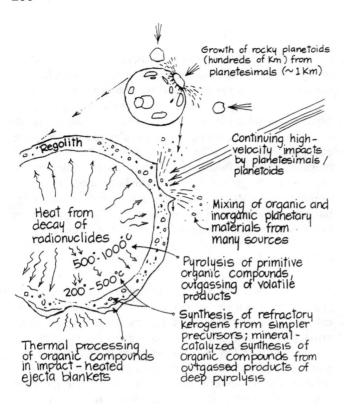

Fig. 4 Early planetary formation involves both the destruction and synthesis of prebiotic organic compounds.[23]

histories of those bodies, ranging from very mild in the case of (unimpacted) comets, to extreme in the case of differentiated meteorites and formed planets. The nature, abundance, and distribution of the biogenic elements and compounds within these bodies are related to these thermal effects.

In particular, the distribution of the biogenic elements and compounds in the solid bodies of the solar system inward of the giant planets is determined during this stage (Fig. 4). This distribution must have been one of the important factors in providing the set of conditions necessary for the origin of life on Earth. As the planets form, extreme temperatures would pyrolize primitive organic compounds, and result in the outgassing of volatile products that could later recondense, or alternatively, be lost to the solar environment. Slightly lower temperatures would result in the formation of refractory kerogens from simple precursor molecules, including recondensed volatiles. To complicate matters, in the later stages of planetary accretion organic materials delivered by the infall of primitive bodies could survive with only a minimum of processing, depending on the nature of the impact that accompanied their arrival. It is this compelling mix of materials and conditions that provides the environment for prebiotic evolution in the planetary environment, and the subsequent origin of life.

B. Prebiotic Evolution

The epoch of Prebiotic Evolution begins with the formation of planets and ends with the emergence of living systems.

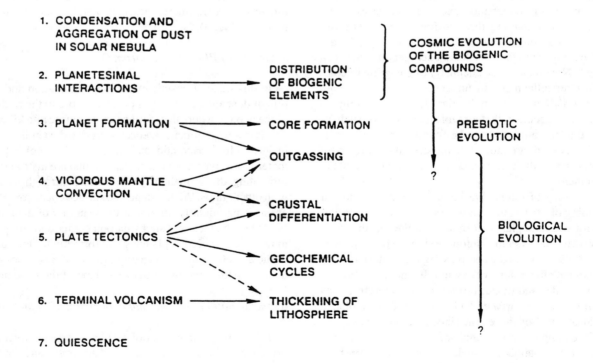

Fig. 5   Stages of planetary evolution (after Kaula, 1975).[8]

For present purposes this period can be viewed from the perspective of two kinds of processes: planetary and chemical evolution.

Planetary evolution occurs on global or regional scales as a consequence of the origin and development of planets. This process provides the primary driving forces for setting, maintaining, and altering the physical and chemical conditions of a planet's various environments within which living systems may be realized. Processes of chemical evolution occur on macro- or micro-environmental scales. These processes consist of interactions and reactions of inorganic and organic molecular systems driven by sources of free energy that establish the physical-chemical mechanisms and pathways used by primitive life forms developing from the materials of the prebiotic environment. In this environment, the initial stages of chemical evolution leading to life may be associated with the synthesis and transformation of organic compounds.

Planetary properties and processes involving the biogenic elements have made possible the conditions conducive to the origin and evolution of life on Earth, and perhaps elsewhere. At the most general level, these conditions have allowed the persistence of bodies of liquid water on Earth, and the development of a hydrologic cycle that interweaves with the geochemical cycles of the biogenic elements.

Planetary processes thought to be related to the origin of life may be viewed within the context of the stages of planetary evolution as described by Kaula.[8] Figure 5 shows the relationships between these stages, the processes involved, and the epochs of evolution they are thought to influence.

For example, core formation and accretion play major roles in determining the early thermal history of a planet, influencing the time of origin and the compositions of the crust, the early atmosphere, and the oceans. These, in turn, determine both the global and local planetary conditions in which life can form. Recent evidence, as well as theoretical considerations, suggests that residual impact events that form the tail-end of the accretion process may cause the reformation of these planetary properties for hundreds of millions of years after the initial formation of a planet. These impacts could tend to "reset" the conditions required for the origin of life, and could severely affect the potential for life, once formed, to survive. In the case of the Earth, initial formation of the planet 4.5 billion years ago may have been followed by the formation of the crust, the early atmosphere, and the oceans, one or more times. This process would considerably shorten the amount of time available between the achievement of a stable Earth and the emergence of the first life, which happened more than 3.5 billion years ago. Under these circumstances, the origin of life may have taken place very quickly (by geological standards), requiring less than 400 million years.

1. Planetary Conditions for the Origin of Life

The nature of biological systems is to be far from equilibrium with their environments, a characteristic that may pro-

vide insight into the processes that could have resulted in the first living systems. The interfaces between different planetary domains can provide a flux of matter and energy through the boundary regions, and gradients in the physical and chemical properties that are established. It is there that physics, chemistry, and biology can interplay to provide an environment that can drive a system away from equilibrium, yet not be so energetic as to disrupt self-assembled chemical structures that must have been the initial steps toward the living state.

Conditions far from equilibrium have certainly occurred throughout the history of Earth at solid-liquid-gas phase boundary regions. These regions include, among others, fumarolic and volcanic vents on continents and continental shelves, deep-sea plate spreading centers, submarine and island-arc volcanic vents, the land surface, and the sea surface. These regions may have provided the locations for the formation of the first living systems, and under conditions quite different from those generally found today. These conditions are fundamentally distinguished from current ones by the lack of biological competition for the substrates from which they formed.

To characterize the conditions under which life formed on the early Earth, and potentially could form elsewhere, researchers into the origin of life require the perspective of comparative planetology that is provided by space exploration as well as a detailed knowledge of the Earth. An encapsulation of this knowledge should allow the development of prebiotic epoch models of specific geophysically active boundary regions in which chemical evolution could have occurred, providing limits for the range of variations in temperature, pressure, nature, and intensities of fluxes of energy and matter, and the chemical and mineralogical compositions of the boundary regions as a function of time. In addition, the role of the biogenic elements and compounds in influencing specific geophysical and geochemical processes that established, maintained, and altered physical-chemical conditions in these regions must be characterized as a function of time. Such models will allow a greater appreciation of the contributions of cosmic processes to the establishment and maintenance of the conditions for the origin of life, and their interplay with processes unique to planetary bodies.

The period of interest for the characterization of prebiotic planetary processes leading to the origin of life is bounded by the onset of accretion of Earth and the earliest known occurrence of life about 3.5 billion years ago (although preserved isotopic signatures suggest that life may have existed as long ago as 3.8 to 4 billion years ago). Planetary processes that have been important include: 1) the flux of intact organic compounds supplied to the atmosphere and surface waters by the accretion of cometary and/or carbonaceous chondritic material; 2) the energetics and dynamics of accretion and core formation; 3) surface cooling and atmospheric formation to allow the occurrence of liquid water; 4) atmospheric formation, and the redox state of the atmosphere; 5) minerals available as potential chemical catalysts in the boundary

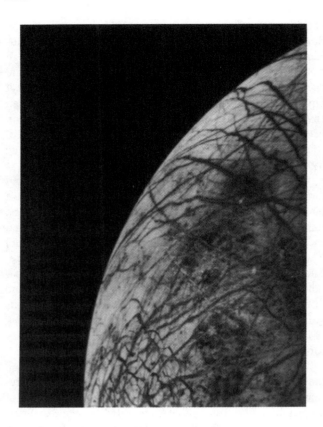

**Fig. 6 Voyager 2 view of the jovian moon Europa.
The complex array of streaks indicates that the crust
has been fractured and filled by materials from the
interior. The lack of relief or any visible mountains
or craters is consistent with a thick crust of ice.**

regions; 6) solar radiation of different wavelengths reaching
the surface; 7) photochemical processes occurring in the
atmosphere, at the interfaces of the atmosphere with oceans
and land, and in surface waters; 8) the interaction of liquid
water, atmospheric gases, or both with crustal rocks; and 9)
geochemical cycles of the biogenic elements. Unfortunately,
the known record of these processes on Earth is limited. The
3.8 billion-year-old igneous rocks and metamorphosed
volcanogenic sediments in Greenland (the Isua Formation)
provide the earliest record currently available.

Thus far the study of these sediments indicates the existence of bodies of liquid water, carbon dioxide in the atmosphere, volcanism, higher heat flow, a relatively stable differentiated crust, and emergence of continental shelf environments, from which the occurrence of weathering, a hydrologic
cycle, and a carbon geochemical cycle can be inferred. Beyond these, the record is mute. Limited as they are, these
characteristics and processes provide boundary conditions on
planetary environments that are consistent with those of
environments recorded in 3.5 billion-year-old sedimentary
rocks in western Australia (the Warrawoona group) which
contain the earliest apparent evidence of life. This circumstantial evidence suggests that life could have existed on the

Earth 3.8 billion years ago, but it does not provide any
definitive evidence about the environment in which life first
formed. Because of the recycling of the Earth's crust caused
by plate tectonic processes, such evidence may no longer exist
on Earth.

Further knowledge of the environments of an earlier Earth
may have to be derived from theoretical models that can be
applied to the scant data that remains on Earth, and to the
abundant data available on the other planets of the solar
system. Other planets are interesting because of their own
unique histories, but in the search for knowledge about the
origin of life they are also important because of the relevant
information they can supply. The study of lifeless planets can
provide examples of environments where chemical or biological evolution ended, or never even began. On such bodies
it may be possible to learn how planetary or solar system
processes may have broken the thread of chemical or biological evolution, or may have maintained it in ways that we
cannot now predict, and do not now understand. All of the
major planets and/or their moons can tell us more about the
events that led to this planet, and to life.

Clues to the history of water and its interactions with
planetary environments are to be found on Venus, with its
water-containing atmosphere, and the Galilean satellites,
Callisto, Ganymede, and Europa (Fig. 6), with their surfaces
of water ice. Understanding whether Venus has lost an initial
endowment of water comparable to Earth's, or has always
been strongly depleted in water, may help to characterize the
mechanisms that distributed the biogenic elements and compounds among the terrestrial planets. The Galilean satellites,
if built up from planetesimals resembling carbonaceous chondrites and comets, may also contain a frozen record of the
organic matter that survived planetary accretion.

Saturn's moon Titan is of great interest as a natural laboratory in which to study aspects of the organic chemistry on a
planetary scale. Although the atmosphere of Titan (Table 2)
is more reducing than the most likely atmosphere on the
primitive Earth, with methane as the dominant carbon source,
the full range of complexity that is possible in planetary
organic chemistry and the processes responsible for the compounds observed on Titan are poorly understood. Even
though conditions on Titan are much different than those on
the early Earth, Titan's low temperatures and abundant organics should provide clues to prebiotic organic chemical evolution and its relationship to the formation of planetary bodies.

Even without the prospect of life on Mars, the evidence of
liquid water and a more clement epoch early in martian history
at the time when Earth may already have had a thriving
microbial biosphere has exceedingly important implications.
Nonetheless, the possibility that life arose on Mars early on in
the course of planetary evolution must be kept open and
investigated whenever the opportunities to send missions to
Mars arise. The chemistry of the martian surface soils, as seen
in the biomimetic responses of the Viking biology experiments, continues to be intriguing and inadequately understood; it may reveal important clues to the role of minerals and

Table 2   Composition of Titan's Atmosphere

Species	Name	Abundance
	Major Components	
N_2	Nitrogen	73-99%
Ar	Argon	10-15%
CH_4	Methane	1-6%
H_2	Hydrogen	0.1-0.4%
	Hydrocarbons	
C_2H_6	Ethane	20 ppm
C_3H_8	Propane	20-50 ppm
C_2H_2	Acetylene	2 ppm
C_2H_4	Ethylene	400 ppb
C_4H_2	Diacetylene	30 ppb
	Nitriles	
HCN	Hydrogen cyanide	20 ppb
HC_2CN	Cyanoacetylene	10-1000 ppb
C_2N_2	Cyanogen	0-100 ppb
	Oxygen Compounds	
CO_2	Carbon dioxide	10 ppb
CO	Carbon monoxide	60 ppm

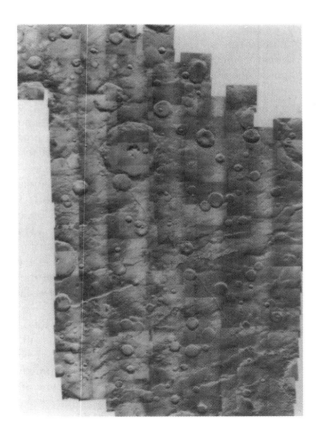

Fig. 7 Cratered terrain of Mars. This is a mosaic of photographs of a 1000 kilometer portion of the planet's surface taken by NASA's Viking orbiter in June 1980.

inorganic chemistry in prebiotic evolution before the development of a planetary organic chemistry or a hydrosphere or both. Elucidation of this chemistry and its relationship to the mineralogy and surface processes on Mars remains to be accomplished, a goal that will await the availability of fresh samples from Mars for detailed study.

Because it lacks plate tectonic activity of the sort that has destroyed Earth's ancient crust, Mars may contain abundant clues to the history of the formation of the terrestrial planets. Two-thirds of the surface of Mars, mainly in the southern hemisphere, is covered by an ancient, densely cratered terrain (Fig. 7) bearing a superficial resemblance to the lunar highlands, and which may be as much as 4 billion years old. The remainder of the planet is covered by much younger, sparsely cratered plains that include major volcanic units such as Olympus Mons, a massive, extinct volcano 27 km tall, and the Valles Marineris, a network of steep-walled canyons that stretch across the equatorial regions for a distance of over 4000 km.

In the ancient terrain and elsewhere on the surface is evidence that Mars has not always been cold and dry. The large valley networks and outflow channels suggest the past existence of copious amounts of liquid water on or near the martian surface, and it seems clear from the length and size of the valley networks that liquid water once would have been fairly stable at the surface. This, in turn, implies that martian surface temperatures and atmospheric pressures were once considerably higher than they are today. Some of the martian fluvial features occur in terrain that is heavily cratered, indicating that this more clement climatic regime may have occurred 3 to 4 billion years ago. Under these conditions, 4 billion years ago the surface of Mars could have been much

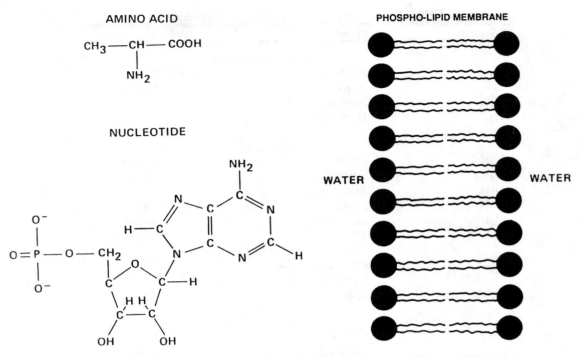

Fig. 8 Structure of some key biological materials.

like that of Earth's, and perhaps conducive to life as well.

This view is supported by theoretical considerations that suggest that during the first 800 million years after the formation of Mars and Earth, the atmospheric composition and pressure on these planets were determined primarily by outgassing of juvenile material and the delivery of volatile materials from extraplanetary sources. During this period the surface may have been dominated by volcanism and the processes involved in crust formation. Higher heat flow immediately after formation ensured more rapid recycling of atmospheric elements, particularly carbon. In fact, Earth, Venus, and Mars may have all undergone initial periods of outgassing and crust formation resulting in similar surface conditions on these three terrestrial planets. Thus, it may be that some of the best clues to the prebiotic evolution and origin of life on Earth are to be found, today, on Mars.

2. Chemical Evolution and Life

On the prebiotic Earth, sources of free energy provided the driving force for the emergence of physical and chemical energy-using systems that ultimately acquired the combination of attributes we now recognize as "living." Such systems owe their existence to the complexity of the matter and energy that make up the universe, and can be viewed (as can we!) as eddies in the great river of energy flow that began with the "Big Bang" that started the universe. As such, the formation of living systems from nonliving precursors is not antientropic, but appears to have been a result of properties that are integral to the structure of existence.

Although it is not possible to specify a universally accepted paradigm for the sequence of transformations that led to the origin of life, it is likely that the process began with simplicity and moved toward complexity. It is also likely that the path of prebiotic chemical evolution was neither direct nor sequential. Parallel development of various steps in the process doubtless occurred, and if present-day biological systems are any clue to the prebiotic systems, then progress towards life was likely made by a serendipitous combination of unrelated functions that resulted in novel capabilities. Although it is true that amino acids and phospholipids have amazing properties of self-organization, it is also true that nucleic acids can encode a great deal of information and catalyze certain important chemical reactions. Each of these groups of molecules has unique capabilities that we now associate with life on Earth, and each must have been involved to some degree in the origin of life (Fig. 8).

Whatever the sequence of events that led to the origin of life, it appears to have taken place within the first 700 million years of Earth history, perhaps the period of greatest change on Earth, encompassing planetary accretion, core formation, and the emergence of oceans and continents. Because of the planetary disturbances that resulted from large impact events during those years, it is also possible that this sequence of events had to be repeated one or more times. The result of these events was the formation of systems that we call "living," which had acquired the capability for self-replication and metabolism. How the mechanism of self-replication

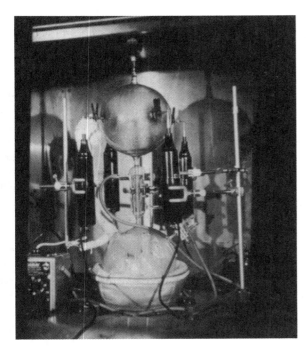

Fig. 9 Apparatus used to produce amino acids from methane, ammonia, and water by electric discharge. (Courtesy of Cyril Ponnamperuma.)

arose on the primitive Earth stands as a central problem for the origin of life. To reconstruct this process conceptually, the answers to two fundamental questions are sought by exobiologists: 1) How structurally and functionally complex can a system become without a genetic capability? And conversely, 2) How structurally and functionally simple can a system be and still carry out self-replication?

In suggesting answers to these questions it is important to recognize that the very nature of prebiotic systems that resulted in life remains unknown; their composition may have been inorganic, organic, or some combination of the two. Most research has been focused on organic structures because all known life forms are based on a restricted but universal set of organic compounds. Yet studies of the cosmic origin of the biogenic compounds, the Miller-Urey experiment, and its many successors convincingly demonstrated the ease with which biochemically relevant organic compounds could have been delivered to or synthesized in the Earth's prebiotic environment.

Largely due to the work of Oparin and Haldane, in the early 1950s the early Earth's atmosphere was perceived as a strongly reduced or CH_4-containing gas mixture. As a consequence, considerable weight was given to the view that the first organisms were organic and heterotrophic, that is, capable of utilizing organic compounds already in the environment as their energy source and cellular building blocks. To test the hypothesis that these organic compounds could have been directly synthesized on the early Earth, Harold Urey and his graduate student Stanley Miller devised a simulation experiment in the laboratory (Fig. 9). Starting from an atmosphere

of methane, ammonia, and water vapor, Miller and Urey were able to use their apparatus to produce a variety of organic compounds associated with life. These included glycine, alanine, and aspartic and glutamic acids—amino acids commonly found in proteins. Further research using similar apparatus but with different starting mixtures has resulted in considerable progress toward the synthesis of other organic structures—e.g., peptides, microspheres, coacervates and nucleic acids—under putative prebiotic conditions.

In contrast to a reducing Earth, however, the geochemistry of Earth's oldest sediments from Greenland's Isua Formation, evolutionary models of the atmospheres of Venus, Mars, and Earth, as well as new ideas about the energetics of planetary accretion and the timing of core formation have since resulted in an alternative view. This view holds that carbon in Earth's early atmosphere took the form of CO_2 and that the prebiotic atmosphere was in a more or less neutral redox state, much like it is today. In this context, the synthesis of organic compounds in the atmosphere is much less fruitful in terms of both abundance and molecular diversity of products than under the conditions postulated by Oparin and Haldane. Under these conditions the role of inorganic mineralic structures may have been more important, leading along lines of argument derived by Bernal[9] to the postulation of crystal genes and a mineralic rather than an organic chemical nature for the first living systems.

In another departure from the original hypothesis of Oparin and Haldane, the fossil record in the sediments of western Australia and South Africa and the record derived from the molecular phylogeny of contemporary organisms holds open the possibility that the universal ancestor to all life on Earth was an autotrophic organism. An organism that is capable of extracting free energy from its environment to manufacture its structural components. This could have been accomplished by either photo- or chemo-autotrophy. Whether the universal ancestor was also the original living organism remains an open question. If it was not, then the question concerning the organic or mineralic or mineral-organic make-up of the archetypal life form must also remain open.

Perhaps the most compelling areas that have been identified as possible locations for the origin of life on the early Earth are geophysically active regions such as undersea volcanic vents, hot springs, and perhaps the atmosphere-sea interface. Phase boundaries occur in these regions with enhanced gradients in temperature, pressure, chemical composition, and energy that would have created the domains far from equilibrium within which life could have emerged. Despite questions as to the composition of the early atmosphere, strong arguments can now be made for the existence of reduced oceanic waters containing ferrous iron and other materials at these locations. Contemporary researchers are now investigating pathways for synthesis of either inorganic or organic geochemical structures at these locations in the context of reduced oceans and neutral atmospheric compositions (CO_2, N_2, H_2O), as well-reduced atmospheres (CH_4 or CO, N_2 or NH_3, H_2O and H_2).

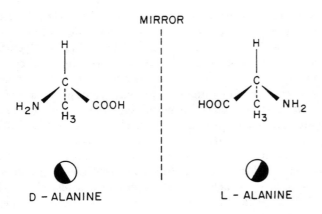

Fig. 10 Two forms of alanine, L (levo-) the left-handed, and D (dextro-) the right-handed versions. The L-amino acids predominate in terrestrial biology.

Regardless of the bulk conditions of the early Earth, other data about the potential modes for the origin of life are accessible through experimental or theoretical approaches. These include the energetics of physical forces that govern interactions among molecules and the rates at which physical-chemical changes occur under specified conditions. Of considerable importance are the intrinsic physical and chemical properties of organic matter, for these properties would predispose or limit the ability of particular organic compounds (e.g., peptides, polynucleotides, carboxylic acids) or minerals (e.g., salts, clays) to fulfill certain critical functions (e.g., catalysis, replication, and phase separation from the environment).

Direct evidence of the steps in chemical evolution that led to the origin of life has been lost, but some of those steps may be inferred from the complex physical and chemical phenomena observed in even the most primitive living organisms. Clues may be found in the sequences of reactions in metabolic and biosynthetic pathways or in the structure and composition of the enzymes and co-enzymes that catalyze or regulate them. Another record resides in the evolutionary divergence of structures and functions among microorganisms based on amino acid and nucleotide sequences in proteins and nucleic acids, respectively.

Among the functions attributable to the first living systems are: a) the capture, storage and use of energy from the environment; b) synthesis of structures capable of function; c) catalysis; d) maintenance of a micro-environment distinct from that of the ambient environment; e) self-replication; f) translation. Functions a-d contribute to a primitive metabolism, although e-f comprise a genetic system.

Capture, storage, and use of energy from the environment. Organic, inorganic and mineral-organic complexes have the potential to absorb and store energy from sunlight and then release it under physical or chemical stimulation. The fixation of N_2 and conversion of CO_2 to organic compounds and structures by sunlight under conditions consistent with neutral

atmospheric compositions or reduced Fe^{2+}-containing seas may have been possible on the prebiotic Earth because of these complexes. Heterogeneous gas-solid and gas-liquid systems containing clays and other geochemically plausible minerals have been identified as potential candidate systems. Photochemical systems containing organic or inorganic substrates may be capable of synthesizing energy-rich compounds for use in condensation reactions or able to create ion-gradients or drive species transport across a phase boundary. Through such systems photochemical or hydrolytic or exothermic geochemical redox reactions may have been coupled to endothermic reactions to drive otherwise energetically unfavorable processes in prebiotic reaction sequences.

Synthesis of structures capable of function. The synthesis of amino acids, nucleic acids, lipids, and condensing agents necessary to convert monomers to polymers may have occurred on the early Earth, as well as in interstellar and pre-solar space, as previously discussed. The specific prebiotic synthesis pathways that were important on the early Earth are not well-understood today, though the existence of Fe^{2+}-containing oceans suggests that photo-reduction could have been an important process, although the sulfides present in hot springs and ocean vents have also been suggested as possible CO_2 reductants. Pathways of specific interest include those that would lead to the formation of the constituents of ribonucleic acid (RNA). For example, appropriate nucleosides might be formed by Miller-Urey synthesis, but all known prebiotic synthesis pathways that form ribose form a wide range of other sugars as well. Once formed, the condensation of ribose with the appropriate bases under most conditions yields complex mixtures of products other than RNA. In addition, one intriguing and important problem surrounding the development of these synthesis pathways involves the possible origin of optical chirality in bio-organic structures. Why modern biological systems incorporate only left-handed amino acids remains a mystery (Fig. 10).

The adequacy of selective condensation as a means of providing the building blocks for life from complex heterogeneous mixtures of organic compounds remains to be established. Under some conditions a developing polymer chain of amino acids or nucleotides can add subsequent monomers at the "direction" of the existing polymer, but this may not happen under the most plausible conditions that would have occurred on the prebiotic Earth. Future experiments must involve the design and operation of a laboratory scale reaction chamber modeled after a geophysically active aqueous environment, complete with geochemically reasonable reactants and fluxes of energy. Such environments may have been widespread on the early Earth, and may have led to the multiple production of functional structures of this sort.

Catalysis. Catalysts are crucial to biological systems because the molecules that interact in cellular processes are generally quite stable, and therefore quite slow to react. Such sluggishness was probably not as much of a problem in the

Table 3 Codon Assignments for RNA Triplets

Second Base

		G	C	A	U	
	G	gly gly gly gly	ala ala ala ala	glu glu asp asp	val val val val	G A C U
First Base	C	arg arg arg arg	pro pro pro pro	gln gln his his	leu leu leu leu	G A C U
	A	arg arg ser ser	thr thr thr thr	lys lys asn asn	met ile ile ile	G A C U
	U	trp term cys cys	ser ser ser ser	term term tyr tyr	leu leu phe phe	G A C U

Third Base

time before the proliferation of biological systems, because the competition for substrates would have been much less severe. The catalysis of reactions important to biochemistry are today handled almost exclusively by highly efficient proteins, but in the earliest living systems catalysis by polysaccharides and coenzyme-like compounds may have been significant. Nonetheless, the existence of relatively simple condensation catalysts capable of acting selectively (e.g., on protein rather than nonprotein amino acids) on a mixture of substrates to yield a restricted set of products has not been demonstrated. Other mechanisms of catalysis have also been suggested, and catalysis by the exposed surfaces of clays and other minerals in CO_2 reduction, nitrogen fixation, redox reactions, and amino acid or nucleotide oligomerizations has been investigated. These sites would seem to have been important if only because of their potential abundance on the early Earth. Perhaps the most important discovery in catalysis, with respect to the origin of life, has been the discovery of catalytic sites within RNA molecules that promote self-splicing.[10] Whether RNA catalysis was ever significant with respect to other molecular types, however, is an open question.

Maintenance of a micro-environment distinct from the ambient environment. Despite the potential for the production of organic molecules under the conditions on the early Earth, the destruction of those molecules would have also taken place. Without some mechanism for separation from the environment, the "primordial soup" would have been very dilute indeed. Concentrations of reactants could have been enhanced by the evaporation of water from tidal pools, or in

areas where water circulation was restricted to an area of high reactant concentration. However, inevitably more direct means of sequestration would be needed for life to exist.

In today's living systems this general function is carried out by membranes, and they make other functions possible. These functions include energy generation, protection against harmful variations in the external environment, maintenance of intracellular pH and ionic composition within ranges favorable for catalytic activity, and the concentration of biochemical fuel and building blocks inside while eliminating toxic waste products to the outside. Some if not all of these requirements would also have been necessary for self-replicating chemical systems.

Modern membranes are composed primarily of lipids, and membranes have also been formed in water by organic extracts of lipid-like materials from meteorites—a source that certainly would have been available on the primitive Earth. In addition, membrane-like enclosures have also been experimentally formed from amino acids after thermal condensation. Combinations of peptides, carbohydrates, and nucleic acids when mixed together in water also spontaneously organize themselves into clusters called coacervates. Each of these mechanisms could have provided an important sequestering function during the course of chemical evolution. The ability to form "internal" micro-environments is not restricted to organic systems. Clays and other minerals that may have been important for catalysis also form crystalline shapes and interlayer regions that are capable of at least partial separation of an internal realm from the ambient environment.

Self-replication. Several hypotheses for the origin of self-replicating systems have been advanced over the years. These have involved concepts such as: proteins replicating directly, nucleic acids replicating independently of proteins, nucleic acids and proteins coevolving, and self-replication in clays or other mineral catalysts that eventually incorporate nucleic acids and proteins. Up to now, only a nucleic acid model for a self-replicating system has received experimental support. Although no progress has yet been reported on direct self-replication, significant progress in the nonenzymic template-directed synthesis of complementary polynucleotides has been achieved. The discovery of catalytic RNA molecules[8] has significantly altered what has been a central paradigm of origin of life theory: that both nucleic acid and protein were required to initiate a self-replicating system. The concept of a self-catalytic, self-replicating system is now being fully explored experimentally with RNA systems, and an "RNA-world" has been conceptualized where all life would have been based on RNA rather than on DNA nucleic acids.

Translation. Even if a self-replicating RNA system formed the basis for the first life on Earth, one of the most difficult problems in our understanding of the origin of life is understanding how such a system might have developed the ability to express information coded in the RNA into the synthesis of proteins. The accurate translation of the coded genetic message into the amino acid sequence in a protein (Table 3) depends today on the ribosomes, transfer RNAs, and aminoacyl-tRNA synthetase enzymes that are present in the cell. The complexity of their interactions obscures the origin of the translation system. Nonetheless, the ubiquitous presence of this system in living organisms suggests that it arose early in the history of life on Earth. To understand how a process of such complex nature may have developed, however, clues may be found in the nature and extent of interactions between peptide and nucleic acid surfaces, and in particular in the interaction between the amino acids and their respective codonic and anti-codonic nucleotides. With data of this sort, we will be able to begin to understand the development of an essential step in the origin of life, one that enabled the conversion of information to action.

C. The Early Evolution of Life

Though life may plausibly have arisen from physical and chemical conditions that would be reproducible today, it is clear that the emergence of life changed the nature of the planet irrevocably. Living systems may be thought of simply as complex physical-chemical processors, but in their capacity to reproduce themselves and to evolve in response to environmental changes they changed the direction of planetary evolution. The story of the Earth as a living planet is inextricably bound to the ever-changing story of life.

In a multitude of ways, the early Earth was a different planet than it is today. Biological change has been particularly marked. Unlike the early Earth, the major contribution to biomass today is no longer from microorganisms, but rather from vascular land plants, and the bioenergetic strategy of primary producers is oxygenic photosynthesis rather than anaerobic processes. During these and similar changes, the evolving biota were active participants in processes that have changed the nature of the surface of the planet over time, ranging from the deposition of major formations of the biogenic elements as carbonate, petroleum, coal, gypsum, and phosphorite, to the production of an oxygen atmosphere and an oxidized ocean, and to the widespread distribution of life on land.

When Charles Darwin's work, *On the Origin of Species*, appeared in 1859,[11] the broad outlines of the history of plants and animals were rapidly coming into focus. The familiar plants and animals encompassed by his work, however, have existed for less than 600 million years—less than 15 percent of the age of the Earth. What came before, during the first 85 percent of geologic time? The first multicellular organisms of any kind appeared in the fossil record only about 1 billion years ago. What can we learn about the antiquity of life, the attributes of the earliest organisms, and how those attributes changed over time? Darwin realized that answers to these questions would permit the successful extension of his theory of evolution by natural selection to the entire history of life on Earth.

Only within the past three decades, however, has there been dramatic progress in making these issues amenable to scientific inquiry. In recent years, the known fossil record has been extended up to 3.5 billion years in the remote past, making the oldest known fossil microorganisms nearly as old as the Earth. The age of these microfossils shows that the history of life on Earth is largely the history of microscopic and unicellular, rather than multicellular, organisms.

In their time, with its lack of knowledge of the ancient Earth and the nature of the other planets, Darwin and his supporters were unlikely to have given much thought to Mars or other extraterrestrial bodies having a geological record pertinent to his theories. Yet today it seems that the history of Mars should be replete with clues bearing on the origin and evolution of the early Earth, and perhaps its earliest biosphere. In this age of planetary exploration, the continuing assessment of the role of natural selection in biological evolution can be extended to other planets, as well as to the ancient Earth. It is the perspective of planetary exploration and comparative planetology that allows us the proper perspective about what life can do to a planet.

The evolution of Earth life may be viewed in this context as the diversification of a heterogeneous catalyst that mediates the cycling of the biogenic elements between reservoirs, sources, and sinks that may be found in the atmosphere, hydrosphere, and lithosphere. From this perspective the earliest interplay between biology and the physical environment represents the beginning of interlocked tectonic, biogeochemical and meteorological cycles, forming feedback loops on a global scale, which may have regulated climate, the habitability of environments, and biological productivity over time. Clues drawn from astrophysics, geology, microbial biology, and ecology must be integrated to inform us about the origin of Earth's biosphere. These may contribute to an understanding of the forces that shape the nature and distribution of life on other planets.

In seeking to understand the early evolution of life, it is important to keep in mind the key questions that need to be answered and to identify approaches that will make answers to those questions a possibility. Some of the key questions include: Were the first organisms autotrophic or heterotrophic? What physical and chemical driving forces were operating on microbial evolution? When and under what circumstances did various physiologic and metabolic innovations arise? When and using what biochemical strategy did microbial life colonize soils? Two approaches have been adopted to provide answers to these questions. One approach is to examine those ancient rocks that bear testimony on early evolution, both biological and geological. The other is to examine modern-day microorganisms as "living fossils" in which the layered mask of evolution has hidden clues to early life in biochemical and biophysical vestiges of an earlier time.

1. The Geologic Record

Remarkably few fossils have been found in rocks older than 2.5 billion years—currently there are only five microfos-

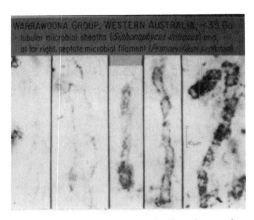

Fig. 11 Filamentous, prokaryotic (i.e., bacterium-like) microfossils in petrographic thin sections of carbonaceous chert from the Early Precambian (ca. 3.5 b.y. old) Warrawoona Group in the North Pole Dome region of the Pilbara Block, northwestern Western Australia. (Photo courtesy of J. W. Schopf.)

sil and eight stromatolite localities of that age that are known. (Stromatolites are layered, often mound-shaped structures formed by microbial communities.) This paucity underscores the importance of the recently discovered 3.3 to 3.5 billion-year-old stromatolites and microfossils in South Africa and western Australia (Fig. 11). The wide variety of cellular shapes in these fossils indicates a diverse biota with origins even deeper in antiquity.

In addition to preserving valuable biological fossils, ancient rocks also have recorded the environmental contexts and time scales within which ancient organisms evolved. These records reveal how developments in biological evolution were related to changes in global and local conditions over time. From these records we have seen that the early evolution of unicellular life was an integral aspect of the development of the planetary environment.

The available evidence suggests that the origins of Earth and of life were not separated greatly in time. Only a few traces of Earth's passage through its earliest billion years remain, but it must have been marked by great changes in its physical environment from an intense thermal regime that was hostile to life to one that sustained a diverse microbiota. Its next 3 billion years, a period of less dramatic change, has left behind a more substantial and decipherable record of events.

What, then, is known about the Earth prior to 3 billion years ago? Despite the uncertainties inherent in the fossil record, an attempt has been made to establish a geological time scale for major events in biological evolution. Of these major events, the advent of oxygenic photosynthesis and the development of planktonic eukaryotes, multicelled organisms, and skeletons occurred between 3 and 0.6 billion years ago. Over this period the rocks also record periodic increases in production of igneous rocks and an increase in mountain-

building. Glaciations, apparently rare before 1 billion years ago, became more frequent.

Current understanding of the Sun's development suggests that it was only 70 to 80 percent as luminous 4 billion years ago as it is today, though some astronomers have suggested that the early Sun was brighter and more massive than today. There is also evidence that the oceans existed in liquid form during this time, and even with a hot Sun and the higher heat flow from the Earth's interior this implies that the early atmosphere must have been better able to retain the incoming solar radiation. Theoretical models of the Earth under cool-sun conditions indicate that keeping the oceans' liquid would have required about 100 times the present atmospheric level of carbon dioxide, acting as a greenhouse gas, whereas a hotter sun would have required less of a greenhouse effect. In either event, we can be assured that early life proliferated under a much different set of environmental conditions than exists today.

Together, the 3.8 billion-year-old Isua metasediments of Greenland and 3.5 billion-year-old rocks from South Africa and western Australia record a marine environment dominated by volcanic islands. Black cherts, some of them microfossiliferous, were apparently deposited during relatively quiescent periods between cycles of volcanic eruptions. Pervasive volcanism would have injected dissolved minerals as well as gases containing carbon, hydrogen, and sulfur into the ancient seas.

In addition to high levels of carbon dioxide, the early atmosphere must have had little oxygen, as evidenced by the apparent ubiquity of ferrous iron in the surface environment. The presence of ferrous iron is reflected in the widespread occurrence of iron formations, in the relatively high iron concentrations of the oldest marine carbonates, and in ancient soils by its depletion attributable to loss by leaching. Iron formations were deposited almost exclusively between 3.8 and 1.8 billion years ago. Although the end of these deposits was once believed to mark the rise of oxygenic photosynthesis, the true paleobiological significance of iron formations remains uncertain.

In the early history of the Earth, physical changes in the planetary surface environment would have influenced both the rate and the direction of early microbial evolution. The Sun gradually attained its present-day luminosity, major accretionary impacts declined, the Moon's separation from the Earth increased, volcanism declined, and the continents grew in volume and wandered across the face of the planet. It is difficult, however, to find unequivocal evidence of these influences in the fossil record. Nonetheless, a major increase in the abundance of fossils coincides with the growth of continents and the emergence of wide, "modern" continental margins between 2.8 and 2.2 billion years ago. More than 150 microfossiliferous deposits have now been found in rocks between 2.5 and 0.6 billion years old. It may be that environmental change somehow triggered biological innovations that dramatically increased the abundance and diversity of life, but it also may be that the expansion of these new

Table 4 Comparison of Early Earth and Early Mars

Property	Early Earth	Early Mars
Water	Oceans	Evidence for Surface Liquid Water. Hydrological Cycle(?)
Temperature	> 273 K	$\simeq$ 273 K
Atmosphere	CO_2, N_2, H_2O > 1 atm	CO_2, N_2 (?), H_2O $\simeq$ 1 atm
Geochemical Carbon Cycle CO_2 --> Carbonate Rocks	Reactions in Water	Reactions in Water
Carbonate Rocks --> CO_2	Continued Subduction and Volcanism	Early Volcanism Only
Duration of Thick Atmosphere b.y.(?)	4.5 b.y. --> Present	4.5 b.y. --> 3.5
Preservation of Rock Record b.y.	Highly Altered and Reworked	~ 2/3 Surface is > 3.8
Biology	Diverse Life at 3.5 b.y.	?—?

NASA Technical Memorandum 82478, 1983

environments merely improved the preservation of the rock record and its fossils.

Recent geochemical concepts and analytical methods have also been applied to Precambrian studies of microfossiliferous, stromatolitic and organic-rich samples. In addition, studies have been made of the chemical and isotopic features of ancient rocks, which make them different from rocks deposited in more recent times. These features include rocks with organic molecular markers that differ from those in recent sediments, rocks with unusual isotopic compositions of the biogenic elements, and rocks with unusual metal contents (e.g., iron formations). Such contrasts can signal the imprint of discrete, major evolutionary events, either biological, geological, or both.

Elemental ratios in materials in ancient rocks (including biogenic, major, minor and trace elements) that are characteristic of biochemical fractionation patterns can be attributed to specific biochemical processes (e.g., photosynthesis, sulfate reduction, and methanogenesis). These patterns, coupled with isotopic patterns and molecular markers, may be found in the kerogenic and other components of ancient and modern sediments and provide evidence for these processes. The simultaneous acquisition of chemical, isotopic, microfossil, and paleoenvironmental information on a common set of rocks constitutes the most effective way of determining the geologic relationships between the rock components of Precambrian sedimentary basins.

Stable isotope patterns of some of the biogenic elements (e.g., $^{13}C/^{12}C$, $^{34}S/^{32}S$) in rocks supplement the microfossil and geochemical records in ancient rocks. Oxygen isotope patterns also can reveal changes in the temperature of sedimentary environments over time. Unfortunately, it is difficult to interpret the isotopic record in terms of the nature of the biota that deposited the record and the occurrence of events of evolutionary significance, either biological or environmental. These efforts are hampered by the overlay of diagenetic or metamorphic alteration and a paucity of isotope fractionation data from modern ecosystems and organisms that can be used as a baseline for ancient data.

Although rocks of Archaen age have the potential to contain direct clues of the earliest forms of life, rocks of Proterozoic age are also important to our understanding of early evolution. Many excellent sections of rock with well-preserved samples are available. From these, considerable detailed information about the depositional environments, population dynamics, organic chemistry, and stable isotopic compositions of the fossils can be extracted. These rocks not only hold many clues to the rise of multicellular life and the modern biosphere, they also can teach us how to examine the older, more poorly preserved Archaen rocks.

In addition to information gained by trace fossils and chemical signatures of early life, evidence about the nature of the Earth's evolving biota can also be gained from the evidence of how this biota, in turn, has modified and modulated the gross features of the Earth's biosphere over time. Certainly, early life played a major role in the processes that have modulated the long-term evolution of atmospheric carbon dioxide and oxygen levels on Earth. Early life may have had a distinct role in the deposition of the iron formations mentioned previously and in the evolution of the oxidation state of the atmosphere and ocean through time, as revealed by the analysis of paleosols. These changes suggest a powerful role for living organisms.

To fully understand the interplay of early organisms and their environment, exobiologists study modern analogs of ancient microbial communities to see how the abundance, physiology, and environment of the microorganisms influence the specific morphological, chemical and isotopic features preserved in rocks. Microbial mats growing in hypersaline lagoons or on the bottom of restricted lakes, for example, are accessible, modern-day phenomena whose features are still controlled almost exclusively by unicellular life. These mats are thought to be analogs of ancient stromatolite-forming microbial communities. In particular, mat communities are ideal for studying the transition between anoxygenic and oxygenic photosynthesis, a critical aspect of the evolution of photosynthesis, and can provide additional insight into the origin of the stable isotope distributions observed in stromatolites preserved from the early Earth.

Ultimately, the amount of new knowledge that can be gained from the rock record about the early evolution of life is limited by the availability of a fossil record preserved in ancient rocks. On Earth, the search for older rocks and primitive organisms is being actively pursued, but the amount of this material remaining on Earth will always be extremely limited. In the future, exobiologists hope to extend the search for evidence of the early evolution of life to Mars, where the record of the earliest billion years of planetary history may yet be preserved intact.

The potential for a warmer, wetter, Mars early in the history of the solar system has been alluded to earlier in this chapter with respect to the prospects for chemical evolution leading to the possibility of life on that planet. With or without ancient life, the apparent similarities between Mars and Earth during that time frame make Mars important in comparative studies of planetary evolution. Table 4 summarizes contemporary estimates of the properties of early Mars and the primordial Earth. In general, the environment on Mars was probably comparable to that of the early Earth in all of the biologically important parameters over the time period encompassing the origin and early evolution of life on Earth.

Without doubt the discovery of even extinct microbial life on Mars would have a profound impact on planetary and biological sciences because it would provide evidence of life elsewhere, but such a discovery might also provide insight into the evolution of life on Earth. For example, there is currently much discussion about the role that a global-scale biology can play in controlling the environment of a planet, and the so-called Gaia hypothesis that life, once established, controls its planetary environment. It has been argued that life on early Mars would have been dependent on the existence of geochemical cycles over which it had no influence (as was probably true on the early Earth). If it is found that life did evolve on Mars, reached a fair degree of microbiological

sophistication (e.g., stromatolites), and subsequently became extinct, this would certainly limit the application of that hypothesis.

2. The Biological Record

If life on Earth is the result of physical and chemical processes inherent in the make-up of the planet, it could very well be that the *first* living organism failed to survive the rigors of the early Earth and left no descendants. Life could have started numerous times, and failed. At some point, however, life as we know it today began and spread over all of the Earth. The descendants of that ancient life are alive today, and the structures and functions of contemporary organisms can be studied for the evidence of their evolutionary history that forms a fundamental part of their make-up. Some of this evidence may have been masked by more recent events in evolution and some may have been lost entirely, while other evidence has been preserved practically unchanged over vast periods of time. The trick, for exobiologists, is to determine which evidence is which.

Certain guiding principles help simplify the task of making sense of the vast puzzle of evolution. One such principle, parsimony, assumes that there is an economy of nature that conserves nature's innovations. Thus, if several organisms share a certain trait, in the absence of evidence to the contrary it is assumed that that trait was inherited from a common ancestor rather than evolved independently on several separate occasions. Traits or attributes can be addressed interchangeably in this context, whether specific physical characteristics (e.g., topography of an enzyme) or chemical compositions (e.g., base sequence of a nucleic acid) of the structures involved in carrying out the functions essential to life. At another level, the principle can refer to the functions themselves (e.g., replication, nitrogen-fixation).

In tracking nature's parsimony it is important to trace the broad generalities that link all living things on Earth. Certain important traits are shared in identical form by every living organism. For example, all life utilizes essentially one set of amino acids for the building blocks of proteins and one set of nucleotides for the building blocks of RNA and DNA. Fundamental features of the very complex genetic information system are shared by all organisms (e.g., enzymes, nucleic acids). Comparative biochemistry suggests, then, that all life currently on Earth is descended from early common ancestors that contained nucleic acids that spelled out a genetic code for proteins, and that these structures and functions had a common origin in ancient times.

This approach to the study of evolution possesses considerable power and promise, but it is still far from being able to describe the first simple, living cell. If we assemble a list of those traits that we now know are shared by all living organisms—and many of these traits are remarkably complex—we can construct a "profile" of a common ancestor of all extant life. Such an exercise, however, confronts us with a dilemma. The attributes of such an organism, its mechanisms for repro-

Table 5   Major differences between prokaryotes and eukaryotes[13]

Prokaryotes	Eukaryotes
Mostly small cells (1-10μm). All are microbes	Mostly large cells (10-100 μm). Some are microbes: most are large organisms
DNA in nucleoid not membrane-bound. Genophores not chromosomes. DNA not coated with protein*	Membrane-bound nucleus containing chromosomes made of DNA, RNA, and proteins
Cell division direct, mostly by binary fission. No centrioles, mitotic spindle, or microtubules.	Cell division by various forms of mitosis: mitotic spindles (or at least some arrangements of microtubules)
Sexual systems rare: when sex does take place, genetic material is transferred from donor to recipient	Sexual systems common: equal participation of both partners (male and female) in fertilization. Alternation of diploid and haploid forms of meiosis and fertilization.
Multicellular forms are rare. No tissue development	Multicellular organisms show extensive development of tissues.
Many strict anaerobes (which are killed by oxygen) facultatively anaerobic, microaerophilic, and aerobic forms	Almost all are aerobic (they need oxygen to live): exceptions are clearly secondary modifications.
Enormous variations in the metabolic patterns of the group as a whole	Same metabolic patterns of oxidation within the group (Embden-Meyerhof)glucose metabolism. Krebs-cycle oxidations, cytochrome electron transport chains.
Mitochondria absent, enzymes for oxidation of organic molecules bound to cell membranes (not packaged separately	Enzymes for oxidation of three-carbon organic acids are packages within mitochondria
Simple bacterial flagella composed of flagellin protein	Complex 9 - 2 undulipodia composed of tubulin and many other proteins
In photosynthetic species, enzymes for photosynthesis are bound as chromatophores to cell membrane not packaged separately. Various patterns of anaerobic and aerobic photosynthesis including the formation of end products such as sulfur sulfate and oxygen	In photosynthetic species, enzymes for photosynthesis are packaged in membrane-bound plastids. All photosynthetic species have oxygen eliminating photosynthesis

*"Bacterial chromosome" a term used by molecular biologists to refer to the genome is confusing and should be avoided

duction, energy transduction, and metabolism, are far too sophisticated to have existed at the time life began. This "common ancestor," as we can now define it, must have already experienced considerable biological evolution. The greatest challenge, then, is to elucidate that earlier phase of evolution and to characterize the nature of the simpler and more primitive organisms, for which there are no living analogs, by extrapolation from the evolutionary study of the traits of contemporary life forms.

Deciphering the earliest evolutionary events requires an understanding of the origins of the diversity of form and physiology that exists among microorganisms. This diversity is reflected in two major subdivisions among microorganisms: the prokaryotes and the eukaryotes (Table 5). Prokaryotic cells—all bacterial—are generally small and relatively undifferentiated. Eukaryotic cells—which make up all the plants, animals, fungi, and many microorganisms—are gener-

ally larger, more complex, and internally differentiated. These cells contain several types of internal organelles, such as mitochondria and chloroplasts, which themselves are related to the free-living bacteria. The currently accepted theory of the origin of these cells stipulates that they arose by symbiotic association between pre-eukaryotic cells—the urkaryotes—and certain types of formerly free-living prokaryotes.[11]

At another level, life on Earth today can be divided into three major groups. Studies of a particular trait, the nucleotide sequences of the so-called 16S-portion of ribosomes (16S-RNA), in a large number of bacteria have revealed three major groups of prokaryotes: eubacteria, urkaryotes, and archaebacteria. The urkaryote is represented by that part of the eukaryotic cell that is external to the organelles. There are a great number of extant eubacterial species, but relatively few known archaebacterial species. Nonetheless, the archaebacteria appear to be an ancient group that exhibits as much diversity

PRIMITIVE OXYGEN CYCLE

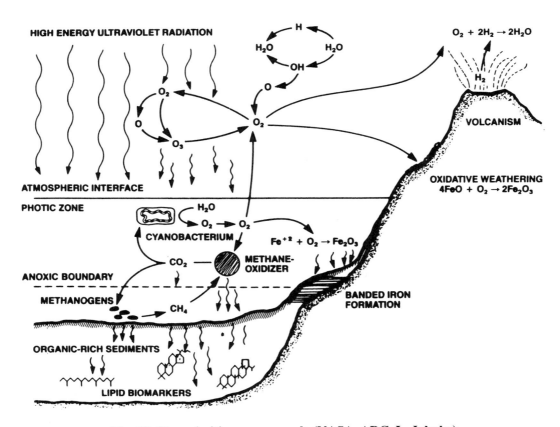

Fig. 12 The primitive oxygen cycle (NASA, ARC, L. Jahnke).

as the eubacteria. Traits held in common by all three groups, if derived from a common genetic basis, are likely to have been possessed by early living organisms. Some of those traits would have been developed to help early organisms deal with the rigors of the early environment. Therefore, studies of such evolutionary relationships also hold the promise of providing a biological perspective on the environmental conditions of the early Earth. To pursue these studies, exobiologists reconstruct the geneology of ancient, key biochemical traits of microorganisms, using phylogenetic studies based upon either sequences of RNA, DNA, proteins, or chemotaxonomic markers.

For example, eubacteria have been examined to seek an origin for photosynthesis as a cellular trait, and it appears that photosynthesis is indeed ancient. Major eubacterial groups are photosynthetic. Furthermore, nonphotosynthetic phenotypes have arisen several times from lines that were already photosynthetic (e.g., the gut organism *Escherichia coli* most likely arose from purple photosynthetic bacteria). The discovery that halophilic archaebacteria use a retinal pigment to transduce light into chemical energy suggests an alternative model for a photosynthetic system at least as primitive as the extremely complex chlorophyll-based one employed by the eubacteria. As such, it seems strange that retinal light transduction has only been found in halophilic bacteria, and so

porphyrin-based transduction systems are being sought in other archaebacteria.

The reduction of carbon dioxide to organic matter is also an ancient capability, and it is a process for which organisms have devised alternative strategies. Ribulose bisphosphate carboxylase (RuBPC), a key carbon dioxide-fixing enzyme of the Calvin cycle, is itself an ancient protein shared by many diverse organisms. Studies correlating composition and structure with the functional mechanisms of enzymes that carry out such fundamental roles as carbon dioxide fixation, nitrogen fixation, capture and transduction of energy from sunlight, among others, are being conducted to understand the nature of the simplest biochemical systems capable of exhibiting function. These functionally irreducible systems may eventually be able to serve as target models for synthetic chemists to use in their attempts to reconstruct the prebiotic evolution of such systems.

The biological utilization of molecular oxygen, a seminal development for life, may be correlated with evidence of changes in atmospheric composition. As mentioned earlier, geological evidence indicates that atmospheric oxygen levels were orders of magnitude lower on the early Earth than today. Because significant quantities of oxygen very likely first accumulated as a result of oxygen-producing photosynthesis, and the subsequent burial of reduced-carbon biomass, the first

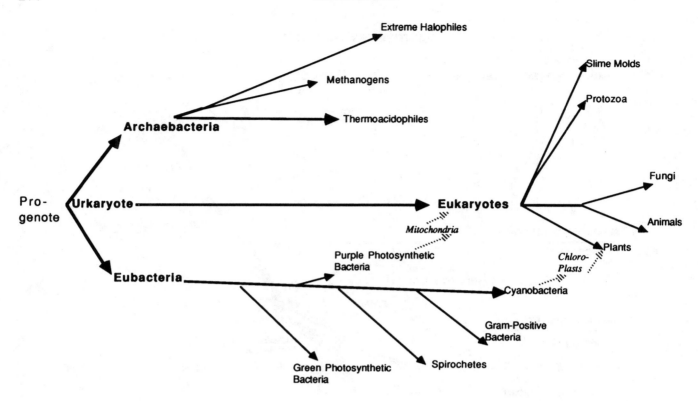

Fig. 13 Relationships among modern-day organisms, as deduced from rRNA sequence comparisons.[15]

organisms must have been anaerobes. The biochemical record supports this conclusion: anaerobic eubacteria are ancient compared with their aerobic counterparts. The evolution of oxygen respiration is an area of particular interest to exobiologists because of its planet-altering effects. It is not presently known if it evolved from an anaerobic system by acquiring individual steps that involved reaction with oxygen, albeit with low efficiency, or if it evolved from a system originally designed to transfer reducing equivalents to molecules other than oxygen (e.g., nitrate, sulfate, etc.)? An examination of the process of denitrification suggests that the components of nitrate respiration could have been precursors of oxygen respiration.

The development of a phylogeny of respiration systems holds great promise for charting the origin of this process, as well as for documenting the rise of atmospheric oxygen in the biological record, a record that should be concordant with the geochemical record. An understanding of the evolution of the biological processes involved in developing the oxygen cycle on Earth (Fig. 12) also will provide clues to chemical or structural fossils in the geological record that are characteristic of organisms with well-defined oxygen requirements. Given the host of biochemical adaptations to the rise of oxygen that can be studied, together with continuing progress in defining oxygen levels using the geologic record, it should be possible to synchronize large stretches of microbial evolution with the geologic time scale.

It is now generally accepted that a series of symbiotic

associations is responsible for the unique features of eukaryotic cells. From the study of modern eukaryotes it has been possible, in part, to reconstruct the evolutionary steps and the biochemical mechanisms involved in this process. Studies of the ultrastructure of eukaryotes coupled with molecular phylogenetic approaches have yielded insight into the evolution of these cells, and the identification of the relationships between living things on Earth.[14] These relationships (Fig. 13) resulted from the interplay of living organisms during the first several billion years of life on Earth, and laid the basis for the tremendous rise of complexity and variety that followed, only 1 billion years ago.

In the future, exobiologists will study the record of evolution found in rocks and cells to discover fundamental questions about life on the early Earth. They will try to determine the biochemical and genetic properties of the universal ancestor of all life and the characteristics of its environment, to trace the evolution of physiology and metabolism among the eukaryotes as well as the major groups of prokaryotes by means of molecular phylogeny, and to deduce the simplest biochemical mechanisms and structures that can carry out various of the necessary functions of a living system.

D. The Evolution of Advanced Life

The history of the early evolution of life on Earth (Fig. 14) is dominated by the story of unicellular organisms—their evolution, ecology, and planetary effects. It can be said that

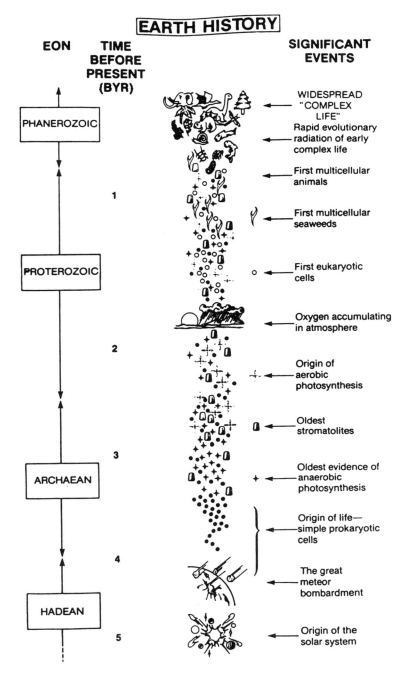

Fig. 14 Early Earth history.[16]

unicellular organisms continue to dominate the natural world, and that they are the dominant organisms on Earth even today. Nonetheless, biological evolution did not stop with the rise of complex unicellular organisms, and from the human point of view the last billion years of evolutionary innovation has been dominated by the evolution of complex multicellular organisms. From present evidence, this phase in the evolution of life on Earth appears to have been dominated by three major processes: 1) the evolution of complex ecological relationships between organisms, as constrained by biotic mechanisms; 2) mediation of those relationships by a planetary environment that has fluctuated due to intrinsic planetary processes; and 3) the recurrent destruction of existing planetary environments and organisms by events whose origins were found in outer space.

1. The Marine Record

Complex organisms first arose in the sea, and indeed all lineages of which we have knowledge, living or extinct, originated in marine environments. The record of basic evolutionary patterns that best illustrates the development of

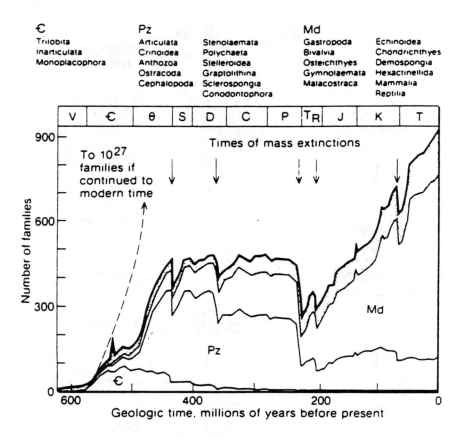

Fig. 15 Changes in the number of marine taxonomic families over geologic time. Upper curve depicts total number of families. Other curves subdivide the total among three major faunas (Cambrian = "C", Paleozoic = "Pz", Modern = "Md") that dominated the seas in succession, and a few other organisms (stippled area). Curves refer mostly to "shelly" forms that leave fossils; about 1900 modern marine families are known, many of which are not shelly.[22]

organic complexity is, therefore, that of the marine fossil biota. The trends found in the marine fossil record appear to be paralleled by those seen in the continental record, although the lessons of continental events are seen at lower taxonomic levels than those of oceanic events.

Multicellular marine plants were probably extant over 1 billion years ago, and the best evidence now available indicates that metazoans (multicelled animals) first appeared about 680 million years ago. Within the next 100 million years they gave rise directly to organisms that lacked digestive tracts, but which lived in the water column and on sediment surfaces. Organisms that arose during this time and had digestive tracts are known chiefly by their burrows in sediments. If these animals all originated after 680 million years ago, and we cannot yet be sure that they did, then the earliest metazoan radiation must certainly be judged as rapid. Beginning about 600 million years ago, an immense evolutionary radiation occurred among marine metazoans. Within the span of 100 million years, nearly all of the present-day phyla whose members have mineralized skeletons appear in the fossil record. In addition, several now-extinct phyla with skeletons also appeared. It is generally believed that the mineralized skeletons functioned as adaptations to life upon (as opposed to

within) the sea floor. Most of the lineages that possess digestive tracts and which dwelled upon the sediments seem to have descended from sediment-burrowing ancestors.

The latest Precambrian and early Cambrian periods (between 600 and 550 million years ago) witnessed the origin and use of novel body plans on a scale that was unprecedented and that has not been repeated. The enormous development of biological innovation within this period defined the shape of life on Earth, and was chiefly responsible for the complexity and diversity of modern body architecture in all metazoans. With the exception of the origin of eukaryotic cells, this radiation represents the most critical step in the development of a fauna that led to life as we know it, and eventually to the development of intelligent life on Earth.

To a lesser extent, the major bursts of evolution, such as those seen in the early Cambrian period, were repeated at other times during the Phanerozoic eon (the most recent 570 million years of Earth history). These bursts were characterized by the establishment of major body plans, by rising diversity among the various evolutionary lines of descent, and then by the extinction and replacement of biological groups at all taxonomic levels as biological diversity was partially reduced. Accordingly, the marine life of the Phanerozoic can be di-

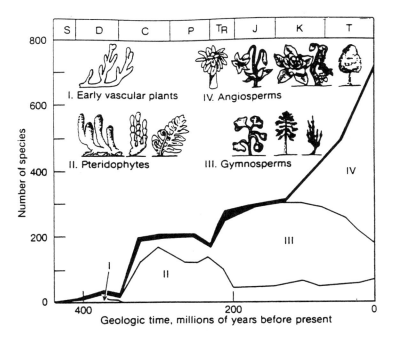

Fig. 16 Four groups of vascular plants have successively dominated terrestrial flora. The transition from group **II** to group **III** is unique in its coincidence with an interval of major change in the physical environment. Solid black line at the top of the graph represents nonvascular land plants and plant fossils whose affinities are uncertain.[22]

vided into three major faunas or compositional phases.

The first such phase was established between 600 and 500 million years ago, with its tremendous radiation of biological forms. Trilobites and inarticulate brachiopods were prominent members of this early fauna.

The second phase, lasting until the end of the Paleozoic Era (some 230 million years ago), saw the dominance of articulate brachiopods, crinoids, and some other newly abundant taxa in benthic (sea floor-dwelling) communities. The change from the first to the second phases was evidently accompanied by a restructuring of benthic ecosystems; these became significantly more complex. The late Permian extinctions (250 to 230 million years ago) brought the second phase to a close.

The third phase is represented by the fauna that rose to dominance following the Permian extinctions. This fauna was characterized by gastropods, bivalves, crustaceans, fish, echinoids, etc. Despite the revolutions in benthic community composition and structure that occurred during changeovers between phases, there was no dramatic increase in the types of anatomical complexity of organisms to rival the increase that occurred early in the first phase. This third compositional phase has continued to the present day, as seen through the lens of the fossil record (Fig. 15).

In summary, the record of the marine fauna is characterized by the diversification of the major taxa, involving partial or complete replacement of previously dominant taxa, followed by the periodic elimination of taxa during episodes of mass extinction. One central lesson is that the pattern of evolution

that has emerged cannot be viewed as a linear progression from simpler to more complex organisms.

2. The Land Record

The record of life on the land before multicellularity arose is nearly nonexistent, though it has been speculated that the land surface may have been used as a temporary refuge for marine metazoans before the arrival of land plants. The oldest known record of vascular plants on land is from the Silurian period, some 440 million years ago and 200 million years after the development of the first true marine metaphytes. The subsequent radiation of land plants and the rise of groups of plants based on new basic innovations in reproduction and vasculature is not dissimilar in its broad outlines from the appropriate phase of the marine record (Fig. 16). Of particular note is the mass extinction that took place at the end of the Permian period.

Like the plant record, the record for land animals is much less complete than that for the marine species. In particular, soft-bodied land fauna such as the arthropods are subject to irregular patterns of fossilization that tend to obscure real trends in their diversification or extinction (Fig. 17). As a result, the mass extinction events that appear significant in the marine record are often difficult to discern in the spotty land record, except when those events result in the loss of particularly distinctive groups of organisms. The demise of the dinosaurs at the end of the Cretaceous period is one such discernible extinction event.

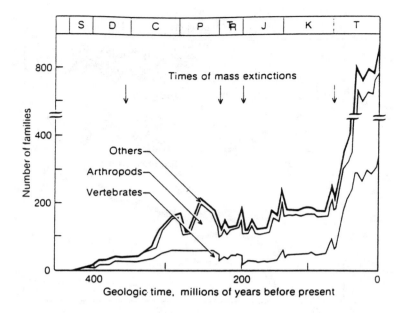

Fig. 17 Increase in diversity of nonmarine animals with time. Lower curve depicts vertebrates; width of center area represents arthropods. Upper curve shows total number of families, including protozoans and mollusks.[22]

3. Evolutionary Influences

The record of evolution that is reflected in the fossil record depicts a biota that has been tremendously affected by events in the solar system and on the planet itself. Earth has changed continuously throughout its history and continues to be active today. Such activity has caused environmental changes that have affected the course of biological evolution. Movements of the continents have caused long-term sea-level fluctuations, changes in the areas of shallow marine and continental habitats, regional climatic shifts, alteration of the geographic continuity of oceans and continents, and uplifts of mountain ranges. Other environmental changes have included the onset of glacial and thermal intervals, effects due to perturbations of the Earth's magnetic field, and variations in atmospheric and ocean chemistries. The causes of many of these environmental fluctuations are not well understood. Some, including the movements of the continents, are due to internal Earth dynamics, and still others are probably related to feedback mechanisms involving life processes themselves.

To understand more fully the relationship between geological change and evolution on Earth, a number of approaches are being developed to determine the environmental factors affecting evolution. For example, although plate tectonics has repeatedly isolated and then reunited biogeographic regions over geologic time, we do not know the actual evolutionary impacts of these changes except in a few instances. In addition, even though biological activity has had a profound effect upon the Earth's atmospheric composition, we still do not know the magnitude or impact of such effects. We do not know how much oxygen was present when multicelled organisms evolved, or if the evolutionary radiation of plants altered atmospheric CO_2 levels and thus world climate.

Extensive questions remain to be answered.

Extraterrestrial phenomena can also produce environmental changes, which in turn may influence the course of biological evolution. Asteroidal and cometary impacts are the foremost among these in terms of their potential effect on evolution, while long-term orbital effects in the Earth-Moon-Sun system[17] can also lead to climatic changes that may have had a profound effect on Earth environments. The likelihood that an impact event was responsible for mass extinctions at the Cretaceous-Tertiary boundary[18] dramatically underscores the need to assess the importance of such phenomena in the history of life.

To assess the importance of extraterrestrial phenomena to the evolution of advanced life it is necessary to identify unambiguous signatures of global perturbations to the terrestrial environment in the geological record. For example, in the future, statistical evaluations will be carried out to correlate epochs of climatic instability with the various periods of the Milankovitch cycles involving Earth's orbital and precessional changes, and the history of solar fluctuation will be obtained from measurements of ^{14}C, ^{10}Be and ^{18}O in polar ice as a function of time. Meanwhile, the presence of an anomalously enriched layer of iridium and other platinum group elements at the Cretaceous-Tertiary boundary has been shown to signify the redeposition of dusty debris from the impact of an extraterrestrial body. Additional evidence such as shocked quartz grains has been used to suggest a location for at least one likely impact crater in the Caribbean Basin, on the Yucatan peninsula in Mexico.[19]

To better evaluate the nature and frequency of terrestrial impacts as agents of global ecological change affecting evolution, it is necessary to better understand the prevalence of such events. Impact craters on Earth, the Moon, Mars, and

Venus are being located and measured, and those on Earth are being dated and geochemically characterized. This approach is currently being pursued with remote sensing techniques from satellites, but in time the direct analysis of samples from such craters would provide extensive and detailed corroborating evidence about the nature of impact events in the inner solar system.

If we assume that disruption is the natural state for the Earth as a home for life, it remains true that the nature of the relationship between environmental disturbance and evolution is an open question. With too much disruption organisms might remain small (even unicellular) to reproduce rapidly and there would be no advantage to an adaptation to novel environments that might disappear all too rapidly. Alternatively, with too little disturbance, a suite of well-adapted organisms could eventually occupy a static planet, thereby competitively suppressing the expression of novel biological innovations such as multicellular complexity. Perhaps an "intermediate" level of disturbance (as perhaps occurred on Earth) permits advanced, and ultimately, intelligent, life to arise. A detailed alignment of the biological and geological histories of the planet Earth can help to address these issues, but ultimately a comparison to some other evolutionary history will be needed to understand this phenomenon.

An initial understanding of how astrophysical, solar system, and planetary events have influenced the evolution of advanced life on Earth has provided the basis for predicting the distribution of advanced life among other solar systems throughout the galaxy. If, when we have completed our study of life on Earth we find that none of the important facets of evolution that have shaped the nature of Earth's life are unique to this planet, then the prospects that life may be found elsewhere are increased.

III. Life in Extreme Environments

An understanding of the immense range of environments occupied by life defines the Earthly limits of pressure, temperature, duration and quality of sunlight, and other factors that advanced organisms can tolerate. The absolute limits on environmental conditions within which advanced life on Earth can exist define the nature of biochemical, morphologic, physiologic, and behavioral responses by which life adapts to these extremes, and may provide insights into possible environmental limits on the distribution of advanced life, as we know it, elsewhere in the universe. As members of the species *Homo sapiens*, we are limited in our natural exposure to environmental extremes, but other organisms are continually being found that are extending the envelope that contains life.

Whereas vertebrate and higher plant life are relatively susceptible to extremes, microbial life forms have inhabited nearly every accessible habitat on Earth. Living bacteria have been isolated from water (at high pressure) where temperatures are about 150 °C, and they can grow at temperatures greater than 100 °C when pressures are sufficient. Spores and

other dormant microorganisms can survive temperatures of −240 °C for long periods, although some organisms can grow at temperatures near −25 °C. Similar varieties of organisms are preserved in conditions of vacuum, grow at pressures up to 1300 bars, and can survive pressures up to 20,000 bars.

Organisms exposed to ultraviolet radiation can survive up to doses of 50,000 ergs/mm^2, and ionizing radiation up to 2-4 Mrad. Still other microorganisms grow in solutions with pH of from 1 to 12, and survive for a time at pH near 0 and 14. Some microorganisms are adapted to high concentrations of heavy metals (e.g., 1 percent copper solutions). Many organisms can survive for long periods without external energy sources, without nutrients, and with very little water. Only a few microorganisms can grow at water activity values of 0.6, but many can survive at water activity values near 0. A requirement for water seems to be the most universal limitation on the growth of Earth organisms.

IV. The Search for Evidence of Life Elsewhere

Understanding the origin and evolution of life on Earth, and its adaptations to challenging conditions, may provide exobiologists with information about the potential for life elsewhere. But even the most in-depth knowledge of Earth life can only provide circumstantial evidence about that question. Understanding the distribution of life in the universe requires additional data that cannot be gained on a single planet, or indeed, in a single solar system.

Although the discovery of life forms on other worlds would provide an extraordinary opportunity to generalize our knowledge of the origin and evolution of life, we will also benefit from understanding other worlds where life *could* exist, but is not to be found. For a small handfull of worlds (both planets and moons) in this solar system we could conduct the search for this life directly, but most of the worlds of interest will be attached to other stars and therefore beyond the reach of direct examination for the proximate future. Nonetheless, indirect methods may be able to provide us with critical clues about life on other worlds using technology becoming available today.

A. Studies In Situ—The Direct Search for Evidence of Life

The early history of solar system exploration using spacecraft was dominated by reconnaissance of the Earth's neighbors. The Moon, Venus, Mars, and eventually Jupiter and the outer planets were surveyed by "flyby" missions. The Moon, Venus, and Mars were later visited by orbiting spacecraft and landers. At least initially, all of these early reconnaissance missions were intended to provide information about the prospects of life on these other worlds. Uniformly, they returned a verdict about the solar system that had been previously suspected by some—there was no place like home.

Unlike its nearest neighbor, the Earth, the Moon was shown by the Ranger and Luna spacecraft, and their successors Surveyor and Lunokhod, to be airless, dry, and devoid of

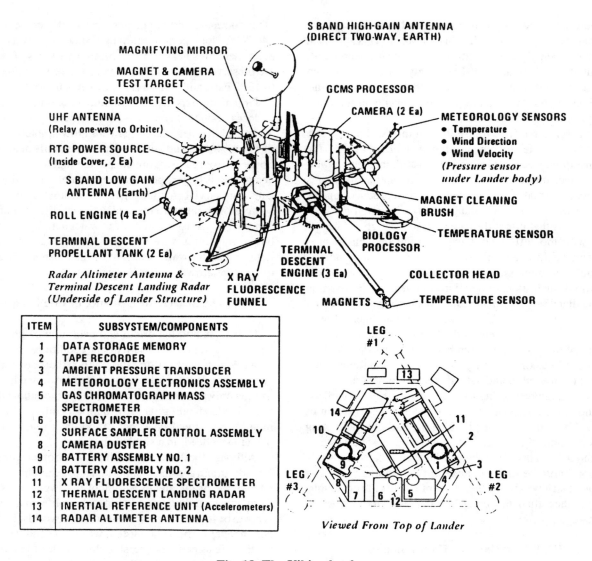

MAGNIFYING MIRROR

MAGNET & CAMERA
TEST TARGET

SEISMOMETER

UHF ANTENNA
(Relay one-way to Orbiter)

RTG POWER SOURCE
(Inside Cover, 2 Ea)

S BAND LOW GAIN
ANTENNA (Earth)

ROLL ENGINE (4 Ea)

TERMINAL DESCENT
PROPELLANT TANK (2 Ea)

*Radar Altimeter Antenna &
Terminal Descent Landing Radar
(Underside of Lander Structure)*

S BAND HIGH-GAIN ANTENNA
(DIRECT TWO-WAY, EARTH)

GCMS PROCESSOR

CAMERA (2 Ea)

METEOROLOGY SENSORS
• Temperature
• Wind Direction
• Wind Velocity
*(Pressure sensor
under Lander body)*

MAGNET CLEANING
BRUSH

TEMPERATURE SENSOR

BIOLOGY
PROCESSOR

TERMINAL
DESCENT
ENGINE (3 Ea)

X RAY
FLUORESCENCE
FUNNEL

MAGNETS

COLLECTOR HEAD

TEMPERATURE SENSOR

ITEM	SUBSYSTEM/COMPONENTS
1	DATA STORAGE MEMORY
2	TAPE RECORDER
3	AMBIENT PRESSURE TRANSDUCER
4	METEOROLOGY ELECTRONICS ASSEMBLY
5	GAS CHROMATOGRAPH MASS SPECTROMETER
6	BIOLOGY INSTRUMENT
7	SURFACE SAMPLER CONTROL ASSEMBLY
8	CAMERA DUSTER
9	BATTERY ASSEMBLY NO. 1
10	BATTERY ASSEMBLY NO. 2
11	X RAY FLUORESCENCE SPECTROMETER
12	THERMAL DESCENT LANDING RADAR
13	INERTIAL REFERENCE UNIT (Accelerometers)
14	RADAR ALTIMETER ANTENNA

LEG #1
LEG #3
LEG #2

Viewed From Top of Lander

Fig. 18 The Viking lander.

sites for life. With surface temperatures ranging from -173 °C to +127 °C on the Moon, it was not surprising that none of these spacecraft revealed any signs of life on the Earth's natural satellite; nor did examination of the samples returned by the Apollo missions.

Still other spacecraft, the Soviet Union's Venera and Vega series and the United States' Mariner and Pioneer probes, provided a picture of the planet Venus that has ruled out the hope of finding life there. A thick carbon dioxide atmosphere laced with sulfuric, hydrochloric, and hydrofluoric acid, and surface temperatures of over 450 °C make Venus an unlikely place to look for, let alone find, signs of life. Venus stands, instead, as an example of what a runaway greenhouse effect can do to a planet that may have been originally much like Earth.

As a result of planetary exploration, our view of Mars has changed considerably since the first observations were made by early astronomers. The first telescopes revealed a planet that appeared, in many respects, similar to Earth. In 1877,

two small moons were discovered; these were named Phobos and Deimos—Fear and Terror. It was determined that the martian solar day was approximately 24 hours. The tilt of Mars's axis—with the poles alternately oriented toward the Sun—suggested the presence of seasons. These and other early Earth-based observations led many, particularly Percival Lowell, to believe that life was abundant on the red planet. However, advancements in technology and the advent of spacecraft exploration have extended our vision, forever changing our view of Mars. Because of the U.S. Mariner and Viking missions and the Soviet Union's Mars flybys, the Lowellian image of a lush, vegetated planet survives only in the annals of imaginative fiction. In some aspects, contemporary Mars bears a closer resemblance to our own Moon.

The barometric pressure at the surface of Mars is less than 1 percent that of the Earth. This thin atmosphere is composed mainly of carbon dioxide (95 percent), nitrogen (2.5 percent), and argon (1 percent). Because of the nature of its atmo-

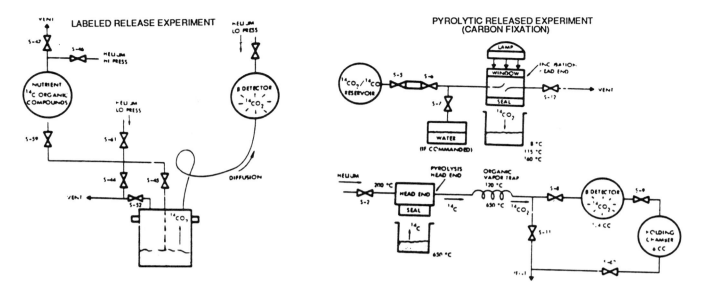

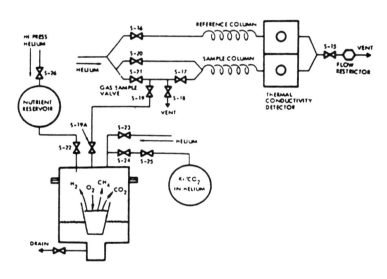

Fig. 19 Schematic drawings of Viking biology experiments.

sphere, Mars lacks a protective blanket of ozone like that surrounding Earth. Therefore, ultraviolet radiation is able to penetrate to the surface, producing strong oxidants in the top-regolith. It is the presence of iron oxides formed by these oxidants that imparts the red color to the planet.

The low atmospheric pressure also precludes the existence of liquid water on the present-day surface of the planet. This is significant, since one requirement for life seems to be water in the liquid form, or at least water activity such that a cell can incorporate it in or near this state. If our current paradigm for life is correct, the unique properties of water make it likely that extraterrestrial life forms would also be dependent on its availability. Mars is dry. Besides the residual water-ice cap discovered at its north pole and some water vapor in the

atmosphere, abundant water has not been observed on contemporary Mars. Nonetheless, the water that once flowed on the martian surface in the past is not likely to be the only water that the planet possesses. Other surface features and crater morphology indicate that water is present on Mars, and much of that water may be buried as permafrost ice.

1. The Viking Missions and Life Detection Experiments

Mars is the first (and so far the only) other planet where we have directly sought to detect life. A major goal of the Viking missions was to determine the presence or absence of life on Mars.[20] The Viking lander carried the most complex set of instrumentation that has ever been landed robotically on

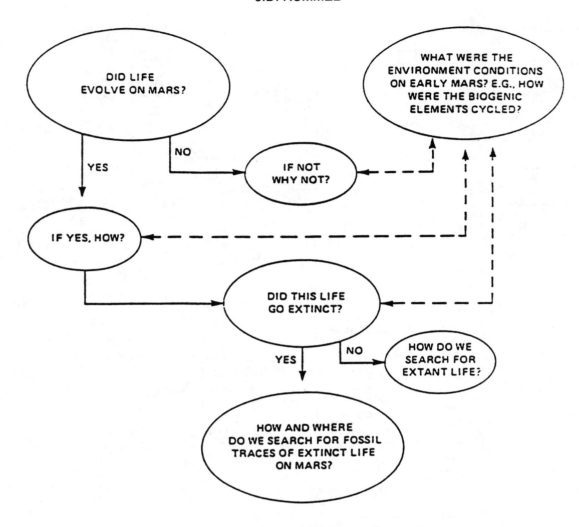

Fig. 20 Logic diagram for the approach to the questions regarding life on Mars. (Courtesy of C. P. McKay, NASA, ARC.)

another planetary surface (Fig. 18).

In addition to the lander cameras, which were expected to show the presence of any obvious macroscopic life forms, and the Gas Chromatograph/Mass Spectrometer (GCMS), designed to detect the presence of organics in the martian soil, the Viking landers contained three experiments (the Viking Biology Package, Fig. 19) specifically designed to search for indications of life. The first of these was the Gas Exchange Experiment (GEx), designed to determine if martian life could metabolize and exchange gaseous products in the presence of a nutrient solution. The second was the Labeled Release Experiment (LR), which sought to detect life by the release of radioactively labeled carbon initially incorporated into organic compounds in a nutrient solution. The third was the Pyrolytic Release Experiment (PR), based on the assumption that martian life would have the capability to incorporate radioactively labeled carbon dioxide in the presence of light (photosynthesis).

The results of these experiments showed definite signs of chemical activity, which was later judged by the Viking Biology Team as probably nonbiological in origin.[21] Of the three instruments in the Viking Biology Package, all produced results consistent with a highly reactive soil. Unlike the GEx and PR experiments, the results of the LR experiment were altered by heat treatment of the soil sample, which suggested to some a biological effect. Nonetheless, the results from the Biology Package were not judged independently, but in the context of the other lander instruments. Of all of the results gained by the Viking lander, by far the most surprising result was the failure of the GCMS to find organic material at the parts-per-billion level of detectability. The lack of organics, coupled with the extreme dryness of the planet, severely constrains the possibility of life existing in the martian surface soils. Therefore, results of the biology experiments were interpreted as being consistent not with life on the surface, but with a highly reactive martian soil. The oxidizing nature of these soils appears to preclude the existence of any unprotected organics at the surface.

The Viking results, although not at all conclusive, suggest that life does not currently exist in the surface soils of Mars, though life might be found in a cryptic niche that cannot be found using presently available data. The Viking biology experiments were a gamble that life would be widespread, and relatively easy to detect. The Viking data provide the evidence that this is not the case, but those data do not address the overall question of the existence of life on Mars. As a result of the Viking mission, the questions of interest to exobiology have been more explicitly framed, and can be addressed anew. The main questions, therefore, are: What was the course of chemical evolution on Mars (and did organics survive long enough to form biologically significant molecules)? Did such a process ever result in the formation of replicating systems and life on early Mars? And if so, what was the fate of that life? A conceptual scheme for the arrangement of these questions is given in Fig. 20.

In the future, sampling of the ancient surfaces of Mars will allow a detailed understanding of the extent to which chemical evolution occurred and biological evolution was possible. Three possible scenarios for the evolution of Mars have been suggested, based on our current understanding of the early environments of Earth and Mars:

1) Life arose on Mars and conditions were suitable for its maintenance for over a billion years. In this scenario, life on Mars developed to a stage that may be comparable to the stromatolites observed in ancient sediments on Earth. On Earth, the record of biological evolution from the earliest ancestor to the formation of well-developed communities has been hidden by plate tectonic recycling of the crust. Mars has not undergone this recycling. If a complete fossil record could be found on Mars and organically preserved microfossils identified, then such a study could yield unique insight into the evolutionary process of early life on Earth. Using isotopic and geochemical means to understand the environmental context in which these earliest organisms lived would provide powerful constraints for theories of the energy generation mechanism of the earliest life (autotrophy vs. heterotrophy) and the biological cycling of essential elements in the earliest biosphere. If extant life forms could be found, then the record of evolution could be traced through living systems as well.

2) Prebiotic evolution on Mars led to the development of the first organisms, but conditions became unsuitable for life at a very early stage (approximately 3.8 billion years ago). Martian sediments may provide a glimpse of the planetary conditions that precede life. Current models of prebiotic synthesis exist for virtually all of the basic building blocks of life, including sugars, amino acids, and nucleotides. In this scenario, life originated much as Oparin perceived it—in an organic-rich primordial soup. A competing hypothesis argues for an "inorganic" origin to the first self-replicating system, possibly based on clay minerals. Mars appears to be rich in clay minerals, and any abiotic sources of organic material that may have been operative on the early Earth should have been operative on early Mars as well. Thus, if evolution on Mars

was arrested very early in its biological development, a detailed examination of the organic and inorganic geochemistry of the martian sediments may help to resolve key questions on prebiotic evolution.

3) Neither life nor any relevant variant of prebiotic evolution occurred on Mars. If we find evidence that neither life nor prebiotic evolution occurred on the primordial Mars, then our present model of the physical evolution of the martian environment may be incorrect—an environment suitable for life may never have existed there—or our understanding of prebiotic chemical evolution could be severely flawed. Such a finding would increase our knowledge of Mars and our understanding of the origin of life. It would certainly prompt a more in-depth comparison of early Earth and early Mars in an effort to determine exactly which critical environmental or planetary characteristics could account for their disparate biological histories.

Beyond the search for life, past and present, a goal of exobiology on Mars is also to study the distribution and evolution of the biogenic elements (C, H, N, O, P, S) and compounds (e.g., H_2O, CO_2, NO_x) as an exercise in comparative planetology. The cycling of these elements is a key to the sustenance of a biosphere. Even in the absence of life, studies of these cycles will provide points of comparison and contrast to the biogeochemical cycles of the biogenic elements on Earth.

Information on the global-scale cycling of the biogenic elements can be collected, to a large extent, by robotic spacecraft. Human presence, however, would greatly facilitate the collection of more specific information on fine-scale gradients, isotopic variations, and elemental ratios. Interesting mineral phases, such as clay, can play an active role in processing the biogenic elements and compounds. Areas of rich salt concentration may be sites of enhanced water activity. The study of this natural cycling of biogenic material would be useful in establishing the role of abiotic synthesis in the origin of life on Earth.

Planetary evolution and the interaction of global reservoirs of volatiles are areas of interest for the study of evolution of life on planetary surfaces. If life did originate on Mars and subsequently became extinct, this process would certainly be associated with changes in the cycling of the biogenic elements. Evidence for such changes may still be gleaned from a study of the detailed elemental and isotopic structure of the layered terrain. Relatively recent information on the global cycles of carbon dioxide and water on Mars may be obtained from studies of the polar laminated terrain.

2. Indirect Evidence About Life's Origins—Cosmic Dust Collection

Whereas further understanding of the prospects of life on Mars will have to await the launch of future missions to that planet, the Earth is constantly receiving samples of extraterrestrial materials that can shed new evidence on the nature of

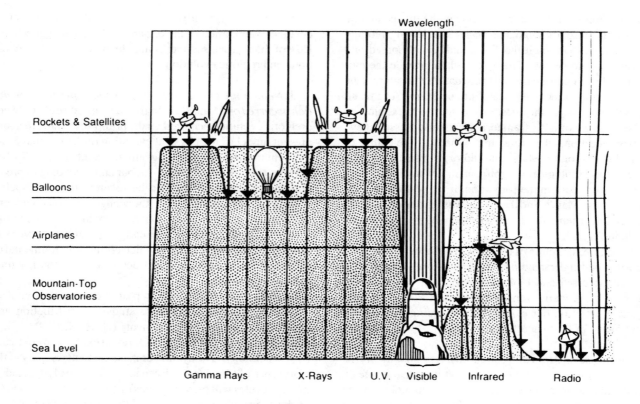

Fig. 21 Observatories in space, high above the Earth's absorbing atmosphere, can provide new vistas of the universe.[24]

the rest of the solar system. Many of these samples, such as meteorites, can only safely be collected after they have fallen to Earth, but smaller samples of "cosmic" or interplanetary dust particles (IDPs) are constantly impinging on the Earth and can be collected in the atmosphere or in space.

IDPs are 1-100+ micron sized particles that travel in space at hypervelocity speeds (~8-50+ km/s). These IDPs represent "fossils" of early solar system development and are of importance to exobiology because they provide important clues concerning the chemical, temperature, pressure, and radiation environments during planetary formation and evolution. IDPs may be of cometary, meteoritic, planetary, or interstellar origin. In the past, IDP collection has been actively pursued in the atmosphere via collection devices mounted on U-2 and ER-2 aircraft, and by space flight experiments such as those on the Long Duration Exposure Facility. Improved space collection techniques are desired because IDPs collected by aircraft are contaminated by atmospheric constituents, and the space collection techniques used so far cause the volatilization of organic components and considerable structural damage to the particles. In addition, trajectory information on the intact particles is needed to trace their source.

A number of flight opportunities for cosmic dust collection are under study. Since the average flux density of IDPs in space is approximately 1 per square meter per day, on-orbit collection requires long duration experiments. One concept under study is to place a Cosmic Dust Collection Facility in

space as an attached payload on Space Station Freedom. This would allow both the intact captures of IDPs in space and the collection of trajectory information to correlate the chemistry and petrology of IDPs with their parent bodies.

B. Remote Observations of Natural Phenomena

Most of our information about extraterrestrial conditions and objects has come from the analysis of electromagnetic radiation. With the exception of those planets that can be visited by spacecraft and those rare occurrences when accessible extraterrestrial material such as meteorites can be traced to their origin, observational methods remain the most successful way to learn about conditions in deep space and on other worlds.

Before the beginning of the space age, limitations on the electromagnetic radiation available at the Earth's surface limited our ability to observe the universe (Fig. 21). Access to the space environment for observatories above the Earth's atmosphere has provided a greatly expanded window through which to learn about processes important to the origin, evolution, and distribution of life in the universe. Through this new window the universe can be viewed at all wavelengths to answer questions about the biogenic elements and their compounds in stars, the interstellar medium, and on the planets and small bodies of this and perhaps other solar systems. Concurrently, important research is being carried out using a combination of ground-based and airborne observatories at those wavelengths that do penetrate the atmosphere.

Perhaps the most important objective in the search for natural phenomena that give evidence about life beyond our own solar system is the search for planets around other stars, because life as we know it is a planetary phenomenon. Only on planets o r large moons are we likely to find the liquid water and minerals that appear to be required for life, and only on such bodies are we likely find the gaseous atmospheres, local volcanism, hydrothermal vents, lightning strikes, etc., that appear to have been important to the origin of life on Earth.

Observations of other stars and the interstellar medium can also provide information on the abundance and distribution of the biogenic elements in the universe, and tell us about the conditions under which complex organic molecules form or are destroyed. Additional observations of planets, asteroids, and comets will focus and complement the future direct examination of those objects by spacecraft. Of particular importance are observations that can be made in the infrared and radio regions of the electromagnetic spectrum. Evidence from these astronomical observations can help to explain the processes in circumstellar, interstellar, and nebular stages of physical-chemical evolution that govern the composition and distribution of the biogenic elements from stage to stage of their transition from their birth in stars to their incorporation into planetary bodies and their later evolution on those bodies. Coupled with laboratory experimentation on Earth, and later in space, we can use this information to help us understand how we arrived at the prerequisite conditions for life.

Eventually, observational technology might advance to the point where we will be able not only to detect planets around other stars, but to analyze their composition. If we hypothesize that advanced life on planets in other solar systems might have the same requirement for oxygen respiration as it does on Earth, then this assumption could lead to searches not only for other planets, but for oxygenic planetary atmospheres. Conducting such a search will require further technological development of space-based optical interferometers with a large collecting area and capability for high angular resolution, but could take place within the next 20 years.

C. Observations of Indirect Phenomena Associated with Life

There are several basic constraints on our ability to look for life elsewhere in the universe that are tied to the inadequacy of our technology. Despite the achievements of the last few decades, other worlds are still difficult to reach. Thus we are limited in our selection of worlds to explore for life. And once we arrive on a distant world, we are limited in our ability to conduct the search. In many respects, we have no more direct knowledge about the conditions for life under the surface of Mars, which we have reached, than we do about the prospects for life on Europa, which we have not.

Moreover, current prospects for reaching worlds around

other stars are very dim. The energy requirements for humans to complete such a trip within a single lifetime are enormous, and well beyond our forecast capabilities. Only photons currently are making the journey. As noted above, we might eventually be able to detect the planetary effects of living organisms by direct observation of planets around other stars, but now even that is out of the question. How then, do we sample the hundreds of billions of other stars in our galaxy for signs of life?

One method is to look for indirect indications of life from technologies associated with intelligent life elsewhere. Based on what we know about life on Earth, there is no reason to believe that what happened here is unique. Given the correct circumstances there is no a priori reason to believe that life elsewhere would not first develop intelligence and eventually technologies capable of spanning the distance between the stars. The detection of life by looking for signs of technology associated with extraterrestrial intelligent life is the basis of the search for extraterrestrial intelligence (SETI) approach to finding life in the universe, and the details of the approach are dealt with elsewhere in this volume.

If the means for interstellar travel were to exist elsewhere in the universe, the arrival of visitors from another solar system would, of course, provide the surest sort of proof of the existence of life elsewhere. Unfortunately, there is currently no evidence for a technology that would make interstellar travel feasible, and no evidence of visitors to Earth. Despite numerous reports of unidentified flying objects (UFOs), there are no unequivocal cases nor any replicable evidence that suggest an extraterrestrial origin for UFOs. Without such evidence, the UFO question is one that will have to be dealt with outside of the confines of the science of exobiology. Efforts within exobiology are instead focused on a search for evidence of known technologies and repeatable phenomena. As such, the search for extraterrestrial intelligence/technology is a short-cut in the search for life in the universe, and today is the only credible means for looking for life outside our own solar system.

D. Future Mission Prospects for Exobiology

Although hypotheses about life in the universe have been proposed on the basis of ground-based research and space-flight data, there are critical gaps in our understanding that can only be filled by more extensive space exploration. Combined with the prospects of conducting simulation experiments aboard Space Station Freedom and the capabilities of future space observatories, these new planetary missions will provide essential pieces to the puzzle of life in the universe.

1. Inner Planet Missions

Present-day planning by the spacefaring nations of the world has focused on the Moon and Mars as the next targets for extensive exploration.

Missions to the Moon will permit a broadly based research

program on questions of fundamental exobiological significance. The collection and subsequent analysis of interplanetary and perhaps interstellar dust particles will reveal additional information about the cosmic history of the biogenic elements and compounds. Simulations of dust-grain chemistry, studied in the lunar environment, will further our understanding of the synthesis of complex organic molecules in space. Exposure of terrestrial organisms on the Moon will allow extensive studies of the survivability and adaptation of life in the space environment, and constrain hypotheses about the spread of living organisms through space.

As our lunar capabilities expand, analyses will be performed on samples from the polar regions and the deep subsurface for possible prebiotic molecules delivered by cometary impact. Analysis of samples from a variety of lunar craters will significantly improve our understanding of the timing and nature of the impact events that have affected the evolution of complex life on Earth. Perhaps the most important benefit of lunar exploration will be the use of the lunar surface as a platform for astronomical observations of organics in planetary atmospheres and interstellar environments.[23] Eventually, the use of the radio-quiet lunar farside for a search for radio signals from intelligent species beyond the solar system will extend similar terrestrial observations into domains that are inaccessible from Earth.

Current capabilities in exobiology need to be extended to realize the potential of the lunar opportunity. Earth-based microanalytical techniques for detection of minute amounts of organics in individual dust grains need to be further developed to acquire information from lunar collections and experiments. Existing devices for exposing samples to the space environment need to be modified to allow the use of the lunar environment for studying the synthesis of complex organics on grains and for studying the survivability of microorganisms. To make optimum use of lunar-based telescope facilities, existing observatory instruments will have to be modified to optimize their use for the detection of the biogenic elements. Depending on the astrophysical objectives that are pursued, exobiology-specific telescope facilities may be required for observations of extraterrestrial radio signals of intelligent origin.

Future exploration missions to Mars will provide a unique opportunity to understand the role that life plays in evolution of the terrestrial planets. The U.S. Mars Observer mission is scheduled for launch in 1992, while Russia is currently envisioning missions in both 1994 and 1996. Concepts under study in the U.S., Europe, and elsewhere include a Mars network of geochemical and seismological stations, extensive rover missions and the prospect for a Mars sample return mission, and the eventual human exploration of Mars.

Exobiology capabilities will need to be extensively augmented to study the question of life on Mars. Understanding the history and distribution of water on Mars is a key requirement for finding sites where biological activity may have occurred in the past, and where a chemical or morphological record of that activity may have been recorded. Analysis of

the Mars Observer data, for example, will reveal information about water, mineralogy, and the surface and subsurface structure of the planet. This sort of remote sensing data will be used to locate specific sites of biological interest such as paleolakes, hydrothermal sites and springs, and sites of episodic water activity, whereas later, in situ measurements will be used to verify that the target sites had liquid water habitats suitable for life. In addition, if water currently exists near the surface of Mars, those sites would be focal points for a search for present-day life. Instruments need to be developed for penetrators and surface stations to be used on a follow-on to Mars Observer, a Mars network mission, with emphasis on in situ analytical capability to include instruments to measure evolved gases, electrical properties of the soil, and chemical, elemental, and isotopic composition. These capabilities will be needed to search for organic material below the surface, to characterize the proposed soil oxidant and its role in organic destruction, and later to guide sample collection for detailed analysis on Earth. Rover and sample return missions will need to be equipped with specific instruments to search for and select samples for terrestrial analysis for extinct and extant life. These will include imaging devices, mass spectrometers, and increasingly capable sample acquisition devices.

An Earth-based research capability must be maintained to permit effective understanding of the data returned from the exploration missions, and to test concepts for future missions. Extensive research is needed using terrestrial analogs of the Mars environment (e.g., the Antarctic, simulation chambers, etc.) to develop microanalytical instruments and laboratories for exobiological analysis of returned samples, to better understand the chemical properties of the soil and its biological potential, to learn how to detect fossils in sediments that once harbored life, and to apply the lessons learned on Mars to our questions about how life originated on Earth.

Sometime in the next century, human operations on the Mars surface will allow the establishment of basic experimental and field support capabilities at a Mars outpost. Humans will be able to conduct both direct and robotically assisted investigations of local sites for exobiology. Aided by teleoperated robots and able to react to new discoveries on a real-time basis, human presence may be essential to an eventual understanding of Mars exobiology. Having the capability on Mars for an iterative analysis of elements, organics, oxidants, and gases, and the ability to do extensive microscopy on a range of selected samples will significantly enhance a thorough search for signs of life on Mars. Concurrently, it will also be necessary to monitor the nature and extent of human-associated microbial contamination of the martian surface and subsurface, which could serve to confound exobiology efforts if not closely scrutinized.

2. Outer Planet Missions and the Exploration of the Small Bodies of the Solar System

After the stunning successes of the Pioneer and Voyager spacecraft on their reconnaissance missions to the outer planets, a series of follow-on missions has been planned to explore further these awesome worlds. As of this writing, NASA's Galileo mission is on its way to Jupiter, where it will conduct an extensive tour of the jovian system and send a probe into the atmosphere of the planet itself. The Cassini mission is currently being built for a 1996 launch to the saturnian system, where a similar tour is planned, but the moon Titan, rather than Saturn itself, is the target of the European-supplied Huygens probe. Each of these missions will also enhance our knowledge of asteroids by conducting short-range encounters with individual asteroids on their way to the outer solar system. A future comet nucleus sample return, a mission concept that is called "Rosetta," is under consideration by NASA and the European Space Agency. Together with the asteroid flybys, these missions promise to revolutionize our knowledge of the comets and small bodies of the solar system.

E. Planetary Protection

Understanding the potential for life elsewhere in the universe is a difficult task. Within this solar system we are faced with the prospect that, unlike Earth, most other locations are devoid of life. To satisfy our scientific interests in the rest of the solar system, we need to make sure that Earth life does not become artificially established on other solar system bodies. To satisfy the people of the Earth that their interests are being considered during the process of solar system exploration, we need to guard against the inadvertent importation of possible extraterrestrial organisms to Earth. Our activities in the biological quarantine of spacecraft, or as it is now known, "planetary protection," spring from these two considerations.

Since the earliest days of the space program, NASA has been concerned with the protection of the planets and other solar system bodies from biological contamination. As early as 1959 the Agency had adopted a policy calling for the sterilization of payloads "which might have an impact on a celestial body" in response to concern expressed a year earlier by the U.S. National Academy of Sciences.

Such concerns on the part of the international community eventually culminated in the 1967 Outer Space Treaty, which codified the principle that states should pursue studies of solar system bodies "... so as to avoid their harmful contamination and also adverse changes in the environment of the Earth...".[24] The recommendations of COSPAR, the International Council of Scientific Unions Committee on Space Research, were considered to be a key factor in guiding the conduct of these studies.

In the period since 1967, NASA policy has matured in an interactive process that has included the recommendations of the Space Studies Board of the U.S. National Academy of Sciences as well as COSPAR. The intent of the policy, however, has not changed. Today, the basic NASA policy is expressed in the following statement:

> The conduct of scientific investigations of possible extraterrestrial life forms, precursors, and

remnants must not be jeopardized. In addition, the Earth must be protected from the potential hazard posed by extraterrestrial matter carried by a spacecraft returning from another planet. Therefore, for certain space-mission/target-planet combinations, controls on organic and biological contamination carried by spacecraft shall be imposed, in accordance with issuances implementing this policy.[25]

This policy was adopted by COSPAR in 1984. The basic policy is also intended to be applied to manned missions. The application of this policy can best be understood in the context of actual space-flight missions. Two such missions to which the policy has been applied are the upcoming Galileo mission to Jupiter, and the Mars Observer mission. Galileo is an example of a mission that has generated a low level of concern because of the extremely low probability of growth for terrestrial organisms on Jupiter. Nonetheless, Jupiter and its system of moons are of considerable interest in relation to studies of organic material in the solar system. The planetary protection plan for this mission ensures that adequate documentation about the eventual location of the spacecraft will be available to future investigators of the jovian system. In addition to this documentation, an additional provision in the mission's planetary protection plan will enable a future decision by NASA to avoid specific portions of the jovian system that might warrant greater protection when disposing of the spacecraft at the end of the mission. This provision builds into the mission an ability to respond to potential new discoveries about Jupiter and its moons by the Galileo spacecraft.

Despite the extreme nature of the surface conditions discovered by the Viking spacecraft, Mars is still a potential home for indigenous life. Thus, the Mars Observer mission's planetary protection plan requires clean room assembly of flight hardware, limitations on the orbital dwell time in the lower atmosphere of Mars, and an eventual placement of the spacecraft into a high and stable orbit at the end of the mission to preclude the spacecraft from impacting the surface of Mars before 2038. These measures, although not too intrusive, do have cost and operational impacts on the mission. Future information about Mars may either relax or tighten such requirements. In the case of a future Mars rover or sample return mission, our lack of concrete knowledge about the martian subsurface environment might be considered a limitation that will dictate a conservative posture in protecting Mars. Deciding the hazard posed by a returned sample in the absence of solid data will not be possible in the absolute sense, a problem that might dictate that such a sample will be handled in a very cautious manner. In addition, the science needs of a sample return may dictate that the spacecraft not carry any biological contamination that could alter the characteristics of the returned sample. Such a requirement would be more stringent than required for planetary protection alone, but would guarantee the protection of the scientific value of a martian sample.

Acknowledgments

The preparation of this chapter has been aided greatly by the assistance of Dale Andersen, Sherwood Chang, Don DeVincenzi, and the members of the Exobiology Discipline Working Group, who have taught me much, but are not responsible for my interpretation of their lessons. Jill Tarter and Bob Wharton were kind enough to read earlier drafts. As an author, I thank my fellow editors of Volume 1 for their patience.

References

[1] Lederberg, J. Exobiology: Approaches to life beyond the Earth. *Science,* 1960, Vol. 132, p. 393.

[2] Metrodorus of Chios. 4th century B.C.

[3] Darwin letter to Hooker, February 1871. Courtesy of Prof. Melvin Calvin, University of California, Berkeley. In: Hartman, H., Lawless, J.G., and Morrison, P. (Eds.) *Search for the Universal Ancestor*, 1985, NASA SP-477.

[4] Oparin, A.I. *The Origin of Life*, Moskovskiy Rabochiy (in Russian). Moscow, 1924.

[5] Haldane, J.B.S. The origin of life. *The Rationalist Annual*, London, 1929.

[6] Wood, J.A., Chang, S. (Eds.) *The Cosmic History of the Biogenic Elements and Compounds*, NASA, Ames Research Center, 1985.

[7] Space Studies Board. The Search for Life's Origins, National Academy Press, Washington, D.C., 1990, p. 24

[8] Kaula, W. 1975. In: Space Studies Board. The Search for *Life's Origins*, National Academy Press, Washington, D.C., 1990, p. 57

[9] Bernal, J.D. The Origin of Life, World Publishing Co., Cleveland, Ohio, 1967.

[10] Cech, T.R. RNA as an enzyme. *Scientific American*, 1986, vol. 255, pp. 64-75.

[11] Darwin, C.R. *On the Origin of Species by Means of Natural Selection*, John Murray, London, 1859.

[12] Margulis, L. *Symbiosis in Cell Evolution*, W. H. Freeman, San Francisco, 1981.

[13] Margulis, L., Schwartz, K.V. *Five Kingdoms: An Illustrated Guide to the Phyla of Life on Earth.*, W. H. Freeman, New York, 1989, 2nd edition, p. xvi pp. 1-376.

[14] Woese, C. Archaebacteria. Scientific American, 1981, vol. 244, pp. 98-100

[15] Adapted from Woese, C. Archaebacteria. *Scientific American*, 1981, vol. 244, pp. 98-100

[16] Milne, D., Raup, D., Billingham, J., Niklaus, K., Padian, K. (Eds.). *The Evolution of Complex and Higher Organisms*, NASA SP-478, 1985, pp. 1-197.

[17] Milankovich, M. Kanon der Erd*bestrahlung und sein Andwendung auf das Eiszeitenproblem*, Roy. Serb., 1941, Acad. Spec. Publ. 132.

[18] Sharpton, V. I., Ward, P.D. (Eds.) *Global Catastrophes in Earth History: An Interdisciplinary Conference on Impacts, Volcanism, and Mass Mortality*, 1990, Geological Society of America Special Paper No. 247.

[19] Pope, K.O., Ocampo, A.C., Duller, C.E. Mexican site for K/T impact crater? *Nature*, 1991, Vol. 351, p. 105.

[20] Soffen, G.A. The Viking Project. *Journal of Geophysical Research*, 1977, Vol. 82, pp. 3959-3970.

[21] Klein, H.P. The Viking biological experiments on Mars. *Icarus*, 1978, Vol. 34, pp. 666-674.

[22] DeFrees, D., Brownlee, D., Tarter, J., Usher, D., Irvine, W., Klein, H. *Exobiology in Earth Orbit*, NASA, Ames Research Center, 1989.

[23] Mumma, M.J., Smith, H.J. (Eds.) *Astrophysics from the Moon,* American Institute of Physics Conference Proceedings 207, New York, 1990.

[24] Treaty on principles governing the activities of states in the exploration and use of outer space, including the moon and other celestial bodies, Article IX, U.N. Doc. A/RES/2222/ (XXI) 25 Jan. 1967; TIAS No. 6347, 1967.

[25] NASA Management Instruction 8020.7C, 1991.

Chapter 7

Earth and the Biosphere:
Planetary Metabolism as a Paradigm for Global Biology

Berrien Moore III and David S. Bartlett

I. Introduction

Viewing the Earth from space has greatly stimulated "holistic" concepts of the important processes that control and respond to changes in the global environment. From this perspective the Earth functions as a "metabolic" system of linked parts in which changes in one part affect the others in complex ways. In this global context it is useful to envision Earth as encompassing several distinct but interrelated "spheres." The physical-chemical environment is divided into the lithosphere, consisting of the solid Earth and soils; the hydrosphere, consisting of surface waters in oceans, lakes, rivers, and streams; the cryosphere, the frozen water in polar ice caps, glaciers, ice, and snow; and the atmosphere, the gaseous environment above the Earth's surface. Current environmental concerns encompass all of these spheres. Some concerns include the loss of arable soils by erosion and degraded fertility; management of the supplies and quality of fresh water for human consumption and agriculture; the potential for expansion or contraction of polar ice masses resulting in sea-level changes; and observed changes in atmospheric composition, with possible consequences ranging from risks for human health to unprecedented impacts on global climate.

The unique characteristics of the Earth system, as well as much of the potential for major environmental perturbations, rest with the fifth major sphere, the biosphere, consisting of all living things. Virtually all of the aspects of the Earth's physical-chemical environment are quite different from those that would be observed on an "abiotic" world. Plants and animals consume and produce various compounds, altering the chemical composition of the other spheres. Plants alter the physical environment by changing the reflectivity, or albedo, of the surface and by transporting water from soils to the atmosphere. The human component of the biosphere is responsible for well-documented changes in the distribution and composition of plant and animal life, in the chemical composition of the atmosphere, and in the distribution and quality of water, among many others. However, human activities take place in the context of major interactions and feedbacks among the various spheres that have controlled and altered the Earth system since its origins. Consequently, if we are to predict the consequences of human activities, we must understand the Earth as a system, and in particular, we must understand the biosphere and its behavior under both natural and perturbed circumstances. Inquiries in pursuit of this understanding have been called "Earth system science," and life scientists clearly have a major role in identifying, monitoring, and predicting the changing characteristics of the biosphere and its interactions with the physical-chemical environment.

A science that chooses the globe as its fundamental biogeophysical unit faces extraordinary conceptual difficulties. The questions that can be asked about biology at this level are not immediately obvious. It is also not clear how to formulate theories or experiments for a biological system of this size. From the viewpoint of the physical sciences, the scale is not particularly grand; geophysics, meteorology, and astrophysics often measure systems of planetary magnitude and larger. However, the consideration of biological systems on a planetary scale is new, and appropriate paradigms are needed to understand ecosystem dynamics at the global level.

The primary dictum of global biology is that "energy flows and matter cycles." The first part of this statement is a consequence of the second law of thermodynamics. Energy must move from low entropy sources to high entropy sinks; sustained reversal of this direction of flow will result in a violation of one of the most universal laws that has emerged within science. The second part of the primary dictum, dealing with the global cycling of matter, also follows from the laws of physics, but in a less well understood way which would be appropriate to clarify.

A closed system is defined as one through which there is no flow of matter. The Earth approximates such a system, although the hydrogen leak to space and arrival of cosmic debris are not negligible on a geological time scale. In any case, an abstract closed system conserves atoms but allows for variation in molecular composition and spatial distribution. When electromagnetic energy flows into a closed system, its subsequent flux is determined by the spectral distribution of the radiation and the molecules present in the system. Energy that enters the system can be converted into chemical potential, heat, or macroscopic configurational energy, which is largely gravitational in the case of the Earth. For chemical or

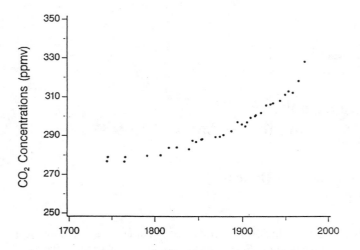

Fig. 1 Atmospheric CO$_2$ concentrations since about 1750 derived from the Siple ice core in West Antarctica.[1]

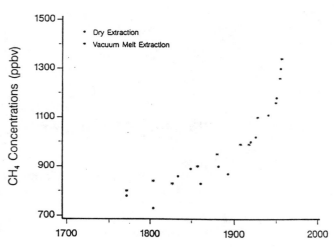

Fig. 2 Atmospheric methane concentrations since about 1770 derived from the Siple ice core. Two methods of extraction are compared, showing excellent agreement.[1]

gravitational energy the second law's tendencies toward degradation limit the accumulation and result in a constant flux from these low entropy forms to the higher entropy form of thermal energy. The flow of heat from the system to a thermal sink is the final stage in energy processing.

All closed systems with an energy flux from a source, whose spectral distribution is very different from the system's own black body distribution, are subject to an energy pumping to high levels of chemical potential and a second law relaxation to thermal levels. The existence of geochemical cycles is the inevitable result of the energy flow in a closed system. In a planet devoid of life this can be seen in high and low chemical potential compounds such as those observed on Mars. When biota are present they are of necessity involved in the flows that lead to biogeochemical cycles. The form of the cycles depends on biological and geological factors, but their existence is deeply embedded in the physical-chemical properties of closed systems subject to energy flux. A consideration of chemical thermodynamics makes possible one further conclusion. One component of the chemical cycle will be the molecular form of the element with the largest enthalpy of formation, given the other atoms present and other boundary conditions such as temperature and pressure. The second law tells us that the system is constantly drawing toward a chemical equilibrium in which all of the elements are combined in their lowest energy states, such as carbon dioxide, phosphate, sulfate, and so forth. The most efficient cycles will be able to operate with these chemical forms.

The critical role of living systems in all of the Earth's geochemical cycles is a relatively recent discovery. The recognition of biotic factors as potential homeostatic controls of biogeochemical cycles has allowed for significant advances in our understanding of the natural metabolism responsible for the compositions of the atmosphere, oceans, and sediments on the surface of our planet. Since such a planetary metabolism is now, and has been for some time in the past,

interactive, wherein physical, chemical and biological processes are inextricably linked, quantifying the contribution of the biota, as we noted earlier, is essential for a better understanding of global processes. The recognition of living organisms as a global homeostatic control factor can be attributed to the fact that, even though biological reactions allow for extremely high chemical fluxes globally, such fluxes are characterized by high turnover rates in some instances, and are thus underestimated because of what appears to be a very modest net synthesis on a global scale. Because of the restricted elemental make-up of biological systems, the possible chemical transformations that are directly mediated by the biota are limited in number and dominated by the elements carbon, nitrogen, phosphorus, and sulfur.

In sum, the varied dynamic patterns reflected in various states of the biogeochemical cycles are the consequences of a myriad of biological, chemical, and physical processes that operate across a wide spectrum of time and space scales. In the absence of significant disturbances, these processes define a natural cycle for each element with approximate balances in sources and sinks that result in a quasi-steady state for the cycle, at least on time scales less than a millennium.

This quasi-steady state no longer exists on Earth. Although humans have always modified natural systems, the signature of our collective activities has only begun to become evident during the last 300 years. In particular, since the beginning of the Industrial Revolution, human activity has significantly altered biogeochemical cycling at the planetary scale. The magnitude of human disturbance of biogeochemical cycles now may be approaching a critical level. The values of important state variables, such as the concentration of atmospheric carbon dioxide (CO$_2$) and methane (CH$_4$), as well as their derivatives, are moving into a range without historical precedent. For example, during the 30 years between 1957 and 1987, the pool of carbon in the atmosphere (in the form of CO$_2$) has increased from 670 to more than 740 Pg (10^{15} g) C

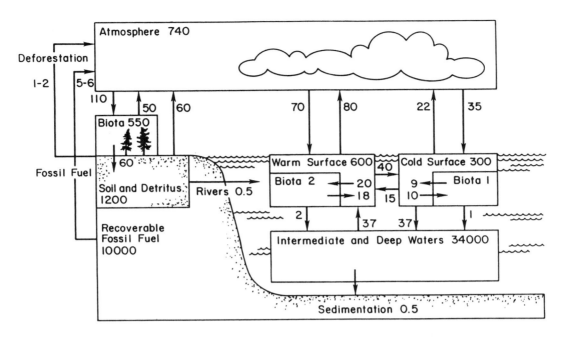

Fig. 3 The global carbon cycle.[3] Units are Pg (10^{15} g). Reprinted with permission from Academic Press, Inc.

as a result of fossil fuel burning and forest clearing. The annual rate of increase of CO_2 is currently about 3 Pg C (equivalent to roughly 0.4 percent); CH_4 is increasing by 1 percent per year. From ice core records we know that the concentrations of both CO_2 and CH_4 were relatively constant for several thousand years before 1700. Since 1700 the concentrations of CO_2 and CH_4 have increased by more than 25 percent and 100 percent, respectively (Figs. 1 and 2).

The increase in the atmospheric CO_2 and CH_4 concentrations, as well as in other greenhouse gases, due to human activity has produced serious concerns regarding the heat balance of the global atmosphere.

II. Biogeochemical Cycles

The principal material cycles relevant to the biosphere's role in the Earth system are those of carbon (C), nitrogen (N), phosphorus (P), sulfur (S), and water. There are numerous excellent descriptions of these biogeochemical cycles in the literature including, most recently, the one by Schlesinger.[2] For our purposes we will summarize the general aspects of these important cycles as background for the following discussion of major issues for Earth system science and studies of the biosphere.

A. Carbon Cycle

Carbon, as the major component of organic compounds, and its cycling are of critical importance in the Earth system. The major reservoirs through which carbon is cycled on time scales less than millennia are the atmosphere, terrestrial biota and soils, and the oceans. Figure 3 shows these elements of the carbon cycle from the perspective of CO_2 and the esti-

mated flows between them in schematic form. In the atmosphere carbon is present in trace concentrations, primarily as CO_2 (approximately 355 ppmv), secondarily as CH_4 (1.7 ppmv), and in very small amounts of other compounds. As described above, concentrations of CO_2 and CH_4 are increasing by approximately 0.4 percent/yr and 1.0 percent/yr respectively. The mass of carbon in the atmosphere (approximately 740 Pg) is comparable to that in each of the compartments at the Earth's surface: terrestrial biomass (550 Pg), soil and detritus (1200 Pg), and the surface ocean (900 Pg). By far the largest pool of carbon is found in the intermediate and deep waters of the world ocean (34,000 Pg) as dissolved inorganic carbon, primarily as the carbonate (10 percent) and bicarbonate (90 percent) ions. The size of the dissolved organic pool is uncertain, but there is a general agreement that the pool is about 1000 Pg C. Within the terrestrial pool carbon is largely incorporated into organic molecules in living and dead biomass.

Atmospheric CO_2 is consumed by the biosphere through photosynthesis and returned to the atmosphere through autotrophic and heterotrophic respiration. The seasonality of these processes in the large ecosystems of the temperate and boreal Northern Hemisphere produces an annual oscillation in the atmospheric concentration of about 5 ppmv (10.6 Pg/yr). However, this seasonal net change masks what must be a very much larger amount of carbon that is cycled annually through the biosphere (Fig. 4). The magnitude of the global biospheric pool as well as the total and net amounts of carbon cycled through this pool are poorly known, and the values shown in Fig. 3 are estimates subject to large uncertainties.

A current estimate of total carbon fixed annually by photosynthesis (total primary production) in the terrestrial biosphere is 110 Pg. Of this amount, approximately half (50 Pg)

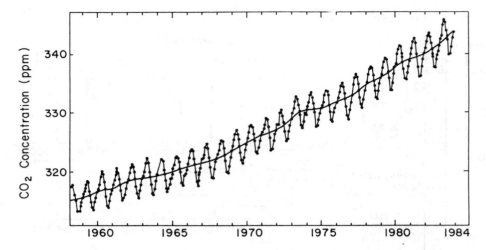

Fig. 4 Changes in atmospheric CO_2 concentration from 1958 to 1984 measured at Mauna Loa Observatory, Hawaii.[4]

is believed to return quickly to the atmosphere through autotrophic respiration, whereas approximately another half (60 Pg) is returned each year through decomposition of dead material. This leaves the terrestrial biosphere in approximate steady state with respect to net accumulation of carbon. However, the annual increase in atmospheric CO_2, attributed to human activities, is about 3 Pg (less than 3 percent of estimated total annual production). Therefore, a relatively small deviation from steady state in the balance of total production and respiration/decay could have a major impact on the change in atmospheric composition. Interestingly, ice core records indicate that the pre-industrial carbon cycle was essentially in balance for several thousand years, but large changes in the atmospheric concentration occurred in earlier times.

In the ocean, the pool of particulate organic carbon is quite small relative to that on land (approximately 3 Pg). Yet the dynamics of growth and decay in marine phytoplankton produces very rapid turnover, so that the total annual production by marine biota is relatively large (estimated at 30 Pg/yr). As on land, very small deviations from the approximate balance between total production and respiration could therefore have large consequences for the small net change in atmospheric concentration. The fact that the ice core record reveals a relatively constant atmospheric CO_2 concentration for several thousand years before 1700 indicates that biological activity was relatively constant. There is little reason to believe that it is responding to the increase in atmospheric concentration today; therefore, it is unlikely that marine biota are serving as a net sink for the excess CO_2 now entering the atmosphere.

The major sink for the "excess" CO_2 is simple diffusion at the sea surface and subsequent downward mixing into the vast pool of dissolved inorganic carbon in the world ocean. Exchange between this inorganic pool and atmospheric CO_2 is governed by ocean circulation and physical-chemical exchange rates across the water surface and is believed to result in a net sink for atmospheric CO_2 of about 3 Pg/yr. This

accounts for about half of the amount added to the atmosphere annually through fossil fuel burning (6 Pg). Added to the observed annual increase in atmospheric burden of 3 Pg, the results are in a rough balance between estimated fossil sources and sinks. However, there is compelling evidence that changing land use, principally forest clearing for agriculture (deforestation), results in a net flux of carbon to the atmosphere.[5-15] The current net flux is estimated to be between 1 and 2 Pg C as CO_2 per year. If correct, this means that an additional sink for 1-2 Pg C per year remains to be identified, and/or that the net ocean sink may have been underestimated.

A possible additional long-term sink for carbon may be the terrestrial biosphere. It has been suggested[16] that the terrestrial biosphere is consuming the excess carbon and storing it in increasing biomass, particularly in the temperate/boreal Northern Hemisphere. In effect this means, as discussed above, that in these areas the annual total production is slightly larger than the sum of respiration and decomposition, resulting in a net carbon sink. It is possible that increasing CO_2 concentrations have "fertilized," and thus enhanced, the growth of temperate forests although other nutrients, in particular nitrogen, generally are limiting to growth in these environments. It is also possible that regrowth in deforested areas is compensating for most of the source produced when existing vegetation was cleared; however, this was considered by Moore et al.[5] and Houghton et al.,[6,12] and discounted. Whether or not the balance is currently providing a net carbon sink, it has been proposed that such a sink could be created by a large program of forest replanting.

Processes producing and consuming CH_4 are also important elements of the global carbon cycle. The amounts of carbon present as CH_4 are small relative to CO_2 (only 1.7 ppmv in the atmosphere). However, CH_4 is very active both chemically and radiatively (its "greenhouse" activity is approximately 20 times that of CO_2 on a per molecule basis) and it therefore plays an important role in atmospheric chemistry and radiative transfer. In addition, its concentration in the atmosphere is increasing at roughly double the rate of increase

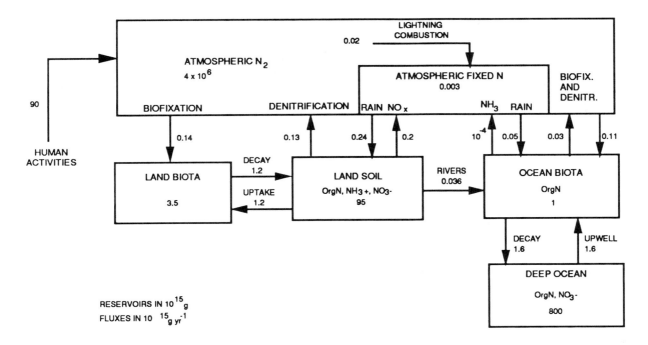

Fig. 5 Global nitrogen cycle.[17]

of CO_2. Fossil CH_4 is released to the atmosphere from coal mining and natural gas recovery and distribution, but the major sources of CH_4 are related to microbial decomposition of organic material under anaerobic conditions.

Suitable methanogenic circumstances of abundant organic detritus and anaerobic conditions are found in natural swamps and marshes and in rice paddies (where wet soils restrict transport of oxygen), and in landfills and the guts of termites and ruminant animals. These are the principal sources of CH_4 to the atmosphere, with wetlands and paddies thought to contribute about half the estimated total annual source of .54 Pg C per year. The annual increase in the atmospheric CH_4 burden is .04 Pg C per year. The .5 Pg C per year as CH_4 not accounted for by increasing atmospheric burden is believed to be lost primarily in reactions with the hydroxyl radical (OH) in the atmosphere, a process that produces water vapor (an important "greenhouse gas" in its own right). It consumes OH stocks that would otherwise be available for reaction with other atmospheric trace elements.

Given the large natural sources of CH_4, it is not clear what drives the rapid increase in concentration observed in recent atmospheric measurements and in ice core records. Like the increase in CO_2, atmospheric CH_4 concentrations began to rise from prehistoric levels at the beginning of the 19th century, implicating anthropogenic origins (Fig. 2). Current theory is that rapidly increasing human populations dating from that period expanded the magnitude of rice cultivation and of domestic ruminant animal herds. More recently, increases in coal mining and natural gas recovery, as well as in sources from landfills and biomass burning, have added to the anthropogenic contributions. It is also possible that, as concentrations of CH_4 and other reactive species in the

atmosphere have risen, increased competition for the relatively small pool of atmospheric OH has reduced the magnitude of that sink. The magnitudes of the sources, sinks, and transfer rates for CH_4 are subject to great uncertainty and the only reasonably constrained value is that of the atmospheric burden and the annual increase in that burden.

Many aspects of the global carbon cycle are not well understood. Uncertainty centers on the role of terrestrial ecosystems, in which at least two factors govern the level of carbon storage. First and most obvious is the alteration of the Earth's surface, such as the conversion of forest to agriculture that results in a net release of CO_2 to the atmosphere. Second and more subtle is the possible change in net ecosystem production resulting from changes of global cycles. Measuring such changes will require a much clearer understanding of the nitrogen and phosphorus cycles, since they (not carbon) are the limiting nutrients in most terrestrial ecosystems. Unfortunately, our knowledge of the way these biogeochemical cycles relate to each other compares poorly even with our general understanding of the individual cycles themselves. In addition, although large quantities of carbon do not pass through the CH_4 cycle, production and consumption of this radiatively and chemically important gas are dominated by biospheric processes that are not well quantified. These uncertainties about the global carbon cycle are important and must continue to receive intense scientific attention.

B. Nitrogen Cycle

Nitrogen is essential for many biological processes, and like carbon, is cycled through atmospheric, terrestrial, and oceanic pools—both organic and inorganic (Fig. 5). The largest pool of nitrogen, unlike carbon, resides in virtually-inert molecular form in the atmosphere. Biologically and chemically active forms of nitrogen are created through "fixation," in which molecular nitrogen is broken into individual atoms and recombined with other elements forming, for example, nitrite, nitrate, nitrous and nitric oxide, and ammonia. In these fixed forms, nitrogen is a critical nutrient that is the limiting factor for growth in many biological systems. In the atmosphere, nitrous oxide is a potentially significant greenhouse gas and an important constituent in the production/destruction cycle of stratospheric ozone. Nitric oxide is a major contributor to urban "smog."

A small amount of nitrogen fixation takes place in the atmosphere when lightning dissociates molecular nitrogen. A larger amount is fixed by soil (.14 Pg N per year) and marine (.03 Pg N per year) microbes that are often living a symbiotic existence with photosynthetic organisms that use the fixed nitrogen. An estimate of the annual uptake of nitrogen by terrestrial biota is 1.2 Pg; much larger than the amount of newly fixed nitrogen available. The deficit is made up through recycling of nitrogen released from decomposing organic detritus. Similarly, in the oceans, the majority of nitrogen sustaining biological production is recycled within the water column with 10 percent or less supplied from a combination of biological fixation, rainfall, and run-off from land. Highly specialized terrestrial and marine microbial communities also return molecular nitrogen to the atmosphere as a by-product of their unique metabolism—a process called "denitrification"—closing the cycle between molecular nitrogen and fixed forms. Except for the size and rates of change of atmospheric nitrogen pools, the pools and flows within the nitrogen cycle are poorly quantified.[2, 18]

Human activities have had significant impacts on the nitrogen cycle, particularly concerning atmospheric concentrations of fixed nitrogen and through the fertilization of agricultural systems and run-off to freshwater and nearshore marine environments. For example, the pool size of atmospheric N_2O, which is about 1500 Tg (10^{12} g) nitrogen, is increasing by 0.2 to 0.3 percent per year. A large portion of this increase may be due to accelerated fossil fuel and biomass burning over the past 40 years. There have also been large increases in the application of nitrogen fertilizer and in the discharge of sewage. Much of the nitrogen in fertilizer and sewage is reaching recipient aquatic systems such as groundwater, wetlands, rivers, estuaries, and the coastal ocean. Estimates of the N_2O generated as a result of this eutrophication show that total releases have increased by 50 percent over the past 50 years.

When humans burn fossil fuels, they not only release large amounts of carbon to the atmosphere, but they may also increase the input of nitrogen. Some of this nitrogen may enter terrestrial ecosystems in precipitation. This rise in available nitrogen may stimulate both carbon fixation and storage in, for instance, forest ecosystems. Conversely, wood harvests can reduce not only the carbon stock for forest ecosystems, but the nitrogen stock as well. First, nitrogen exits the forest in harvested material. Second, erosion, accelerated by the harvest, carries off nitrogen-bearing soil. Third, forest cutting can dramatically raise losses of inorganic nitrogen, principally nitrate removed in solution by streams that drain cutover areas. A fourth pathway may also exist: wood harvests may stimulate denitrification. In addition, there is another possible coupling between carbon and nitrogen through fire. Rapid oxidation of carbon in litter with a high C:N ratio reduces the amount of nitrogen that can be immobilized by microorganisms during decay, thereby increasing the amount of nitrogen available to plants. Further understanding of these cycles will require a clearer picture of the coupling between the two elements.

C. Phosphorus Cycle

Phosphorus, like nitrogen, is a critical nutrient that is in short supply in biologically available form and so is a limiting factor for production of terrestrial and marine biota. Its relative insolubility limits its availability to organisms in soils, rivers, and oceans; sedimentary deposits provide its major reservoirs. Phosphorus is nonvolatile, a quality that restricts its role in atmospheric chemistry. Phosphorus is transported, primarily in particulate form, in rivers from the large terrestrial pool into the oceans, where much of it is deposited in bottom sediments. To an even greater extent than nitrogen, therefore, recycling of organic phosphorus provides the stocks needed for production in the biosphere.[2] In the absence of human activity, these characteristics limit this element's role in global biogeochemical cycling.

Human activity, however, has altered the availability of phosphorus in direct and indirect ways. For example, most major rivers and estuaries have undergone eutrophication due to the addition of phosphate from agricultural, urban, and industrial sources. The application of phosphorus fertilizer is a direct perturbation, but subtler alterations of the phosphorus cycle may influence the dynamics of other cycles. Fire, either natural or as a management technique, may increase the available stocks of phosphorus into "more available" forms. Increased levels of available phosphorus can, in turn, raise the rate of nitrogen mineralization in soils.

D. Sulfur Cycle

The sulfur cycle is similar to that of the nitrogen cycle in that this important biological nutrient is cycled through the biosphere and atmosphere in a variety of forms, several of which are biogenic in origin.[2, 19] Unlike nitrogen, the largest sulfur pool is in the lithosphere, with a secondary but important pool in the oceans in the form of sulfate. A large amount of sulfate is emitted directly to the atmosphere from the surface ocean in wind-blown spray. Anaerobic sulfates reducing bacteria in the oceans and terrestrial wetlands produce sulfides, primarily hydrogen sulfide but including others such as dimethyl sulfide and carbonyl sulfide, which are emitted to the atmosphere. In the atmosphere sulfur is present as sulfur

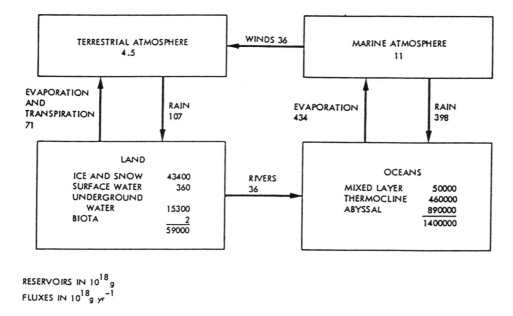

Fig. 6 Global hydrologic cycle.[17]

dioxide and lesser amounts of hydrogen sulfide. Beyond these general characteristics, the sulfur cycle is poorly understood, with less quantitative information on pool sizes and transfer rates than any other element.

What is quite certain is that anthropogenic activities must be exerting major impacts on the sulfur cycle, particularly in the atmosphere. Human activity has increased the present total global flux of sulfur to the atmosphere from a pre-industrial level of about 228 Tg S yr[-1] to a current flux of approximately 340 Tg S yr[-1], a 50 percent increase. Indirect calculations suggest that emissions of gaseous sulfur to the atmosphere from fossil fuel combustion are already on the same order of magnitude as discharges from natural systems. Some of the largest changes have occurred over continental regions where present anthropogenic emissions account for 70 percent of the total sulfur released to the atmosphere. In industrial areas sulfur dioxide (SO_2) is the major sulfur compound emitted. Sulfur dioxide is rapidly hydrolyzed to sulfuric acid (H_2SO_4), which is then deposited back to terrestrial and aquatic ecosystems in the form of acid rain.

E. Hydrologic Cycle

Since the surface of our planet is dominated by water and is subject to energy flow, the existence of water cycles also follows in a very natural way. Meteorology, hydrology, and biogeochemistry are all ultimately mediated by the ubiquitous cycling of water. Water cycles involve all of the possible energy storage modes. At the macroscopic (meteorological) level, we have the primary evaporation-precipitation cycle in which energy goes from electromagnetic (solar radiation) to thermal (heating, evaporation, and condensation) to gravitational potential (precipitation and ocean density gradients). At the molecular level we can describe the flow from H_2O to

O_2 and biological reducing power, then back to H_2O. Here the energy goes from electromagnetic to chemical to thermal.

It is important in discussing water to remind ourselves of the obvious: ordinary water is a compound of the most extraordinary macroscopic and molecular properties. We have come to understand most of these in terms of hydrogen bonds, electric asymmetry, and proton mobility. It is nonetheless remarkable that these molecular features render water such a fit substance for all its varied roles in biogeochemical and energy cycles.

Water, of course, forms the basis for all life. The cycles of all of the important elemental nutrients discussed above are therefore connected with, and ultimately controlled by, the hydrologic cycle. In addition, water is the major transporter of energy on global scales. Ocean currents carry warm tropical waters towards both poles, moderating the Earth's climate in higher latitudes. Evaporated water carries latent energy in atmospheric winds until it is released by precipitation, transporting heat away from the equator and water away from the oceans and onto land. This cycle of energy in turn drives atmospheric circulation. Density changes in the surface ocean produced by net evaporation/precipitation is a major driver of ocean circulation. In turn, circulation in the atmosphere and ocean, as well as evaporation/precipitation dynamics, controls global climate, creating a complex web of feedbacks between the hydrologic cycle and climate dynamics. An important additional factor in these interrelated hydrologic/climatic processes is that water vapor is an atmospheric greenhouse gas, and when condensed in clouds has a shading, "anti-greenhouse" effect.

The global cycle of water is summarized in Fig. 6. In simple terms, water is evaporated from its dominant pool, the oceans, and then falls as rain either back into the oceans (about 90 percent) or on land (about 10 percent). The cycle is closed over decadal time scales by river flow from land back into the oceans. On land, water may be cycled through a number of pools—ice and snow, surface water, underground water, biota, and the terrestrial atmosphere—before its ultimate return to the sea. Much of the rain falling on land is cycled back to the atmosphere in the vapor phase, where it is available for reprecipitation. This process is enhanced by vegetation that can transport water from below the soil surface and exchange it with the atmosphere through the large surface area created by leaves (evapotranspiration). Thus, as in virtually all other biogeochemical relationships, the biota are not simply passive respondents to the climatic environment, but actively change it, thus resulting in important feedbacks when human activity or other factors change the distribution or character of the biospheric elements. Deforestation, for example, can reduce local rainfall by breaking the evapotranspiration/precipitation cycle and result in permanent changes in local climate, reducing the potential for regrowth of the preexisting ecosystem.

There are major uncertainties in several elements of the hydrologic cycle, in particular in the size of the ice/snow and groundwater pools and the magnitudes of the net evaporation/precipitation balances for both the marine and terrestrial systems. In addition, the net fluxes of water from the marine to the terrestrial atmosphere and from land to the ocean in run-off are estimates accurate only to within a factor of 2. Human activities have altered the cycle in significant but poorly understood ways, both directly as in agricultural use and management of surface and groundwater, and indirectly as when clearing of natural vegetation changes evapotranspiration rates. In addition, a major concern related to the greenhouse effect and global climate changes are their consequences for the hydrologic cycle. Changes in the amount and geographic distribution of rainfall are predicted by models simulating global warming. These changes have the potential for more catastrophic consequences than increased global temperatures by themselves.

III. Important Questions

Today, major questions need to be answered regarding not only the details of global budgeting of individual cycles, but more importantly, the interactions of such cycles with each other for which very little, if any, experimental data exist. Whereas carbon (in the form of CO_2) has clearly been accumulating in the atmosphere for at least the last 20 years at the rate of 1 ppm yr^{-1}, attempts to balance the sources and sinks of atmospheric CO_2 remain elusive. Postulated carbon sinks in terrestrial and marine biota are difficult to reconcile with the limitations on primary production that are presumed imposed by nitrogen and phosphorus stocks. One difficulty lies in the higher C/N, and C/P ratio in fossil fuels as compared to organic carbon. Increases in atmospheric CO_2 stocks via fossil fuel burning are thereby not accompanied by balanced increases in availability of nitrogen and phosphorus from these sources.[20, 21] This magnifies the imbalance in the car-

bon budget by compounding the uncertainties discussed earlier regarding in estimates of the of net CO_2 release from terrestrial systems due to land use change and CO_2 uptake by the oceans.

Changes in global and regional hydrologic cycles will profoundly affect production and consumption of CH_4. The abundance and distribution of freshwater wetlands, a major source of CH_4, will be altered by modified rainfall. Further, changes in primary production in the terrestrial biosphere resulting from altered nutrient cycles will affect the pool of organic carbon available for decomposition through methanogenic pathways.

Important issues remain unresolved with respect to nitrogen cycling on land as well as in the oceans. The notion of a steady-state concentration for oceanic nitrogen (on time scales of 10^4 years) appears to be difficult to support due to the apparent imbalance between the sources of oceanic nitrogen (transport from land, input from the atmosphere, and in situ fixation) and oceanic losses (due to denitrification and removal to sediments). It has been proposed that if the present sources and sink terms are to be relied upon, oceanic nitrogen would undergo a gradual depletion on a time scale of 10^4 years followed perhaps by major deposition of nitrogen into the oceans during the onset of ice ages.[22] This problem is of profound importance, especially from a climatic point of view, since it is believed that both nitrogen and phosphorus could limit the fixation of carbon in the oceans, which in turn could profoundly affect atmospheric CO_2. The nonsteady-state condition of oceanic nitrogen rests on existing global data for sources and sinks that are meager at best, and better global data have to be acquired to validate any such hypothesis.

For terrestrial ecosystems, a major dilemma exists as to why, even though nitrogen is abundant in the atmosphere and soils, fixed nitrogen is generally the element that limits the growth of plants in both natural and agricultural ecosystems. Once again, some insights with respect to the recalcitrant nature of the nitrogen bound to organic carbon in the soil are gained by achieving an understanding of the relationships and linkages between carbon and nitrogen cycling. Considerable microbial immobilization of soil nitrogen could occur due to the much lower C:N ratios (6 to 12:1) of microbial decomposers as compared to their substrates, whose ratios are as high as 120:1 (for fresh litter) and 500:1 (for wood). In addition, the coupling of nitrogen fixation to carbon fixation is reciprocal due to their biochemistry. For example, nitrogen fixation is biochemically a very expensive process (to fix 1 mole of N_2 requires anywhere from 25-50 moles of ATP) and generally occurs at the expense of oxidation of fixed carbon. Finally, there are basic global biological issues: Why are there so many species that can fix carbon, but so few that can fix nitrogen? Is it related to the energy cost and source or other factors?

There are major questions concerning the role of phosphorus and its relationship to nitrogen and carbon cycling, particularly in aquatic systems. For example, fertilization of lakes with phosphorus increases production and seems to be

Table 1   Comparison of orbital Earth survey sensor characteristics

Sensor	Spectral Bands	Ground Resolution	Swath Width (km)	Coverage Frequency	Scene Area (km²)
AVHRR	1 VIS, 2 NIR, 2 TIR	1-4 km	2700	24 hrs (12 hrs for TIR)	126×10^5
MSS	2 VIS, 2 NIR, 1 TIR (Landsat-3)	80 m	185	16 days	34×10^5
TM	3 VIS, 3 NIR, 1 TIR	30 m	185	16 days	34×10^5
SPOT	2 VIS, 1 NIR	20 m	60 (80 in max off-nadir mode)	26 days (1-4 days in off-nadir mode)	036×10^5

VIS = Visible (400-700 nm)   NIR = Near-infrared (700-5000 nm)   TIR = Thermal infrared (8000-13,000 nm)

the major factor controlling eutrophication, despite laboratory studies suggesting that other nutrients should limit system production before phosphorus does.[23]

Our understanding of the global sulfur cycles is at an even more primitive state than that of carbon, nitrogen, or phosphorus. It is generally accepted that most of the reduced sulfur gases (hydrogen sulfide, dimethyl sulfide, etc.) are biogenic in origin, but no data exist regarding the nature of the sources or source strengths and their spatial and temporal distributions. Furthermore, such reduced gases are oxidized to SO_2, whose mechanisms and rates of reaction remain poorly understood. As many as half of the oxidized sulfur gases could be accounted for by such oxidation reactions, the other half being acquired by combustion of fossil fuels.

Clearly, the many uncertainties regarding global biogeochemical cycles require an intense research effort that links field and laboratory investigations of the underlying cycling processes, collection of large data sets that quantify pools and transfer rates on global scales, development of simulation models to fill in gaps in empirical observations and provide predictive capabilities. Space technology, in the form of remote sensors of various kinds, has revolutionized our ability to observe and measure global scale phenomena. In the following section we present examples of the development and use of orbital sensors for studies of the terrestrial carbon cycle.

IV. Global Data Collection: Remote Sensing and the Terrestrial Carbon Cycle

Terrestrial carbon cycling is mediated primarily by living vegetation and microbial transformations of dead plant material.

Vegetation assessment is one of the best-established applications of remote sensing, dating from the period when aerial photography was the only means of obtaining large area data sets. The availability of orbital multispectral scanner data, beginning with the 1972 launch of Landsat 1 (then called ERTS 1), has stimulated many further applications to mapping and assessment of land cover, land use, and vegetation.

Today, orbital scanner imagery is used routinely for vegetation inventories on regional scales. The Landsat Multi-

spectral Scanner (MSS) has two visible and two near-infrared spectral bands and images the surface with approximately 80-m resolution cells (see Table 1 for sensor descriptions). For Landsat 3, launched in 1978, a thermal infrared channel was added for detection of surface temperatures. In 1981, the Thematic Mapper (TM) instrument was added to the Landsat system. The TM has three visible, three near-infrared, and a thermal channel and improved ground infrared resolution of 30 m. The more recent French SPOT sensor has two visible and one near-infrared spectral bands and 20-m resolution. Although all of these instruments produce detailed and valuable results in studies on regional and smaller scales, they produce so much data that continental or global-scale inventories are difficult. Moreover, the associated narrow swath width often makes coverage of rapidly changing phenomena impossible over large scales. As a result, the Advanced Very High Resolution Radiometers (AVHRR) carried on meteorological satellites of the National Oceanic and Atmospheric Administration have been applied to larger area studies of vegetation dynamics. The sensors were designed primarily to focus upon the dynamics of clouds. Consequently the spectral bands are not optimized for vegetation coverage, but the wide area coverage and rapid repeat times have made the AVHRR an unexpectedly valuable sensor of vegetation dynamics (see Table 1). Specifically,

• AVHRR has 1-4 kilometer resolution and therefore reduces by more than two orders of magnitude the number of picture elements ("pixels") per unit ground area produced by the higher resolution sensors. This greatly reduces the cost of data acquisition and analysis for large areas.

• AVHRR's wide ground swath and orbital characteristics permit imaging of the entire Earth surface at least once per day. This allows much more detailed time sequences of surface changes than, for example, the 16-day coverage intervals of the Landsat sensors.

The daily coverage of AVHRR frequently allows more rapid accumulation of cloud-free data over much of the Earth's surface. In the tropics, however, cloud cover resulting from convective activity more often affects the afternoon crossing times of AVHRR than the morning overpasses of Landsat, mitigating the advantage of AVHRR at these latitudes. The SPOT sensor can be pointed off-nadir to acquire data over a particular area more frequently than its 26-day orbital cycle. Such coverage is not continuously available, however, and analysis is still burdened by large quantities of data.

In one of the first terrestrial applications of AVHRR, Tucker et al.[24] produced a map of major vegetation types for the entire continent of Africa. Three weeks of AVHRR data were composited to obtain virtually cloud-free (less than 2 percent) imagery on which to base spectral discrimination of surface cover types. It was estimated that approximately 1100 Landsat-MSS scenes would be required to cover this area; several times this number would be needed to provide cloud-free imagery. The accumulation of clear, continent-wide AVHRR data every 3 weeks permitted a detailed time course of changes in surface spectral response during a sequence of 28 three-week periods, during which expansion and contraction of zones of vigorous growth in response to changing rainfall were observed. Subsequent monitoring has documented variability in the size of the North African arid zone over a period of several years. Long-term data sets of this kind illustrate significant year-to-year variability and have the potential to identify longer term trends related, for example, to anthropogenic "desertification." However, to achieve the full value from such time series we will need to insure that the sensor is very well calibrated and that the atmospheric effects on the data are well understood.

Tucker et al.[25] have also demonstrated the use of AVHRR data in documenting the extent of tropical forest clearing in a region of Brazil. This information is particularly important if we are to evaluate fully the biotic source of CO_2 since existing estimates of the rate of Amazonian forest destruction vary widely.[26] In testing the applicability of AVHRR to determination of land use change in the tropical forests, a test of remote mapping was conducted within a 40,000 km^2 area in Rondonia, Brazil. The results indicated that disturbed forests could be measured with AVHRR, even when substantial regrowth had occurred. More recently, evidence has emerged that the higher resolution and other capabilities provided by Landsat and SPOT may be more appropriate for studies of deforestation in the tropics.[27] As noted above, the morning data acquisition times of Landsat encounter much less cloud cover in the tropics than the afternoon overpasses of AVHRR. In addition, the spectral characteristics of AVHRR are not optimal for accurate detection of clearing in many tropical environments. Finally, even where large areas are being cleared, as in western Brazil, the small size of individual clearings and large perimeter-to-area ratios of complex clearing patterns can produce large errors when using the relatively coarse spatial resolution data provided by AVHRR.[27]

Landsat has also proven particularly valuable in providing information about vegetation condition based upon the analysis of the spectral characteristics of the reflectance data. For example, a wavelength region of particular interest for high-spectral resolution study is located between the strong chlorophyll absorption at approximately 680 nm and the strong reflectance of the near infrared (NIR) plateau characteristic of

vegetation reflectance curves. This sharp rise in reflectance is known as the red edge, and previous studies have related subtle 5-15 nm shifts in its position to changes in chlorophyll type and amount.[28-32] A diagnostic shift of the chlorophyll absorption feature and the red edge to slightly shorter wavelengths (known as the blue shift) has been shown to characterize in situ and airborne spectral data acquired from trees undergoing forest decline in both the U.S. and Germany.[31-34]

What is particularly valuable in these studies is that not only can we begin to map and thereby document the extent of forest decline throughout the world, but we may be able to probe the connections between changing biogeochemical cycles. For instance, changes in the nitrogen cycle may be leading to nitrogen saturation of boreal and temperate forest ecosystems. This saturation may lead to acidification of soils and increased mobility of aluminum in surface waters, and to pathological imbalances of essential nutrients such as carbon, nitrogen, phosphorous, and sulfur in plants. Remote detection of nitrogen saturation through measurement of changes in nitrogen and lignin content of canopies shows great promise.[35]

In addition to the impact of nitrogen saturation on temperate forests, phytotoxic effects of elevated tropospheric ozone on sensitive boreal forest species appear to act as a predisposing factor that adversely affects total chlorophyll concentration in those species. This, in turn, may affect carbon allocation of fixed carbon compounds such as lignin and tannins, which influence decay rates, nutrient cycling, below-ground biomass, and other factors affecting the vigor and growth of the ecosystem. High-spectral resolution sensors can provide precise details of the red chlorophyll absorption maximum and adjacent red edge reflectance texture in the visible/near infrared that may be used to monitor subtle changes in total chlorophyll concentrations of forest canopies.

Potentially, major fluxes of carbon can also be quantified using remote sensing. Using AVHRR data, Tucker et al.[36] have shown the existence of an important correlation between the Normalized Difference Vegetation Index (NDVI—a linear combination of reflectance in the red and NIR spectral regions) derived from AVHRR data and atmospheric CO_2 concentrations, and therefore global net primary production (NPP). This extends to a global scale the work of Goward et al.,[37] which related NPP and NDVI for temperate ecosystems.

Such large area monitoring of changes in vegetative mass has obvious application to studies of the cycling of carbon between atmosphere and biosphere. The decreases in atmospheric CO_2 during spring/summer periods of intense plant growth and subsequent increase of CO_2 during the high-latitude winter were clearly associated with observed changes by Tucker et al.[36] in their use of remotely measured vegetation indices.

Although these and other studies have shown remote measurements to be responsive to relative changes in vegetation amount, there is no current way to calibrate large area measurements to permit quantitative calculation of the rate of assimilation of CO_2 by plants. Such calculations are clearly required to address the question of whether terrestrial vegetation is serving as a net source or sink for CO_2.

Recent research in the field has indicated that such rate measurements may eventually be possible. For example, Bartlett et al.[38] and Whiting et al.[39] have demonstrated a strong relationship between the vegetation index used by Tucker et al.[36] and the net CO_2 consumption in experimental plots of vegetation in temperate wetlands and subarctic tundra. Similar results have been obtained for other vegetation types. The sensitivity of spectral vegetation indices to CO_2 exchange is a result of their relationship with a canopy's chlorophyll density and thus its capacity to absorb photosynthetically active radiation (PAR). Because absorbed PAR is the energy source for photosynthetic fixation of CO_2, its value can be quantitatively converted to a carbon assimilation rate. Remote measurements can therefore be used to construct a summation of PAR absorbed by a canopy through time and to calculate the carbon assimilated. Variable plant physiologies and environmental conditions will, of course, affect both the remote detection of absorbed PAR and the photosynthetic efficiency. More experimental work is required before remotely sensed data can be used to calculate carbon source/sink strengths for large areas of heterogeneous vegetation. Nevertheless, the global multispectral data to accomplish this task are now being acquired by AVHRR and other sensors, and when suitable analysis algorithms are established, retrospective analysis should permit evaluation of temporal changes in vegetative source/sink strengths.

A. Assessing Biogenic Methane Sources

In addition to their direct involvement in global carbon cycling, vegetative processes are of interest as effective integrators of the physical-chemical characteristics of their environment. Temperature, water, and nutrient availability, and soil composition combine to control the worldwide distribution of terrestrial vegetation. These parameters exert critical influences on a number of other biospheric processes that are not as readily observed as the distribution of plant characteristics. Sensing of vegetation can therefore often serve as a substitute for direct observation of important processes and their products.

For example, as we have seen, the global CH_4 cycle is critically dependent on the distribution and magnitude of natural wetland sources. Wetland vegetation is usually distinct from that of drier habitats and displays sensitivity to varying conditions within large wetland ecosystems. Remote vegetation inventories can therefore be expected to provide data on both the extent of wetland habitats and on factors that may modulate the rate of CH_4 emission from these habitats. An experimental inventory of CH_4 missions in the Florida Everglades wetland system has been performed to test these expectations.[40] Landsat TM (Table 1) data were used to map vegetation types within a 1400 km^2 test site. Field measurements of CH_4 flux were used to determine the magnitude of emissions from the various vegetation types identified in Landsat imagery. It was found that several distinct CH_4

emission regimes were present within the test site, and that more than an order of magnitude separated the strongest from the weakest sources even though soils were saturated virtually throughout the site. Vegetation type was a better indicator of these regimes than other observed variables such as temperature, soil depth, and water depth. As a result, a regional CH_4 emission inventory was produced by image analysis and measurement of the area of each CH_4/vegetation regime. Total flux from the test site estimated in this way ranged from 43,000 kg/day during the dry season to 55,000 kg/day during the wet season.

The implication of these results for global assessment of CH_4 fluxes is clear. Although direct observation of CH_4 emissions from space is not currently possible, *existing* orbital imagery has the potential to provide estimates of source strengths through mapping of relevant vegetative communities and their hydrologic status.

V. Developing the Earth System Models: A Possible Strategy for Global Biogeochemical Studies

The Earth system can be viewed as being composed of two interacting subsystems: the physical-climate subsystem and the biogeochemical subsystem, linked by the global hydrologic cycle. Progress in understanding the Earth as a system requires a better quantitative understanding of the global biogeochemical subsystem.

We have made significant progress in gaining insight into the dynamics of the physical-climate subsystem; however, progress in developing a firm quantitative understanding of the planet's biogeochemical subsystem is less satisfying. Models of the physical-climate subsystem, so-called general circulation models (GCMs), exist at a variety of institutions around the world; prognostic global biogeochemical models are at a relatively primitive stage. The challenge to those who study the planet's metabolic system is to develop a suite of global biogeochemical models. These models need to be comparable in prognostic dynamics to the current GCMs and in time would be linked, partly through the hydrological coupling, to GCMs, thereby providing models of the Earth system.

There has been recent progress on putting chemistry (and in the case of the oceans, biology) into the general circulation components: the atmosphere and oceans. For example, the addition of simple (though increasingly complex) biological-biogeochemical models into ocean GCMs (e.g., the Princeton-GFDL effort) could allow for the study of biological changes under a forcing of changing climate and ocean circulation fields. Of particular interest would be the species shifts and other ecological transitions that likely would occur in a changing climate. These issues are not yet considered in this complex modeling environment (within a GCM) and therefore changes in the biogeochemical system that might result from ecological changes are not treated. Also in this context, though there is no true coupling (the physics drives the biology; there is no feedback from the biology such as effects

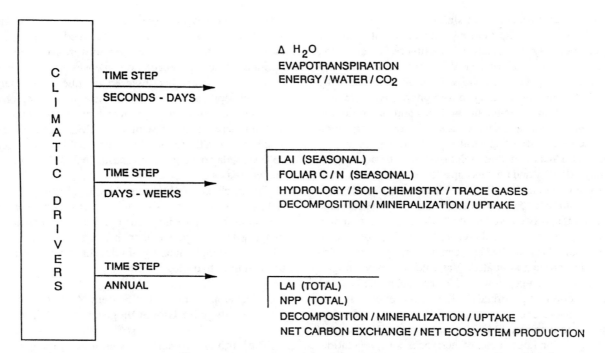

Fig. 7 Time constants associated with various physical and biological processes. Reprinted with permission from *Research Strategies for the U.S. Global Change Research Program*, 1990. Published by National Academy Press, Washington, DC.

on mixed layer depth), the structure certainly has the potential of allowing a biological feedback on the circulation.

Recently, some exploratory attempts have been made to study the response of the model-coupled climate system to realistic time-evolving scenarios of the greenhouse forcing. However, coupling oceanic and atmospheric models introduces new problems of long-term drift and instabilities that are not exhibited by the uncoupled models. Further, adding biogeochemical processes to coupled ocean-atmosphere GCMs is a prerequisite for complete description of the effect of CO_2 removed from the atmosphere by the ocean. Adding biology and chemistry to GCMs is a nontrivial exercise: the complexity of the fine-scale response of uncoupled ecological models, if proven necessary, could potentially overwhelm available and foreseen computing resources.

The next major effort needs to occur in terrestrial systems, wherein we develop the proper treatments of the exchange between terrestrial systems and atmospheric biogeochemical compounds, including water and energy. In addition, terrestrial models need to incorporate ecosystem dynamics.

VI. Developing the Terrestrial Component of Earth System Models: The Next Step

The possibility of major changes in the global environment presents a difficult task to the scientific research community: to devise ways of analyzing the causes of and projecting the course of these shifts as they are occurring. Purely observational approaches are inadequate for providing the needed predictive or anticipatory information, because response times

of many terrestrial ecosystems are slow and there is much variability from place to place. Furthermore, many important processes cannot be measured directly over large areas, such as those processes that occur in soil. We need models to express our understanding of the complex subsystems of the Earth and how they interact with, respond to, and control changes in the physical-climate and biogeochemical subsystems.

The primary research issues in understanding the role of terrestrial ecosystems in global change is the analysis of how processes with vastly differing rates of change, from photosynthesis to community change, are coupled. Representing this coupling in models is the central challenge to modeling the terrestrial biosphere as part of the Earth system.

Terrestrial ecosystems participate in climate and in the biogeochemical cycles on several temporal scales. The metabolic processes that are responsible for plant growth and maintenance and the microbial turnovers associated with decomposition of organic matter, move carbon and water through rapid as well as intermediate temporal scale circuits in plants and soil. Moreover, this cycle includes key controls over biogenic trace gas production. Some of the carbon fixed by photosynthesis is incorporated into plant tissue and delayed from returning to the atmosphere until it is oxidized by decomposition or fire. This slower carbon loop through the terrestrial component of the carbon cycle, which is matched by cycles of nutrients required by plants and decomposers, affects the increasing trend in atmospheric CO_2 concentration and imposes a seasonal cycle on that trend (Fig. 4). The structure of terrestrial ecosystems, which responds on even

LEVEL 1

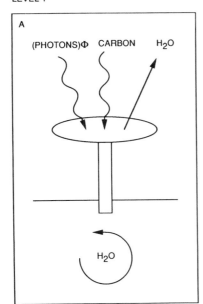

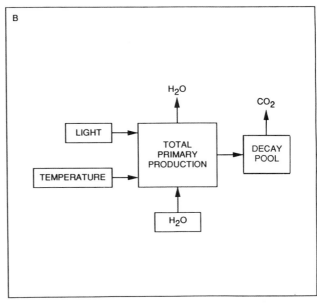

Fig. 8 Schematic representation (A) and model configuration (B) for processes with time constants of seconds to days (level one models). (A) shows a conceptual model of a land plant with an input of photons (or photosynthetically active radiation, PAR) and carbon, and an output of water vapor. Reprinted with permission from *Research Strategies for the U.S. Global Change Research Program*, 1990. Published by National Academy Press, Washington, DC.

longer time scales, is the integrated response to the intermediate time-scale carbon machinery. The loop is closed back to the climate system since it is the structure of ecosystems, including species composition, that sets the terrestrial boundary condition in the climate system from the standpoint of surface roughness, albedo, and to a great extent, latent heat exchange.

These separate temporal scales contain explicit feedback loops that may modify the system dynamics. Consider again the coupling of long-term climate change with vegetation change. Climate change will drive vegetation dynamics, but as the vegetation changes in amount or structure, this will feed back to the atmosphere through changing water, energy, and gas exchanges. Biogeochemical cycling will also change, altering the exchange of trace gas species. The long-term change in climate, driven by chemical forcing functions (CO_2, CH_4) will drive long-term ecosystem change. Modeling these interactions requires coupling successional models to biogeochemical models to physiological models that describe the exchange of water and energy between the vegetation and the atmosphere at fine time scales. There is no obvious way to allow direct reciprocal coupling of GCM-type models of the atmosphere, which inherently run with fine time constants, directly to ecosystem or successional models, which have coarse temporal resolution, without the interposition of a physiological model. This is equally true for biogeochemical models of the exchange of CO_2 and trace species. This cross-time-scale coupling is nontrivial and sets the focus for the modeling strategy.

Intuitively, we might develop a global model of terrestrial ecosystem dynamics by combining descriptions of each of the physical, chemical, and biological processes involved in the system. In such a scheme, longer term vegetation changes are derived by integrating the responses of rapidly responding parts of the model. But we cannot simply integrate models that describe the rapid processes of CO_2 diffusion, photosynthesis, fluid transport, respiration, and transpiration in cells and leaves to estimate productivity of whole plants, let alone entire ecosystems. The nature of the spatial averaging implied in the selection of parameters and processes is difficult to consider because of nonlinearities, which means that the choice of scale influences the calculation of averages.

To progress in the development of terrestrial ecological models, we choose processes to treat in different models based on the phenomenological scales involved. As is common in physical models, terms in fundamental equations can be included or ignored depending on the temporal and spatial scales or interest (e.g., ignoring gravitational effects in quantum physics, including Coriolis effects in large-scale fluid motion, etc.). Careful organization of a suite of models, each describing processes that operate at different rates, is crucial to the practical development of terrestrial ecosystem models for use in Earth system models of global change.

Atmosphere-biosphere interactions can be captured with simulations operating with three characteristic time constants, based on current model structures (Fig. 7). The first level represents rapid (seconds-days) biophysical interactions between the climate and the biosphere (Fig. 8). The dynamics at this level result from changes in water, radiation, wind, and accompanying physiological responses of organisms. They

LEVEL 2

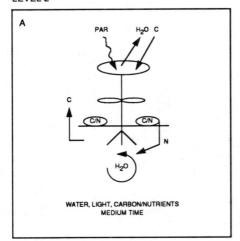
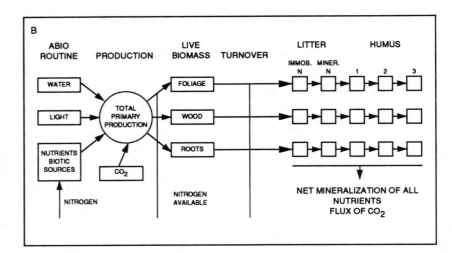

Fig. 9 Schematic representation (A) and model configuration (B) for processes with time constants of days to weeks (level two models). (A) again shows a conceptual model of a land plant with an input of PAR and carbon, and an output of water vapor. In addition, soil reservoirs of carbon and nutrients (C/N) are shown. Reprinted with permission from *Research Strategies for the U.S. Global Change Research Program*, 1990. Published by National Academy Press, Washington, DC.

also occur rapidly relative to plant growth and nutrient uptake, and far more rapidly than species replacement. Simulations at this level are required to provide information to climate models on the exchange of energy, water and CO_2. Tests of this level of model can be accomplished using experimental methods, including leaf cuvettes, micrometeorological observations, and eddy correlation flux measurements.

The second level captures important biogeochemical interactions. This level captures weekly to seasonal dynamics of plant phenology, carbon accumulation, and nutrient uptake and allocation (Fig. 9). Most extant models at this level use integrative measures of climate, such as monthly statistics and degree-day sums. Changes in soil solution chemistry and microbial processes can be captured at this level for calculation of trace gas fluxes. Primary outputs from this level of model are carbon and nutrient fluxes, biomass, leaf area index, and canopy height or roughness. This level of model is usually tested in field studies with direct measurements of biomass, canopy attributes, and nutrient pools or fluxes.

A third level of model represents annual changes in biomass and soil carbon (net ecosystem productivity, carbon storage), and in ecosystem structure and composition (Fig. 10). Inputs are calculated indices summarizing the effects of climatic conditions on biomass accumulation and decomposition. The outputs include ecosystem element storage, allocation of carbon and other elements between tissue types, and community structure. These types of models currently represent individual organisms or populations, and are difficult to apply at large scales because of computational and data requirements. Considerable work will be required to develop large area implementations. This type of model is validated using a combination of process studies, as described above, but integrated to derive annual fluxes, and comparative stud-

ies. The community composition and population dynamics aspects of these models are often validated using paleo-data.

An approach to this coupling is highlighted in Fig. 11. A level three model converts annualized indices of climatic conditions and the current ecosystem state into total leaf area and structure for the next year. Within these total values, the second level calculates the phenology of leaf production and loss, the rate of nutrient mobilization and uptake, and therefore the seasonal pattern of ecosystem dynamics. Using these seasonal patterns, the first level converts climatic data into energy and water balances over very short time steps.

Decomposition calculations can be driven by level two vegetation modules and integrated to set nutrient availability in level three vegetation calculations. Inorganic soil chemistry routines can operate on almost any time scale, as they tend to be somewhat independent of temperature and linear with time, but may be nonlinear with concentrations. Nutrient cycling and soil chemistry modules can run under altered climatic drivers for some time, and then predictions can be made of the consequences of changes in ecosystem state for surface-atmosphere interactions and trace gas fluxes.

Several issues must be resolved to develop and implement such terrestrial modeling schemes in an Earth system model of global change.

•*Calculation of indices of climatic effects on biological activity:* There are several different ways to summarize the effects of climatic conditions on biological activity. These range from very simple calculations of estimated evapotranspiration, water deficits, and drought indices to physiologically sophisticated and computationally demanding models of water, energy, and carbon balances at the leaf and canopy level. Which of these provides the most accurate depiction of climate-biotic interactions, and which can be parameterized

LEVEL 3

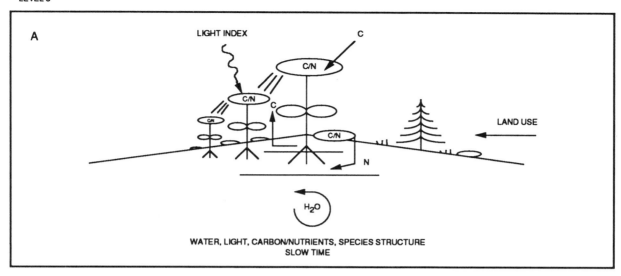

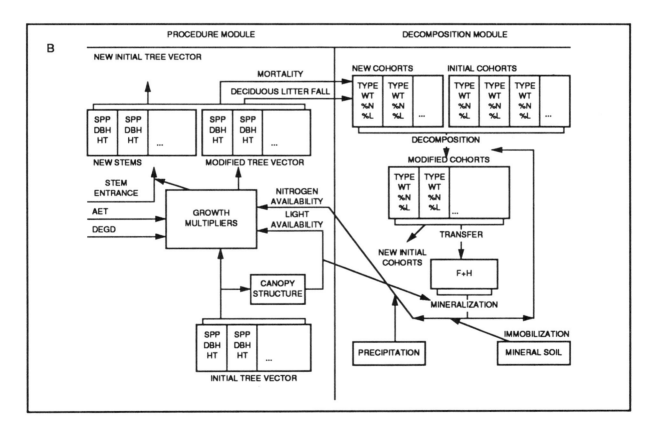

Fig. 10 Schematic representation (A) and model configuration (B) for processes with time constants of years (level three models). (A) again shows a conceptual model of land plants, including shading effects, and with an input of light and carbon. Soil reservoirs of carbon and nutrients (C/N) are also shown. Reprinted with permission from *Research Strategies for the U.S. Global Change Research Program,* 1990. Published by National Academy Press, Washington, DC.

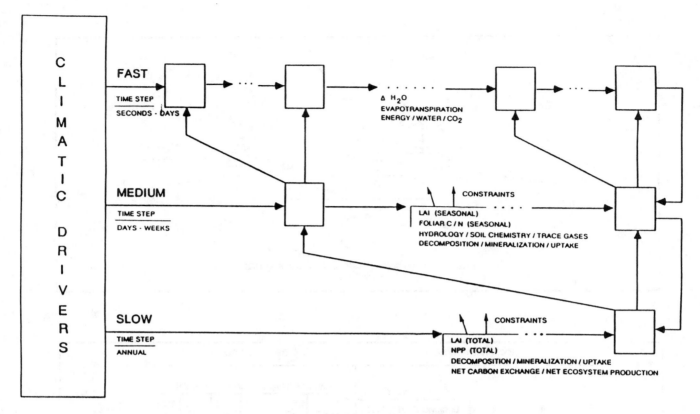

Fig. 11 Conceptual linkages of models at different time levels, showing interaction of different levels of constraints (see text). Adapted from _Research Strategies for the U.S. Global Change Research Program_, 1990. Published by National Academy Press, Washington, DC.

most easily from existing or obtainable field data?

•_Spatial scale of the level three ecosystem module:_ Models of forest ecosystem dynamics are of two types: stem-oriented models that enumerate all individuals within the modeled area, and aggregated models that deal only with biomass compartments such as foliage, wood, and root (e.g., see Fig. 10). Grassland models are generally of the species-aggregated type. The stem models are valuable for examining gap-phase dynamics within a landscape and can predict changes in species composition explicitly. They are tied to a spatial scale at which canopy gaps occur. The aggregated models are independent of spatial scale and are computationally much simpler, but do not capture the successional dynamics or species-specific characteristics of ecosystems. At some cost, the stem models can be aggregated spatially by subsampling and geographic information system (GIS) technology to reach GCM spatial scales. Alternatively, the aggregated models can be parameterized to include successional changes.

•_Linking processes across spatial scales:_ Models need to be organized for use at several levels of geographic detail, with the rapid and slow modules running in concert or separately. At the most detailed geographic level, underlying data are organized on a grid of land cells, and models are solved for each grid cell or with a sampling strategy. Both data and model solutions can be mapped and managed by a geographic information system. The data requirements and implementa-

tion logistics are very demanding at this level. In regional studies, data and model results are tabulated against biome or ecosystem extends, although in some applications it is useful to average or lump data and model results to global scale (see Fig. 11).

An added complexity is that human activities affect a large fraction of the world's terrestrial ecosystems. These disturbances—which range from total management, harvest, and land-use change to subtle pollutant impacts—cannot be ignored in any analysis of changes in the role of land systems. Two aspects of the land-use perturbation and other human activities must be treated: 1) the rates and distributions of the disturbances per se must be described, perhaps by using a GIS; 2) the more difficult issue is the effects—the redistribution of carbon and nutrients in the compartments, as well as the setting in motion of successional patterns. This effect of land use change is perhaps best initiated at level three and allowed to move upward through the constraint structure (Fig. 11).

VII. Summary

The Earth is changing in ways not yet understood, but we do know that the changes are partly the result of human activity. These changes are most evident in the altered states of the various biogeochemical cycles. These cycles represent the integration of physical, chemical, and biological processes; they reflect the metabolic state of the planet. Consequently, their alterations are clear signals that our activities are now affecting fundamental aspects of the Earth system. It is unlikely that human activity will change quickly enough to slow significantly these global changes; therefore, we must begin quickly to gain the needed understanding to foresee better the consequences of these changes.

This understanding will rest upon new insights into the dynamics of terrestrial ecosystems in a changing chemical and physical environment, and more generally, into the coupling of the physical-climate subsystem to the biogeochemical subsystem. Fortunately, the time is now ripe to couple models of ecological and biogeochemical processes to climate models. Global data sets are being acquired with the promise of significant advances in the next 10 years. What is needed is the commitment of scientists to the development of the appropriate models and paradigms to use this information and thereby to detect the shoals and reefs that are before us and to help guide our planet into safe harbor.

References

[1] Boden, T.A., Kanciruk, P., and Farrell, M.P. *TRENDS '90: A Compendium of Data on Global Change,* U.S. Dept. of Energy, Oak Ridge National Laboratory, ORNL/CDIAC-36, 1990.

[2] Schlesinger, W.H. *Biogeochemistry: An Analysis of Global Change,* Academic Press, Harcourt, Brace, Jovanovich, Publishers, 1991, p. 443.

[3] Moore, B., Gildea, M.P., Vorosmarty, C.J., Skole, D.L., Melillo, J.M., Peterson, B.J., Rastetter, E.B., Steudler, P.A. Biogeochemical cycles. In: Rambler, M.B., Margulis, L., Fester, R. (Eds.). *Global Ecology: Towards a Science of the Biosphere,* Academic Press Inc., 1989.

[4] Keeling, C.D. Atmospheric CO_2 concentrations—Mauna Loa Observatory, Hawaii 1958-1986. NDP-001/R1 Carbon Dioxide Information Center, Oak Ridge National Laboratory, Oak Ridge, Tennessee, 1986.

[5] Moore, B., Boone, R., Hobbie, J., Houghton, R., Melillo, J., Peterson, B., Shaver, G., Vorosmarty, C., Woodwell, G. A simple model for analysis of the role of terrestrial ecosystems in the global carbon budget. In: Bolin, B. (Ed.). *Carbon Cycle Modelling. SCOPE 16,* Wiley and Sons, New York, 1981.

[6] Houghton, R.A., Hobbie, J.E., Melillo, J.M., Moore, B., Peterson, B.J., Shaver, G.R., Woodwell, G.M. Changes in the carbon content of terrestrial biota and soils between 1860 and 1980: A net release of CO_2 to the atmosphere. *Ecological Monographs,* 1983, Vol. 53, pp. 235-262.

[7] Houghton, R.A., Boone, R.D., Melillo, J.M., Palm, C.A., Woodwell, G.M., Myers, N., Moore, B., Skole, D.L. Net flux of CO_2 from tropical forests in 1980. *Nature,* 1985, Vol. 316, pp. 617-620.

[8] Palm, C.A., Houghton, R.A., Melillo, J.M., Skole, D.L. Atmospheric carbon dioxide from deforestation in Southeast Asia. *Biotropica,* 1986, Vol. 18, no. 3, pp. 177-188.

[9] Houghton, R.A., Boone, R.D., Fruci, J.R., Hobbie, J.E., Melillo, J.M., Palm, C.A., Peterson, B.J., Shaver, G.R., Woodwell, G.M., Moore, B., Skole, D.L., Myers, N. The flux of carbon from terrestrial ecosystems to the atmosphere in 1980 due to changes in land use: Geographic distribution of the global flux. *Tellus,* 1987, Vol. 39B, pp. 122-139.

[10] Houghton, R.A., Skole, D.L., Lefkowitz, D.S. Changes in the landscape of Latin America between 1850 and 1980. II. A net release of CO_2 to the atmosphere. *Forest Ecology and Management,* 1991, Vol. 38, pp. 173-199.

[11] Detwiler, R.P., Hall, C.A.S. Tropical forests and the global carbon cycle. *Science,* 1988, Vol. 239, pp. 42-47.

[12] Melillo, J.M., Fruci, J.R., Houghton, R.A., Moore, B., and Skole, D.L. Land-use change in the Soviet Union between 1850 and 1980: causes of a net release of CO_2 to the atmosphere. *Tellus,* 1988, Vol. 40B, pp. 116-128.

[13] Houghton, R.A. The future role of tropical forests in affecting the carbon dioxide concentration of the atmosphere. *Ambio,* 1990, Vol. 19, pp. 204-209.

[14] Houghton, R.A., Skole, D.L. Carbon. In: Turner, B.L., Clark, W.C., Kates, R.W., Richards, J.F., Mathews, J.T., Meyer, W.B. (Eds.). *The Earth As Transformed by Human Action,* Cambridge University Press, Cambridge, U.K., 1990, pp. 393-408.

[15] Skole, D.L. Acquiring global data on land cover change. In: Turner et al. (Eds.). *Land Cover and Land Use Change,* Proceedings of the 4th Global Change Institute, OIES, UCAR, in press.

[16] Tans, Pieter P., Fung, Inez Y., Takahashi, Taro. Observational Constraints on the Global Atmospheric CO_2 Budget. *Science,* 1990, Vol. 247, pp. 1431-1438.

[17] McElroy, M. Global change: A biogeochemical perspective. NASA—Jet Propulsion Laboratory Publication #83-51, 1983, p. 33.

[18] Rosswall, T. The global biogeochemical nitrogen cycle. In: Likens, G.E. (Ed.). *Some perspectives of the Major Biogeochemical Cycles,* John Wiley and Sons, 1981, pp. 25-49.

[19] Ivanov, M.V. The global biogeochemical sulfur cycle. In: Likens, G.E. (Ed.). *Some Perspectives of the Major Biogeochemical Cycles,* John Wiley and Sons, 1981, pp. 61-78.

[20] Peterson, B.J., Melillo, J.M. The global carbon-nitrogen-phosphorus cycle; A key to solving the atmospheric CO_2 balance problem? In: Moore, B., Dastoor, M.N. (Eds.). *Interaction of Global Biogeochemical Cycles,* JPL Publication 84-21, Pasadena, CA, 1984, pp. 97-139.

[21] Moore, B. The oceanic sink for excess atmospheric carbon dioxide. In: Duedall, I., Kester, D.R., Park, P.K. (Eds.). *Wastes in the Ocean, Volume IV: Energy Wastes in the Ocean,* John Wiley & Sons, 1985.

[22] McElroy, M. Marine biological controls on atmospheric CO_2 and climate. *Nature,* 1983, Vol. 302, pp. 328-329.

[23] Schindler, D.W. Interrelationships between the cycles of elements in freshwater ecosystems. In: Likens, G.E. (Ed.). *Some perspectives of the Major Biogeochemical Cycles,* John Wiley and Sons, 1981, pp. 113-123.

[24] Tucker, C.J., Townshend, J.G.R., Goff, T.E. African land-cover classification using satellite data. *Science*, 1985, Vol. 227, pp. 369-375.

[25] Tucker, C.J., Holben, B.N., Goff, T.E. Intensive forest clearing in Rondonia, Brazil, as detected by satellite remote sensing. *Remote Sensing of Environment*, 1984, Vol. 15, pp. 255-261.

[26] Skole, D.L., Moore, B. Global land cover conversion and deforestation: Evaluation of estimates, effect on the environment, and the development of a monitoring program. In: United Nations Environment Programme, State of the Environment Report, for presentation at the United Nations World Conference on Environment and Development, June 1992, in press.

[27] Skole, D.L. Personal communication.

[28] Chang, S.H. Collins, W. Confirmation of the airborne biogeophysical mineral exploration technique using laboratory methods. *Economic Geology*, 1983, Vol. 78, pp. 723-736.

[29] Horler, D.N.H., Barber, J., Barringer, A.R. Effects of heavy metals on the absorbance and reflectance spectra of plants. *International Journal of Remote Sensing*, 1980, Vol. 1, pp. 121-136.

[30] Horler, D.N.H., Dockray, M., Barber, J., Barringer, A.R. Red edge measurements for remotely sensing plant chlorphyll content. Committee on Space Research Symposium on Remote Sensing and Mineral Exploration Proceedings, Pergamon Press, Oxford, 1983, Vol. 3, pp. 273-277.

[31] Rock, B.N., Hoshizaki, T., Lichtenthaler, H., Schmuck, G. Comparison of in situ spectral measurements of forest decline symptoms in Vermont (USA) and the Schwarzwald (FRG). Proceedings of the International Geoscience and Remote Sensing Symposium (IGARSS '86), IEEE 86CH2268-1.3, 1986a, pp. 1667-1672.

[32] Rock, B.N., Hoshizaki, T., Miller, J.R. Comparison of in situ and airborne spectral measurements of the blue shift associated with forest decline. *Remote Sensing of Environment*, 1988, Vol. 24, pp. 109-127.

[33] Rock, B.N., Williams, D.L., Vogelmann, J.E. Field and airborne spectral characterization of suspected acid deposition damage in red spruce *(Picea rubens)* from Vermont. Proceedings of the 1985 Machine Processing Remotely Sensed Data Symposium, LARS. Purdue, West Lafayette, Indiana, 1985, pp. 71-81.

[34] Rock, B.N., Vogelmann, J.E., Williams, D.L., Vogelmann, A.F., Hoshizaki, T. Remote detection of forest damage. *Bioscience*, 1986b, Vol. 36, pp. 439-445.

[35] Waring, R.H., Aber, J.D., Melillo, J.M., Moore, B., III. Precursors of Change in Terrestrial Ecosystems. *Bioscience*, 1986, Vol. 36, pp. 433-438.

[36] Tucker, C.J., Fung, I.Y., Keeling, C.D., Gammon, R.H. The relationship of global spectral vegetation indices and atmospheric CO_2 concentrations. *Nature*, 1986, Vol. 319, pp. 195-199.

[37] Goward, S.N., Tucker, C.J., Dye, D.G. North American vegetation patterns observed with the NOAA-7 advanced very high resolution radiometer. *Vegetation*, 1985, Vol. 64, pp. 3-14.

[38] Bartlett, D.S., Whiting, G.J., Hartman, J.M. Use of vegetation indices to estimate intercepted solar radiation and net carbon dioxide exchange of a grass canopy. *Remote Sensing of Environment*, 1990, Vol. 30, pp. 115-128.

[39] Whiting, G.J., Bartlett, D.S., Fan, S., Bakwin, P.S., Wofsy, S.C. Biosphere. Atmosphere CO_2 exchange in tundra ecosystems: Community characteristics and relationships with multispectral surface reflectance. *Journal of Geophys. Research.*, in press.

[40] Bartlett, D.S., Bartlett, K.B., Hartman, J.M., Harriss, R.C., Brannon, D.P., Clark, C., Pelletier, R., Sebacher, D.I. Methane emissions from the Florida Everglades: Patterns of variability in a regional wetland ecosystem. *Global Biogeochemical Cycles*, 1989, Vol. 2, pp. 363-374.

Chapter 8

SETI:
Search for Extraterrestrial Intelligence

John Billingham and Jill Tarter

I. What is SETI?

A. Definition

SETI is an acronym that stands for the Search for Extraterrestrial Intelligence. The acronym was first proposed during the NASA Science Workshops on Interstellar Communication in 1976, and is now widely used. The first published reference work on SETI was the report generated by these Science Workshops.[1] The term SETI has largely replaced two earlier descriptions of the subject: Interstellar Communication[2] and Communication with Extraterrestrial Intelligence (CETI). [3,4] The reason for the change is that most current activities deal literally with attempts to *search* for evidence of the existence of extraterrestrial intelligent life, whereas the term "communication" can be taken to mean two- or many-way communication between civilizations in the universe. One day that might happen, and our civilization on Earth might be one of the communicating parties. However, it is not likely to happen until we have first uncovered evidence of the existence of extraterrestrial intelligence (ETI) as a result of a *search*. So the word "search" better describes what SETI programs are trying to do, namely *detect* evidence of the existence of extraterrestrial life. If successful, SETI will achieve *one-way* communication, from them to us. An analysis of the many possible methods of conducting searches is given in Section III of this chapter.

B. History of Ideas About ETI and SETI

Space contains such a huge supply of atoms that all eternity would not be enough time to count them and the force which drives the atoms into various places just as they have been driven together in this world. So we must realize that there are other worlds in other parts of the universe, with races of different men and different animals.

Lucretius
1st Century BC [5]

Ideas about the possible existence of extraterrestrial intelligent life go back at least 2000 years. During the Dark Ages we find little evidence of any further insights, perhaps because of the prevailing belief that the Earth was the center of the universe. When this Ptolemaic view was overthrown in the 15th and 16th centuries by Galileo and Copernicus, we find the reemergence of ideas about ETI. These ideas were not accepted at first. Giordano Bruno was burned at the stake in Rome in 1600 for postulating a plurality of inhabited worlds in the universe. A couple of centuries later, the concept had gained much more acceptance, even though scientific knowledge of the universe and biological evolution was still primitive. In the middle of the 19th century great excitement was caused by newspaper articles about ETI on the Moon. They turned out to be hoaxes. At the end of the century, the astronomer Percival Lowell believed that he had observed canals on Mars (he had not) and Marconi even listened (without success) for radio signals from Mars. Ingenious schemes were proposed for heroic engineering activities to create patterns on the Earth's surface that would be visible to Martians or other extraterrestrials (for example, the creation of huge geometric patterns in ditches in the Sahara Desert, filled with burning kerosene). The first proposals for detecting extraterrestrial civilizations by listening for their radio transmissions were made in the 1920s.[6]

In 1938, Oparin published his classical paper on the origin of life.[7] Rapid improvements in astronomical, planetary and biological sciences over the next few decades, and the first experiments on chemical evolution in 1954[8] provided the background for a growing realization that the great story of the origin and evolution of life on Earth might, in some form, be repeated on other planets in other solar systems in the universe. In 1960 Lederberg[9] coined the term "exobiology" to denote the study of the origin, evolution, and distribution of life beyond the Earth, and the stimulus of the space age led to the actual search for life on Mars as part of the NASA Project Viking Mission.[10]

In parallel with the growing realization that the origin and evolution of life might be a universal phenomenon, there was an appreciation that intelligent life might also have emerged in many places in the galaxy and the universe. In 1959, G. Cocconi and P. Morrison published their seminal paper in *Nature*.[11] They proposed the use of frequencies at or near that of the hydrogen line, 1420 MHz, searching for other civilizations, and achieving interstellar communication. One year later[12] Frank Drake conducted the first definitive search for ETI signals over a 2-month period using a small radiotelescope at Green Bank, West Virginia. Drake did not know of Morrison's paper. He detected no signals, but the modern age of SETI had begun.

Ideas about SETI now began to proliferate. The first review of the new thinking, the results of a meeting of a small group of U.S. experts in 1961, was published by A.G.W. Cameron under the title *Interstellar Communication* in 1963.[2] The book *Universe, Life, Intelligence* by I. Shklovsky was published in 1962.[13] The joint Soviet-American book *Intelligent Life in the Universe* was published later by I. Shklovsky and C. Sagan.[14] The first symposium on the problem of extraterrestrial intelligence took place in 1964 at the Burakan Astrophysical Observatory in the U.S.S.R. Its proceedings were published in Erevan in 1965.[15] The book by Soviet scientists entitled *Extraterrestrial Intelligence: Problems of Interstellar Communication* was published in 1969 under the editorship of S. Kaplan.[16] In 1971 NASA entered the field when they published *Project Cyclops: A Design Study of a System for Detecting Extraterrestrial Intelligent Life*, by B. Oliver and J. Billingham.[17] In 1971 a Soviet-American conference on CETI was organized in Byurakan by the Academies of Sciences of the U.S.S.R. and U.S.A. A shorthand report of this conference was published under the editorship of C. Sagan in 1973.[3] A Russian edition of the proceedings of the conference was published in 1975.[4] In 1975 and 1976 Philip Morrison led a series of U.S. science workshops resulting in the publication of the first book called *SETI*.[1]

II. Scientific Basis of SETI

The previous section gave a brief review of the historical evolution of ideas about ETI. The current hypothesis is that the origin and evolution of life and intelligence are natural phenomena throughout the universe. It is postulated that life is not now and never has been confined to the Earth. Given the vast number of galaxies and stars it is not unlikely that life and intelligence are widely distributed in the universe. This theory is the scientific basis for the search for extraterrestrial life. It was the rationale for the biological experiments on Project Viking,[10] where two unmanned spacecraft carried out a remote search for microbial life on the surface of Mars in 1975 and 1976. No extraterrestrial life was found on Mars. The theory is also the basis for past and present searches for extraterrestrial intelligence, SETI. Given that our return to Mars to look again for evidence of microbial life could be decades away, the only significant search for extraterrestrial life currently under way is SETI.

It is now important to ask about the number of civilizations that might currently be co-existing with us in the universe. If this number is small, say 1 in every 10 galaxies, then the average distance to our neighbors is measured in millions of light years, and the chance of our detecting them is small. (Note, however, that even in this case the total number of

civilizations in the universe would be large: there are perhaps 100 billion galaxies, so there would be 10 billion civilizations.) If, on the other hand, the number of civilizations in our own galaxy is large, say one million (out of 400 billion stars), then the nearest is only 200 light years away, and much more easily detectable.

A. The Drake Equation

In 1961, astronomer Frank Drake devised an expression for representing the possible number of currently co-existing communicative civilizations in the galaxy as a function of the key variables involved in their genesis.[18] He presented it to the U.S. scientists who gathered at Green Bank in the same year. It is widely known as the Drake Equation:

$$N = R_* f_p n_e f_l f_i f_c L$$

where

N = the number of currently co-existing communicative technological civilizations in the galaxy

R^* = the rate of star formation averaged over the lifetime of the galaxy, in units of number of stars per year

f_p = the fraction of suitable stars that have planetary systems

n_e = the mean number of planets within such planetary systems that are ecologically suitable for life

f_l = the fraction of such planets on which life actually begins

f_i = the fraction of such planets on which life then gives rise to intelligence

f_c = the fraction of such planets in which the intelligent beings evolve to an advanced communicative technology

L = the mean lifetime of such civilizations

The formula contains many probabilistic estimates. Our confidence in these values gets progressively worse going from left to right in the equation. There are also major differences among those who have studied the Drake Equation on what the individual values are. So we are dealing with an expression containing values that are subjective probability numbers. In the discussion that follows, the authors have given their own assessments.

1. Stars and Planets: R, f_p, and n_e

The rate of star formation in the galaxy R is now reasonably well known. It is about 20 per year. Stars vary in mass and composition all of the way from the giant O stars that use up their nuclear fuel rapidly and explode as supernovas after a short time (10 to 100 million years), to small M stars that are only just big enough to have nuclear reactions and which can last for hundreds of billions of years. The massive stars have lifetimes too short to support the origin and evolution of life. The M stars may not have enough energy to irradiate planets to temperatures suitable for life. In the middle are the F, G, and K stars with masses close to that of our Sun. They have intermediate lifetimes. Our Sun will have lasted about 12 billion years before running out of nuclear fuel and becoming a red giant. One planet in our solar system has spawned life. It is called Earth. So it would seem natural, if we are to search for life elsewhere in the galaxy, to focus our attention on other F, G, and K stars. Some 20 percent of all of the stars are in this category.

Many such stars, perhaps 80 percent, belong to binary or multiple star systems, some with complex orbital dynamics that have yet to be understood. A major unknown is whether planetary systems will form around such stars. Another unknown is the degree to which planetary orbits around such stars are sufficiently stable to allow the planets to have long lifetimes and comparatively stable environments. It is likely that widely separated binaries could each have a retinue of planets in stable orbits. It is also possible that close binaries could have planets that orbit both stars. A reasonable estimate of the number of F, G, and K stars having planets with stable orbits is 50 percent. These have been called "good Suns."

We now have another question to ask. What fraction of these good Suns do have planetary systems? Modern astrophysical theory says that the birth of intermediate mass, main sequence stars is accompanied by the birth of a retinue of planets that form from the protoplanetary disc of dust and gas surrounding the star. Furthermore, the theory says that this process is the rule, and therefore that most, if not all, such stars will have planetary systems. When Drake first conceived his equation 30 years ago there was little direct evidence of the existence of extrasolar planetary systems. Today we have rapidly increasing numbers of tentative detections of such systems, either as flattened discs of dust and gas, detected with modern telescopes operating at infrared and optical wavelengths, or as indirect detections by astrometry and radial velocity studies. These measure the wobble of the parent star caused by the gravitational influence of the planet in orbit around it. For our estimates of reasonable values in the Drake Equation we shall assume that all solar-type stars have planets.

The next question is how many planets, on average, are suitable for the origin of life. We would expect that a suitable planet would be another "Earth." It would have a mass, composition, atmosphere, and temperature something like our own planet, and that it would offer some reasonable environmental stability over periods of billions of years. We would expect it to have a metallic core, an atmosphere with a reasonable density, healthy concentrations of the biogenic elements, liquid water, and equable temperatures. It could be at different distances from its parent star, depending on the mass of the star and all the planetary characteristics, and still be suitable for life. The distance between the maximum and minimum orbital radii is known as the "ecoshell." There is much argument about its thickness. Some say it is very thin, which would mean that the likelihood of a terrestrial planet being at the right distance from its star is small. Others believe that it could be

thick, extending in our own solar system, for example, all of the way from the orbit of Venus to the orbit of Mars. (Note that it is possible that life did begin on Mars at the same time that it began on Earth, and has subsequently become extinct. It is also conceivable that life may still be present on Mars.) The value of n_e in the Drake Equation depends on all the factors discussed above. In the case of our solar system, n_e is 1 or just possibly 2. Our estimate for the mean value of n_e in the galaxy, lacking good astronomical measurements, is 1.

Now we are able to estimate the values of the first two factors in the Drake Equation, f_p and n_e. F_p is made up of the fraction of all of the stars that are good Suns, 0.2, times the fraction of stars that can have reasonably stable planetary orbits, 0.5, times the fraction of solar-type stars that have planets, 1.0. So $f_p = 0.1$. Since we have taken n_e to equal 1, the first two items in the Drake Equation now give us a combined estimate of 0.1. If this were correct it would mean that one tenth of all of the stars has, on average, one planet suitable for life.

2. The Origin and Evolution of Life: f_l

With regard to the Drake Equation the question is, "On what fraction of suitable planets does life actually begin and evolve into complex forms?" About the origin of life, most exobiologists now believe that the evolution of a good Sun and a good Earth will probably facilitate the formation of those organic molecules that are the building blocks of life and their subsequent self-assembly into the first self-reproducing systems. In other words, the process would seem to be a natural consequence of having the right planet in the right place orbiting the right type of star. On Earth it seems as though life began soon after it could possibly have begun, that is, after the end of the great meteorite bombardment about 4 billion years ago. It is possible, of course, to envisage situations where life might have difficulty getting started because the combination of solar and planetary conditions is at one end of what must be a distribution curve of suitability for life. Our Sun-Earth combination must be near one end of the distribution curve, since life originated so rapidly. We shall assume that f_l, the number of "good Earths" per planetary system where life does begin, is so close to 1 that for the Drake Equation we shall use 1.

3. Intelligence, Cultural Evolution, Civilization, Science and Technology: f_i and f_c

The next step is much more difficult to assess. On Earth there was a period of some 4 billion years during which life slowly evolved into millions of separate individual species through the processes of mutation and natural selection. Since we do not yet know of any extraterrestrial life, we do not know where Earth fits on the distribution curve of the pace of evolution through time in all those solar systems that harbor life. It is easy to imagine extrasolar planetary circumstances less hospitable than those of Earth, where life may remain in a comparatively simple state for 4 billion years. (It is also possible to imagine that life only progresses so far, and is then threatened by adverse physical circumstances. For example, life may have begun on Mars and then became extinct as the planet lost its atmosphere.) It is also possible that the 4 billion years it took us to reach a level of biological complexity that spawned intelligence is unusually long. Perhaps it usually happens much more rapidly. Some critics of SETI have argued that the vast number of separate, unlikely, individual steps in biological evolution mitigates against any comparable process elsewhere. It is of course true that the *exact* process could not be repeated elsewhere. It is also true that every species of complex life on the Earth is unique. The probability of the existence of any one specific genome, identical to that on Earth, in the extraterrestrial realm, is so close to zero that for all practical proposes it can be taken as zero. There is only one *Drosophila melanogaster* and only one *Tyrannosaurus rex* in the universe. So, the critics argue, complex life elsewhere cannot exist. They are mistaken. What is clearly possible, perhaps probable, is that the process of Darwin-Wallace evolution is universal, and that a huge variety of species can perfectly well emerge on other planets of other solar-type stars given enough time. We might expect that certain anatomical, physiological, biochemical, behavioral and social characteristics of complex extraterrestrial life will be similar to those we find here on Earth, and just as with the genome, they will not be identical, but they could perfectly well be *similar*. After all, similar characteristics appear in widely separated animal and plant groups on Earth even when the genetic heritage is different. This is known as convergent or parallel evolution. It is interesting to ask why evolution should not converge between planets in the galaxy as well as between continents on the Earth. Perhaps we should expect higher organisms of other worlds to have eyes (they appeared 40 separate times on Earth), and limbs, and sexual reproduction, nervous systems, and cooperative group behavior. They may have more characteristics than the sum of those on Earth. They may have less. For SETI all that matters is that in some cases there will appear, as an important case of parallel evolution, the phenomenon of intelligence.

"Intelligence" is hard to define, or even adequately describe. Is a frog intelligent? For SETI such questions are academic. SETI has its own definition, which is "the ability to construct and use large radiotransmitters and radiotelescopes." The basic hypothesis of SETI is that this type of intelligence occasionally arises in the universe, as it did here on Earth. In many locations there will be complex life, of varying ages, but without any trace of intelligence. Indeed, the conventional wisdom in the evolutionary biology community is that there is no "trend" towards the human type of intelligence. Occasionally it may appear as one of a huge number of possible outcomes associated with the variability of diverse life forms in the universe. However, it is not preordained.

There has been some discussion in the evolutionary biology community about the unique nature of *Homo sapiens*. The arguments are persuasive. No other organism in the universe will have 3 billion basic pairs arranged in identical genes in an identical sequence on identical chromosomes. ETI and *Homo sapiens* would not be able to interbreed. As with *Drosophila melanogaster* and *Tyrannosaurus rex*, human beings are unique. This argument has been used by critics of SETI to say that we should not waste our time looking for human beings elsewhere because they do not exist. Their argument is flawed. SETI is not looking for extraterrestrial versions of *Homo sapiens*. SETI is looking for intelligence of the human type. Creatures with the power of abstract thought, who can construct and act on at least partly successful internal models of the external world, who can use their skills to build complex structures, and are able, to some degree, to predict the future. They may look something like us, a little like us, or nothing like us. They will never be the same as us. To emphasize the point, SETI is not looking for hominids, hominoids, or humanoids. These are all creatures of Earth. SETI is looking for the *cognitive* type of intelligence possessed by Homo Sapiens, but embodied in extraterrestrial beings having a variety of different body plans, function, genetic make up and social organization. Given billions of years of evolution we will estimate that 1 in 20 complex extraterrestrial biologies spawns cognitive intelligence. So f_i is .05.

Of all these cases, how many now go on to develop civilization, science and a communicative technology that would allow SETI to detect them? Some authors have argued that the rapid advances in technology since the beginning of recorded history some 10,000 years ago, and particularly in the Western World in recent centuries, are very special cases and not generally applicable. Some have argued that many different subgroups of *Homo sapiens*, for example, the aborigines, have not developed a sophisticated technology. True enough, but they may simply have not had time. Different manifestations of technological advance have been developed on Earth by different civilizations. Although civilizations have risen and fallen, technological knowledge has in aggregate advanced very rapidly when viewed on the scale of geological time. The attribute of cognitive intelligence seems likely to lead to civilization, science and technology, given a few hundred thousand years. So we take the emergence of communicative technologies from intelligence to be a very high probability: $f_c \approx 1$.

4. The Longevity of Civilizations

The last factor in the Drake Equation, L, is the mean longevity of a technologically communicative civilization. If L is a few tens of years, there will be almost no chance of success for SETI. If L is a billion years, the universe will be teeming with civilizations. There is less we can say about L than any of the other factors in the Drake Equation because we are not able to look far into our own future. At least for f_l, f_i and f_c we have one example here on Earth. All we can really say is that any civilization that develops a stable society could achieve great longevity. Doubtless many civilizations will not, and will destroy themselves or wither away. Some

Table 1

Calculation of the number of currently co-existing communicative civilizations in the Milky Way Galaxy, and the mean distance between them, for different values of the mean longevity in the communicative phase.

Mean Longevity (years)	Number of Civilizations	Mean Distance Between Civilizations (light years)
10^2	10	10,000
10^3	10^2	4642
10^4	10^3	2154
10^5	10^4	1000
10^6	10^5	464
10^7	10^6	215
10^8	10^7	100
10^9	10^8	46
10^{10}	10^9	21

authors have proposed a bimodal distribution of longevity with two large peaks, one at the low end, with lifetimes of a few hundred years, and one at the high end, with lifetimes of hundreds of millions of years. In SETI what matters is the mean.

Since our level of ignorance of the values in the right-hand side of the Drake Equation is so profound, it is not surprising that there is a wide range of guesses, and much argument, among those who have studied this question. Some remark that it takes only one factor on the right-hand side to be close to zero for the number of civilizations to be close to zero. Others point out that the origin and evolution of life appears to be a natural process and that the immense number of life sites and the enormous extent of geological time argues for a widespread distribution of life at all stages of evolution.

Since the universe is perhaps 20 billion years old, life could have begun on the planets of Population I stars (with heavy elements) as much as 10 billion years ago. Taking 5 billion years to reach cognitive intelligence after the birth of a solar system, which has happened once, there may today be civilizations that are 5 billion years old. So any ETI species that we discover will be between our own stage of evolution and 5 billion years into the future. We will not detect any ETI less advanced than we are because they will not have the technology that would allow us to detect them. Therefore, on a statistical basis, those civilizations we detect will be much older than we are. This has some profound implications.

Even if we should detect only a faint carrier signal with no message, we would know at once that in at least one other case a civilization has in some way achieved stability and longevity. This could be a powerful stimulus for us to do the same. If there is a message, the gain in knowledge for our own civilization could far exceed the sum of all of our knowledge today. Further, it is not conceivable that the ETI species that we detect could be the only other civilization in the universe. If we detect one, there will be many. No doubt a much more intense search would follow the first discovery.

Let us now put in the estimates that we have made for the different factors in the Drake Equation:

$$N = R_* f_p\, n_e f_l f_i f_c L$$
$$= 20 \times 0.1 \times 1 \times 1 \times 0.05 \times 1 \times L$$
$$= 0.1\, L$$

So, in the opinion of the authors of this chapter, the number of currently co-existing communicative technological civilizations is equal to one-tenth of the mean longevity of a civilization in years. The importance of L becomes clear. What does it mean in terms of the number of civilizations in the galaxy and the mean distance between them? Table 1 shows the number of L calculated for different values.

The difficulty of making the detection obviously goes up with the distance. So our task could be comparatively easy if there are 1 billion civilizations in the galaxy. The nearest would be close. However, if the number is 10, then the nearest is so far away that detection becomes very difficult.

There is another way to look at the numbers. If we suppose that there are 400 billion stars in our galaxy, and that civilizations are associated with only 1 in 100,000 of these stars, then there are today 400,000 ETI species in our own neighborhood in the universe. Life can at the same time be rare per stellar system, but abundant in the galaxy.

The Drake Equation is largely concerned with subjective probabilities. Although it illuminates so clearly all the factors that determine the density of civilizations in the galaxy, it does not provide a concrete solution. We seek the real solution by carrying out the experiment, SETI, to test the hypothesis that intelligent life is widespread in the universe. A thorough search must be carried out, perhaps over a long time, to detect the first signal of ETI origin.

There are a large number of different ways in which a search could be conducted. Extensive analyses over the last

Table 2   Some trace gases in the Earth's atmosphere

	Thermodynamic Equilibrium Concentration (Mole Fraction)	Actual Concentration Mole Fraction	Atmospheric Enhancement	Source
Methane (CH_4)	10^{-145}	1.7×10^{-6}	a 10^{139}	Biology/ Volcanism
Ammonia (NH_3)	2×10^{-60}	10^{-10}	a 10^{50}	Biology
Nitrous oxide (N_2O)	2×10^{-19}	3×10^{-7}	a 10^{12}	Biology/ Combustion
Carbon disulfide (CS_2)	0	10^{-11}		Biology

30 years, beginning with the seminal paper of Cocconi and Morrison in *Nature* [11] and some 60 actual searches beginning with Project Ozma by Drake[12] have now laid a firm foundation for future searches.

Sections III though V of this chapter describe the technical approaches to SETI that have been made, are being made, and will be made in the future. Clearly we have reached that stage in our own technological evolution where we now have sophisticated engineering capabilities to enable us to detect the existence of other technologies over the immense distances between the stars.

It is also clear that the expected value of an unambiguous detection is very high.

The basic rationale for conducting SETI can now be summarized as the conclusion to this section. We now have a good scientific basis for putting forward the hypothesis that cognitive intelligence is widespread in the universe. We have the technological capability to undertake comprehensive searches, and we believe that the value of the discovery would be high.

Taken together, these three factors argue for the devotion of some small fraction of the resources of our own civilization to the search for other civilizations.

B. Summary

Ideas about the possible existence of extraterrestrial intelligent life began surfacing more than 2000 years ago. Since the Copernican revolution these ideas have developed in parallel with the gradual increase in knowledge of astronomy, planetary science, and evolutionary biology. They crystallized in 1959 with a specific proposal to conduct a search for ETI in the microwave region in the spectrum[11] and with the first actual search.[12]

The scientific basis of SETI is encapsulated in the Drake Equation.[18] The basic hypothesis is that intelligent life is widespread in the universe. This hypothesis is based on the following postulates: 1) There are a huge number of star systems in the universe that include one or more planets capable of supporting life; 2) Given a "good Sun" and a "good Earth," the origin of life will occur as a natural process; 3) Given billions of years of comparative stability of the planetary environment, life will evolve by Darwinian evolution into a wide variety of different forms; 4) Occasionally one evolutionary line may lead to the appearance of cognitive intelligence, cultural evolution, civilization, science and technology; 5) If the mean lifetime of civilization is long, there will now be a very large number of ETI species in the galaxy and the universe; 6) Whereas the number of extraterrestrial civilizations is unknown, the intrinsic value of detection of the existence of even one other civilization would be very high; 7) If we detect one other, there will be many; 8) Progress in technology now allows us to engineer systems that can achieve radio communication over immense distances in the galaxy (see succeeding sections); 9) The confluence of these factors, our scientific knowledge of the evolution of cognitive intelligence, our modern technological capabilities, and the expected value of the unambiguous detection of a signal, together constitutes the rationale for SETI.

III. Technical Approaches to SETI

The acronym SETI is in some sense a misnomer. As of today, we have no means for directly detecting Intelligence over interstellar distances. What we can do is to attempt to detect manifestations of a Technology, produced by that intelligence. On some water-covered planet circling a nearby star, there just might exist extremely intelligent beasts that are analogous to our dolphins and whales; we have no way of attempting to find them. Intelligent as they might be, such creatures do not possess manipulative appendages, and therefore they do not modify their environment in ways that are detectable by us at a distance. The term SETI is historical, and it is more pleasant to the ear than SETT, but we should not forget that for the immediate future it is technology, born of intelligence, that we seek to detect.

This will not always be the case. Considering the advanced technology development now underway, it seems fairly safe to assert that within a few generations of space-based astronomical instrumentation, we should be able to detect putative evidence for the existence of life itself on a distant planet, whether or not that life has developed a technology. The development of large, orbital or lunar, single-dish or interferometric, telescopes at optical or infrared wavelengths holds out the promise of an inferential detection of extraterrestrial life. Once a terrestrial-type planet at a nearby star can be directly imaged (an incredibly difficult task because of the huge contrast in brightness between the faint reflected light from the planet and the luminosity of its nearby parent star), then it may be possible to make a chemical assay of the trace gases in the planetary atmosphere. If one were to find, for example, spectroscopic lines that indicated the simultaneous presence of the reactive gases CH_4 and O_2, one would have very strong evidence for an exobiological source function at the base of the atmosphere. Such non-equilibrium chemical profiles cannot be explained by any known combination of ion-molecule or Fischer-Trophe, gas-grain chemistry driven by the energy from a solar-type star. Table 2 shows the actual, non-equilibrium concentration of some biological trace gases in the present terrestrial atmosphere. These data are taken from a paper[19] that proposes to include the frequency range from 3 to 10 microns as part of an infrared detector being considered for a future Mars Observer mission. At the proposed infrared frequencies, detection of such trace gases as CH_4, NH_3, and N_2O, in concentrations more than thermodynamic equilibrium values, could give evidence of an extant microbial biota somewhere on the Red Planet! Because of the Aeolian circulation on Mars (or on a distant terrestrial planet), any atmospheric investigations such as these necessarily sample the entire planet and are thus not dependent upon a fortunate choice of landing site.

The fact that these measurements have yet to be made on a body in our own solar system should indicate to the reader just how difficult a task it will be to extend such studies to an extrasolar planet. To date, no fundamental limitations in optics or positional control for the necessarily large imaging telescopes have been uncovered. Both optical and infrared systems can search for the presence of O_2 and O_3. Methane and other biological trace gases are more readily detected in the infrared, but it is far too early to conclude whether either wavelength will eventually live up to this tantalizing promise.

In the event that such a chemical assay eventually uncovers a non-equilibrium admixture of trace gases, what will it mean? It will provide putative evidence for some form of exobiology on the planet, but it will probably not be able to tell us whether it consists of blue-green algae or intelligent species. In summary, we can anticipate the detection of life and technology elsewhere in the universe and infer the existence of intelligence, but we cannot directly search for intelligence, so SETI is a bit of a misnomer.

Given that, for the present, we are limited to searching for evidence of a distant technology, what should we search for? We cannot imagine what we cannot imagine, and therefore we are forced to extrapolate from terrestrial experience and practices. This forward extrapolation is based on the fact that any extraterrestrial technology we are capable of detecting will likely be far in advance of our own technology. The Milky Way Galaxy is some 10 billion years of age, and our Sun and the planet Earth are about 4.5 billion years old. By contrast our relevant technology is less than 100 years old. Statistical probability strongly argues that life on other planets may well be found in the microbial state that characterized billions of years of our own planet's evolution; however, if that life has developed a technology, then that technology will likely be older than our own. The chances that another technology would be younger than the Earth's are roughly given by the age of our technology divided by the age of our galaxy or 10^{-8}.

Today, the most visible artifacts of our technology have to do with our needs for transportation, energy production, manufacturing, and information exchange. We can make a modest forward projection of these activities to a more advanced technology. Several astronomical searches have been conducted over the past three decades based on models from such extrapolations. It is extremely difficult to analyze the significance of the negative results from any of these searches. It is impossible to say whether nothing was found because nothing exists to be found, or whether the model was flawed and the search did not achieve adequate sensitivity. Ideally, the benchmark of any systematic search should be whether the strategy could detect a current Earth-analog somewhere within our galaxy. This at least removes the possibility of a faulty extrapolation, but as we shall see, the resources required for such searches are nontrivial.

A. Interstellar Travel/Astroengineering

The simplest of all of the search strategies is the passive approach, where one simply waits for an extraterrestrial spacecraft to land on Earth and make its presence known. The many reports of such events notwithstanding, there is not any incontrovertible evidence that we have ever been or are being visited by extraterrestrial vehicles.[20] The term UFO stands for Unidentified Flying Object and refers to (primarily) visible sightings of phenomena that cannot be readily explained by the observer in terms of their known experience base. UFOs have nothing to do with little green men (or women) in flying saucers, and indeed the most frequently reported UFO is the planet Venus.[21] The fact that many members of the general public continue to choose to believe otherwise, in spite of the lack of physical evidence, stems from the financial incentives available to promoters of this concept (including the entertainment media) and the ingrained human need to believe in some form of being which is more lofty than ourselves. It was once a widespread belief that the aurora borealis was the result of light reflecting off the wings of angels or the swords of heavenly armies on high[22]; not everyone was pleased when scientists provided a verifiable, but more mundane, explanation of the Northern Lights in terms of high energy particles interacting with the Earth's magnetic field lines near the magnetic pole.[23]

There is an absolute distinction between the fields of SETI and UFOlogy; SETI requires repeatable and independently verifiable proof of the existence of another technology. Belief will not suffice. It is also legitimate to require such proof for the unanticipated arrival of a body from outer space. This is not forthcoming in the case of UFOs. In contrast, every few years the Earth is nearly struck by a bolide or meteor that enters the atmosphere at a shallow angle and produces a fiery display visible over a large area (the arrival of an extraterrestrial spacecraft into our atmosphere should be at least as energetic as this). Nobody has predicted its arrival, nobody anticipated the event, and yet the aftermath of these spectacles always finds hundreds, if not thousands of still photos and video tapes; incontrovertible evidence of the happening. Somehow, the purported arrival of the little green men always manages to escape detection except by one or a handful of individuals, and they never seem to have cameras with them!

The absence of extraterrestrial spacecraft is not surprising, given our current understanding of the laws of physics. Einstein's special law of relativity illustrates that the energy of any particle with mass increases rapidly as the speed of light is approached. To travel over interstellar distances therefore requires that spacecraft go extremely slowly or pay an extraordinary energy bill for the trip! Let M_o be the mass of a particle at rest. When that particle moves at a velocity v, its total energy E is given by

$$E = M_o c^2 \left(1 - v^2 / c^2\right)^{-1/2}$$

Clearly as v approaches c (the speed of light) this energy becomes infinite. The most efficient relativistic rocket is one that leaves its ejected propellant at rest with respect to the original inertial frame from which the rocket was launched, and the rocket having the smallest mass ratio (mass of delivered payload divided by the total mass of payload and fuel) is one whose exhaust consists of photons only.[24] In either case, and even granting that the advanced extraterrestrial technology can deal with the in-flight hazards posed by collisions with interstellar dust particles and the containment of anti-matter fuels, either the energy bill or the trip time will be huge. Travelling at a velocity of 71 percent of c, so that the time lapse on board the spacecraft will appear to be 1 year per light year travelled, a one-way trip to a star 20 light years away will age the crewmembers by 20 years and require the energy equivalent of a millennium's worth of current world energy consumption (assuming the final ship's payload weighs 3600 tons).[25] An advanced technology presumably must have energy resources far more than current terrestrial measures. Even so, the energy bill for this one-way jaunt amounts to 1 millisecond of the total luminosity output of the Sun or 15 1/2 days worth of all of the solar energy falling on the Earth. There are a number of ways to reduce this energy bill, but there is no magic. As previously mentioned, the trip could be made at slower speeds and involve multiple generations of crew. The penalty for carrying the on-board fuel for annihilation could be eliminated if the needed fuel were harvested en route or the propulsion were provided from an external source, as in the case of Robert Forward's rocketless rockets.[26] The mass of the payload could be reduced until it consists of only a small probe that would send back information. Finally, the spacecraft could be eliminated altogether and the exploration could be accomplished by using massless photons for remote sensing and listening.

Although this latter strategy is the basis for almost all of the recent and ongoing SETI observational programs, there have been a few legitimate attempts to search for evidence of extraterrestrial spacecraft. Freitas and his coworkers have looked for probes in stable "parking orbits" within our solar system.[27] Since technologies will not be coeval in the galaxy, the strategy of sending a small probe to a distant stellar system will most probably incorporate the ability to await the emergence of a life form and/or its development into a technological civilization. In the multi-body dynamical gravitational field of a planetary system, energy will need to be expended on "station keeping," the process of keeping the probe in the same relative position or orbit with respect to the object of interest. In the case of the Earth-Moon-Sun system, there exist several Lagrangian points where gravitational forces nearly cancel out and a probe might remain situated for a long time with relatively little energy expenditure. Indeed it is known that these locations are natural collection places for interplanetary debris. Optical searches by U.S. researchers as well as active radar searches by Suchkin et al. of the Soviet Union[29] have ruled out the presence of any large, shiny (radar or visible light reflecting) space probes near many of the terrestrial Lagrangian points. Although we have argued that space travel is energetically unfavorable, at least one search has been made for large interstellar spacecraft. Gamma ray bursters (GRB) are extremely energetic short-lived phenomena that to date have no universally accepted explanation (although most models invoke some sort of interaction between an orbital disk of material and a superdense neutron star or black hole). If one assumes instead that they represent the annihilation of matter and anti-matter during a spacecraft mid-course acceleration maneuver, they could conceivably provide evidence for interstellar travel. An analysis of existing data on the GRB sources failed to turn up a spatial and temporal relationship between these events that could provide evidence for any plausible interstellar trajectories.[30]

Another manifestation of advanced technology might be the astroengineering projects in which it engages closer to home. Although there may be other motivations for such projects, energy production is one that is a direct extrapolation of terrestrial behavior. On a large scale, it is possible to envision the use of nuclear fission, fusion, and stellar luminosity to meet the energy requirements for an advanced civilization. Observational searches (with negative results) have been conducted to look for the dumping of fissile waste material into the host star's atmosphere,[31] short-lived, radioactive tritium resulting from the leakage of orbital fusion reactors[32] and excess infrared emission from solar-type stars surrounded by Dyson Spheres to capture and convert all of the stellar luminosity into usable energy.[33] Indeed, Nikolai Kardashev[34] developed a classification scheme for advanced civilizations according to whether they could control an amount of energy equivalent to current terrestrial values (Type I), the output of their star (Type II), or the output of their entire galaxy (Type III). Independently, Arthur C. Clarke referred to the mysterious and vastly energetic Seyfert Galax-

Table 3   Searches to date

61	Documented searches since Ozma (1960)		
52	Radio	9	Dedicated
6	Optical	38	Directed
1	IR	14	Commensal
1	UV		
1	g-Ray		

ies as "the industrial accidents of the universe"![35] As mentioned before, negative results from searches based upon such extrapolations are impossible to interpret.

B. Information Transfer/Particle and Electromagnetic Radiation (Except Microwave)

For the purposes of short-range or local transfer of information, an advanced technological civilization might well make use of exotic modulation schemes or particles that we cannot yet comprehend. However, if the goal is to transmit information over large interstellar distances for a communication network or to create a beacon that will attract the attention of another distant technological civilization, the rules of the game change. The laws of physics as we now know them, and our current understanding of the nature of the universe, suggest that the suitable options for long-distance communication may be limited.

Consider what qualities would make a good information carrier over vast interstellar distances. The particles carrying the encoded information should: a) have minimal energy per quantum, other things being equal; b) have as high a velocity as possible; c) be easy to generate, modulate, launch, and capture; d) should not be appreciably absorbed or deflected by the interstellar or interplanetary medium.

Item b) argues for massless particles, whereas c) argues against known or postulated "inos" (particles for which the mass bounds are uncertain, but which have exceedingly small capture cross-sections, e.g., the neutrino), item d) mandates a particle without electric charge (to avoid being deflected by the intervening galactic magnetic field); *photons* fit all of these criteria. Items d) and a) together argue in favor of *microwave* photons, but that argument is somewhat dependent on the specifics of extraterrestrial engineering practices (such as whether they build diffraction limited telescopes at all wavelengths), and whether or not the signal is broadcast, or beamed directly at us.

It was Cocconi and Morrison who first suggested a microwave search 32 years ago[11] and Drake who independently conducted the first microwave search, known as Project Ozma, in 1960.[12] The majority of the searches since then (Table 3) have concentrated on microwave frequencies, where the background radiation from astrophysical sources is at a minimum. Microwaves will form the basis for the next major advance in search techniques, as described in a later section of this chapter. For the moment, we consider some of the search concepts based on photons other than microwaves.

Lasers offer the ability to transmit extremely wide band-

widths of information-bearing signal. It has been argued that an interstellar communications network would use visible or infrared lasers. The problem with interstellar laser communications is the luminosity of the stellar spectrum, which provides an extremely bright background against which to detect the desired signal and/or the extinction of the signal caused by absorption and scattering on interstellar dust grains. One can beat down the thermal contribution from the star in three ways: by using a very narrow bandwidth for transmission and reception; by so tightly beaming the transmitter and receiver that the signal is spatially resolved from the star; or by transmitting in one of the deep absorption lines of the stellar spectrum, where the contribution from thermal emission is reduced. In the first instance, one loses the high data rate communications advantage; the second solution requires gigantic systems with extraordinary accuracy and the ability to target the signal exactly where the receiver will be years in the future when the signal arrives; and the third technique offers only an order of magnitude improvement that scarcely helps.

Lasers seem more appropriate to the later, CETI phase (C for communications) than to the search or SETI phases. Nonetheless, they have been suggested since the very inception of this field,[36] and have recently been inaugurated into a search[37] using single elements of the world's first infrared interferometer at Mt. Wilson. One justification for this search lies in the fact that the atmospheres of Venus and Mars demonstrate nonthermal emission lines associated with CO_2. An advanced technology might install large mirrors on orbit to induce natural CO_2 laser emission along a long, multiply-reflected, pathlength, which in turn could form the basis for an interstellar beacon.[38] Such technological feats are trivial compared with those recently suggested[39] for an optical laser communications system. Such a system might be rapidly pulsed to increase the signal-to-noise ratio, without melting the physical components that must transmit the enormous powers required for detection at a distance. Shvartzman and his colleagues pioneered the MANIA system, an optical detector for rapid pulses (pulse durations of 3×10^{-7} to 300 seconds), which operates on the 6 meter optical telescope of the Special Astrophysical Observatory in the Soviet Union.[40] This system would be capable of detecting the sort of Type II civilization that could engineer the optical laser communications. The MANIA detector was developed for more classical astronomical research, but solar-type stars are included as targets for SETI whenever the schedule permits.

C. Microwave Radiation/The Cosmic Haystack

In the last section, the terms visible, infrared, and microwave were used to describe different wavelength regions of the electromagnetic spectrum. It was assumed that the reader has a qualitative, if not quantitative, understanding of these terms. The wavelengths of visible light are measured in nanometers, those of the infrared are measured in micrometers, and microwave wavelengths span the millimeter to centimeter range. Figure 1 represents the energy density per

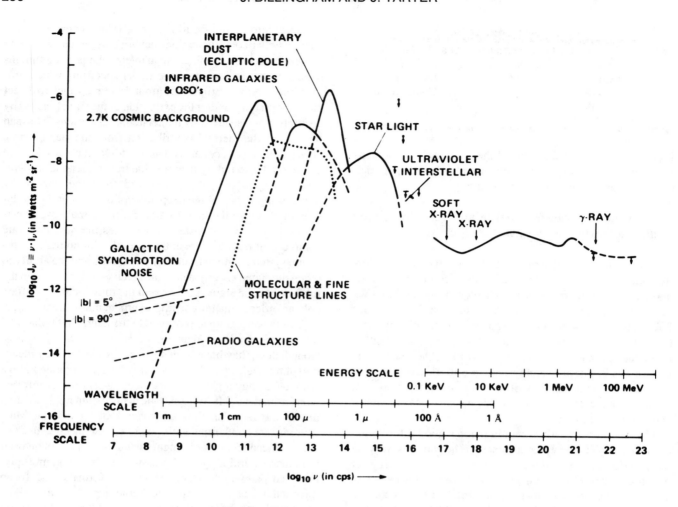

Fig. 1 Cosmic background radiation (NASA Ames Research Center)

steradian on the sky of all of the different types of natural astrophysical emission over all of the wavelengths to which our instruments are sensitive. This is the same sky emission seen by any civilization inhabiting our galaxy, almost independent of location. This is the background noise, above which a signal must be detectable, if SETI is to succeed. As mentioned previously, the microwave portion of the spectrum is much quieter than the higher frequencies (shorter wavelengths). In free space, above the terrestrial atmosphere, an ideal microwave receiver would experience a natural contribution to its noise temperature, as shown in Fig. 2. This defines the free-space microwave window. The low frequency (long wavelength) edge of the window is set by the synchrotron emission from relativistic electrons spinning around the magnetic field lines in the halo of the Milky Way Galaxy. Long before the contribution from glowing infrared dust and gas begins to close the window at the high frequency edge, another contribution to the receiver noise temperature is encountered in the form of quantum noise. This instrumental noise is proportional to the frequency and is negligible at the lower end of the window. For a space-based technology, the range of frequencies from 1 to about 60 GigaHertz (30 cm to

5 mm) is the quietest region of the spectrum and a promising candidate for establishing an interstellar signpost or beacon. However, for a technology, such as ours, that has not yet set up housekeeping above its own atmosphere, the quiet window closes rapidly at higher frequencies due to the presence of molecular oxygen and water vapor. Figure 3 illustrates the terrestrial microwave window covering about 1 to 10 GHz. In any search for evidence of extraterrestrial technologies, we shall be constrained by cost, by how much the general public and their elected representatives are willing to spend on this exploration. Therefore, it makes sense to begin a systematic search for signals by confining ourselves to the terrestrial microwave window, and operating on Earth, using existing ground-based facilities. We can consider the more expensive options of building dedicated telescopes and operating in space (or on the Moon), if our first efforts are not successful.

Frequency is not the only dimension that must be explored to look for signals. The time of arrival of any signal, the amount of power contained in the signal, and the directions from which it comes are also unknown. Until it is detected, the nature of the signal itself is unknown, and this strongly impacts the design of the receivers needed to detect it. If we

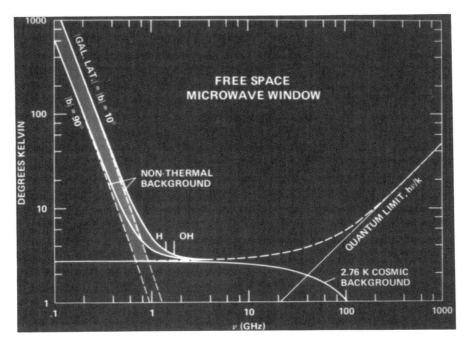

Fig. 2 Free space microwave window (NASA Ames Research Center)

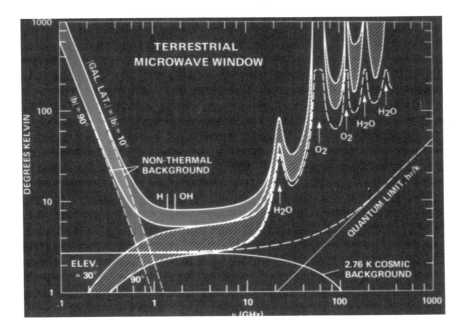

Fig. 3 Terrestrial microwave window (NASA Ames Research Center)

nevertheless assume that the receiver is matched to the signal being sent, then it is possible to depict the parameter space that must be searched for a signal using only three axes.

The first axis represents the unknown direction from which the signal might come. It can be either the number of specific "targets" that one must search to be successful, or the total number of antenna beams it takes to tesselate the entire sky in an all sky survey. There is no unit associated with this axis, since it is a pure number. The second axis is the unknown frequency of the signal. The unit chosen for this axis is GigaHertz (GHz), where 1 GHz represents 1 billion cycles per second. The last axis combines the unknown power of and distance to the transmitter. This axis is the sensitivity that the receiver must achieve to detect the signal. Here the units are square meters per watt (the number of square meters of collecting area that one watt of signal power can be spread across and still be detected); sensitivity improves as this unit increases. Figure 4 has been constructed if the search is

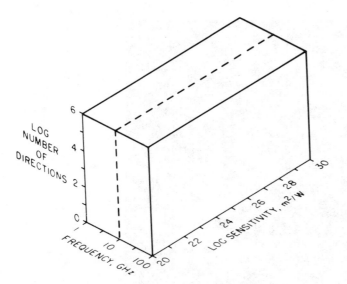

Fig. 4 Open checkbook volume of search space (NASA Ames Research Center)

conducted simultaneously in two orthogonal senses of polarization so that no energy from the signal is missed, and so that the receiver is well matched to the signal type.

The boundaries of the three-dimensional volumes of Fig. 4 represent what would be required to search the entire sky or the million closest solar-type stars, over the free-space microwave window, with sufficient sensitivity to detect the leakage radiation from the current Earth's television and radio transmissions (average transmitter power about 1 megawatt), assuming the analogs were somewhere within the Milky Way Galaxy (within 100,000 light years).[41] Such a search would require vast resources, and an orbiting or lunar platform for its execution. The volume represented is about a factor of a million greater than that which will be searched by NASA's ambitious High Resolution Microwave Survey (see Section V). It is worthwhile remembering that SETI is a truly vast exploration. Even the search through the microwave window could take many decades, and there is always the possibility that the arguments for microwave frequencies are not as compelling as they seem today. This research bears the uncomfortable burden of not being able to promise success with any one search effort, and having to argue for future, more capable systems on the basis of previous failure. How far our species will decide to take this search ultimately will depend upon the perceived worth of answering the age-old question, and our civilization's "threshold of pain" beyond which it will not go, preferring instead to adopt the profound conclusion, "we are alone." There is a long way to go before such a conclusion becomes warranted (if indeed it ever does), but the exciting thing is that we have commenced, at first in hit-or-miss fashion, and soon on a very systematic and well defined comprehensive search, perhaps the first of many. Having started, we have removed that age-old question from the realm of priests and philosophers and placed it within the framework of scientific exploration where it properly belongs.

IV. SETI as an Observational Science

The authors are aware of 61 SETI observational programs since the first Project Ozma search in 1960. The pace at which searches are added to this archive has increased substantially over the past decade, as SETI has gained credibility and respectability within the international scientific community. Frank Drake was indeed a bold pioneer when he conducted his 1960 search.[12] Early on, many of the scientists who got involved in SETI were those with previously established reputations and stable employment, who could afford to indulge in something that was considered "questionable." This was not the way to insure that the vast amount of searching that might be required actually got accomplished, and it perhaps explains why the systematic exploration of the microwave spectrum that has been endorsed for over 30 years is just now commencing. The other reason for the long delay in the conduct of large-scale searches has been technological limitations. Radio astronomy developed as a science very rapidly following World War II, producing nearly perfect receivers for the longer microwave frequencies early on. However, the computational capacity needed to make a systematic search has only recently become affordable. For the most part, the past 30 years of searching has used what the radio astronomical community could provide, and invoked specific hypotheses to limit the scope of the search being conducted to a scale manageable by one or a few researchers. These limiting hypotheses have revolve around "magic" frequencies, preferred directions, and or times and plausible extrapolations of terrestrial technologies (as in Section III.A). In different countries, at different times, the hypotheses have been widely divergent.

A. History of SETI Searches

Frank Drake's Project Ozma carried out on the Tatel telescope of the National Radio Astronomy Observatory in Green Bank, West Virginia, was a so-called "targeted search." He preselected the two nearest stars that resembled the Sun in terms of mass and luminosity (Tau Ceti and Epsilon Eridani). To distinguish between natural astrophysical emission and a technological signal, he built a special receiver having a single narrow channel of width 1 Hz (see discussion below for rationale) that he tuned across 400 KHz of the spectrum near the "magic" frequency associated with the 21-cm line of neutral hydrogen that was also favored by Cocconi and Morrison.[42] It would be nearly two decades before another search was conducted with such fine resolution (primarily because researchers were using existing radio astronomy equipment rather than building their own). This very first search experienced most of the trials and excitement that were to become part of all of the searches that followed. Drake and his collaborators had initially planned to keep the details of the search secret until it was concluded, since they realized that it might be difficult to analyze meticulously any tentative results if the public and the media were present. However, the publication of the Cocconi and Morrison paper took the Green Bank scientists by surprise. Feeling a certain amount of institutional pride, and chagrin at being "scooped," Otto Struve, the director of the observatory, inserted the news about the impending search into an otherwise traditional astronomical presentation. This indeed brought the press and other sightseers to Green Bank and complicated the task of conducting the search in a scientific manner. Drake and his coworkers also got to experience the full range of emotions that accompany the detection of any "false alarm." Having finished the initial series of observations on the first star, the telescope was steered onto the second star. Immediately, the chart recorder began going off scale, recording a very regular signal that was not present on the other target star. Drake recalls thinking, "can it really be this easy?"[43] It was some time before he could arrange to connect the detection apparatus to a hand-held omnidirectional antenna that he extended out the window of the control room. Detection of the same signal on this omni confirmed that the signal had nothing to do with the star being observed, and the researchers' adrenaline flow returned to normal. This, then, was the first encounter with terrestrially generated radio frequency interference (RFI), a problem that continues to increase in severity each year.

As a result of Project Ozma, publication of the Cocconi and Morrison paper and the interest and influence of I.S. Shklovsky, Russian scientists in the 1960s began an observational program of quite a different character. Impressed by the work of Kardashev, who predicted the likely shape of the continuous emission and variability of any advanced technical civilization, Sholomitskii and his coworkers detected the variability of CTA102. Journalists from *Tass* overinterpreted the data on this powerful radio source as being the signature of an advanced technology. This sensational news made *The New York Times*[44] before U.S. scientists measured the redshift of the source in question and identified it as a quasar. (Note that others also took the notion of Kardashev's predicted spectral signature of an advanced civilization seriously. Ken Kellermann working in Australia concluded his paper on the radio galaxy 1934-63 with the statement that no "notch" of ETI origin had been found in its spectrum.[45]) Troitski and his colleagues used a narrow "picket-fence" filter bank spectrometer, with 13 Hz channels spaced 4 kHz apart, to observe 11 stars and our neighboring galaxy M31 (Andromeda Galaxy) at 927 MHz.[46] With this search, the Soviet scientists added the idea of searching an entire galaxy at once, hoping for not just a Type II civilization, but a Type III civilization that would emit a signal so powerful it could be detected over intergalactic distances. Next, the concept of episodic or pulsed events was added to the criteria of potential signals from intelligent extraterrestrials. The Russians constructed broadband (dipole) receivers and deployed them to different sites throughout the Soviet Union for a survey of the sky visible from those latitudes. A single dipole receiver had little or no spatial discrimination. Their scheme was that the detection of the same powerful event at the different sites, with time delays

characteristic of a point source on the sky, would identify the nature of the signal and discriminate against local interference seen at the individual sites. In addition to lacking spatial resolution, dipoles also lack sensitivity, so any signal detected in this manner would have to be intrinsically strong. Given the power believed to be at the disposal of Type II and Type III civilizations, this was not considered a limitation. These searches appear to have been conducted at least sporadically (with different sites participating) from 1968 through 1983.[47] The Soviets also made the first SETI observations at another "magic" frequency, that associated with the natural maser emission from the OH masers (four frequencies near 18-cm wavelength). In 1970 and 1972, Slysh and coworkers used the newly constructed Nancay telescope in France to study 5 OH maser sources and the 10 nearest stars to try to find evidence of an intelligent signal.[48] For a decade following Project Ozma, it was the Soviets who dominated the field of SETI observations.

In 1971 an impressive array of Soviet and American scientists met at the Byurakan Astrophysical Observatory in Soviet Armenia, under the sponsorship of the U.S. and U.S.S.R. Academies of Science. They discussed the searches made to date and the engineering studies of dedicated systems required not only for the systematic searches of the future, but for the communication that would follow.[3] The prestige and recognition afforded by the joint sponsorship of the national academies of science seems to have made SETI an acceptable science. During the next decade, searches increased in frequency and the Americans dominated the field, with one Australian and one West German contribution. Searches used radio astronomical equipment in ways never intended by its designers. Likewise, stored data were reanalyzed with SETI in mind. "Magic" frequencies increased in number and "magic" places (such as the galactic center) and times (synchronization of sender and receiver by means of novae or supernovae) were also explored. By 1981, when another meeting under the sponsorship of the U.S.S.R. and Estonian Academies of science again brought together U.S. and U.S.S.R. scientists, the state of Soviet observational programs was diminished. The only new and exciting Soviet development throughout the decade had been the construction of a system for searching for rapid optical pulses called MANIA (described in Section III.A). Although mainly intended to study unusual radio objects, stellar targets for SETI were inserted into the observing list, whenever possible.[50]

The 1980s saw a new turn in SETI observations: the construction of equipment optimized for detecting technological signals rather than astrophysical ones. Many of these systems, or their descendants, are in use today and are discussed in the next section. Attempts to detect evidence other than intentional radio beacons became more numerous, and most of these have already been discussed in Section III.A. The one thing that remained a cornerstone of the observational programs of the 1980s was the inability of researchers to recognize the presence of an interesting candidate signal, although it was still within the beam of the telescope. Either raw data were recorded on site and laboriously analyzed after the fact, or data exceeding some preset threshold were identified as interesting and recorded for later follow-up. To date, this later follow-up has failed to reacquire the candidate signals, or when it has, the signals were shown to be due to interference. But what about all those other cases? Most probably they were caused by interference as well, but RFI is intrinsically time variable and cannot be positively identified as such without real-time detection and analysis. The recent advances in computational speed and the decrease in the cost of computer memory will soon make this real-time analysis possible. This will be the hallmark of searches in the 1990s and beyond.

B. SETI Today

1. U.S. SETI Programs

There are four SETI observing programs currently in operation in the U.S.: at the Ohio State University Radio Observatory (OSURO), at Mount Wilson, the SERENDIP II program, and META SETI. Each of these takes a different approach, and together they represent the range of possible search strategies. In addition, the NASA High Resolution Microwave Survey, planned to be 10-billion times more comprehensive in its coverage of the search space than all previous searches combined, got under way beginning in late 1992.

a. Ongoing searches. In the early 1970s, the Ohio State University Radio Observatory (OSURO) completed the radio survey of the sky and the catalog for which it had been constructed. Government funding for the telescope operations was withdrawn. In 1973 the telescope began a sidereal survey of the sky, looking for evidence of ETI at a frequency corresponding to the 21-cm line in a frame of reference at rest with respect to the galactic center. It is necessary to define this special frame of reference; the rotation of the galaxy, the peculiar motion of the Sun, our orbital velocity and the rotation of Earth means that at any moment sender and receiver are moving with some relative velocity and that signals transmitted from one will arrive Doppler shifted by some amount at the other. This shift (and indeed a drift in frequency due to any relative accelerations) could be compensated for, if the velocities of the transmitter were known. In a sky survey such as this one, there are multiple candidate targets, at different distances, within the telescope beam at one time, and so it is not possible to compensate for each of them. However, if sender and receiver know their own velocity with respect to a special frame of reference, both could compensate for their own motion to transmit and receive a signal that will appear at the "magic" frequency in that special rest frame. In 1973, OSURO adopted the galactic center rest frame, and commenced its search. It continues this task today with inadequate funding and volunteer labor supplied by a consortium of small colleges that find the instrument an ideal vehicle for providing students with "hands-on" experience. Because

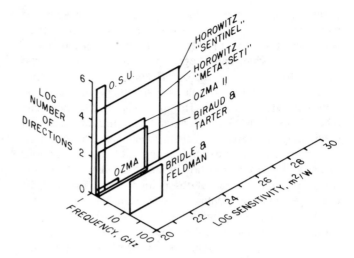

**Fig. 5 Some current SETI searches
(NASA Ames Research Center)**

of the low level of support, this aging telescope has very limited backend electronics, and is more often "off" the air than "on." Nevertheless the collecting area is large (equivalent to a 53-m parabolic dish), and this facility is planning to become the first to implement an automated "real-time" detection scheme. Whenever a signal with the right response pattern is detected above threshold, the telescope will interrupt its programmed sky scan. It will then track and record data on the source as long as it remains above the horizon, then it will resume its scan of the sky. Although the recorded data must still await the arrival of a human at some later time to discover the event, it is hoped that the tracking of the source will provide enough information to distinguish between RFI and possible ETI. In the latter case, reacquisition must be possible if the candidate is to be considered believable. OSURO has been motivated to implement this real-time approach in part because of a now infamous "wow" signal discovered by a researcher early in the search, and never found again. The data available suggest to some that this signal came from a great distance and not from terrestrial interference. A good deal of telescope time has been spent trying to reacquire this signal with no success.[51]

The most recent entry to the list of ongoing SETI searches involves the infrared spectrum, not microwaves. Charles Townes, who early on suggested lasers as devices for interstellar communication, has recently completed construction of an infrared interferometer, operating on flatbed trucks on top of Mount Wilson. Albert Betz, a colleague of Townes, has built a tunable 1000-channel acousto-optical spectrometer with high spectral resolution (relative to what is needed astronomically) to search for 10 micron CO_2 laser emission from the vicinity of 150 nearby stars. He used one of the 1.5-m telescopes of the interferometer as a collector. This search has just begun. The ability to achieve high gain, at these shorter wavelengths, with modest size antennas might provide a useful interstellar communications network of highly collimated, beamed signals, if indeed advanced technologies can manipulate the CO_2 in the atmosphere of their own planet or some other body in their planetary system and by so doing create powerful laser emission.

The first SERENDIP system consisted of a 100-channel spectrometer functioning at the Hat Creek Radio Observatory. It was the first example of the so-called commensal searches, because it shared the radio waves being collected by an astronomer using the telescope for astronomical research and simply analyzed the data stream for evidence of artifacts. The challenge for this type of approach is to keep track of what direction on the sky the antenna is being pointed and at what frequency the sky is being observed. In the original SERENDIP, this operation depended upon observing logs and comments from the primary observer and was often undetermined. Although the spectrometer functioned in real-time, recording data in any channel that exceeded a preset threshold, the process of trying to determine whether any recorded events represented multiple detections of the same signal at the same frequency coming from the same direction on the sky took much more time than the data acquisition. SERENDIP was replaced by SERENDIP II, which had a spectrometer with 65,536 channels of 1 Hz resolution, and when deployed on the 300-foot telescope in Green Bank, it also had a direct data line to the computer controlling the telescope. The position of the telescope and the values of the local settings (which then provided the frequency of the observation) were automatically recorded along with the data above threshold. In all, about 12,000 hours of commensal observing was accomplished before the 300-foot antenna collapsed. The observations spanned the frequency range from 18 to 21 cm and covered much of the sky visible from Green Bank with varying sensitivity depending on the nature of the primary observations being conducted. Several dozen candidate signals were subsequently reobserved using the Green Bank 140-foot antenna during time requested by the SERENDIP observers. No signal was reacquired.[52] SERENDIP II has recently been upgraded by the addition of an optical disk in order to allow it to record all 65,536 channels of spectral data, not just those few channels above threshold. In this configuration it has been used to study the statistics of RFI at a number of sites being considered as dedicated sites for SETI observations in the future.[53] Soon SERENDIP II will be replaced by SERENDIP III, which will provide millions of channels of spectral resolution and will be deployed at Arecibo in the same commensal fashion.[54] The main drawback of this type of observation is the large amount of post-processing necessary to understand whether any detections represent recurrences of the same signal, and the necessity to develop filters that recognize and disregard local interference. This latter impediment has been very instructive and has provided an opportunity to learn lessons needed by future real-time search systems.

META SETI stands for Megachannel Extraterrestrial Assay, and is by far the most capable of any system on the air today. In order to create a system that could conduct a significant search with modest resources, Paul Horowitz has made a number of simplifying assumptions. He has assumed that the signal is being beamed directly at us and nowhere else. Given that line of sight, the senders can compensate for all of their motions with respect to some standard of rest, and we can do the same with respect to ours. Then a "magic" frequency transmitted by the sender will be detected by the receiver at exactly the right frequency and that frequency will not change in time, even though our Earth is rotating and moving through the galaxy at high speed. Further, he assumes that the signal will be monochromatic (that is it will occur at only one specific frequency) and that he can use spectrometer channels that are extremely narrow to find it with the highest possible signal to noise ratio (Section V.A discusses the rationale for this choice). All that remains is to pick the right "magic" frequency and the right frame of reference. Since 1985, when META first began searching the sky visible from Harvard, Massachusetts, with a 26-m antenna, it has searched the 79 percent of the sky visible from that site, at three different magic frequencies relative to each of three different inertial reference frames in each of two circular polarizations, with eight million spectral resolution channels, each 0.05 Hz wide.[55] The magic frequencies are the 1420 MHz line of neutral hydrogen, twice that frequency and an 18-cm line associated with the OH radical. The three frames of reference adopted are a frame associated with the motion of the center of mass of the Earth and Sun, the galactic center frame of rest, and the inertial frame in which the 2.73 K cosmic background radiation is at rest. The uncertainty in the velocity of this last reference frame is the reason META must be conducted with so many channels, even though it is a "magic" frequency strategy. The eight million channels of 0.05 Hz width just cover the 400 kHz needed to account for the possible velocity errors.

The search is fairly automated, scanning a strip of sky 1/2 degree wide for 1 day before moving the telescope. Information about any channels that contain accumulated power in excess of 20 times the expected rms noise level are automatically recorded to tape. Tapes are analyzed at the end of each week. Use of such narrow binwidths, and compensation for the Earth's motion with respect to a particular reference frame provides a side benefit; the technique automatically discriminates against terrestrial interference. Since a local oscillator in the system must be shifted many times per second to properly remove the effects of the Earth's motion and permit the detection of an ETI signal at a fixed frequency, any fixed frequency signal on the Earth will appear to drift in frequency by the rate the local oscillator is changed. It requires 20 seconds for a 0.05 Hz wide bin to fully register the presence of a signal. Thus, a terrestrial interfering signal that is made to drift through a number of channels in less than 20 seconds will be poorly sensed by the META spectrometer.

In his selection of a number of magic frequencies (HI line, $2 \times$ HI line, OH lines) and a number of inertial reference frames (heliocentric, galactic barycenter and cosmic background rest frame), Horowitz is trying to expand the simplifying assumptions that make his search strategy tractable. To

WHY SEARCH FOR NARROWBAND SIGNALS ?

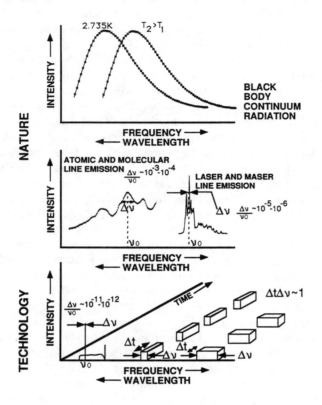

Fig. 6 Tutorial on narrowband signals (NASA Ames Research Center)

acquire full sky coverage, the META system has recently been duplicated by two young engineers from Argentina. META II has been operating since October 1990 on a 26-m antenna near Buenos Aires, providing the only continuing search of the southern sky.[56] Like SERENDIP, META can be expected to grow in the future, perhaps as large as 100 million channels. In this way it will attempt to remove the limiting "magic" frequency hypothesis and undertake a more systematic search of the sky.

b. NASA high resolution microwave survey rationale. To be readily detectable, any signal must appear to be distinct from the natural emissions that are studied by astronomers. Its degree and sense of polarization, and its modulation scheme must not make the signal look like other sources of cosmic noise, or it will be missed. Natural emissions are broadband; that is, they occur over a wide range of frequencies. The top panel of Fig. 6 illustrates the typical black body radiation that is generated by celestial bodies of all of the temperatures from the 2.73 degrees Kelvin cosmic background remnant radiation from the Big Bang, to the visible light radiated by stars whose atmospheres have temperatures of thousands of degrees, to X-rays generated by turbulent gas that has a temperature of many millions of degrees. The middle panel illustrates

the fact that sometimes the smooth black body curve is punctuated by emission or absorption features that are indicative of the presence of various atoms and molecules in the gas. These spectral line features are still relatively broadband; the frequency width of such a feature divided by the central frequency of the feature is about 10^{-3}. The narrowest known natural spectral features belong to astrophysical masers created from molecules such as the OH radical and H_2O. For masers the fractional bandwidths of the features can reach 10^{-5} to 10^{-6}. In contrast, the bottom panel of Fig. 6 illustrates the results of a technologically generated signal. In order to generate easily detectable signals that require a minimum of transmitted power, engineers often compress that power into a very narrowband continuous wave or CW signals having a fractional bandwidth as small as 10^{-12}. This spectral purity is something that appears to be impossible in nature, and therefore any signal exhibiting this characteristic provides strong evidence for a technology. On the left of the bottom panel, the transmitted power associated with a television signal is illustrated. The modulated signal that represents the information-bearing picture is spread over 6 MegaHertz (MHz) and to any receiver other than a tuned TV receiver, this power would look like random noise. However, embedded in the signal are both video and audio CW carriers that have a much higher spectral energy density and are readily detectable (indeed this is how your TV locates the information-bearing signal associated with a particular station). Although it is amusing (or distressing) to think of our early TV and radio broadcasts leaking away from the planet Earth and now enveloping nearby stars, it is the carriers and not the pictorial content that are the most detectable. Unless the receiving civilization chooses to build planet-size collectors, the information content associated with the picture will probably go undetected because the signal-to-noise ratio is so low. The lower panel of Fig. 6 illustrates something else that can be done to minimize the transmitted power necessary to convey a certain amount of information; the power can be concentrated in time as well as in frequency. It is very economical to broadcast regular, narrowband pulses, whose width in the frequency dimension is no greater than that required by the duration of the pulse. The Uncertainty Principle demands that the product of pulse duration and bandwidth exceed unity. Technology strives to come as close as possible to this lower bound, whereas naturally produced pulses (the pulsars) are characterized by a product that exceeds unity by many orders of magnitude. Taking the approach that searches for evidence of extraterrestrial technology should concentrate on those types of signals that (as far as we know) Nature cannot generate, leads us to a search strategy that looks for narrowband signals compressed in frequency and perhaps also in time. Here "narrowband" means anything appreciably narrower than 300 Hz, the width of the narrowest known OH maser feature. As opposed to natural signals, we expect a technologically generated signal to be highly polarized, and although we suspect it will be circularly polarized, the detection equipment should be able to match any arbitrary sense of polarization. Having defined the type of signal to be

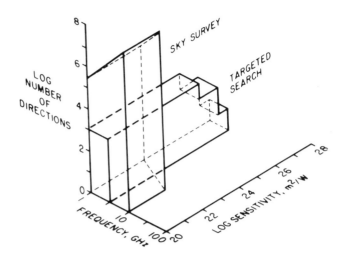

**Fig. 7 SETI MOP search volume
(NASA Ames Research Center)**

sought, it is now possible to devise search strategies and instrumentation that are optimized for its detection.

c. Technical approach. In order to optimally detect a narrowband signal, it is necessary to use a receiving system with individual channels whose frequency width is exactly matched to that of the signal itself. Broader channels sense more noise without detecting any additional signal power, and narrower channels exclude some of the available signal power. This has led Horowitz to build his META SETI system with ultra-narrowband channels of width 0.05 Hz. However, such a system is limited to detecting only those signals that remain constant in frequency for at least 20 seconds; there can be no uncompensated relative accelerations between sender and receiver and the signal must be a narrow CW carrier, narrowband pulses are too broad to be detected. The most likely source of acceleration between sender and receiver is planetary rotation or the spin of an orbital satellite. The frequency drift introduced by either of these will be proportional to the frequency of the signal itself. Using our own solar system as a model, we find that the fractional rate of change of frequency with time $(\dot{v}/v)$ will be less than 10^{-9} per second, or about 1 Hz per second at a frequency of 1 GHz. In order to remove the limiting assumption that any signal will be intended for us and therefore Doppler compensated, the NASA High Resolution Microwave Survey has adopted 1 Hz as a minimum channel binwidth for its instrumentation and has incorporated signal detection algorithms that search for all of the possible drifts in frequency up to +/- 10^{-9} Hz per second/Hz. In addition, the NASA High Resolution Microwave Survey will also make use of channels as wide as 30 Hz to permit a search for narrowband pulses and to allow for a rapid survey of the sky.

The survey will use existing radio telescopes around the world. To these telescopes it will bring the special purpose digital signal processing equipment required to divide the incoming radio signal into tens of millions of narrow chan-

nels, and the dedicated special purpose computers needed to sift through the outputs of all of those channels seeking patterns that would indicate the presence of narrowband CW or pulsed signals. These systems will run in an unattended mode, automatically attempting to determine in real-time whether detected signals are due to RFI or whether they might be coming from a distant extraterrestrial transmitter. The requirement for real-time or near-real-time signal detection and RFI recognition demands extremely fast computational capability. Scientists are alerted and brought into the process whenever a signal passes the automatic verification process. Additional tests will be performed depending on the nature of the signal itself, and independent confirmation will be sought for those candidate ETI signals that continue to pass these tests. If and when it becomes clear that the most probable explanation for the detected signal is in fact an ETI transmission, the results will be publicly announced and the relevant data will be made available for inspection. (See Section V.)

Two different strategies have been employed by SETI researchers for deciding the directions in which to look for a signal. One can select targets, such as stars like our Sun, that have an a priori higher probability of hosting planets like our Earth and evolved life. Or one can search the entire sky (inevitably at lower sensitivity) in case the appropriate target is so far away that we are not yet aware of it and we would fail to look in the proper direction if we restricted the search to the known targets. Both these search strategies will be employed simultaneously by the NASA High Resolution Microwave Survey. The Targeted Search will use some of the world's largest radio telescopes that routinely conduct radio astronomical observations, and the Sky Survey will make use of smaller antennas that are part of NASA's global Deep Space Network (DSN). The observational phase of the NASA High Resolution Microwave Survey commenced in October 1992 and will last through the end of the century.

Together these two search strategies should accomplish a search that is millions of times more comprehensive than what has been possible over the past 30 years. Figure 7 illustrates the volume to be searched and should be compared with Fig. 5 to appreciate what an improvement the special purpose digital signal processing equipment and the use of large antennas will permit. However, one should remember that as impressive as this progress will be, the volume searched by the NASA High Resolution Microwave Survey will still be about a factor of a million less than the volume of Fig. 4, which represented the effort to systematically search the Milky Way Galaxy for an Earth analog. Success cannot be guaranteed, but unless we search, failure is assured.

d. Targeted search. Antennas and RF Systems: The current list of target stars contains 773 stars chosen from the "Royal Greenwich Observatory Catalogue of Stars Within 25 Parsecs"[57] as being similar to the Sun. The list is now being optimized to remove unsatisfactory multiple star systems or stars that are too young to have permitted the billions of years that seem to be necessary for evolution, or stars that are too far from the exact spectral classification of our Sun. Stars that are removed will be replaced by other good candidates, and when the task is completed the target list will contain about 1000 solar-type stars within 100 light years of Earth. These nearby stars will be approximately uniformly distributed on the sky and will require telescopes in the northern and southern hemispheres to complete the observations.

Antenna size is the most critical factor in determining the sensitivity that can be achieved in a given observing time. Therefore, the Targeted Search would like to utilize the largest available antennas. The Project expects to use a small percentage of the available time on the 1000-foot Arecibo telescope in Puerto Rico and around 1995 it will take over the operation of the Green Bank 140-foot telescope as a dedicated facility for SETI observations. Time has been requested on the 70-m telescope in NASA's DSN complex in Tidbinbilla, Australia. In addition, it is possible that the 91-m telescope in Nançay, France and the 64-m CSIRO telescope in Parkes, Australia will be utilized to complete the observations. The efficiency of these large antennas decreases at higher frequencies because of irregularities in their surfaces, and therefore the Targeted Search will concentrate on the 1 to 3 GHz portion of the terrestrial microwave window, where the best sensitivity can be achieved. Higher frequencies will be observed where the opportunity exists at particular observatories. Each target will be observed for at least 300 seconds at every frequency. Stars closer than about 20 light years and all of the stars observed with the dedicated SETI facility will be observed for at least 1000 seconds at each frequency. This not only increases the sensitivity for those stars near enough to have detected and responded to our early television transmissions, but it allows for the detection of pulses with longer pulse repetition periods. In all, about 50,000 hours of observing time are required to complete the Targeted Search, including the dedicated site.

Radio astronomy observatories build feeds and receivers for their telescopes that are optimal at the natural emission line frequencies of interesting atoms and molecules. The DSN builds feeds and receivers that cover the precise frequencies that are emitted by the spacecraft being tracked. SETI is thus unique in its desire to study the entire terrestrial microwave window. Covering a wide range of frequencies and yet achieving a very low system temperature in order to maximize the sensitivity of the observations is a difficult technical challenge. For the Targeted Search, the Project expects to be able to cover the 1 to 3 GHz portion of the spectrum with only two dual polarization wideband feeds followed by low-noise cryogenic amplifiers and receiver systems, although attaining a system temperature of better than 25 K at all frequencies. This represents an improvement of about a factor of 2 in the current system temperatures for some of the observatories mentioned above. It is anticipated that these so-called RF systems will be useful additions for traditional radio astronomical observations. The requirements for detecting drifting and non-drifting CW signals demand very good phase stability from these systems, and the overall gain stability will

be good enough for radio astronomical usage.

Spectrum Analysis: The Targeted Search will utilize a multichannel spectrum analyzer (MCSA) that has a 10 MHz input bandwidth and simultaneously provides six narrowband resolutions as output. These outputs are:

14,370,048 channels of resolution binwidth 1 Hz,
7,185,024 channels of resolution binwidth 2 Hz,
2,592,512 channels of resolution binwidth 4 Hz,
2,052,864 channels of resolution binwidth 7 Hz,
1,026,432 channels of resolution binwidth 14 Hz, and
513,216 channels of resolution binwidth 28 Hz

The MCSA is a discrete Fourier Transform device that implements a Fast Fourier Transform (FFT) based on a prime factor algorithm using a custom VLSI chip developed for the Project.[58] It is being implemented by Silicon Engines, Inc., in Mountain View, California. The processing is done in real-time and the output data rate from each of the resolutions is 20 megabytes per second. The architecture of the MCSA is based on two sets of special filters (to limit the effects of any strong RFI signal in the input band) followed by a Fourier Transform to produce a power spectrum. The input data are oversampled both in frequency and time in order to avoid a loss of sensitivity to signals with frequency between two channels or pulses spanning two time samples. There is an MCSA to operate on each of the circularly polarized data streams delivered by the RF system. Output from the 1 or 2 Hz resolution binwidths goes to a CW detector and data above threshold from each of the six resolutions go to a pulse detector.

Signal Detection, Verification, and Confirmation: Two separate dedicated hardware processors are used to identify nearly straight line patterns in the frequency-time domain that could be the result of narrowband CW or pulsed signals that may or may not change frequency with time. The CW detector must achieve a processing speed of 1200 MIPS and contain 20 gigabytes of temporary memory in order make a detection in less time than it took to acquire the input data. After a 1000 second observation the CW detector can find a signal that is 6 dB below the noise in any single sample. The pulse detector operates on each of the six output resolutions in an attempt to match the unknown width of the pulse. Because the input data rate is lower, the pulse detector requires only about 60 MIPS of processing capability and 2 gigabytes of memory. The signal detection algorithms were developed by Cullers and his colleagues[59] and the hardware is being implemented at NASA Ames Research Center and by Reykjalin, Inc., in Berkeley, California.

Any signal detected by the CW or pulse detector is reported to the computer that controls the entire system. Here the reports are compared with a database of known RFI and a decision is made as to whether or not the target needs to be reobserved at that frequency. Reobservation consists of moving the telescope and local oscillators back to the same target and frequency. If the signal is reacquired, the telescope is moved off source. If the signal disappears, the telescope is

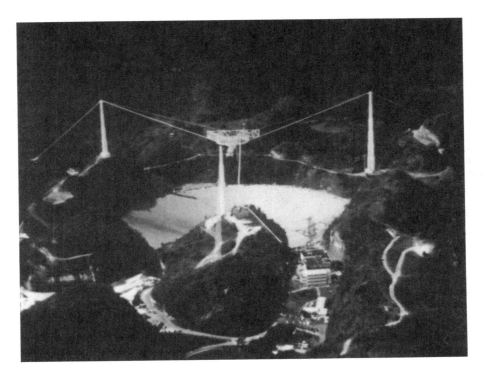

Fig. 8 Arecibo, Puerto Rico: National Astronomy & Ionosphere Center, Cornell University, Space Sciences Building, Ithaca, New York

moved back on source and a small map is made to determine the peak position of the signal. A signal that is not reacquired when the telescope is moved back on source or one that persists when the telescope moves off source, is labeled as interference and added to the database. Following any successful outcome from this automated verification process, a scientist will be alerted and will continue tests that may ultimately lead to an independent confirmation of an ETI signal.

e. The sky survey. Antennas and RF Systems: The area of the sky seen by a radio telescope (its half-power beamwidth) becomes smaller as the diameter of the antenna increases. For an antenna of given size, the beamwidth decreases as the frequency of the observation increases. In a search for faint ETI signals, large antennas are desirable because of the increased sensitivity they provide. However, in a search strategy that covers the entire sky, smaller antennas with larger beamwidths must be used in order to cut down the time required to complete the search. Furthermore, these smaller antennas have smoother surfaces than the larger ones used for the Targeted Search, and therefore can be used at higher frequencies to explore the entire terrestrial microwave window. The NASA High Resolution Microwave Survey will make use of new beam-waveguide 34-m antennas now being constructed at the DSN stations in the United States, Australia, and Spain. These are extremely efficient and frequency agile devices that provide the ability to change the observing frequency by changing the position of a large mirror to redirect the RF signal to different receivers. The Project will provide the continuous frequency coverage from 1 to 10 GHz that is needed for SETI with six packages containing dual-polarization feed horns, low-noise amplifiers and receivers. Two will be identical to those used in the Targeted Search and four more will be needed to cover the 3 to 7 GHz range. At the present time the Project is requesting 16 hours per day of time on one of the 34-m antennas in the DSN for a period of 6 and a half years to complete the search. The first half of the time will be at Goldstone, and then the southern sky will be observed from Tidbinbilla. In order to complete the search in this length of time the antennas will be driven across the sky at a rate of 0.2 degrees per second, in an oval pattern that attempts to keep the elevation angle (and therefore the interference) roughly constant.

Spectrum Analysis: The Sky Survey will utilize a digital FFT spectrum analyzer unit having an instantaneous bandwidth of 320 MHz and a channel resolution of 20 Hz. Four 80 MHz modules are used side by side to implement the full 320 MHz in a single unit. Two units are provided in order that both right-hand and left-hand polarizations can be observed simultaneously. A real-time, post processor accepts data from the spectrum analyzer, and stores data that exceed a specified threshold. Signal detection is carried out by comparing these above-threshold data to data collected along a nearby scan path, as described below. This wideband spectrum analyzer has been designed by the Jet Propulsion Laboratory.

Signal Detection, Verification, and Confirmation: In order to scan the entire sky, the celestial sphere is divided into

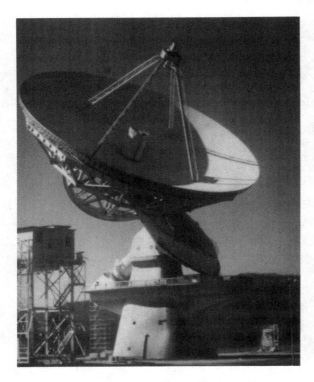

Fig. 9 140-foot antenna at National Radio Astronomy Observatory, Green Bank, West Virginia

elongated frames approximately 45 degrees wide by 1 degree high. The sky frame width (except near the celestial poles) is oriented along the nearly constant elevation direction in which the beam is scanned. An oval-shaped scan pattern is used to scan each frame. Signal detection is carried out by comparing data taken along adjacent scan lines separated by one half-power beam width. Candidate signals, identified in the adjacent scan detection algorithm, are reobserved under software control. If any candidate signals are reacquired in the follow-up process, a scientist will be summoned to the control station, although additional data on the candidate signal continue to be collected and recorded.

Detection of a verifed signal by either the Targeted Search or the Sky Survey will then be followed by procedures similar to those outlined in the section on post-detection protocols, discussed at the end of this chapter.

2. U.S.S.R. SETI Programs

In the last few years, new Soviet SETI observational programs have begun. The OBZOR program first proposed by Troitskii in 1981[46] to use 100 small antennas to continuously monitor the sky at 565 MHz seems to have permanently stalled, but a new generation of experimentalists are beginning to implement observational programs. V. Strelnitsky has recently published a new search strategy based on the idea that extraterrestrial intelligence would communicate using shorter wavelengths at which it would be possible to transmit very narrow beams (10^{-10} - 10^{-11} degrees). Such narrow beams will create enormous signal-to-noise ratios, but will not be able to illuminate the habitable zone (region where planets with surface temperatures suitable for liquid water might exist) of a distant star. Instead, it has been argued that the transmitting civilization would aim its narrow beam directly at the central star of a potential receiving civilization. If the receiving civilization (us in this case), chooses to observe a potential transmitting civilization only when that star is at opposition (i.e., our Sun, the Earth, and the distant star are all in a line), then the transmission will be successful, assuming that the frequency is correct and the sensitivity of the receiver is adequate. This is, in fact, another "magic" time strategy. Strelnitsky and Filippova have identified a list of 29 solar-type stars that are near the ecliptic plane (those for which the linear alignment is possible) and have begun a program of observations called ZODIAC using existing Soviet radio and optical telescopes. Moreover, Strelnitsky has urged all of the other observers having these stars among their targets to observe them at times surrounding their opposition.[60]

In addition to this ZODIAC program of observations scheduled at opposition, the Soviets began a small observing program known as Aelita at the Orlyonok Young Pioneers camp on the Black Sea coast. Local astronomers and engineers donated an existing 3-m antenna and constructed a new receiving system for the camp, and it will be used by the youngsters to conduct a 21-cm survey of the equatorial region of the sky between declinations of +/- 23 degrees.

Plans for building a sophisticated signal processing back end for the Bears' Lake 64-m antenna near Moscow are just now coming to maturity. An active SETI observing program using this large, dedicated antenna can be expected to commence within a few years.[61] The largest millimeter radiotelescope with a mirror diameter of 70 m is being built in the Soviet Union. It will operate at wavelengths longer than 1 mm. This facility is erected in the mountains near Samarkand (Plato Suffa). This telescope will be used for the search of communicative signals at the frequency of positronium main transition (1.5 mm). A full sky survey to search for astroengineering constructions will be carried out as well. The Soviets have also extended an invitation to U.S. observers to bring SETI-specific receiving equipment to a number of Soviet telescopes for an extended series of joint SETI observations. This program is expected to materialize sometime in 1992.

3. SETI in France

The largest radio telescope in France belongs to the Observatory of Paris and is located in the middle of the country at Nançay. This is a larger version of the Kraus telescope at Ohio State University and has a collecting area equivalent to a 91-m parabolic dish. In 1980, this facility finished building a 1024-channel autocorrelator with variable resolution to conduct spectral line radio astronomical research. Some of the staff were interested in SETI, and so they included an option for achieving a narrow resolution of 48 Hz for such studies.

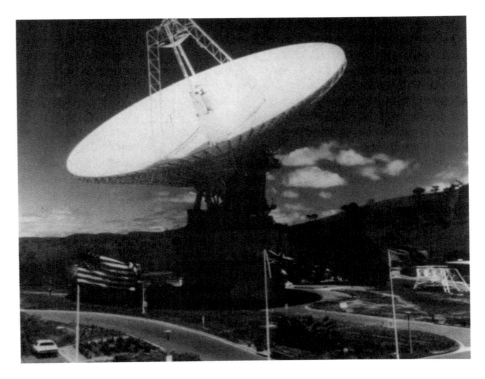

Fig. 10 70 m antenna in Australia (NASA Ames Research Center)

From 1981 through 1988 the Nançay Radio Observatory hosted a collaborative U.S. (Jill Tarter) and French (Francois Biraud) SETI observational program.[63] This was also a targeted search at "magic" frequencies, but it attempted to remove the uncertainty in reference frames by searching nearly 1 MHz of the spectrum surrounding the 21-cm hydrogen line and 2 MHz surrounding the 18-cm OH main lines. The telescope has limited tracking capability, and whereas each of 343 target stars were in view, the autocorrelator was shifted in frequency in order to cover as much of the desired frequency range as possible. Observations were recorded and analyzed in the 24-hour period before the target was again visible, and any required reobservations of candidate signals were made at that time. The long running program provided good statistical data on the prevalence of interference at the site and its seasonal variation, but no verifiable ETI signal. In 1989 Jean Heidmann joined the collaboration and suggested another way of selecting magic "frequencies" for stars within 100 light years, based on the periods of known pulsars.[64] The basic frequency of a nearby pulsar (<500 light years) is multiplied by some "remarkable" number such as pi or e to generate a frequency that is within the quiet region of the microwave spectrum. For each target, the pulsar closest to the line of sight is used, and "magic" frequencies from 1 to 6 GHz are generated and observed. This program has yet to be completed because of the increased incidence of interference when investigating frequencies that fall outside of the "protected bands" of radio astronomy.

4. SETI Programs in Australia

As of this writing, there is one SETI observing project ongoing in Australia. It is being conducted by a collaboration of scientists from various universities, led by David Blair of the University of Western Australia,[65] and uses the large 210-foot CSIRO antenna at Parkes. This is a targeted search of 100 nearby solar-type stars, many of them visible only from the southern hemisphere. This search is being conducted at yet another magic frequency; 4.462336275 GHz = pi times the hydrogen line frequency. Three inertial reference frames, the target star barycenter, the solar barycenter, and the geocenter are assumed. Observations to date have utilized the observatory's correlator and an HP spectrum analyzer to achieve 512 channels of binwidth 100 Hz for each of the three choices of inertial reference frame. The observers continuously studied the accumulated outputs of the three spectrum analyzers so that any signals could be detected and reobserved in near-real-time. One star yielded a tentative detection that was later attributed to time varying interference. These researchers plan to make more observations using systems with narrower binwidths and covering the rest frame set by the 3K cosmic background radiation as well.

After 30 years of searching, it should not be surprising that no signals have yet been found. Figure 5 represents those recent and ongoing searches that have explored the largest volume of parameter space to date. It is impossible to graphically depict just how gossamer thin are the slices of

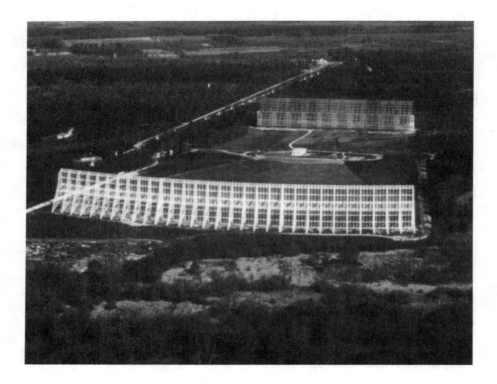

Fig. 11 Nancay Observatory, Station de Radioastronomie, Nancay, France

frequency space that have been explored thus far. In all, the volume explored by Fig. 5 is a factor of 10^{-11} of the volume depicted in Fig. 4. Much effort and energy has been expended over 30 years, but without the proper tools, the total effect has been miniscule with respect to the job yet to be done. In reality, we have not yet begun to search.

V. Other Aspects of SETI

This section deals with aspects of SETI that are separate and distinct from the science and technology covered in the previous chapters. They are interstellar languages, the cultural aspects of SETI, including post-detection protocols, and last but not least, the side benefits of SETI to other areas of human endeavor.

A. Interstellar Languages

The previous chapters have referred to the detection of signals of ETI origin, and have described a variety of different signal types that we look for. However, in all of the cases these have been treated basically as carriers, usually narrowband, which may be continuous or pulsed. The transmission of complex information, in contrast, requires some combination of wider bandwidth, greater signal strength, and more time. It also requires some type of language.

For signals that are intended only for internal use by the transmitting ETI species, it may be very difficult for us to decode complex information. However, in the case of signals that are intended to be detected there could be simple instruc-

tions on frequency, bandwidth, signal strength, polarization, and time for picking up a separate signal containing the message. In constructing such a message it is often assumed that the transmitting civilization will use the principle of anti-cryptography, that is, they will make it as easy as possible to decode. Since they will obviously have a language of their own, the first part of the signal could be instructions on how to read their language. Two authors have tackled the task of developing interstellar languages. In each case they have assumed that we are developing one to use in transmissions from Earth to ETI. How would we do it? In fact, we would be the recipients of a message, but the exercise surely helps us to think about the decoding process.

Freudenthal developed such a language in great detail in 1960.[66] He started by making no assumption about the scientific and technological capability of the other civilization, and built up a lengthy and laborious tutorial beginning with simple mathematical concepts. DeVito[67] took a somewhat different approach in 1990. He made the assumption that the other civilization would be at least as advanced as us in science and technology, and proceeded rapidly through a logical exposition of the basics of science, with emphasis on explaining those quantities that we on Earth have defined in an arbitrary manner. Numbers come first, followed by Mendeleev's periodic table, atomic number, atomic weight, Avogadro's number, the gram, the meter, the degree, the calorie, time as derived from radioactive decay, astronomical concepts, geometry, the differential and integral calculus, acceleration, electricity and magnetism from Faraday's law of electrochemistry, black body radiation, Boltzman's constant,

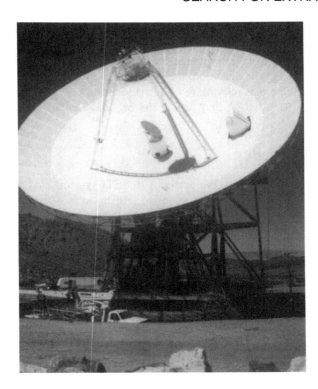

Fig. 12 New 34-m antenna at Goldstone: Jet Propulsion Laboratory, Pasadena, California

Wein's law, and so on. Descriptions of the physical and chemical structure of our planet follow. Biology is more complicated, but can be enhanced by descriptions of biochemistry. When it comes to the physiology and behavior of intelligent beings, and their history and sociology, things become much more difficult. DeVito proposes, as have others, to combine the language with pictures, which are sometimes literally worth a thousand words. Pictures are particularly helpful when describing complex engineering projects. In this way a fairly complete interstellar language can be built up. If we detect a signal, and it incorporates a message, we can expect from them a similar type of interstellar language tutorial, always assuming the transmission is intended for us.

B. Cultural Aspects of SETI

It is generally agreed that the discovery of an extraterrestrial civilization, probably much in advance of our own, would be a major achievement for mankind. Some have compared it to the Copernican revolution. We would be dealing with new knowledge that might greatly exceed in its complexity and importance that which emerged some 500 years ago. The great discoveries of Copernicus and Galileo showed that the Earth was not the center around which everything else in the universe revolved, as Ptolemy believed. The discovery of an advanced extraterrestrial civilization would at once prove that mankind is not the pinnacle of creation, but perhaps just a lowly form of intelligent life. The rich panoply of achievements of the ETI species might be difficult to absorb.

We now ask two questions. First, what is the outcome of the discovery for our own civilization, both in the short term and in the long term? Second, what actions should we take following the discovery? Together these questions embrace the topic of the "cultural aspects of SETI." They embrace many disciplines, especially sociology, psychology, political science, religion, international affairs, and space law. History and cultural anthropology will contribute. Studies on these aspects of SETI have only recently begun.

In the area of the social sciences, much remains to be done. There are really two components. The first deals with the situation today, that is, before the detection is made. The second deals with the situation after detection. The very fact that different nations are slowly but surely putting more effort into carrying out SETI observations will have some cultural effects. At the very least people will become aware of this new endeavor for mankind, and begin to think about the implications of the discovery for our own civilization. The possibility of the existence of ETI is already widely known in the more literate nations, because of education and communications. This is in striking contrast to the situation at the time of Copernicus. At our present stage the ideas embodied in SETI need to be more widely understood, and the implications of success more widely debated. There is a long list of questions. To give some examples: What is the legal status of ETI? How will different religions absorb the discovery into their belief structures? What international organization is best suited to deal with the sociological issues raised by the discovery? Note that the signal may be more than just a carrier, and may contain additional information. The amount of this additional information can vary from small to very large. It is possible that we may be privileged to learn the total knowledge of an advanced civilization, the "Encyclopedia Galactica." This might take a long time to send, and even longer to digest, absorb, and assimilate. In such cases the number of questions we ask is obviously vastly increased, for example: Does the civilization know of other ETI species? What is their history? What is their present social structure? How can we best disseminate the new knowledge? Is there anything to fear? Can the new knowledge be helpful in overcoming some of the pressing problems of our own civilization? How did they overcome similar problems in their past?

These implications can be divided loosely into two parts. The first deals with the absorption of the new knowledge into our own culture. It is clear that there would be an immediate worldwide impact because of the enormous importance of the discovery. But after several weeks or months, with only slow decoding of a long message, if there is one at all, will people go back to watching football games? So we should study near-term and long-term outcomes. The second part deals with actions taken as a result of the discovery. One of the most common questions about SETI is "what do you do if you detect a signal?"

Over the last 10 years a few individuals have begun to think about the specific actions that we might indeed take upon detecting a signal. Recommendations for action are being gathered together in "SETI Post-Detection Protocols."

C. SETI Post-Detection Protocols

Over some years, the SETI Committee of the International Academy of Astronautics, together with the International Institute of Space Law, has developed a document called "The Declaration of Principles for Activities Following the Detection of Extraterrestrial Intelligence".[68] The purpose of this document is to make available to all SETI observers and organizations a common code for a series of logical steps that should be followed after a signal is detected. The Declaration makes the following points about the dissemination of information about the discovery:

1) Verify that the signal is indeed of ETI origin.

2) Notify other observatories to attempt independent confirmation.

3) Then, notify all of the other observers, and appropriate national and international organizations.

4) Disseminate the discovery widely through scientific channels and the media.

5) Make available all of the data through normal scientific channels.

6) Confirm, monitor and record the signal.

7) Seek protection for the ETI signal frequency from the World Administrative Radio Council (to reduce radio frequency interference that might degrade the signal).

8) Do not reply until appropriate international consultations have taken place.

9) Form a committee of specialists to consult on technical aspects of the discovery.

These principles have been endorsed by five international space societies. They are common sense recommendations for action by SETI observers, and they deal with near term actions to be taken after the discovery.

A second Declaration of Principles is now in preparation. It deals with some of the long term questions which we would face after detection, namely those referred to in item 8 above. Should Earth reply? Who decides? Are there reasons why we should not reply? If so, what are they? If we decide to reply, what should we say? Who decides? In what language? Who decides? It could be argued that these questions cannot be answered until we know the content of the signal. Perhaps. But there is one situation that we can begin to examine now, namely, the detection of a signal that has no message, for example an ETI radar or carrier. In view of the lengthy international consultations that must take place before decisions on a reply are reached, it is best to start the process now. Studies will be conducted, analyses performed and a second Declaration of Principles developed on which detailed answers can then be based. It is likely that the final steps will have to take place in the United Nations Committee on the Peaceful Uses of Outer Space.

It should be noted that many of the first papers on cultural aspects of SETI are collected in a special issue of *Acta Astronautica* on SETI Post-Detection Protocol, edited by Tarter and Michaud.[68] The papers are divided into groups dealing successively with receipt and verification of a signal, announcing the detection, the impact of the announcement, legal principles relating to ETI, a discussion on "Who will speak for Earth?", and finally the original Declaration of Principles.

D. Side Benefits

The observations conducted with SETI systems, and the systems themselves, may be of benefit in areas other than SETI itself.

In the domain of astronomy, it has been suggested that any new instruments that open up multidimensional search space by some three orders of magnitude may lead to the discovery of an unexpected major new astronomical phenomenon. On average this has been true over the last 50 years. In the case of the NASA SETI system, the High Resolution Microwave Survey will achieve an opening up of the fine resolution dimension of astronomy by a factor of about 2.5 orders of magnitude. SETI may thus discover some astronomical or astrophysical phenomenon other than ETI.[69] This is serendipity. But the SETI machines can also be used for planned radio astronomical projects. The SETI Sky Survey could be a good vehicle for continuum source surveys at minimum extra cost. Other possibilities are spectral line surveys and use of the "dwell mode" to produce an adequate signal-to-noise ratio for radio astronomy. Further details can be found in the 1983 SETI Science Working Group Report.[70]

Last but not least, the NASA SETI spectrum analyzer and signal processors hold some promise for use by other disciplines. Any field that can benefit from the high resolution detection of unknown signals in complex noise backgrounds should be examined. Examples could be radar astronomy, aircraft radio transmission analysis, geology and geophysics, mass spectrograph or gas chromatograph design, computer-aided tomography, magnetic resonance imaging, neurophysiology, electroencephalography, remote sensing systems, and perhaps many more.

VI. The Future of SETI

No ETI signal has yet been found. We postulate the existence of such signals and do our best to detect them. As we gradually explore more and more of astronomical search space, we will be able to say that signals of a certain strength and frequency did not exist on the day we looked for them. The volume of astronomical search space we have examined so far is minute. In the first few minutes of the NASA High Resolution Microwave Survey (HRMS) in 1992, more astronomical search space was covered than in all of the sixty previous searches over the past 30 years. During the HRMS itself, through the decade of the 1990s, we will cover millions more times of search space. For the sake of convenience, call this period SETI I.

A signal may be detected during SETI I. Remember that if we detect one other, there will be many. So there will be a powerful stimulus to expand the search, to conduct SETI II. It can be predicted that many nations will put considerable resources into an extended series of further searches, SETI II. Some tentative plans can be drawn up today. It is likely that a great number of searches will be undertaken to further expand the dimensions of microwave search space. Searches will be carried out in other frequency domains, such as the infrared[37] and optical.[39] Powerful new spectrum analyzers and signal detection systems will be built. Large new antennas will be constructed to increase sensitivity, the better to detect faint signals. SETI II antennas may be built in space or on the farside of the Moon.

As this great increase in SETI activity is occurring, the people of planet Earth will have to absorb the blunt fact that we are but one of many civilizations, perhaps mediocre or even primitive in comparison with our long-lived elders. At the same time we may be learning unimagined new things about the universe, life, intelligence and society. We will face all of the questions asked in section V under the heading of cultural aspects of SETI. It may be easier for us to achieve unity on Earth. It may not. It would certainly change the lives of our descendants for ever. As Oliver has said, there may be two classes of civilization; those which attempt SETI, succeed, and prosper in a stimulating era of interstellar communication; and those which do not, and which wither away as lonely galactic recluses.[71] We do not know, of course. The questions are profound and surely deserve some intensive study, beginning now.

There is another scenario, not unlikely. SETI I will be completed at the end of the decade without detecting a signal. Note that only a small part of the total of all astronomical search space will have been covered. So there is a different type of stimulus to conduct SETI II, namely the desire to succeed in the quest. Under these circumstances it will be more difficult to obtain support for a continued search. But it will surely happen. As technology continues to improve it will be easier to search deeper and deeper into the dimensions of search space. SETI II may succeed. If no signal is found by 2010, SETI III must be contemplated. It is possible that the search may take us a long time and considerable resources.

We may not succeed for a very long time. We may never succeed. It is possible that the number of civilizations is so small, say one per galaxy, that the odds of a detection are vanishingly small. It is conceivable, though most unlikely, that we are alone. However, it will not be possible to prove that we are alone. Other civilizations may exist but may not be transmitting at all, or they may be transmitting signals so weak that we have a negligible chance of detecting them. All we can do is to try, and if at first we do not succeed, to try and try again.

References

1 Morrison, P., Billingham, J., Wolfe, J. (Eds.) *The Search for Extraterrestrial Intelligence*, Washington, D.C., National Aeronautics and Space Administration, 1977.

2 Cameron, A.G.W. (Ed.) *Interstellar Communication*, Benjamin, New York, 1963.

3 Sagan, C. (Ed.) *Communication with Extraterrestrial Intelligence*, MIT Press, Cambridge, 1973.

4 Billingham, J., Pesek, R. (Eds.) Communication with Extraterrestrial Intelligence. *Acta Astronautica*, 1979, Vol. 6, No. 1-2.

5 Lucretius, 1st Century B.C. Translation by Mary-Kay Gamel, UC Santa Cruz. NASA NP-114 brochure, 1990, p. 2.

6 Barnes, E.W. British Association Symposium on the Evolution of the Universe. *Nature* supplement 128, No. 3234, 1931, pp. 719-722.

7 Oparin, A.I. *Life: Its Nature, Origin and Development.* Oliver and Boyd, London, 1962.

8 Miller, S.L, Urey, H.C. Organic Compound Synthesis on the Primitive Earth. *Science*, 1959, Vol. 130, p. 245.

9 Lederberg, J. Exobiology Approaches to Life Beyond the Earth. *Science*, 1960, Vol. 132, pp. 393-400.

10 Klein, H.P. The Viking Mission and the Search for Life on Mars. *Rev. Geophys. and Space Physics*, 1986, Vol. 17, p. 1655.

11 Cocconi, G., Morrison, P. Searching for Interstellar Communications. *Nature*, 1959, Vol. 184, No. 4690, pp. 844-846.

12 Drake, F.D. Project Ozma. *Physics Today*, 1961, Vol. 14, pp. 40-46.

13 Shklovsky, I.S. *Universe, Life, Intelligence.* Academy of Sciences of the U.S.S.R., Moscow, 1962 (in Russian).

14 Shklovskii, I.S., Sagan, C. *Intelligent Life in the Universe.* Holden-Day, New York, 1966.

15 Extraterrestrial Civilizations: Proceedings of the First All-Union Conference on Extraterrestrial Civilizations and Interstellar Communication (Byarakan, U.S.S.R., May 20-23, 1964). Tovmaryan, G.M. (Ed.). NASA Scientific and Technical Information Facility Translation; N67-30330 through N67-30392.

16 Kaplan, S.A. *Extraterrestrial Civilizations: Problems of Interstellar Communication.* NASA Technical Translation TTF-631, 1971.

17 Oliver, B.M, Billingham, J. *Project Cyclops: A Design Study of a System for Detecting Extraterrestrial Intelligent Life.* NASA CR 114445, 1972.

18 Drake, F.D. *Current Aspects of Exobiology*, Mamikiunian, G., Briggs, M.H. (Eds.), Pergamon Press, 1965, Chapter 9, pp. 323-345.

19 Levine, J.S., Rinsland, C.P., Chameides, W.L., Boston, P.J., Cofer III, W.R., Brimblecombe, P. Trace Gases in the Atmosphere of Mars: A Possible Indicator of Microbial Life. 1989 preprint, to appear in *The Case for Mars III, American Astronautical Society Science and Technology Series.*

20 Klass, P.J. *UFO's: The Public Deceived.* Prometheus Books, New York, 1983.

21 Klass, P.J. (Ed.) *UFOs: The Public Deceived.* Prometheus Books, New York, 1983, pp. 75-79.

22 Eather, R.H. *Majestic Lights.* AGU Press, Washington,

DC, 1980, p. 45.

23 Chaisson, E. *Universe: An Evolutionary Approach to Astronomy.* Prentice Hall, 1988, p. 98.

24 Oliver, B.M. A Review of Interstellar Rocketry Fundamentals. *JBIS*, 1990, Vol. 43, pp. 259-264.

25 *Ibid.*

26 Forward, R.L. A Program for Interstellar Exploration. *JBIS*, 1976, Vol. 29, No. 10, pp. 611-632.

27 Freitas, R.A., Valdes, F. A Search for Natural or Artifical Objects Located at the Earth-Moon Libration Points. *Icarus*, 1980, Vol. 42, pp. 442-447.

28 Valdes, F., Freitas, R.A. *Icarus*, 1983, Vol. 53, p. 453.

29 Suchkin, G.L, Tokarev, Yu.V. et al. Lagrange Points in the SETI Problem. In: *The Problem of Search for Life in the Universe.* Moscow, Nauka, 1986, pp. 138-144 (in Russian).

30 Harris, M.J. A Search for Linear Alignments of Gamma Ray Burst Sources. Preprint 1990.

31 Freitas, R.A. Talent. *JBIS*, 1985, Vol. 38, p. 106.

32 Valdes, F., Freitas, R.A. A Search for the Tritium Hyperfine Line from Nearby Stars. Paper #IAA-84-243 presented at the 35th IAF Congress in Lausanne, Switzerland, 1984.

33 Witteborn, F. Private communication, 1980.

34 Kardashev, N.S. *Transmission of Information by Extraterrestrial Civilizations. Extraterrestrial Civilizations*, Tovmasyan, C.M. (Ed.), NASA TTF-438, pp.19-29; *Soviet Astronomy*, Sept. - Oct. 1964, Vol. 8, No. 2, pp. 217-221.

35 Shmidt, S. *The Sins of the Fathers*, U.C. Berkeley, 1976.

36 Townes, C.H. *At What Wavelengths Should We Search for Signals from Extraterrestrial Intelligence?* U.C. Berkeley, November 1982, pp. 1147-1151.

37 Betz, A. Presented at the Fourth Symposium on Chemical Evolution and the Origin of Life, July 1990.

38 Deming, D., Espenak, F., Jennings, D., Kostiuk, T., Mumma. M., Zipoyt, D. *Observations of the 10 mm Natural Laser Emission from the Mesospheres of Mars and Venus.* Infrared and Radio Astronomy Branch, NASA Goddard, Academic Press, Inc., May 1983, p. 347.

39 Rather, J.D. Lasers Revisited: Their Utility for Interstellar Beacons, Communications, and Travel. Submitted for publication in *JBIS*, March 1990.

40 Schwartzman, V.F. SETI in Optical Range with the 6M Telescope (MANIA). *Bioastronomy: The Next Steps*, Marx, G. (Ed.), Kluwer Academic Publishers, 1988, p. 389.

41 *Program Plan for SETI.* Technologically accessible volume, 1983, Fig. 4.1-5, pp. 4-7.

42 Drake, F.D. Historical Perspective - Project OZMA. *The Search for Extraterrestrial Intelligence*, Kellermann, K.I., Seielstad, G.A. (Eds.), NRAO Workshop No. 11, 1986, p. 17.

43 Drake, F.D. Interview in *SETI Pioneers*, Swift, D. (Ed.) University of Arizona Press, 1990, p. 54.

44 New York Times editorial, p. 36. April 13, 1965.

45 Kellermann, K.I. *Australian Journal of Physics*, 1966, Vol. 19, p. 195.

46 Troitsky, V.S., Starodabtsev, A.M., Gershtejn, L.I.,

Kakhlin, V.L. An Experience of Search for Monochromatic Emission from Stars in Solar Vicinity. *Astron. Journal*, 1971, Vol. 48, No. 3, p. 645-647 (in Russian).

47 Gindilis, L.M., Dubinskij, B.A., Rudnitskij, G.M. SETI Investigations in the U.S.S.R., paper IAA-88-544 presented at the IAF Congress in Bangalore, India, 1988.

48 *Ibid.*

49 *Ibid.*

50 Schwartzman, V.F. SETI in Optical Range with the 6M Telescope (MANIA). *Bioastronomy-The Next Steps*, Marx, G. (Ed.), Kluwer Academic Publishers, 1988, pp. 389-390.

51 Kellermann, K.I., Seielstad, G.A. (Eds.) *The Search for Extraterrestrial Intelligence*, NRAO Workshop No. 11, 1986.

52 Bowyer, S., Werthimer, D., Lindsay, V. The Berkeley Piggyback SETI Program: SERENDIP II. *Bioastronomy - The Next Steps*, Marx, G. (Ed.), Kluwer Academic Publishers, 1988.

53 Tarter, J.C. One Man's Signal is Another Man's Interference. Paper presented at XXIII General Assembly of URSI, Prague, Czechoslovakia, 1990.

54 Donnelly, C., Bowyer, S., Herrick, W., Werthimer, D., Lampton, M, Hiatt, T. The SERENDIP II SETI Project: Observations and RFI Analysis. *Bioastronomy: The Exploration Broadens*, Heidmann, J., Klein, M. (Eds.), Springer-Verlag, 1991, pp. 223-228.

55 Horowitz, P. Ultra-narrowband Searches for Extraterrestrial Intelligence with Dedicated Signal-Processing Hardware. *Icarus*, 1986, Vol. 67, p. 525.

56 Horowitz, P. on META II. *The Planetary Report*, November-December 1990, p. 27.

57 Wooley, R., Epps, E.A., Penston, M.J., Pocock, S. Catalogue of Stars Within Twenty-Five Parsecs of the Sun. *Royal Observatory Annals*, 1970, Vol. 5.

58 Duluk Jr, J.F., Jeday, A., Massing, M., Chang, C-K., Nguyen, H. The MCSA 2.1: A Fully Digital Real-Time Spectrum Analyzer for NASA's SETI Project. Paper # IAA-90-577 presented at the 41st IAF Congress in Dresden, Germany, 1990.

59 Cullers, D.K., Linscott, I.R., Oliver, B.M. Signal Processing in SETI. Special joint issue of *ACM/IEEE*, 1985, Vol. 28, No. 11, pp. 1151-1163.

60 Strelnitskij, V. November 17th, 1991 SETI Celebration in Mountain View, CA. Sponsored by the SETI Institute.

61 Likachev, private communication.

62 Gindilis, L.M., Kardashev, N.S., Rudnitskij, G.M. The Program of SETI Studies in the U.S.S.R. Preprint 1990.

63 Tarter, J.C. Statistics of Excess Observatory Noise at the Nançay Telescope and Elsewhere. Paper #IAA-85-473 presented at 36th IAF Congress in Stockholm, Sweden, 1985.

64 Heidmann, J., Biraud, F., Tarter, J.T. Pulsar-Aided SETI Experimental Observations. Paper #IAA-89-642 presented at 40th IAF Congress in Torremolinos, Spain, 1989.

65 Blair, D.G., Norris, R., Wellington, K.J., Williams, A., Wright, A. A Test for the Interstellar Contact Channel Hypothesis in SETI. Preprint 1990.

66 Freundenthal, H. Lincos. *Design of a Language for*

Cosmic Intercourse. North-Holland, Amsterdam, 1960.

67 DeVito, C.L, Oehrle, R.T. A Language Based on the Fundamental Facts of Science. *JBIS*, in press 1991.

68 SETI Post Detection Protocol. Tarter, J.C., Michaud, M.A. (Eds.), Pergamon Press. Special Issue of *Acta Astronautica*, 1990, Vol. 21, No. 2.

69 Tarter, J.C. SETI and Serendipity. *Acta Astronautica*, 1984, Vol. 11, No. 7-8, pp. 387-391.

70 Drake, F.D., Wolfe, J.H., Seeger, C.L. *SETI Science Working Group Report*. NASA Technical Paper 2244 1983.

71 Oliver, B.M. The Interaction of Life in the Galaxy. Unpublished 1973.

Part IV:

Space Exploration

Chapter 9

Access to Space

Konstantin P. Feoktistov and Geoffrey A. Briggs

I. Introduction

The conquest of space is generally understood to mean humanity's venture into this new environment and the performance of exploratory, research, and economic activities in it. This activity may be conducted either by means of robots remotely controlled from the Earth, or through actual human presence and work in orbit or on other planets. The present chapter is devoted to the technology used in space exploration: launch vehicles, unmanned and manned spacecraft, the last of which afford human beings direct access to space.

To travel to space and remain there, a spacecraft must climb to an altitude of not less than 180-200 km above the Earth's surface and attain a rather high velocity relative to the Earth. This velocity must be high enough that the centrifugal force arising through motion around the Earth is greater than or equal to the force of gravity acting on the spacecraft. If orbital altitude is 200 km, this velocity must be approximately 7.8 km/s. Launch vehicles both lift spacecraft to this altitude and impart this velocity.

Getting into space, i.e., launch vehicle technology, is but the first step towards effectiveness in this new environment. The list of additional spacecraft technologies is, of course, very long—communications, attitude stabilization, command and control, data storage and handling, and power are among the most basic requirements. These basics are already quite advanced; in particular, rapid advances in electronics and software capabilities have given us mature technologies in these areas so that robotic spacecraft can now travel to the far reaches of the solar system. Such basic technologies are equally effective for human space flight, but they represent only the beginning of what is needed to support humans in space.

It is not enough to venture into a new environment. Conditions must be created that allow human beings to live and work in a hostile environment, in addition to those that allow equipment to operate. Besides life support (through supply of oxygen, water, food, etc.), space crews must also be protected from the effects of the vacuum of space, solar and cosmic radiation, overheating and freezing, and meteors. In addition, the means must be provided for communicating with the Earth. Last but not least, it must be made possible to conduct research, economic or other applied work, and to carry on construction in this new sphere of activity.

These goals determine the nature, design, and properties of unmanned and manned spacecraft. However, experience with spacecraft design has shown that these limitations are not excessive, since a great deal of variety in design is possible.

The substantially greater mass that must be launched for manned missions places a tremendous premium on heavy lift launch vehicles. Additional challenges are also imposed by the high inherent risk of human space flight—challenges to improve the reliability of every element of the overall system. Such system design, providing both hardware and software fault tolerance, will remain the essence of successful planning for both manned and robotic space flight.

Another fundamental need for all human missions is the safe return of the crew to Earth. Reentry into the Earth's atmosphere has become a well developed capability, even to the point of having reusable systems like the Space Shuttle Orbiter and Buran. High speed entry is also a key requirement for exploration of other planetary bodies that are the targets for both robotic and human missions. The following technologies have, to a limited extent, been developed and utilized over the last two decades (e.g., the Venera and Luna spacecraft, the Vikings, and Apollo): 1) the ability to navigate accurately to these bodies, 2) to enter into orbit about them, 3) to descend to their surfaces (making high speed entry and descent through their atmospheres in the case of Venus and Mars), 4) avoid hazards on landing, and 5) finally take off again and return to Earth. Mobility on a planetary surface (lunar rovers, manned and unmanned) and in the atmosphere (Venus balloons) is at this time a fledgling capability.

Although this broad experience base is generally encouraging, as we contemplate the future our technologies for future human and robotic exploration of the solar system remain inadequate. At the beginning of the 1990s our exploration efforts still have the character of Herculean efforts, expensive, "high wire" acts. We need innovation in all areas to move into an era where human and robotic space exploration is more flexible, affordable, and less risky. We must, in particular, seek radical alternatives to our present approach of bringing all consumables —fuel, oxidizers, air, food—up to space from the Earth's surface through a deep gravity well. We must also move towards the use of propulsion systems that have substantially greater efficiencies than chemical rockets can achieve. Also, life support capabilities must be greatly increased to deal with the long journey times and the isolation of expeditions to Mars.

II. Space Technology Overview

In this chapter, the evolution of the technologies that provide effective access to space will be reviewed by tracing the principal missions, both human and robotic, that have been flown by the spacefaring nations of the world since Sputnik's flight in 1957. First, however, a brief summary will be provided of the technology elements needed for every space mission.

A. Launch Vehicles

Biomedical considerations affect launch vehicles in a number of ways. This was made clear during the earliest period of rocket design. When propellant reactants for future rockets were tested, their aggressive, corrosive, and toxic properties were confirmed. When firing tests were conducted to test engines and their major modes of operation, designers confronted the need to protect participating personnel from explosions (unfortunately, a frequent occurrence during tests) and the effects of the propellant reactants on the skin, respiratory tract, and mucous membranes. Designers also needed to address issues of ecological protection of the environment from the harmful effects of rocket testing associated with successful tests as well as accidents and disasters.

During subsequent periods of rocket development, it became critical to consider the health and safety of space crews and flight support personnel on the launch platform. Such safety issues are crucial in the design of rockets.

Rocket thrust, resulting from jet exhaust, gradually accelerates the rocket and the spacecraft it is carrying to a velocity of approximately 7.8 km/s, which is necessary to lift a spacecraft into orbit. In modern rockets the propellants are located in the rocket itself, and therefore also undergo acceleration during flight. The first rockets capable of injecting spacecraft into orbit used liquid propellants, i.e., those in which both reactants—the fuel and the oxidant—are liquid. These included purely liquid booster rockets of the R7 family, which put Vostok, Soyuz, and other spacecraft into orbit, and the Atlas, Saturn, Proton, and Zenit rockets. All these rockets are multistage. Typically rockets that inject spacecraft into low near-Earth orbit have two or three stages, while those carrying interplanetary spacecraft have three or four stages. Use of multistage rockets makes it possible to solve the problem of reaching orbital velocities by using a relatively simple design. In this design the heavy engines and tanks of the first stages are jettisoned as their propellant is exhausted, so that remaining propellant is not wasted carrying components that are no longer needed. The classic configuration of a multistage rocket is serial. In this configuration, the first stage is at the bottom, the second above it, the third above that, etc. This is also the sequence in which the stages operate: the first stage is fired first, then, after its propellant is exhausted, it is jettisoned and the second stage is fired, etc. This is the configuration, for example, of rockets like Saturn, Proton, and Zenit. This is the simplest and the most elegant configuration.

However, a so-called parallel-serial configuration was also developed. In this configuration, the tanks and the engine of the first and second stages are arranged in parallel. At launch, the engines of both the first and second stages are fired. This configuration makes it possible to save on the weight of the engines responsible for rocket lift, since not only the first stage, but also the thrust of the second engine is used during this part of the flight. It is true that the weight of that portion of the second stage tanks that contain propellant used only during the operation of the first stage has to be carried until the operation of the second stage is complete. However, the weight saved on engines has generally been greater than the weight added by the tanks. After the propellant in the first stage tank is exhausted, the engines are shut down, the first stage is jettisoned, and only the second stage engine continues to operate. This configuration was used in design of the R7 type rockets and the Space Shuttle.

The efficiency of rockets is one of their most important characteristics. Rocket efficiency is measured by the specific impulse (denoted Isp and having units of seconds) of the fuel/oxidizer combination used—in effect, the time that 1 kg of propellants will burn while producing 1 kg of thrust. To take advantage of the maximum specific impulse of chemical fuels—which in practice is produced by burning liquid hydrogen and oxygen together (where the Isp is about 450 seconds)—the designer must be willing to handle cryogenic liquids at extreme temperatures. Although this capability has been mastered, most launch vehicles still use more readily stored propellants such as kerosene, monomethyl hydrazine, nitrogen tetroxide, etc.; such engines have specific impulses ranging up to 350 seconds.

The major components of liquid propellant rockets are the engines, the equipment of the pneumatic and hydraulic systems that deliver propellant to the engines, the tanks, and the control systems and systems for parameter measurement. An understanding of the typical characteristics of rockets, their size, and the problems associated with their use can be gained through a discussion of typical rockets that have been and are currently being used in space flight (see discussion below).

B. Transfer (Upper) Stages

For payloads that need to go beyond low Earth orbit (e.g., to geosynchronous orbit or to a planet), a transfer stage is needed; the technology of such stages is closely related to that of the launch vehicles. To date all transfer stages have been liquid- or solid-fueled chemical rockets, and such vehicles may themselves be made up of more than one stage [e.g., the U.S. Inertial Upper Stage (IUS) is a two stage solid rocket]. However, higher efficiency approaches are under development.

A first large increase in efficiency would come through the

use of thermal nuclear rockets that do not require chemical combustion to achieve the high exhaust gas temperatures (as high as 1500 K for hydrogen-oxygen). Instead they rely on the high temperature of a fission reactor (2 to 3000 K) to heat the liquid propellant that is pumped through the reactor. Specific impulses of about 1000 seconds are achievable. Such nuclear engines were demonstrated between 1969 and 1971 in the U.S. (the NERVA program) and are indeed feasible. Thermal nuclear upper stage rockets have not been used in space by either the U.S. or the Soviet Union and no definitive safety guidelines have been established for their operation. Pending such detailed analysis, it may be sufficient to comment that reactors would be launched cold and therefore would not have accumulated hazardous daughter products. Shielding and physical separation (distance) would certainly be important to ensure the safety of the crew during and after the time the reactor was used as a heat source.

Another approach to achieving the same level of specific impulse as a thermal nuclear rocket is the concentration of solar heat (by a large focussing mirror) on the combustion chamber. No such rockets have been demonstrated as yet.

A yet larger increase in efficiency would come with the adoption of electrically powered ion engines. Here the effluent of the rocket consists of ionized atoms of (typically) xenon or argon accelerated by magnetic and/or electric fields to a high velocity. Specific impulses of 3000 seconds or more are possible. The principal drawback of such engines (which have been tested but have not been used operationally in space) is the extremely low thrust they produce, requiring engine operation over extended periods. Thus, such an engine, if used as a stand-alone upper stage for a spacecraft leaving Earth, would spend a considerable time passing through the Van Allen radiation belts as it spiralled away from Earth.

Another transfer stage often mentioned is the solar sail, which relies on the reflection of sunlight to achieve a tiny propulsive thrust. It is also very low thrust, like the ion engine. The sail would be a gossamer-thin, silvered material of vast area that would be deployed in space and its orientation with respect to the Sun suitably controlled to achieve the desired thrust direction. Visionary in concept and potentially quite simple in design, solar sails are expected to be deployed in space for the first time in 1992 as part of a privately sponsored race to the Moon in celebration of the 500th anniversary of Columbus' discovery of the New World.

C. Communications

The radio link between a spacecraft and its controllers on Earth provides two-way communications for command, control, and data transfer and is also the critical element for navigation. Over the last three decades the communications link has gradually evolved to remarkable strength. The frequencies used have moved to ever higher frequency (from L to S to X, and soon, K band) in order to increase information carrying capability (bandwidth). At the same time, ground-based radio antennas have grown ever larger in aperture (one approach being to network several antennas together), while receivers have achieved ever greater sensitivities, and data encoding schemes have become much more sophisticated (allowing high fidelity compression of the data). Thus, the bandwidth available for the return of data has increased enormously. For example, in 1965, Mariner 4 was only able to send back data at 8 bps from Mars (distance 70 million km). However, in 1989 Voyager 2 was able to transmit at the equivalent of 40,000 bps from Neptune (distance 4000 million km).

Some spacecraft now use antennas that are furled at launch and, later, deployed in space, thereby freeing them from the constraining diameter of the launch vehicle's payload shroud. It is possible that large antennas might be deployed in Earth orbit to receive data from spacecraft in deep space. As communication frequencies move to the optical region (where lasers would be used to transmit the data), receiving stations will probably be needed in orbit to avoid the problems of the Earth's scattering atmosphere.

D. Attitude Stabilization

An appealingly simple approach to attitude stabilization, one that incurs minimal consumable propellant, is to spin the spacecraft about its axis of maximum inertia. Small rocket thrusters are still required to orient the spacecraft for maneuvers, but basically the spacecraft stabilization is passive. Spacecraft like the U.S. Pioneer series have operated successfully for decades in this mode.

Certain kinds of remote sensing instrumentation (e.g., framing cameras) mounted on pointable platforms do not operate effectively from spinning spacecraft. Many spacecraft are therefore designed to be three-axis stabilized using momentum wheels and/or small rocket thrusters to maintain the chosen attitude in inertia space. Some specialized cases of combining spin stabilization and three-axis controls have been built—notably the Galileo spacecraft and some communications spacecraft—and these are termed dual spin spacecraft.

A recent Soviet innovation in the area of attitude control is the system used by the Regatta spacecraft. It has a large circular solar sail and eight rectangular solar rudders that provide attitude control. This system has the advantage that no control thrusters are needed and, thus, no gases are exhausted that could contaminate the measurements of sensitive science instruments.

For human space flight, only three-axis stabilization has been used to date to avoid the disequilibrating effects of the Coriolis force on the crew. In the future, however, spinning spacecraft of appropriate size and geometry may well be used for manned missions to provide artificial gravity for the crew.

E. Command and Control

For robotic spacecraft the command and control functions (for spacecraft attitude control, instrument pointing, propulsive maneuvers, data gathering, storage and playback, etc.) are typically exercised through a central processing computer and its memories. Appropriate software designed for the spacecraft in question resides in these memories, both random-access (RAM) and read-only (ROM). Often relatively little commonality exists from one spacecraft to another, so that software tends to be specially written for each. Three trends have generally characterized the command and control function over the years: 1) the use of ever faster computers with increasing memory, 2) a movement of functions from hardware to software, and 3) the increasing attention to fault tolerance, error detection, and automatic fail-safing through an in-depth defense of hardware and logic checking.

The first trend (to faster and bigger computers) has not been an unalloyed benefit because it has been permitted only by the ever diminishing size of the microcircuitry, and with this has come an increasing susceptibility to cosmic ray-induced changes in digital memory states.

F. Data Storage and Handling

Digital data, mostly from scientific instrumentation, are generated in enormous quantity by modern spacecraft, consistent with the increasing capabilities of the communications system (see above). Much data may be telemetered to ground stations in real time, but often the rate of data acquisition may significantly exceed the available playback rate. Thus, buffering and/or long-term storage of data are required if the data are not to be lost. On Soviet spacecraft, both digital wire and tape recorders have been used. On U.S. spacecraft, digital tape recorders have been the preferred medium of storage. In the case of the Voyager spacecraft, the digital tape recorders can handle about 5×10^8 bits, sufficient to store about 100 images (or equivalent). Lately, large solid state memories capable of storing 10^9 bits are becoming available.

G. Power

Within the inner solar system (i.e., as far out as Mars' orbit), solar illumination is sufficiently intense to allow a spacecraft to generate electrical power using solar (photovoltaic) cells. Most spacecraft also carry batteries to handle peak loads and to take over from the solar panels when in shadow.

The solar panels (typically large in area relative to the spacecraft bus) are frequently folded for launch and deployed in space only after the spacecraft has separated from any required transfer stage. In the case of spinning spacecraft, the bus is often drum-shaped with the panels occupying the sides of the drum. For U.S. spacecraft, the DC power from the panels is generally conditioned to a 28-volt standard; for Soviet spacecraft a 27-volt standard has been more generally used.

For missions to the outer solar system where solar illumination is inadequate to power solar panels, and for specialized applications in the inner solar system (e.g., for long-lived surface landers and instrumentation in the case of the U.S., and

for high powered orbital radars in the case of the U.S.S.R.), it is necessary to use a nuclear power source. Nuclear power sources come in two principal types, radioisotope thermoelectric generators (RTGs) and fission reactors. In both cases the electricity may be generated by thermo-electric conversion (the Seebeck Effect) with great reliability (no moving parts) but relatively low conversion efficiency (up to 7 percent). In the case of the RTGs, the source of heat is the decay of a radioactive isotope having a suitable half life (typically plutonium 238, which has a half life of about 75 years); they are used for operations that may last for a decade or more. In the case of nuclear reactors, the heat is derived from the fission of uranium 235.

Safety issues have made the use of nuclear power sources in space a cause of public concern in the U.S. and great attention has been paid to building devices of remarkable ruggedness (capable of coping with explosions and the heat load of a reentry after an accident in space, for example) and also to analyzing the implications of all possible accident scenarios. RTGs on U.S. spacecraft have in fact been involved in three different space accidents (the last being the Apollo 13 mission) without any environmental impact. Accidents have also occurred with nuclear reactors on Soviet spacecraft, such as Cosmos 402, where radioactive fuel was scattered on the Earth's surface as a result of the atmospheric reentry.

For manned missions another power source has found frequent application—fuel cells that generate electrical power chemically, in effect by the reverse electrolysis of hydrogen and oxygen (which are stored in liquid or gaseous form). In addition to their convenience (relatively high power levels and power density), fuel cells are a valuable source of water for as long as the fuel lasts.

Another power source expected to find future application on the U.S. Space Station Freedom is a solar dynamics power system where solar heat would be focussed, by means of a large mirror, on an engine such as a turbine alternator.

III. Launch Vehicles

Since launch vehicles provide the most basic capability for access to space, some additional details are provided here of the principal vehicles that make up the present inventory of launchers. Many are improved variants of the military rockets that initiated the space age.

A. Vostok

The Vostok rocket, which injected the first spacecraft into orbit, was three-stage. Its design was based on the R7 rocket. The four side-by-side boosters of the first stage were arranged around the core rocket module, which comprised the second stage. The third stage was attached with a girder structure to the upper portion of the second stage (see figure in Part I, "Historical Aspects of Space Exploration").

All three stages used liquid oxygen as the oxidizers, and kerosene as the fuel. The engine thrust for each first stage

stage and covered by an apex cover to protect it from the mechanical and thermal effects of the air stream when the rocket passed through the dense layers of the atmosphere. After the rocket left the dense layers of the atmosphere, the apex cover was jettisoned during operation of the second stage.

The total duration of operation of the rocket engines was 400 s. At lift-off, acceleration was approximately 1.5 g, i.e., at the moment of lift-off the cosmonaut was pressed back into his chair with a force 1 1/2 times his weight. The maximum acceleration, approximately 4 g, was attained at the end of the first stage rocket's operation and at the end of the second stage.

B. Proton

The Proton rocket had a classical three-stage serial configuration (Fig. 1). It used nitrogen tetroxide as the oxidizer at all stages, with unsymmetrical dimethyl hydrazine as the fuel. Both these components are highly aggressive and toxic. The first stage had six engines with a total vacuum thrust of approximately 1000 metric tons. The second stage had four engines with total thrust of approximately 250 metric tons. The thrust of the third stage was approximately 65 metric tons.

The lift-off weight was approximately 700 metric tons. The payload weight on injection into low near-Earth orbit was 21 metric tons. The length of the rocket without payload was 44 m. The maximal cross-sectional dimension (first stage) was 7.4 m. Lift-off acceleration was on the order of 1.4 g, with a maximum acceleration during the active leg of approximately 4 g.

C. Zenit

The Zenit rocket had a two-stage classical serial configuration (Fig. 2). Both stages used liquid oxygen for the oxidizer and kerosene as the fuel. The lift-off weight was approximately 460 metric tons. The weight of the payload injected into low near-Earth orbit was approximately 14 metric tons. The length of the rocket, including the payload, was approximately 57 m, with a diameter of 3.9 m.

D. Energiya

The Energiya rocket is similar in configuration to the Space Shuttle rocket system. It is a two-stage rocket, with parallel operation of the first and second stages (Fig. 3). The four liquid propellant boosters of the first stage are configured around the core rocket, which serves as the second stage. The payload, the reusable Buran or another spacecraft, is attached to the side of the core rocket module. The booster rockets use liquid oxygen as the oxidizer and kerosene as the fuel. The second stage (main rocket) uses liquid oxygen and liquid hydrogen. The weight of the payload (if an unmanned spacecraft is to be put in orbit) may reach approximately 100 metric tons. If the payload is carried within Buran it can reach 30 metric tons.

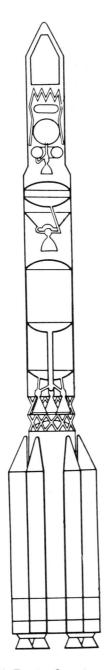

Fig. 1 Proton booster rocket

module was 102 metric tons. The engine thrust of the central module (second stage) was 96 metric tons. Thus, the full thrust of the engines operating on rocket lift-off was: 4 × 102 + 96 = 504 metric tons. The thrust of the third stage engine was 5.6 metric tons.

The lift-off weight of the rocket (with propellant) was approximately 290 metric tons. The weight of the payload injected into orbit, with apogee and perigee of 270 to 200 km, was approximately 4.7 metric tons. The length of the spacecraft was 38.4 m. The maximal diameter of the body of the central rocket module was 2.95 m.

The spacecraft was installed with an adapter on the third

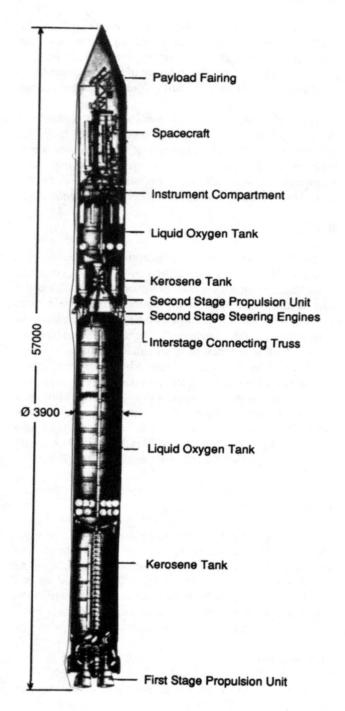

- Payload Fairing
- Spacecraft
- Instrument Compartment
- Liquid Oxygen Tank
- Kerosene Tank
- Second Stage Propulsion Unit
- Second Stage Steering Engines
- Interstage Connecting Truss
- Liquid Oxygen Tank
- Kerosene Tank
- First Stage Propulsion Unit

57000

Ø 3900

Fig. 2 Zenit booster rocket

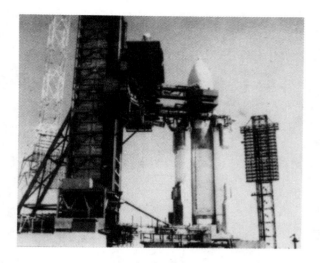

Fig. 3 Energiya booster rocket

E. Ariane 5

The Ariane 5 rocket is designed for launching the Hermes and other spacecraft. It is a modification of the family of Ariane rockets that are scheduled to be used in the mid-1990s. To launch the Hermes it is proposed to use a two-stage version of the rocket. This rocket also uses a parallel system. Two solid propellant blocks of the booster rockets are located to either side of the central main (second stage) rocket. The

second stage uses liquid propellant. The oxidizer is liquid oxygen and the fuel is liquid hydrogen. The Hermes spacecraft is attached with an adapter to the top of the second stage (main rocket).

The total launch thrust of all engines should be on the order of 750 metric tons. The lift-off weight is approximately 600 metric tons. The weight of the Hermes spacecraft the rocket is to launch is approximately 20 metric tons, with the weight of the payload carried by the spacecraft 4.5 metric tons. The overall length is 45 m. The diameter of the solid propellant booster rockets of the first stage is 3.8 m, and the diameter of the main rocket is 2.6 m. Duration of active flight is approximately 10 minutes.

F. Pegasus

The Pegasus is among the newest (1990) and one of the smallest launch vehicles available. It consists of three solid stages and is launched at altitude from under the wing of a converted Boeing B-52 bomber. The first stage has small wings for added performance and the vehicle is capable of launching about 270 kg into a 460-km polar orbit.

The Pegasus first stage develops about 51 metric tons thrust, the second about 13 metric tons, and the third about 4 metric tons. The vehicle is about 15 m in length, 1.3 m in diameter, and weighs about 18.4 metric tons.

G. Delta

The first version of the Delta was flown in 1962. It has been launched in versions having up to three stages, and it uses solid rocket boosters at lift-off. The current commercial Delta 2 employs nine solids with a total thrust of about 450 metric tons. The core vehicle has a single engine (burning RP-1 and liquid oxygen) that produces about 105 metric tons thrust, while the two-engine second stage (burning Aerozine 50 and nitrogen tetroxide) produces about 4.4 metric tons thrust.

Different versions of the Delta can carry between about 4 to 5 metric tons to low Earth orbit. The vehicle has a Star 48 solid upper stage for missions to geosynchronous orbit.

The Delta is about 39 m in length, 2.4 m in diameter, and weighs about 220 metric tons. Maximum acceleration is about 5.7 g.

H. Atlas

The two-stage Atlas has been mated with a variety of transfer stages ranging from the Agena (liquid) to Burner (solid) and the Centaur (liquid hydrogen and oxygen).

The current commercial Atlas has a three-engine first stage that produces about 200 metric tons total thrust (burning RP-1 and liquid oxygen) and is mated to a two-engine Centaur of 15 metric tons thrust (burning liquid hydrogen and oxygen). The vehicle can carry about 6 metric tons to low Earth orbit, 2.5 metric tons to geosynchronous orbit, or 1.5 metric tons to escape. The Atlas is about 46 m in length, about 3 m in diameter, and it weighs about 187 metric tons.

Although the earlier Atlas rockets also had a first stage with three engines, the configuration and total thrust were different—two engines produced about 150 metric tons thrust and the third an additional 27 metric tons. This version, mated with the Agena, was used to launch the early Mariners, Rangers, and Lunar Orbiters. Mated with the Centaur, the early Atlas launched the Surveyor spacecraft to land on the Moon and the Mariner 9 orbiter to Mars.

I. Titan

Having, like the Atlas, started life as an ICBM in the early 1960s, the present Titan has also been produced in many forms. The current Titan 3 comprises two stages together with strap-on solid rocket boosters for launch and an appropriate upper stage.

The two liquid stages burn Aerozine-50 fuel with nitrogen tetroxide. The first stage produces a thrust of about 495 metric tons and the second about 47 metric tons. The two solid rocket motor boosters produce a total thrust of about 1277 metric tons thrust at lift-off.

The Titan can carry about 14.5 metric tons to low-Earth orbit. Its length is about 47 m, its diameter about 3 m, and it weighs about 680 metric tons at lift-off.

The Titan, together with a Centaur upper stage, has been used in the past to launch the Viking landers to Mars and the Voyager spacecraft to Jupiter and beyond. A yet larger version of the Titan—the Titan 4—will be used with the Centaur upper stage to launch future Mariner Mark 2 missions.

J. Saturn

The Saturn family of launch vehicles was developed in the U.S. as the vehicles to test and carry out the Apollo program of lunar landings. After the Apollo, Apollo-Soyuz, and Skylab missions had ended, the remaining Saturn launch vehicles in the inventory were decommissioned.

The Saturn 1B was a two-stage vehicle with an RP-1/liquid oxygen first stage consisting of eight Rocketdyne H-1 engines (745 metric tons total thrust) and with a liquid hydrogen/liquid oxygen second stage consisting of a single Rocketdyne J-2 engine (102 metric tons thrust). This vehicle was about 68 m in length, 6.6 m in diameter, with 587 metric tons mass.

The Saturn 5 (see Figure 25 in Part I, "Historical Aspects of Space Exploration") used for the lunar missions had three stages. The first stage consisted of five Rocketdyne F-1 engines that burned RP-1 fuel with liquid oxygen and produced a total of 3469 metric tons thrust. The five cryogenic J-2 engines of the second stage produced a thrust of 521 metric tons, and the single J-2 engine of the third stage produced 108 metric tons thrust. The length of the Saturn 5 was 111 m, its diameter 10 m, and its mass at lift-off 2910 metric tons.

K. Space Shuttle

The Space Shuttle is a new departure in launch vehicles, having been designed with the capability of reusing its orbital stage and solid rocket boosters.

Compared to conventional launch vehicles, the Space Shuttle has an unusual configuration (Fig. 4). It is a piloted, winged orbiter with three liquid hydrogen/liquid oxygen engines fueled by a large external tank. Two large solid rocket motors are attached to the external tank at launch; after use these are separated at an altitude of 45 km to fall into the Atlantic on parachutes, where they are recovered for refurbishment. After separation of the boosters, the engines continue to power the orbiter with its external tank toward low Earth orbit. The external tank is jettisoned shortly before achieving orbit (it re-enters the atmosphere and burns up), and the orbiter continues under the power of two smaller engines fueled from internal tanks (this propulsion system is termed the Orbital Maneuvering System or OMS). The crew experiences a maximum acceleration of about 3 g after lift-off and the reentry deceleration of about 1.5 g.

At lift-off the three main engines (liquid hydrogen/liquid oxygen) produce a total thrust of about 639 metric tons. The engines are supplemented by the thrust of the two solid rockets, another 2404 metric tons. The smaller OMS engines burn monomethyl hydrazine and nitrogen tetroxide, producing a total thrust of 2.7 metric tons.

Planned maximum payload for the Shuttle is about 29 metric tons to low Earth orbit. The orbiter itself weighs about 84 metric tons and has dimensions of about 37 m (length), 17 m (height), and 24 m (wingspan). The external tank is 47 m long, has a diameter of 8.4 m, and an inert weight of about 33.5 metric tons (fueled, the tank weighs 743 metric tons). The solid rocket boosters are 46 m long, 3.7 m in diameter, and weigh 587 metric tons. In the future, flight duration will be increased to 30 days. Also in the future, the large external tank will be carried into orbit and made available for a variety of applications.

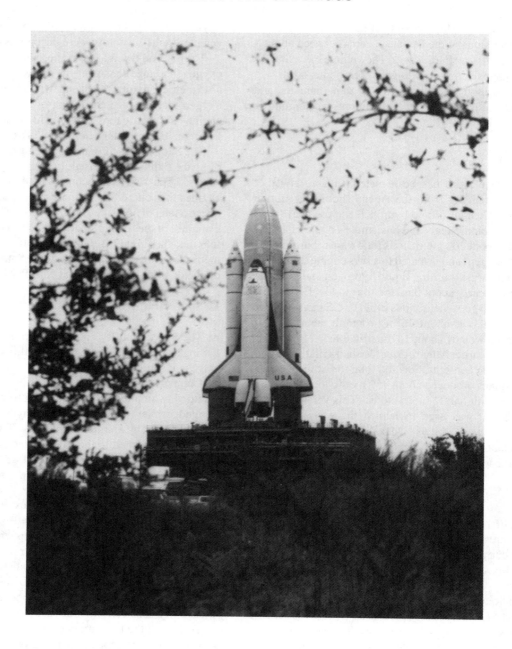

Fig. 4 Space Shuttle launch vehicle and orbiter (NASA 81-R-1)

L. Biomedical Problems and Safety Issues

Biomedical problems and safety issues during launch of rocket systems are predominantly associated with the large quantities of oxidizer and fuel loaded on the rocket. These problems include toxic components, risk of explosion, protection of the service personnel preparing the rocket system for flight and the spacecraft crew from possible emergencies at launch and acoustic effects on the launch platform, and protection of the space crew from acoustic effects due to the rocket engines.

Toxic reactants, if they are used in a given rocket, create significant problems at the launch position. There will always

be the danger of leakage (loss of pressurization) in the fueling systems or in the rocket itself, and this is fraught with the possibility of catastrophic consequences. When such reactants as nitric acid, nitric tetroxide, hydrazine, dimethyl hydrazine, etc. are used, the danger for personnel servicing the rocket is great and stringent safety measures must be taken. Even if the rocket and its launching systems are designed so that no one is on the launching platform from the moment fueling operations begin, until lift-off (because all fueling processes and checking of pressurization have been automated), there is always the danger of a malfunction requiring the presence of experts near the rocket during and after fueling. Gas masks, special protective suits, and highly sensitive devices for monitoring the gases in the atmosphere are essential for personnel located on the platforms for launching such rockets.

Considering the danger to personnel of a launch emergency, fire, or even an explosion, underground shelters, emergency ventilation, and means for decontamination and clean-up of the grounds and facilities must be provided.

Explosion hazard is somewhat lower for rockets with toxic reactants than for rockets with clean reactants. If a decision has been made to use toxic reactants in a given rocket, they are selected to be self-igniting. This, of course, increases the danger of fire, but decreases the danger of explosion. Given the speed with which a fire or explosion would develop, the possibility of emergency situations occurring on the launch platform after rocket fueling makes it essential to provide the means for rapid rescue and evacuation of the crew from the danger area. For rocket systems that are launching manned spacecraft equipped with emergency rescue systems for the active leg of the flight, this is relatively easy to attain: the emergency rescue system must be designed for instant response and diagnosis of the nature of the emergency, and must be highly efficient.

Naturally, given the possibility that an emergency may compel service personnel to be close to the rocket during launch, means for their rapid evacuation has to be provided. An escape system may take the form of a chute or soft gauntlets that will allow those working on high platforms to slide down (e.g., a cable) to the underground shelters.

Even a normal flight of modern rockets is associated with some hazards. The first stage falls on the surface of the Earth. Thus it is necessary to exclude people from the areas (which may reach dozens of kilometers in size) where they are scheduled to fall. For rockets using toxic reactants, this issue is further complicated by the possibility that the first stages may shatter on the surface, with the remaining toxic substances gradually seeping out in these areas, entering ground water, etc.

Moreover, the interaction of the combustion products of the propellant with the atmosphere, particularly in the ozone layer, must be considered. Standard rockets evidently do not present any danger; however, when solid propellant rockets are used, there is a danger of their combustion products interacting with ozone, becoming effective catalysts of its decay.

The very real danger of a rocket accident during the active leg of flight, and thus the danger of rocket fragments falling on the surface of the Earth along the flight path, leads to relatively stringent constraints on the selection of a launch site and trajectory so as to avoid passing over populated regions.

During the active leg of rocket flight, which generally lasts approximately 10 minutes, cosmonauts and spacecraft equipment are exposed to considerable acceleration, acoustic noise, and vibration. Acceleration smoothly increases from 1.4 to 1.5 g at the moment of launch and to 3-4 g at the end of the operation of the first stage rocket. It then decreases to a value on the order of 1 g and then increases again.

When the rocket engine is in operation, there is pulsation of pressure in the ambient air. The power of these air fluctuations is proportional to the power of the engine exhaust (the power of the engine is the power of its exhaust), and range from 1/2 to 1 percent of the power of the engine. This is a large number. For example, for rockets of the Saturn 5, Shuttle, and Buran class, the power of acoustic noise reaches on the order of a quarter million kilowatts.

The level of vibration during rocket flight is not a danger to the cosmonauts; however, it is sometimes a major factor in the design and ground development of instruments and equipment of the spacecraft.

The risk of a fatal accident is always present in rocket flight. This risk is associated with a very high concentration of energy (hundreds of tons of propellant), the power of the rocket engines, structural stress, and the small number of previous flights a given specific rocket model has undergone (compared, for example, to automobiles, aircraft, etc.). This is most strikingly illustrated by the power of the rocket engines. Thus, the power of R7-type booster rocket engines is on the order of 10 million horsepower, while the power of Shuttle engines is on the order of 70 million horsepower. This danger was always clearly perceived by the developers of spacecraft. Even the first American spacecraft—Mercury, Gemini, and Apollo—were equipped with good emergency rescue systems providing for the separation and rapid distancing of the spacecraft from the exploding booster rocket in an emergency. A relatively good emergency crew escape system was developed for the Soyuz spacecraft. This system twice saved the lives of cosmonauts—once during a malfunction of the third stage of the rocket and once during a launch emergency. The absence of completely adequate rescue systems in case of a problem with the booster rocket is unacceptable from a human standpoint and cannot be justified by design considerations.

During injection into orbit, the crew must be protected from more than just booster problems. The completion of the active stage of flight and separation of the spacecraft from the booster is also a critical moment. If the spacecraft does not separate from the booster, it cannot return to Earth and the crew will perish. For this reason, there are back-up systems for separating the spacecraft from the booster rocket.

After separation of the manned or unmanned spacecraft from the booster, the last stage typically remains in orbit and is gradually decelerated by the traces of the atmosphere present at the orbital altitude until it reenters the dense layers of the atmosphere. It then burns up and its fragments fall to Earth. If the altitude of the injection orbit is not high (for example, less than 200 km), this process takes several days. But if the altitude is great, the last stage may remain in orbit for months or years.

It should be stated that this is gradually becoming a problem. At the present time, the number of final stages of rockets, spacecraft that are no longer operational, adapters, and fragments arising from destruction or accidents with equipment in near-Earth orbit is such that the danger of collision is already commensurate with meteor hazard for long-term space vehicles and stations. For this reason, it has become important to find an injection method in which neither the last stage of the rocket nor fragments of the connectors between the booster and spacecraft remain in orbit. This is the advanced system of injection that is now implemented in the Shuttle system. After the termination of operation of the main rocket, the external propellant tank separates from the spacecraft and returns to the atmosphere. The fragments that do not burn up completely do not fall at random, but fall into a scheduled area of the ocean. It is reasonable to have analogous requirements for spacecraft, so that before their operation has ended they leave orbit and no portions or fragments of their structure remain, preventing the gradual accumulation of dangerous debris in near-Earth orbit.

The material presented suggests the following major recommendations for spacecraft and launch vehicles:

• It is extremely undesirable to use rockets with toxic reactants, especially for launching manned spacecraft.

• Rocket systems designed for putting crews in orbit should have completely adequate systems for emergency rescue.

• After a spacecraft has been launched, the last stage of the rocket should not remain in orbit for a prolonged period.

• It is important, if only through calculations, to verify that the products of combustion of the rocket propellant do not present a danger to the ozone layer.

M. Future Directions

The cost of boosting spacecraft is still very great. This is due to the high cost of rocket engines, the complex control systems, expensive materials used for reinforced structures of rockets and their engines, and, mainly, to the fact that they are used only once. It is natural that as early as the 1970s the idea arose of building a reusable system for injecting spacecraft and their crews into orbit.

The first attempt to implement this idea was the creation of the Shuttle system. Despite the excellent work that was accomplished, this experiment can hardly be called successful. The initial projected cost of the launch of the system was that it would not exceed tens of millions of dollars. But this was an overly optimistic estimate: in recent years the cost of launching the system fluctuated within the range of 150-350 million dollars. The main reasons for this were the use of a significant number of nonreusable components and the very complex design requiring complicated preparations for launch and participation of a large number of experts. It is true of course that the analogous Russian system, Buran, is not an improvement over the Shuttle in this respect.

For this reason, the goal of creating a truly reusable and truly inexpensive system for boosting spacecraft has become even more pressing. There are two directions the pursuit of this goal could take.

The first is relatively trivial: the development of reusable one-stage rockets using oxygen-hydrogen propellant with very advanced level of design efficiency. They would inject a spacecraft into orbit, leave it there, then depart from orbit, decelerating in the dense layers of the atmosphere, and land in the launch area. This would be possible if a design could be developed in which the weights of the fuel tanks, engine, thermal shielding, and landing system of the rocket returning to Earth, the control system, and the spacecraft itself do not exceed 10-11 percent of the lift-off weight. This would require extremely strong and extremely light materials, and very light engines, thermal shielding, and landing systems. At present, there are no foreseeable prospects for such a solution.

The second direction is revolutionary. It is suggested by the major shortcoming of modern rockets: their tanks contain not only fuel, but also the oxidizer, which has to be boosted as well. Yet a significant portion of the flight takes place in the dense layers of the atmosphere, which contains oxygen that could reasonably be used for this purpose. There is a good reason why this has not been done. In order to use atmospheric oxygen, aside from the liquid propellant engines (a large portion of the flight still occurs outside the dense layers of the atmosphere), the rocket would have to have air-breathing jet engines, operating at a velocity of no less than 1500-1700 m/s. If it were possible to build a hybrid engine that was light enough and that could operate in an air-breathing mode on take-off and in the dense layers of the atmosphere, and subsequently become a liquid-propellant jet engine, this could produce a considerable savings in the weight of the booster.

These ideas underlay the British design of a reusable HOTOL launch vehicle. It has been proposed that this aircraft would take off from the airport with the aid of a special launch trolley, which would remain on the ground and then would accelerate to an altitude of approximately 25 km running on engines using oxygen from the atmosphere. By this time it would have accelerated to a velocity of approximately 1600 m/s. Then the flight would utilize oxygen stored on board. The fuel for both flight legs would be liquid hydrogen. According to the design, with a lift-off weight on the order of 200 metric tons, HOTOL would be able to inject a payload on the order of 7 tons into orbit and then return to Earth. Judging by reports in the press, work on the projects has been halted at present for lack of financing. It is difficult to judge how feasible this project is, since it depends on the development of a light hybrid engine capable of operating both in air-breathing and in liquid-propellant modes, and virtually no information has been published about the building of such an engine.

Work is being conducted in several promising directions. The German Sanger project presupposes the creation of a completely reusable two-stage system, consisting of two winged vehicles. The first stage is to use air-breathing jet engines, and the second, liquid propellant engines. After the propellant is consumed, the first stage will return to the airfield. The second stage, after injection of the payload into orbit, will return to the Earth and, like the first, be made ready for the next flight.

An even more revolutionary project is currently under development in the United States. It is based on the hypothesis

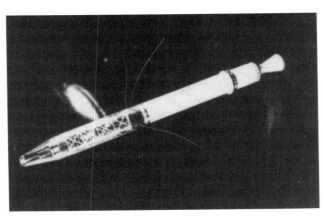

Fig. 5 Explorer 1 satellite

that it is possible to develop an athodyd capable of operating at a velocity on the order of 7.5 km/s.

IV. Robotic Spacecraft

The development of spacecraft has made it possible to focus on research and applied activity in space. The most efficient projects have been those carried out by robotic (unmanned) spacecraft, which made it possible:
- to discover the Earth's radiation belts
- to investigate the Earth's ionosphere and magnetosphere, and the solar wind
- to begin studying the Sun and planets of the solar system
- to begin studying the universe using instruments in orbit and operating on various spectral bands (ultraviolet, infrared, X-ray, gamma)
- to monitor the surface of the Earth using reconnaissance satellites in the interests of national defense and monitoring compliance with international agreements to limit strategic arms
- to create cost-effective satellite communications systems and systems for direct television broadcasting
- to build meteorological satellites that radically increase the quality and reliability of forecasting weather and dangerous hurricanes
- to develop satellite navigation systems, making it possible to determine the position of vessels at sea and of aircraft with accuracy on the order of hundreds and even tens of meters
- to begin regular ecological monitoring of the surface of the Earth, to study natural resources, including surveying the Earth's surface for minerals, detecting and monitoring forest fires, and monitoring crops and cultivated land
- to perform biological research on animals, plants, and biological preparations in microgravity
- to experiment with technological processes to obtain ultra-pure materials and purify biological preparations that are possible only in the absence of gravity on orbital spacecraft.

In the early 1950s, work in all these areas increased

exponentially. Not all the designs for robotic spacecraft proved usable. Many of them are remembered only for the lessons they taught, rather than the results they generated, providing the experience needed for further progress. Below we will discuss selected striking and characteristic achievements in robotic spacecraft, but certainly not all those that are worthy of mention are discussed.

A. Earth Orbit Satellites

1. Sputnik

Sputnik, the first manmade satellite of the Earth, was injected into orbit at a perigee altitude of 228 km and an apogee of 947 km in October 1957. It was spherical, with four whip-type aerials (see figure in Part I, "Historical Aspects of Space Exploration"). The diameter of the sphere was 58 cm, and the weight was approximately 84 kg. The pressurized hull contained a radio transmitter, sensors, and chemical current sources. Sputnik remained in orbit until January 1958. It generated data on atmospheric density (from changes in the altitude of its orbit with time) and dissemination of radio waves in the ionosphere.

2. Explorer 1

The first U.S. spacecraft to reach orbit was Explorer 1 (Fig. 5), launched on January 31, 1958, on a four stage Juno 1 vehicle. An elongated probe only 4.8 kg in mass, Explorer 1 carried a micrometeorite gauge and, most notably, a Geiger-Mueller tube. With its 360 km by 2534 km orbit, the spacecraft passed in and out of the Earth's trapped radiation belts, saturating the tube's counting capability. A correct interpretation of this phenomenon brought lasting fame to the experiment's principal investigator, Dr. James Van Allen, after whom the Earth's radiation belts are named.

Since the early days of Sputnik 1 and Explorer 1, the space environment around the Earth has been investigated extensively by orbiting spacecraft, including many Cosmos, Elektron, Proton and Prognoz spacecraft as well as a series of Explorer, Pioneer, Orbiting Solar Observatory and Orbiting Geophysical Observatory spacecraft. As space research expanded in scope, different types of missions were developed, each of which dictated its own set of specifications for spacecraft.

3. Astronomical Satellites

Impressive successes have been attained with astronomical satellites. Satellites of the type of Copernicus (OSO-3, U.S.), ANS-1 (Netherlands), COS-B (ESA), HEAO 1,2,3 (U.S.), IUE (ESA, U.S., Britain), Astron, Relikt, Granit, Gamma (U.S.S.R.), and many others have provided fundamental new information about our universe.

All of these astronomy platforms are seeking the same general advantage—an unobscured view of the universe free

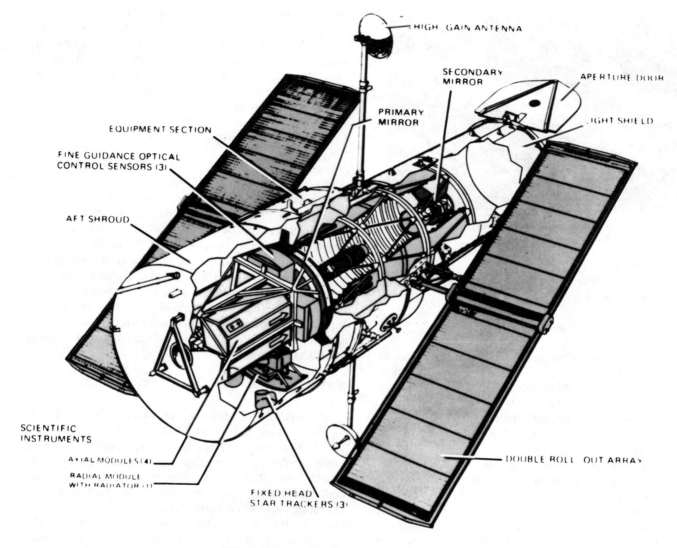

Fig. 6 Hubble Space Telescope (NASA 80-H-230)

of the atmospheric absorptions that entirely block many wavelengths and free, too, of the optical viewing problems associated with the turbulent, scattering atmosphere. Even at radio wavelengths, where excellent observations can be made from the ground, there are benefits to be sought in space, notably to obtain very large baselines for interferometry. Far infrared, ultraviolet, X-ray, and gamma ray astronomy are all possible only in space.   Each of these wavelength bands reveals astrophysical information of great richness.   The opportunity to study the universe at all of these wavelengths, rather than through narrow windows, is revolutionizing science, allowing the discovery and characterization of all of the components of the universe and the determination of its distance scales and age.

This includes discovery of a huge number of X-ray sources, for example, a quasar 10 billion light years away. Work was undertaken to determine the relative amount of deuterium in the interplanetary medium. If only a relatively small amount of deuterium is discovered, this will support a hypothesis of

the relatively low density of matter in the universe, which is compatible with a model of an infinitely expanding universe. Objects were discovered which can with high probability be identified with black holes. New data were obtained on relict radiation developing in the first million years after the Big Bang. Contemporary ideas about the universe and its quantitative characteristics are not only unthinkable without results obtained by astronomical satellites, they are generally based on these results.

Critical information in the search for life's origins remains to be acquired through astronomical techniques, in particular, through elucidation of the cosmic history of the biogenic elements and compounds and in the search for life outside the solar system. Specifically, astronomical techniques are the key to understanding the extent and evolution of molecular complexity in interstellar and circumstellar environments and to determining the composition, structure, and interrelationships among circumstellar, interstellar and interplanetary dust.

On the outside, astronomical satellites appear rather simple, compared with manned spacecraft and planetary probes. But this is only an apparent simplicity. Any satellite is created as a kind of complex, highly organized organism. The characteristics of this organism are:

- the capacity to obtain and process information, exchange information with other organisms and, thus, the presence of organs to obtain information (receivers for scanning space, optical sensors, receiving and transmitting radio lines, etc. instead of our eyes, ears, sense of smell, etc.) and organs for processing it (on-board computers instead of our central and peripheral nervous systems)

- the capacity to exist in a broad and unfamiliar range of environmental conditions while maintaining the internal stability needed for functioning of the organism and, thus, the presence of organs supporting such stability (systems of thermal regulation and sometimes regulation of gas composition, protection from meteors, etc.)

- the capacity to orient in space and, thus, the presence of organs for orientation (optical, gyroscopic and other sensors instead of the vestibular apparatus, eyes, and ears, and power gyroscopes or jet control engines for control of the angular position of the organism's body, instead of our arms, legs, and other muscles)

- the capacity to obtain nourishment to compensate for energy expenditure and, thus, organs to obtain energy (for example, solar panels) or internal stores of energy (for example, radioisotope electrical generators, or chemical batteries)

- the presence of some reserves of strength and performance reserves, in effect, the presence of the sort of reserve that gives a living organism the capacity to combat unforeseen circumstances and disease and that permits it to recover its health and performance capacity even after major injuries and illness (for spacecraft, these are usually test and back-up modes of operation or analysis in on-board computers, back-up elements in instruments, back-ups of the instruments and equipment themselves, etc.)

- automated coordination and synchronization of the operation of internal organs.

In astronomy satellites, of course, the most developed function is the first function—obtaining information—and the means to perform this function have been developed to the level of state-of-the-art science and technology.

The astronomy payloads (Fig. 6) that have been launched in recent years (IRAS, Hipparcos, GRANIT, Hubble, GRO, Rosat, COBE, etc.) or are being readied (AXAF, ISO) all place very heavy demands on our space access capabilities in terms of launch performance (the largest observatories, like Hubble and GRO, weigh tens of tons) and stable orientation (Hubble telescope specifications call for it to be able to point to an accuracy of 0.01 arc sec and hold onto targets for long periods within 0.007 arc sec). Also, inevitably, these space telescopes carry instrumentation of extreme sensitivity and complexity, and also optics in the case of X-ray telescopes, which push the state of the art. Some facilities are specifically designed for in-orbit maintenance, a capability that has already been demonstrated in the case of the Solar Maximum Mission spacecraft, which was repaired in orbit by the crew of the Space Shuttle Challenger in April 1984. A repair mission for NASA's Hubble Space Telescope to fix the well-known optical performance problem is planned for 1993.

At infrared wavelengths, the requirement to cool the detectors to cryogenic temperatures for periods of months or even years has created a need for highly capable coolers. The IRAS satellite, whose 5-month sky survey mission was completed in 1983, cooled its telescope to below 4 K and had a wavelength range of between 8 and 120 μm; the mission duration was limited by the consumption of liquid helium.

The selection of the orbit for any given astronomy payload is a matter involving a number of trade-offs—the desire for a relatively uninterrupted viewing and data return (which argues for a very high, perhaps geosynchronous, orbit), the desire for service capability (which argues for a low orbit accessible to manned spacecraft), and the desire to avoid the Earth's radiation belts in order to minimize sensor noise and degradation. One particularly successful astronomy spacecraft to operate in geosynchronous orbit has been the International Ultraviolet Explorer.

In addition to the long list of robotic observatories that have flown in space, astronomers have also taken advantage of piloted missions, mostly for observations of the Sun. Thus, the Salyut, Mir, Skylab, and Space Shuttle have all been platforms for space astronomy, allowing, among other things, the opportunity to return large quantities of data recorded on film. As human beings further explore space and establish outposts on other bodies, there will be further opportunities for space astronomy. The Moon in particular appears to offer some excellent features for such astronomy, particularly the establishment of long baseline visible and infrared interferometers seeking the ultimate in spatial resolution. Here the rigid platform provided by the Moon's surface offers a unique benefit that, sometime in the next century, will allow the detection and characterization of Earth-sized planets in other solar systems. Indeed, when transportation costs to the Moon have been sufficiently reduced, the Moon may prove to be the ideal site for most space telescopes, including ones with apertures far larger than even the newest generation of ground-based telescopes.

4. Reconnaissance Satellites

The natural desire of governments to derive benefit from new opportunities led to financing of construction of a number of applied spacecraft. Among these are spacecraft with military missions—reconnaissance satellites—the development of which was extensively funded during the period under discussion. Their design is substantially determined by the way images of the Earth's surface obtained by the craft are transmitted to Earth.

If observations rely on photographic cameras, with results recorded on film, then such satellites also must have descent modules or capsules for returning the exposed film. The working life of such spacecraft is relatively short, since it is determined by supplies of film. There was another possibility: to develop the film on board and then transmit images by radio. This made it possible to dispense with descent modules and use the additional carrying capacity thus produced for extra film. But this did not solve the problem in principle.

For this reason, the use of television as a means for observing with high resolution was inevitable, followed by recording of images on video tape for subsequent radio transmission to ground reception stations. To obtain the highest quality information possible, images were recorded in a variety of spectral bands in the visible and infrared portions of the spectrum. To monitor the surface with this technique, large areas are scanned with low resolution followed by selec-tive observation of interesting regions with high resolution. Naturally it is critical for reconnaissance satellites to have maximal resolution. Therefore, they are equipped with long-focus, high diameter lenses, which are virtually telescopes.

For the same goals, attempts were made to put the spacecraft in an orbit that minimized altitude over likely observation areas. However, at low altitudes atmospheric resistance increases rapidly and maintenance of spacecraft at such low altitudes for the requisite period of time required that low-flying reconnaissance satellites carry considerable propellant in the tanks of the propulsion system, which had to be fired regularly to overcome atmospheric deceleration. This was obviously not a promising solution; it was better to use the additional weight for increasing the size of the optical apparatus so the satellite could fly at higher altitudes.

One shortcoming of monitoring the surface in the visible frequency band is that observations are possible only during the day, and then only in the absence of cloud cover with the Sun at a certain height in the observation area. This caused monitoring in "hot" regions to be inadequate. For this reason, it has long been an urgent goal of reconnaissance satellites to enable all-weather observation that are effective night and day. This goal could have been met through the use of on-board side-looking radar with a synthetic aperture. The idea for such radar systems is relatively simple and convincing: the radar sounds the same point during a significant portion of the flight and this is equivalent to observing it with a radio telescope the size of which is equal to the length of the observation interval, which radically improves resolution. This idea was validated on aircraft and spacecraft (side-looking radar in the study of natural resources and scanning the surface of Venus), although resolution remains inadequate for the needs of reconnaissance.

Reconnaissance satellites in their time played a positive role in our divided world, allowing us to conclude the first strategic arms control agreements, since they provided the means to monitor compliance. In the future, such satellites may serve the cause of the safety of mankind, through the development of an international system for monitoring the surface of the Earth and the atmosphere that is available to all countries of the world.

5. Earth Observation Satellites

Reconnaissance satellites have much in common with unmanned spacecraft that observe the Earth's surface and atmosphere. They are used for cartography; monitoring air pollution, areas of vegetation death, and destruction of primary terrain; monitoring ocean pollution, erosion processes, deformation of the shoreline, and the state of the continental shelf; ice reconnaissance; tracking processes of ebb and flow of snow cover and rate of snow melt; predicting river run-off; observing processes in the seas and oceans, plankton and fish resources; soil mapping; monitoring crop growth, distribution of plant biomass on pastures and hay fields, and the state of forests and forest fires; geological cartography and the search for minerals; collecting global meteorological data, etc. All of these spacecraft to various degrees use methods developed for aerial surveys in the 1940s to 1960s.

These methods typically utilize:

• the picture of the surface itself obtained by television cameras in the normal visible band

• images of the surface obtained in a sequential series of spectral bands, permitting, after further processing, spectrometry and photometry of the images obtained

• thermal maps obtained with radiometers operating in the infrared and radio bands

• radar maps obtained using side-looking radar.

Statistical material has already been obtained on the absolute and relative significance of spectral brightness and spectral albedo of various types of surface. For each type of surface (chernozem/black earth, clay, dirt roads, rocks, snow, lakes, rivers, crops in various stages of growth, forests, various types of clouds, etc.), there is a specific function relating the coefficient of spectral brightness and spectral albedo (in absolute and relative values) to the wavelength of the emitted or reflected light. These functions change with temperature, degree of soil moisture, illumination conditions, tree foliage, ripples on the water, etc., and thus make it possible to identify and understand conditions of the surface on the basis of data obtained by satellite. After the satellite data are processed, the equations are solved to enable interpretation of measurement results with respect to the state of crops, signs of pollution, presence of forest fires, etc. It is best to do this on board to ensure the timeliness of information flow and avoid overloading the communications lines with huge amounts of information. Data on the spectral characteristics of various types of surfaces may fall short of statistical significance, requiring additional measurements.

In addition, software and automated information processing devices are needed to process the measurements (weather forecasting, presence of traffic congestion, conditions in areas of construction, geological maps, state of crops, etc.) so as to present results in a form convenient for users and to transmit them directly to the user at his place of work.

Much has already been accomplished—the Landsat, Seasat, Okean, and Meteor systems are already in operation; experiments are being conducted to test methods for studying natural resources using satellites.

Satellites for observing the surface and atmosphere of the Earth can be economically effective only if they operate for prolonged periods. This means they must fly at relatively high orbits, over 500-600 km. (Otherwise, propellant has to be expended on overcoming deceleration caused by traces of the atmosphere at lower orbits.) To obtain a current global picture of meteorological processes on the Earth, at least some meteorological satellites should be in geostationary orbit.

The efficiency of weather bureaus may be increased significantly if the system of meteorological satellites is supplemented by a system of automated ground stations and buoys evenly spaced over the land and sea (for measuring pressure, temperature, air humidity, wind direction and velocity, etc.) that automatically transmit the information gathered by the system of meteorological or retranslator satellites transmitting to meteorological information centers on the ground.

Earth-observing satellite missions of the past 15 years have demonstrated the capacity of remote observations from space to measure virtually all of the parameters of interest to researchers who are trying to understand the complex cycles and interactions that govern the operation of our climate and biosphere. A coordinated international program combined with ground-based observations would be of unprecedented importance.

What has been said about the design of astronomical satellites is also true of Earth-observation satellites. The differences are mainly due to differences in the set of instruments used and the objects observed.

6. Communications Satellites

Communications satellites began to be extensively used in the 1960s. The Intelsat, Molniya, Comstar, Syncom, Ekran, Raduga, Gorizont, and other systems support millions of telephone communications channels and translation of scores of television programs. The major characteristics of these satellites are their large receiver-transmitter antennas and communications radio devices, power gyroscopes for attitude control of the spacecraft, and solar panels for electrical power to the instruments and equipment.

The majority of communications satellites are located in the plane of the equator in geostationary orbit at an altitude of approximately 3600 km above the surface of the Earth. A satellite in such an orbit is motionless relative to the Earth, and seems to hover over a selected point at the equator. This is convenient for communications, since the directed ground-based receiving and transmitting antennas communicating with a given satellite can remain motionless, simplifying the establishment of communications and increasing their reliability.

But the problem of overcrowding of geostationary orbits with operational and defunct satellites has gradually begun to arise. Certain equatorial states have attempted to assert sovereignty over portions of geostationary orbit above their territory. Until now, their demands have been rebuffed, especially since their legal rationale is not obvious and the U.N. agreement on space does not acknowledge sovereignty in space. The related problem of allocating radio frequency bands among individual communications satellites (so that they do not interfere with each other) is closely related to the location of satellites in geostationary orbit. Communications satellites primarily operate in the 4-14 gigahertz (centimeter band of wavelengths) frequency band. According to certain estimates, the satellites will not interfere with each other if they are located sufficiently far apart. For the communication frequency band of 4-6 gigahertz, the critical distance must be no less than 4 angular degrees, and for television retranslator satellites, even those operating at the highest frequency band, this distance must be no less than 8 degrees. Thus, the maximum number of operating slots for communications satellites must not exceed 360/4=90, which is a very small number. For the frequency range of 20-30 gigahertz (millimeter band), the distance between communications satellites evidently may be decreased to about 1 degree, and thus the number of available slots for communications satellites increases to 360. The issue of allocation of slots in geostationary orbit and of communications frequencies will evidently need to be confronted more than once in the future. However, it will probably be possible to find other ways to expand the capacities for using geostationary orbit for communications and television retranslation. For example, large multipurpose communication platforms might be put into geostationary orbit.

Satellite communications is a promising, developing area. Even today satellites are used not only for communications among motionless ground stations, but for communications with ships at sea, aircraft, and even automobiles. Television retranslators already exist that make it possible to receive programs from a satellite directly on one's home antenna, bypassing ground-based retransmitting stations and, thus, ground-based distributors. One can already picture solutions to the problem of communicating with individual tourists on walking tours.

7. Biological Satellites

Research on biological satellites, robotic satellites dedicated to fundamental biological investigations on orbital flights, has played an important role in space biology and medicine.

The first biosatellites (which at that time were not called by that name) were Sputnik 2, carrying the dog Layka (1957), and the recoverable orbital spacecraft (1960-1961) that carried dogs, rats, mice, other animals and plants. The results of research on the flights of such biosatellites, in combination with biomedical laboratory studies, supported the conclusion that human beings could survive space flight. Subsequent research on biosatellite flights has made it possible to study the adaptation of living systems to weightlessness and to improve our understanding of the biological significance of gravity and cosmic radiation.

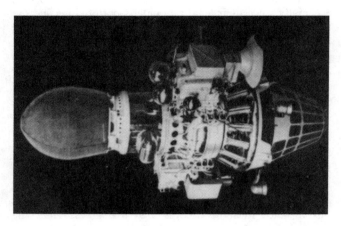

Fig. 7 Luna 9 robotic interplanetary spacecraft

In the U.S.S.R., after the first human flight in space, research was conducted on the following Cosmos series of biosatellites: Cosmos 110 (1965), 368 (1970), 605 (1973), 690 (1974), 782 (1975), 936 (1977), 1129 (1979), 1514 (1983), 1667 (1985), 1887 (1987), and 2044 (1989).

The design of Cosmos biosatellites was dictated by their mission of supporting biological experiments on flights of up to 30 days and returning living creatures to the Earth. The biosatellite consists of three modules: the descent module, an instrument/equipment module, and a pressure vessel containing additional power sources.

The descent module is spherical, with a diameter of approximately 2 m and a volume of 5 m^3. The exterior of the descent module is coated with a substance protecting the body and contents of the module from overheating during descent and reentry. Inside the descent module are the life support system, scientific instruments, and the biological subjects. The scientific instruments and subjects enter the module through two round hatches, 2-3 days before launch. The third hatch serves as the lid of the parachute container. Payload mass is approximately 900 kg.

During orbital flight the biosatellite is not oriented. Acceleration associated with rotation of the biosatellite around its axis is 1.7×10^{-7} g. To dampen angular velocities in flight, the attitude control system is turned on immediately after separation of the biosatellite from the last stage of the booster rocket, an additional two or three times during orbital flight, and also before the retrorocket engine is turned on. Smooth descent and landing of the module is ensured with a parachute system.

Before 1983, Cosmos biosatellites did not have a soft landing system and the magnitude of impact on landing varied from 40 to 90 g (as a function of type of load) with a mean duration of 40-50 ms. At the present time Cosmos biosatellites are equipped with a soft landing system, which significantly increases the reliability and interpretability of the biological experiments.

The United States has flown three biosatellites: Biosatellite 1 and 2 in 1967 and Biosatellite 3 in 1968. In size and payload they were considerably smaller than Cosmos biosatellites. Biological subjects were housed in a cylindrical volume 80 cm in diameter and 50 cm long. One side of the cylinder was a hemisphere. Total free volume was 180 liters.

Soviet and American biosatellites carried the equipment necessary to support life and perform scientific experiments on biological subjects ranging from one-celled organisms to rats and primates.

Unfortunately, Biosatellite 1 did not return to Earth, and the monkey on board Biosatellite 3 became ill in flight and was returned to Earth ahead of schedule. Eight hours after completion of the 8-day flight, the animal died. All this had a negative effect on the American biosatellite research program and it was canceled.

At the present time in the United States and Russia, new types of robotic spacecraft are being developed for scientific experiments, including biological experiments, on orbital flights lasting 2-4 months.

Results of research on biosatellite flights are described in detail in another volume of this work.

B. Beyond Earth Orbit—The Moon

1. Luna Series

Not surprisingly, the first successful launch of a spacecraft beyond Earth orbit was to the Moon—an honor belonging to the Soviet Union's Luna 1 spacecraft, which was launched on January 2, 1958, and passed within about 6000 km of the Moon a few days later. Later in the year, in mid-September, a similar Luna spacecraft impacted the Moon.

Approximately a year later, in October 1959, the unmanned Luna 3 photographed the far side of the Moon (approximately 70 percent of its surface) and transmitted the images back to Earth. The spacecraft had an attitude control system, including optic sensors for orientation to the Sun and Moon, a system for jet control of orientation utilizing stores of compressed gas, and control and thermoregulation systems. Its mass was 280 kg.

The development of Luna 3 was a technological achievement for the time, and produced information about the far side of the Moon, demonstrating distinct differences from the near side, specifically, a general lack of lowland mare regions.

The robotic lunar spacecraft Luna 9 (see Fig. 7) was launched in February 1966 and achieved a soft landing on the Moon. It transmitted several panoramic images of the neighboring surface of the Moon—a bleak, rock-strewn desert.

The control system oriented the apparatus and fired the retrorocket propulsion system on command from a radar device at an altitude of approximately 75 km from the surface of the Moon. The lunar probe separated from the retrorocket stage just before reaching the Moon's surface and fell to its surface. Shock absorption was provided by an inflatable rubber balloon. Luna 9 weighed a total of 1800 kg and the station itself 100 kg.

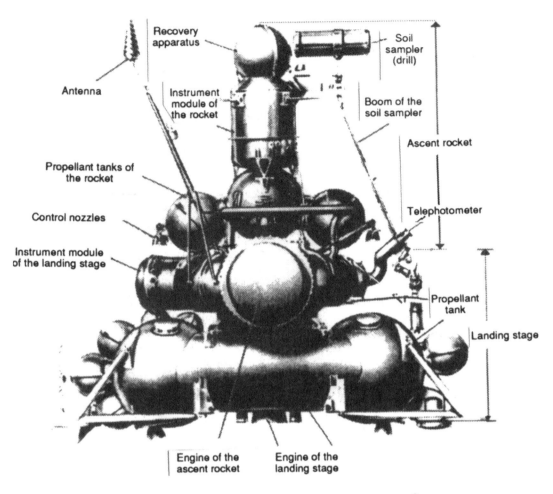

Fig. 8 Luna 16 robotic interplanetary spacecraft

The next step in the Soviet lunar program consisted of the Luna 16 (Fig. 8), 20, and 24 spacecraft, which were designed to obtain soil samples from the surface of the Moon and transport them to Earth. The spacecraft weighed approximately 1900 kg. They included a retrorocket, a four-footed landing stage, a soil-sampling device, and an ascent rocket stage with a recovery apparatus for returning the soil. These spacecraft flew in 1970, 1972, and 1976 and delivered a small amount of lunar soil to Earth.

The automated spacecraft Luna 17 and 21 (1970 and 1973) had a somewhat different mission. They landed Lunokhod rovers (see Figure 31 in Part I, "Historical Aspects of Space Exploration") on the Moon. These rovers were controlled from the Earth on the basis of a stereoscopic television image of the surface. Lunokhod 1 operated for 10 months and traversed a route approximately 10 km long. Lunokhod 2 operated for 5 months and covered a route approximately 37 km long. Aside from panoramic cameras, the lunar rovers carried a soil sampling unit, a spectrometer for analysis of the chemical composition of the soil, and an odometer. The two lunar rovers weighed 756 and 840 kg, respectively.

2. Ranger and Lunar Orbiter

The Ranger spacecraft were designed to return images as they descended to the Moon, beginning at an altitude of approximately 1600 km until reaching several hundred meters above the surface of the Moon. They had a system of three-axis stabilization and were equipped with six television cameras. Since the spacecraft were destroyed on crash landing, they returned their data in real time without recording it. During their three successful flights, they obtained extensive material on the morphology of the lunar surface. The Rangers were the first in the American program to photograph the planets.

The Ranger design was related to that of the first Mariner spacecraft, which had been launched to Venus in 1962. However, the subsequent design of lunar spacecraft did not proceed in this direction. Rather, another type of spacecraft, the Lunar Orbiters, were used to provide detailed information about the surface of the Moon. These spacecraft provided high resolution photographs of the Moon's surface from lunar orbit.

The missions were dedicated to the acquisition of high quality images, at two resolutions, of potential landing sites for Surveyor and Apollo by means of a special film camera system that processed film on board the spacecraft, then photoelectrically scanned the image and telemetered the data back to receiving stations. The number of photographs was constrained by the supply of film (sufficient for 210 frames). There were five successful launches of the Lunar Orbiter in 1966 and 1967. The first three orbiters were placed in similar low inclination, low altitude circular orbits; they each acquired very high resolution near-side stereo coverage of selected areas together with large portions of far side coverage at lower resolution. The fourth orbiter operated from a much higher polar orbit and was devoted to covering all of the Moon's near side, whereas the fifth and final orbiter also observed from a polar orbit, but at lower altitude. Lunar Orbiter 5 provided high resolution coverage of many specific targets on the near side, generally at middle latitudes, together with lower resolution coverage of a significant fraction of the far side. The end result was almost complete coverage of the Moon at moderate resolutions together with targeted coverage that was invaluable both for the planning of lunar landings and for photogeological studies of the Moon.

Additional scientific benefits from the Lunar Orbiters were the precise gravity field mapping that revealed regional mass concentrations (important scientifically and also for purposes of planning accurate landings) and a significant displacement between the Moon's center-of-mass and center-of-figure; radiation and the micrometeoroid flux measurements were also carried out.

The Lunar Orbiters weighed about 390 kg. At the completion of their mapping each was crashed into the Moon to permanently silence their radio transmitters.

3. Surveyor

Planned for the acquisition of scientific data and engineering information (mechanical properties, such as the bearing strength of the lunar soil), the Surveyor missions made many major contributions to understanding the nature of the Moon and to planning the Apollo landings. The automated landings, using closed-loop radar-controlled command sequences, were a major technological development at the time. The Surveyors were launched using the Atlas-Centaur (the cryogenic Centaur upper stage was another major technological development that was brought along concurrently) and placed on a cruise trajectory to the Moon. Landing maneuvers began 30 to 40 minutes before touchdown and the radar initiated the turn-on the main retro engine at a range of about 100 km from the landing point. The final landing, at about 5 mps, was carried out after the main engine had completed its burn and had been ejected at an altitude of 7500 m.

Surveyor mass at launch was about 1000 kg and at landing 285 kg; the main retro engine was a solid fuel rocket of about 4000 kg mass. The spacecraft used three-axis attitude stabilization.

Notable instrumentation included two cameras to provide panoramic views of the site, a small back hoe to dig trenches in the soil, and (for the last three missions) an alpha particle backscatter experiment to measure the elemental chemistry of the material under the lander. Particularly in retrospect, the results of the chemistry experiment were very revealing about the nature of the surface and history of the Moon.

Five of the seven Surveyors were successful, all being targeted to equatorial sites except the last, which landed on crater Tycho's ejecta blanket at 41 S. Surveyor 6 was a pioneer in a small way, too—the first U.S. spacecraft to be launched from another planetary body (but only to a second landing a few feet away).

The manned Apollo missions followed Surveyor in the U.S. program of lunar exploration and are treated below. After Apollo there have been no further manned exploration missions; scientists have had to be content to continue to analyze the data from the suite of robotic and piloted missions of the 1960s and 1970s. Some have anticipated the future exploitation of lunar resources to support permanent bases there and have directed their efforts toward the development of processes that could transform the lunar soil into valuable materials for construction, energy production, and rocket propulsion. Planning for a return to the Moon is underway and both robotic and piloted spacecraft will doubtless find complementary uses.

C. Beyond the Earth and Moon—The Inner Solar System

Venus and Mars are both bodies of exceptional scientific importance in what they may tell us about our own planet Earth. They were formed in the same general region of the solar nebula as the Earth 4 1/2 billion years ago and each is sizable—Venus is almost a twin of the Earth. Yet each has undergone a strikingly different evolution from our own planet, which is an oasis in space, while Venus is a hot desert buried beneath thick clouds and atmosphere, and Mars is a frigid desert under a thin atmosphere; we have a compelling need to know how the wide differences in this planetary triad came about. And in the case of Mars, the possibility of better understanding how life may have originated in solar system has been another key motivation for our exploration of this neighboring body.

Spacecraft missions in the inner solar system have largely neglected the innermost planet, Mercury, even though, as the inner end member of the family of planets, this small body can be expected to provide important insights into the general question of planetary origin and evolution. The scientific priority of Venus and Mars accounts for much of this neglect; technological difficulty—required launch performance and a difficult thermal environment—has played a role, too.

With the availability of large launchers and transfer stages in the mid-1960s, it has been possible to make an aggressive effort to explore first the inner solar system and, more recently, the outer solar system. Designers of scientific instrumentation have exercised great ingenuity in building complex

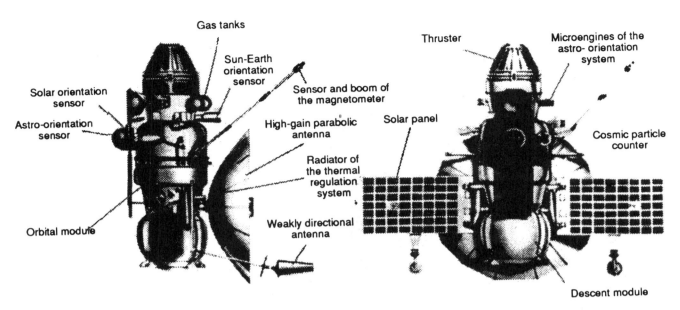

Fig. 9 Venera 4 robotic interplanetary spacecraft

experiments to fit within the tight mass allocations for the payload. The big challenge for the spacecraft designer has been the need to build dependable, long-lived spacecraft capable of looking after themselves when real time operations have been infeasible on account of the substantial round trip light times (up to 40 minutes for Mars, for example). Accurate navigation has also required much effort.

Another challenge has been to design probes capable of high speed entry into the atmospheres of Venus and Mars and, in the case of Venus, withstanding the crushing pressures of the lower atmosphere and the oven-like temperature at the surface. Venus and Mars have been the targets of roughly equal numbers of flyby, orbiter and lander spacecraft. Mercury has received the attention of only one to date, a multiple flyby reconnaissance mission.

1. Mercury

Mariner 10. The first and only spacecraft mission to Mercury was Mariner 10, which entered solar orbit in 1974. Mariner 10 had an unusual trajectory, involving a gravity assist from a Venus flyby. Mariner 10 had a mass of about 500 kg, including a science payload of about 80 kg. Mariner 10 was of the usual three-axis stabilization design and recorded data on a digital tape recorder. In addition to the twin television telescopes, the spacecraft carried ultraviolet experiments, a charged particle telescope, and a magnetometer. The cameras and remote sensing instruments were mounted on a two degree-of-freedom scan platform.

The flyby was designed to shape the spacecraft's orbit about the Sun to ensure repeated encounters with Mercury at about 6-month intervals. Mercury rotates on its axis three times while it circles the Sun twice. A Mercury day is 58.6 Earth days, a Mercury year 88 days. Thus, at each encounter

Mercury was at the same position in its orbit and showing the same illuminated hemisphere; we have as yet seen only half of the innermost planet.

Results from the mission have painted a picture of a planet that most resembles the Moon, but with some interesting differences in terms of its geologic history and present state.

2. Venus

Venera 4, 5, 6, 7, and 8 were robotic spacecraft—sequential modifications of the base design for Venera 3. Their mission was to study the atmosphere of Venus. Each spacecraft consisted of two major components: the orbital module, containing the propulsion system, which orbited the planet, and the descent module (Fig. 9).

The booster rocket placed the spacecraft on a trajectory to Venus. On the way to the planet, parameters of the spacecraft's motion were measured and midcourse corrections were effected by the engine. Electric power for the instruments and equipment was supplied by solar panels and chemical batteries that operated with them.

The weight of the spacecraft was on the order of 1.2 metric tons. The weight of the descent module was 380-475 kg (varying from spacecraft to spacecraft). The shape of the descent module was close to spherical, with a diameter of 1 m.

Because the parameters of the venusian atmosphere were not known in advance, the spacecraft had to be designed to operate in a wide range of conditions, requiring increased thermal protection of the descent module and a very strong body structure, instruments, and the means of attaching them due to the high acceleration (300-g) during deceleration in the atmosphere. Landing utilized a parachute system and shock absorbers.

The flights of Venera 4 and 8 were completed in 1967-

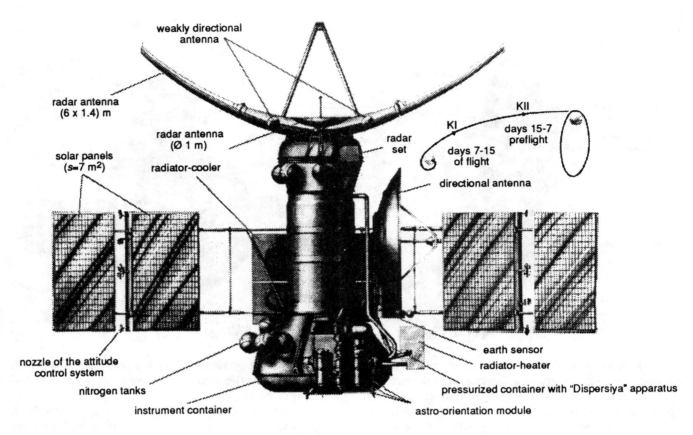

Fig. 10 Venera 15 robotic interplanetary spacecraft

1972. These flights generated nontrivial information concerning the atmosphere of Venus.

Venera 9 to 12. The Soviet spacecraft of the next generation, Venera 9, 10, 11, and 12, continued the study of the atmosphere and surface of Venus in 1975 and 1978. They transmitted to Earth panoramic images of the surface from the landing site, which appeared to be a desert-like rocky area. New information was obtained about the nature of the atmosphere.

Venera 15 and 16. The Soviet Venera 15 and 16 spacecraft (Fig. 10) were launched in 1983 and injected into orbit around Venus at a pericenter altitude of approximately 1000 km above the surface of the planet and an apocenter altitude of about 66,000 km. The inclination of the orbit plane to the plane of the planet's equator was 92.5 degrees, and the period of rotation was approximately 24 hours. The design was based on that of Venera 9 to 12. Instead of descent modules, they had instrument compartments with a side-looking radar apparatus designed for radar mapping of the surface of Venus. The amount of propellant used by the propulsion system was increased to allow the spacecraft to go into satellite orbit, and the solar panels were enlarged.

Mapping operations were conducted from November 1983 to June 1984. Radar sounding of the surface occurred in the area of the pericenter over a period of approximately 16 minutes. During the 24-hour period, Venus rotated by approximately 1.5 degrees relative to the plane of the orbit, so that the next time the pericenter came around mapping could be performed on a new strip of surface, partially overlapping the previous one. Over the 8-month course of the survey, the material obtained made it possible to construct a radar map of the northern hemisphere of Venus (above 30 degrees north latitude) with resolution of 800-2000 m.

The Vega Mission. This mission was designed to study two bodies of the solar system: Venus and Halley's Comet. The mission involved two robotic interplanetary spacecraft, Vega 1 and Vega 2, which were launched in 1984. In June 1985, the descent modules soft landed on the surface of Venus. During descent, balloons separated from them and for approximately 2 days floated freely in the atmosphere of Venus at an altitude of approximately 54 km. During the Venus flyby the robotic interplanetary spacecraft underwent a so-called gravitational maneuver and then a course correction, both of which were meant to alter the trajectories to ensure subsequent encounter with Halley's Comet. This occurred in 1986. Vega 1 passed at a distance of 8890 km and Vega at a distance of 8030 km. During this period, the comet was at a distance of approximately 0.8 AU from the Sun and had just passed the perihelion so that its activity was very high. The rate of approach reached 78 km/s, so that the spacecraft had to be equipped with special shielding to protect them from the impacts of cometary dust. Other than this, the spacecraft preserved the design used earlier for a number of flights to Mars and Venus.

The spacecraft mass was approximately 4.5 metric tons,

including 2 metric tons for the descent module with the balloon probe.

The most important scientific results of the mission were images of the comet's nucleus, determination of its shape, volume, albedo, and temperature, and also measurements of various characteristics of cometary dust, gas, and the processes of interaction between the comet and the solar wind. New data were also obtained on Venus, including accurate measurements of the temperature in the lowest layers of the atmosphere, wind velocity and parameters of turbulence on the balloon's flight path, and the chemical composition at the landing site.

The Vega mission was the first solar system research project involving extensive international cooperation. Scientists and engineers from nine nations participated in development of the scientific instruments and spacecraft systems.

Mariner 2 and 5. Mariner 2, the first of the Mariner spacecraft, was launched to Venus on August 27, 1962, following the earlier loss of Mariner 1 when its Atlas-Agena launcher malfunctioned. The mission was a reconnaissance flyby (at a distance of about 35,000 km) that was successfully executed. The most exciting information that was returned related to the high surface temperatures (on both day and night hemispheres) and the pressures inferred from infrared measurements; the great height and thickness of the clouds; and the observed lack of a magnetic field and associated radiation belts.

The Mariner 5 spacecraft launched to Venus in mid 1967 also made a reconnaissance flyby at a distance of about 4000 km in October 1967 and basically confirmed the data acquired by Mariner 2. The mass of Mariner 5 was about 245 kg, and it was a solar powered, three-axis stabilized spacecraft, like its siblings. It was the last member of the family to visit Venus until the Magellan spacecraft went into orbit about Venus in August 1990.

Pioneer Venus. The philosophy underlying the two-spacecraft Pioneer Venus missions (launched in 1978) focussed primarily on the planetary atmosphere of Venus. For this reason, a spinning spacecraft design was selected. The project called for one spacecraft to be injected into an elliptical orbit around Venus and for the other to send out probes (one large one slowed by parachute and three small ones that fell freely to the planets surface). During the flight, numerous physical and chemical measurements were made of the atmosphere and ionosphere and other experiments were conducted. The large probe and one of the three small ones were targeted to the dayside hemisphere, while the other two probes entered the nightside atmosphere. All of the probes transmitted data at a rate of 256 bits per second directly to two ground stations.

The total weight of the multi-probe spacecraft was 875 kg—585 kg for the four probes and 290 kg for the bus. The large probe weighed about 315 kg and was 1.5 m in diameter (pressure vessel 73 cm in diameter); each small probe was 0.8 m in diameter and weighed 90 kg. They were powered by silver-zinc batteries.

The cylindrically shaped orbiter was 2.5 m in diameter and

weighed 553 kg, including 45 kg of scientific instrumentation and 179 kg of solid rocket propellant for the insertion motor. The high-gain antenna was despun to allow it to be directed at Earth. Most data were returned in real time at rates up to 2048 bits per second; the memory totalled about one million bits.

Magellan. An interval of over 10 years elapsed between the launches of the two Pioneer Venus spacecraft and that of the single Magellan spacecraft in May 1989. The Magellan mission had the goal of mapping Venus using a 20-cm wavelength side-looking radar at a resolution of about 200 m, sufficient to allow a detailed examination of the geological processes that have shaped the crust of that planet. The spacecraft is recognizably of the Mariner class and is three-axis stabilized with a Voyager high gain antenna to provide the very high data rates (about 250 kbps) needed to return the voluminous radar signals.

Magellan's near polar orbit about Venus is highly elliptical with radar data acquisition occurring around the 360-km altitude equatorial periapsis (lasting about 30 minutes) and data return to Earth taking place for the remainder of each orbit.

Two digital tape recorders serve as memories and the data are replayed at X-band frequency. Momentum wheels are used for the three-axis stabilization. The spacecraft mass is approximately 3.5 metric tons. A Star 48 solid rocket engine was used for orbital insertion.

The Magellan spacecraft is notable in having been the first deep space spacecraft launched using the Space Shuttle. The upper stage used for the mission was a two-stage solid IUS (Inertial Upper Stage).

3. Mars

The subject of myth as well as scientific enquiry from time immemorial, Mars remains a compelling target for further exploration by both robots and, potentially, humans.

Mariners 4, 6, and 7. Inevitably, the Red Planet was the planned destination of robotic missions almost from the moment that the space age began. The first opportunity to observe Mars close-up was provided by the Mariner 4 spacecraft on a reconnaissance flyby mission that came within 9600 km of Mars on July 14, 1965. The first views of Mars—21 poor-quality television images—were somewhat misleading in the picture they presented of an ancient cratered planet much more like the Moon than the Earth. The very low atmospheric pressure and temperature values derived from the radio science experiment were, however, definitive measurements that revised downwards some optimistic earlier estimates.

The Mariner 4 spacecraft was launched on an Atlas-Agena and had a mass of 261 kg. Three-axis stabilized, the spacecraft had a modestly sized tape recorder (5 Mbits) which captured images for subsequent playback at a rate of about 8 bps over many days.

In 1969, two heavier (413 kg) and more highly-instrumented Mariner spacecraft were launched to Mars using the

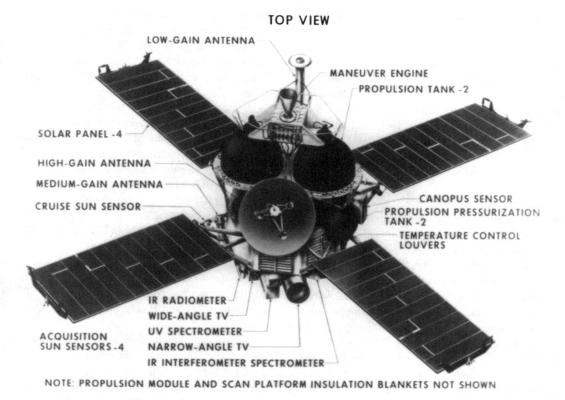

Fig. 11 Mariner 9 robotic interplanetary spacecraft (NASA 69-H-1723)

Atlas-Centaur launcher for further reconnaissance. About 20 percent of the surface was observed, generally confirming the bleak Mariner 4 picture, but also revealing chaotic terrain unlike any seen on the Earth or Moon. Infrared observations of the atmosphere and surface provided evidence of the dominance of CO_2 as the basic atmospheric constituent and of the frigid temperatures that are typical of the nightside surface. The one other planet in the solar system that some had pictured as being potentially hospitable to life assumed a thoroughly hostile character.

Mariner 9. Though similar to the Mariner 6 and 7 spacecraft in design, the Mariner 8 and 9 launched in May 1971 were profoundly different in capability, since they incorporated rocket engines to place them in orbit about Mars for missions that would last many months. Also, they had a full complement of scan platform-mounted remote-sensing experiments—infrared and ultraviolet spectrometers in addition to imaging and radio science—and a powerful telecommunications system able to return data at over 16 kbps. A launch failure of the first Atlas-Centaur eliminated Mariner 8 but the other spacecraft, Mariner 9 (Fig. 11), performed as planned and became the first-ever planetary orbiter in November 1971. Initial operations, however, were disappointing because a global dust storm obscured the surface. After the atmosphere had partially cleared in early 1972, Mariner 9 began to systematically map Mars.

Mars was found to be a planet with two strikingly different hemispheres—a southern hemisphere that is one or two

kilometers higher than the other and highly cratered like the lunar uplands, including two giant impact basins. The terrain of the northerly hemisphere is younger and less cratered. The earlier Mariners had mainly observed the ancient cratered terrain and had not provided even a hint of the giant volcanoes and canyons revealed by Mariner 9 as evidence of a Mars that has experienced dramatic evolutionary forces. Nor had earlier images captured evidence of channels —some giant flood channels, some dendritic in nature—nor the layered sedimentary terrains of the polar regions.

Though all the channels were demonstrably old (as evidenced by the areal density of local craters) and though it is certain (given the low vapor pressure of water in the atmosphere) that liquid water cannot exist at the surface of Mars today, there are few alternatives to explain the origin of the channels other than action of water in the past. This appreciation, together with the evidence of periodic climate change provided by the layered sediments, raises many questions about the early history of Mars in particular. Thus, in the wake of Mariner 9's discoveries the scientific exploration of Mars quickened again, providing renewed motivation to understand the evolution of the planet both in terms of a terrestrial analogue and also as a second planet where life might, at some time, have found a niche.

Mars 2 and 3. Two descent modules of the Soviet Mars 2 and 3 spacecraft descended to the surface of Mars in 1971. Unfortunately, they were unable to return scientific data, most likely due to the consequences of the dust storm. Their orbital

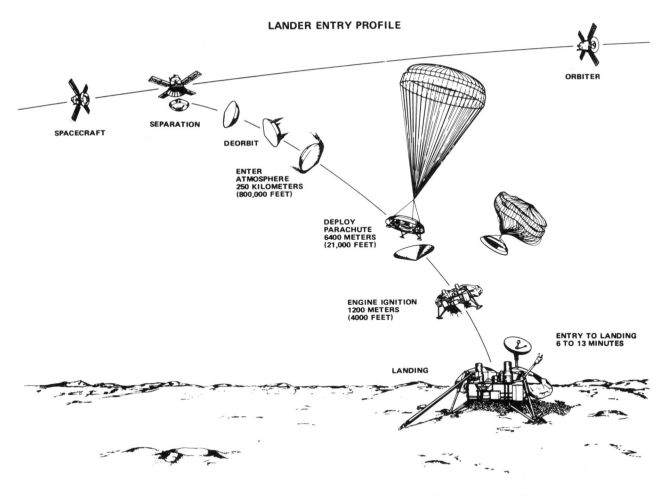

LANDER ENTRY PROFILE

SPACECRAFT

SEPARATION

DEORBIT

ENTER
ATMOSPHERE
250 KILOMETERS
(800,000 FEET)

DEPLOY
PARACHUTE
6400 METERS
(21,000 FEET)

ENGINE IGNITION
1200 METERS
(4000 FEET)

LANDING

ORBITER

ENTRY TO LANDING
6 TO 13 MINUTES

Fig. 12 Viking robotic interplanetary spacecraft (NASA 76-H-448)

modules studied the upper atmosphere and magnetic field, which was found to be very weak. The mass of Mars 2 and 3 was 46.5 metric tons.

Viking. The Viking orbiter and lander mission remains the most ambitious U.S. space project (Fig. 12). In 1975, two robotic spacecraft were launched to Mars, each consisting of an orbiter and a lander. The mission was intended to conduct comprehensive observations of Mars from its surface and from orbit. The orbiters' primary role was to carry the landers into Mars orbit, locate safe landing sites (using television cameras), and, after the landers had separated and landed, to act as relay vehicles for the lander. The landers' primary task was to acquire soil samples, photograph the surrounding terrain, and conduct other experiments. The most important measurements did not have positive results—no signs of life were detected.

The Viking landers each had a mass of 663 kg, including 91 kg of scientific equipment. To reach the surface they were contained within an entry vehicle (378 kg), which in turn was sealed in a bioshield (128 kg). The orbiter had an unfuelled weight of 883 kg; with propellants for orbital insertion it weighed 2328 kg. The orbiter was based on Mariner designs and had a telemetry rate of up to 16 kbps. The landers were

entirely new and were powered by two small radioisotope thermal generators that produced 90 watts of electric power, supplemented by nickel cadmium batteries.

The lander de-orbit maneuver was carried out using a monomethyl hydrazine engine providing a velocity change of 180 m/s. At an altitude of about 5 km, measured by a radar altimeter, the parachute was deployed. Each lander touched down on three legs at a speed of 1.5 m/s controlled by three monomethyl hydrazine thrusters that were used for the terminal descent after release from the parachute at about 1.5 km altitude.

A critical technology issue for the lander was the need to assure that no terrestrial microorganisms would be carried to the martian surface to confound the Viking life detection experiments or other future experiments of this kind. As the only available approach that could provide adequate confidence that the lander was sterile, each vehicle was subjected to 40 hours of baking at temperatures that reached 112 °C. Every component on the spacecraft had to be fully functional after such treatment—a requirement that added substantially to the effort of designing and building the lander and its experiments.

Phobos 2. Though designed primarily to study the inner

martian moon, Phobos, the Soviet Phobos 2 spacecraft has also provided new information about Mars (and about the Sun's activity). In particular, this orbital spacecraft was equipped with a full range of instruments to measure magnetospheric properties of Mars, a subject that had been neglected on earlier orbiters after the early recognition that Mars has only a very small magnetic field. Phobos 2, after being inserted into orbit about Mars in early 1989, made measurements of magnetic field intensity, plasma wave emissions and energetic plasma fluxes.

Interest in the small body, Phobos, remains high—partly because it is an accessible representative of the primitive bodies of the solar system and partly because of its convenient location in the martian gravity field. Potentially, Phobos could be a way-point for human explorers visiting Mars, one that might not only be a suitable base for the operation of automated vehicles on the surface of Mars but also a source of important resources needed for operations in space.

D. Beyond Earth and Moon—The Outer Solar System

Most of the matter in the solar system resides in the outer solar system. It is occupied by the giant planets, which differ from the rocky terrestrial inner planets by being rich in hydrogen and surrounded by dozens of moons and an enormous number of small bodies (asteroids, comets). All these bodies carry information about various phases of the evolution of the solar system. It is thus natural that once it became possible to build and launch reliable spacecraft, there was interest in studying the bodies occupying the outer regions of the solar system.

1. Pioneer 10 and 11

The first spacecraft to venture beyond the orbit of Mars, Pioneer 10 and 11 were tasked to make a thorough reconnaissance (including an assessment of the hazard of micrometeoroids and radiation belts) of the region as far out as Jupiter and, potentially, Saturn. This goal was achieved and laid the groundwork for the later Voyagers.

The identical Pioneers were comprehensively instrumented with particle and field instruments and, although spin stabilized and lacking a scan platform, carried three remote sensing experiments, including a combined photometer-imager. For the first time, spacecraft relied solely on nuclear power, which was derived from four small radioisotope thermal generators mounted in pairs on opposite sides of the spacecraft (providing a total of 155 watts of electrical power at launch). At Jupiter, the 2.74-m diameter high gain antenna, together with the 8-watt S-band transmitters, provided the communications link for the 12 instruments at a rate of 1024 bps.

The spacecraft were launched using the Atlas Centaur vehicle. Pioneer 10 was launched in March 1972 and Pioneer 11 in April 1973. Pioneer 10 crossed the asteroid belt without mishap.

The success of Pioneer 10 at Jupiter provided the confidence for targeting Pioneer 11 in such a way that it would not only acquire more jovian data, but would also use Jupiter's gravity field to swing the spacecraft onto a path continuing to Saturn. This required a much closer passage (43,000 km) by Jupiter, causing Pioneer 11 to penetrate deeper into the jovian radiation belts to assess how large a dose of radiation the spacecraft could survive. As with Pioneer 10, during the closest approach (December 2, 1974) radiation effects induced some spurious commands that interfered with some of the instruments' data gathering, but again the spacecraft survived and provided data upon which Voyager mission planning could be based.

Pioneer 11 made the first measurements of Saturn's magnetic field strength and orientation as well as of the character of the intense belts of charged particles, mainly protons and electrons. Other data were obtained about Saturn and its vicinity.

Long after the historic encounters with Jupiter and Saturn, Pioneer 10 and 11 continue to transmit, still being interrogated regularly as they leave the solar system. Together with the two Voyagers, which also have completed their planetary encounters, the Pioneers are monitoring the charged particle and electromagnetic field environment of the outermost depths of the solar system, making a unique characterization of the heliopause.

2. Voyager

The Voyagers had much in common with the design philosophy of the earlier Mariners. But, cloaked in black insulating blankets for their passage away from the Sun, with three booms (one for three RTGs, one for a magnetometer, one for the scan platform), long radio astronomy antennas, and a 3.66-m high gain communications dish, the Voyagers certainly had the appearance of a new breed. The 825-kg spacecraft are three-axis stabilized and spend most of their time in cruise with the high gain antenna pointing directly at Earth.

The two spacecraft were launched by Titan Centaur vehicles in August and September 1977. Encounters with Jupiter were in March and July 1979, with Saturn in November 1980 and August 1981, with Uranus (Voyager 2 only) in January 1986, and with Neptune (Voyager 2) in August 1989. Following its Saturn and Titan encounter in November 1980, Voyager 1 began to head out of the solar system at a steep 35° angle above the ecliptic.

Identical complements of scientific instruments were mounted on each spacecraft, with two TV cameras (using vidicon tubes), an ultraviolet spectrometer, an infrared spectrometer and a photopolarimeter bore-sighted on the scan platform. The payload weighed a total of 106 kg. The tape recorder capacity was 538 million bits and the X-band communications were sized to be 115 kbps at Jupiter and 45 kbps at Saturn. Major upgrades of the Deep Space Network's large antennas and the use of antenna-arraying allowed the communication data rates to stay above 20 kbps even at Neptune.

The catalog of discoveries made by the two Voyagers as they travelled outward is too extensive to be properly summarized here, for they encountered four major planetary systems, not just four large planets. The comprehensive payload of more focussed instruments then allowed the imaging reconnaissance observations to be immediately extrapolated to a much deeper level of understanding of the phenomena in question.

Voyager 2's passage over Neptune and by Triton placed it on a trajectory that is heading ever outward and downwards relative to the ecliptic. It and Voyager 1 continue to be tracked regularly, and their electrical power and attitude control gas should suffice to allow communications until at least 2015, when they will be well over 100 AU from the Sun.

With the Voyager 2 encounter with Neptune in August 1989, the reconnaissance of the outer solar system was virtually complete; only tiny, anomalous Pluto remains as a planet unseen as yet in close-up. Thus the Grand Tour of the outer solar system, possible only once every 175 years using a series of gravity swing-bys, was completed, even though this original ambitious goal had at one point been abandoned as too expensive.

3. Galileo

The Galileo spacecraft, a combination of a Jupiter orbiter and atmospheric entry probe, was finally launched in October 1989 using the Space Shuttle and an Inertial Upper Stage (IUS). Given the considerable mass of the Galileo orbiter (1138 kg plus over 900 kg of propellant for the propulsion system) and probe (331 kg), and the use of the two-stage solid IUS rather than a more powerful stage like the Centaur (whose development for use in the Space Shuttle was terminated after the Challenger accident), it became necessary to launch Galileo to Jupiter on a complex gravity-assist trajectory involving one Venus and two Earth flybys. Arrival at Jupiter will be at the end of 1995 and will follow up on the discoveries of Voyager. Along the way to Jupiter there will be a first flyby of a main belt asteroid, which the remote sensing instrumentation are well-suited to characterize.

The Galileo spacecraft is a significant departure from the earlier Mariners (including Voyager). First, it has a dual-spin configuration designed to allow the scan platform-mounted, remote sensing instruments to be pointed from a three-axis stable spacecraft while the particle and field instruments sweep out their fields of view from a spinning spacecraft. Second, the spacecraft has a new level of electronic capability contained in 19 microprocessors with a total of about 320 kbytes of random access memory and 41 kbytes of read-only memory. Spacecraft and instrument functions increasingly reside in software and most subsystem programs are completely reprogrammable.

The spinning section has its axis generally pointing at Earth and it is dominated by a 4.8-m deployable high-gain antenna (for both S-band and X-band signals). This section also carries the 5 m long booms upon which are mounted RTGs that provide electrical power. Another boom carries the particle and field instruments. The spacecraft bus is part of the spun section; it contains most of the electronics and, integrally, the retropropulsion system (supplied by Germany). This propulsion system provides all the thrust required for attitude control maneuvers and for velocity changes.

The despun section (connected to the spinning section by a spin bearing assembly that provides both a mechanical interface and an electrical power and data interface) contains the Jupiter entry probe, the scan platform with its four instruments, electronics bays, and the probe's relay radio antenna and hardware.

The Jupiter probe, which will be released 150 days before encounter, is designed to tackle an atmospheric entry velocity of unprecedented magnitude—about 50 km/s! It decelerates to Mach 1 in just a few minutes, during which time peak heating exceeds 40 kw/cm^2. About half of the probe's mass is required for the carbon phenolic heat shield. The descent module itself (containing the instruments) is not a sealed pressure vessel like the Pioneer Venus probes, but is vented to save weight; individual units within the probe are sealed as necessary and the unit is designed to survive to the 20 bar level.

A key instrument on the probe is the neutral mass spectrometer, designed to measure the major constituents of the atmosphere as a function of altitude and also to search for trace constituents.

4. Comet Rendezvous Asteroid Flyby (CRAF) and Cassini Missions—Mariner Mark II

The next missions to the outer solar system that were planned to follow Galileo were to make a long-duration, close-up study of a comet nucleus (CRAF) and to study the saturnian system and its large moon Titan (Cassini).

As of this writing (April 1992), the CRAF mission has been cancelled. Among a long list of specific objectives, both missions were to address goals related to the origin and history of complex organic molecules in solid, icy material, and, in the case of Titan, in a complex atmosphere-surface system.

Both missions were to use a new generation, three-axis stabilized deep-space spacecraft—known as Mariner Mark II —one that is generally more simple than the dual-spin Galileo spacecraft. Cassini will also carry a Titan probe provided by the European Space Agency.

The CRAF mission was to travel to its target—one of the periodic comets, probably Kopff—after launch on a Titan 4 Centaur and after following a gravity-assist trajectory somewhat less complicated than that of Galileo (using only one Earth flyby). The asteroid flyby was to take place on the final outward leg as the spacecraft passes through the Main Belt. The planned rendezvous was to occur when the comet was near aphelion, out towards the orbit of Jupiter. After this maneuver the spacecraft was to stay with its target as the comet entered the inner solar system and became active. Telescopic cameras, spectrometers, and radiometers were to

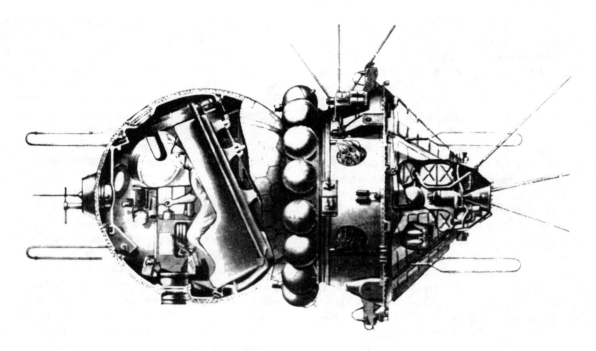

Fig. 13 Vostok spacecraft

map the inactive nucleus at fine resolution and then monitor the transition to full-scale activity. During this phase dust and gases from the comet were to be captured and their inorganic and organic chemistry analyzed. A comprehensive payload of plasma instruments was intended to allow study of the complex interactions of the cometary gases and dust with sunlight and the solar wind.

The Cassini mission, also to be launched on the Titan 4 Centaur, in many ways follows the pattern of Galileo's mission plan at Jupiter. The principal difference is that the probe will be targeted into the atmosphere of the moon Titan, rather than into Saturn's atmosphere. Again, the orbit at Saturn will permit many close flybys of the larger moons, including multiple flybys of Titan. The surface of this moon will be imaged using radar in the manner of Veneras 16 and 17 and Magellan at Venus. For the many other moons and the ring system, conventional imaging and spectroscopic techniques will be used. The Cassini science payload includes a complete suite of plasma instruments to make direct measurements of the complex interaction between the magnetosphere with the rings and with the atmosphere of Titan.

V. Manned Spacecraft

All manned spacecraft must provide humans with adequate living conditions, ensure their return to Earth, and enable them to conduct research and observations. Despite differences in mission, configuration, and design, manned spacecraft have much in common. On the other hand, one can still divide (somewhat arbitrarily) manned spacecraft into four categories:

• manned spacecraft for independent applied tasks (Vostok, Mercury, Voskhod, Gemini, the first version of Soyuz, Space Shuttle)

• transport spacecraft for delivering crewmembers to space stations and returning them to Earth

• interplanetary spacecraft (Apollo)

• space stations (Salyut 1, 4, Skylab, Salyut 2, 3, 5, 6, 7, Mir).

A. Vostok

Vostok was the first manned spacecraft. Its mission was to study the ability of humans to live and work on an orbital space flight in weightlessness, albeit for a very short time (on the order of several days).

The spacecraft consisted of two basic modules (Fig. 13): a descent module and an instrument-equipment module. The descent module housed a single cosmonaut and an ejection seat, a visual attitude control device, a control console, radio telephone communications and direction finding equipment, life support equipment, a parachute system, automatic control equipment, and chemical batteries for operation during descent. Pressure and atmospheric composition in the module were Earth standard. The remaining equipment (everything not required by the descent module during return and not requiring direct access by the cosmonaut during flight) was housed in the instrument-equipment module. This design was dictated by the need to minimize the amount of equipment inside the descent module so as to reduce the size and weight of the heat shielding.

Within the hermetically sealed instrument-equipment module were instruments controlling orientation; program driven, clock-based and switching instruments; radio apparatus for transmission of commands to the automatic equipment on board; instruments for orbital monitoring and telemetry; equipment for the thermal regulation system; and chemical batteries. The propulsion system was located on the exterior of the instrument-equipment module in a cylindrical niche at the bottom.

Mounted on the exterior surface were antennae, the solar and infrared sensors of the attitude control system, and louvers for the thermal regulation system. Above the radiator, which also served as the bottom of the instrument module, were the microjet engines for attitude control, (which operated on supplies of compressed gas). The compressed gas was stored in cylinders hung like a necklace around the instrument-equipment module where it was joined to the descent module.

The spacecraft was launched by the Vostok three-stage rocket. Descent from orbit required joint operation of the liquid-propellant jet propulsion system and the attitude control systems. There were three attitude control systems. One supported automatic orientation of the spacecraft in an orbital system of coordinates and used an infrared local horizon sensor and a gyro-orbitant, an instrument which, after horizon sensing, controlled the spacecraft's heading. The second system also supported automatic orientation of the long axis of the spacecraft in the direction of the Sun. This was sufficient for descent, since the launch was timed so that during the planned descent circuit, at the point when the retrorocket would be fired, orientation toward the Sun approximately corresponded to the orientation needed for the deceleration impulse. The third system utilized manual orientation on the basis of optical instruments, allowing the cosmonaut, using manual control levers, to orient the spacecraft along all three axes relative to the Earth's horizon and flight direction.

The infrared sensor malfunctioned on the first unmanned test flight. The mechanism rotating the horizon-scanning mirror failed to function, since the gear friction was chosen without considering the changes introduced by the need for the mechanism to operate in a vacuum. The same problem occurred during the second unmanned test flight. For this reason, all remaining Vostok flights used solar orientation for descent, with the exception of the sixth and last flight, which used manual orientation.

In the event of a failure of the propulsion system or all the attitude control systems, there was a back-up descent mode utilizing the natural deceleration of the spacecraft by the atmosphere. The spacecraft's orbit had been selected so that time in orbit did not exceed 10 days. Oxygen supplies and power sources were selected to suffice for a 10-day flight.

At that time, the major problem in returning from orbit was protecting the descent module from the effects of the incandescent plasma that would be produced in front of the spacecraft when it entered the atmosphere at a velocity of approximately 7.8 km/s. To address this problem simply and directly, the Vostok's descent module was built in the shape of a sphere.

• A sphere has a minimum surface area (to cover with heat shielding) per given internal volume and thus would require close to the minimum thermal shield weight. This general idea was subsequently confirmed through exact calculations.

• The aerodynamic characteristics of a sphere and the data essential for computing processes of heat exchange on its surface were well known, which made it possible to reduce development time by dispensing with additional experimental aerodynamic and heat-physics research.

• With a sphere, it was easy to provide stability during movement through the atmosphere. The displacement of the center of mass from the center to the forward portion of the vessel ensured that the spacecraft would move with that part first. The increasing ram effect helped ensure stabilization of the spacecraft.by damping the auto-oscillations around the center of mass during deceleration. The latter made it possible to proceed without an active control system during atmospheric flight, which considerably simplified the spacecraft.

Since the spacecraft was spherical in shape, there was only aerodynamic resistance (no aerodynamic lift) and the spacecraft followed a ballistic trajectory. When the spacecraft entered the atmosphere at an angle of 2-3 degrees to the horizon, the maximal acceleration operating on the spacecraft and cosmonaut was 9-10 g. After deceleration to a velocity of 200 m/s at an altitude of approximately 7 km, the hatch cover was jettisoned, and the cosmonaut was ejected, and he landed using a parachute. At an altitude of 4-5 km, the parachute system of the spacecraft was deployed, allowing it to land at a velocity of approximately 7 m/s.

In the event of an emergency during launch or the initial leg of the flight, the rocket engines were to shut down and the cosmonaut ejected (in response to command from an automated rescue device) and landed by parachute. If an emergency occurred during the second or third stage of flight, the engines were also to shut off, and the descent module would separate, descend, and decelerate in the atmosphere. The same landing sequence would then occur as during descent from orbit.

During orbital flight the heat generated in the descent module was transmitted to heat-transport fluid through the gas-fluid heat exchanger and then to the radiator in the instrument module. The heat generated within the instrument module was transmitted to the same radiator by blowing air through the module along the wall containing the radiator.

The spacecraft's mass was 4.7 metric tons, and the diameter of the descent module was 2.3 m.

Between 1961 and 1963, there were six Vostok flights. Duration of the first flight was 1.5 hours (one orbit), and duration of the next five were 1, 4, 3, 5, and 3 days. All were successful. During the flights, technical and medical studies and experiments, observations, and photography were conducted. The flights generated significant information, including the demonstration that a human being can live and work in weightlessness for at least 5 days; and that almost all cosmonauts experience discomfort under conditions of weightlessness. There was insufficient data to determine whether this discomfort was due to individual differences or the period of

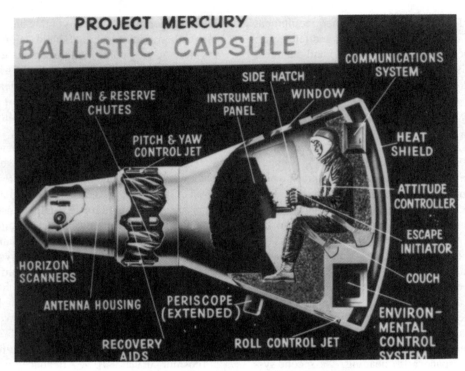

Fig. 14 Mercury spacecraft (NASA 183A)

adaptation to weightlessness. It became clear that it was possible and necessary to move forward.

B. Mercury

The American spacecraft Mercury was developed to obtain information about the human capacity for space flight.

In shape, the spacecraft was a truncated cone, the broad base of which was covered with a heat shield, in the form of a spherical segment (Fig. 14). The conical surface of the sides was covered with a metal casing. On the small base of the cone was a cylindrical recovery (parachute) compartment. The sealed cabin, which had the same contours as the exterior, was protected from overheating in flight by an outer layer of thermal insulation. A three-sided escape tower attached to the recovery compartments contained the solid propellant engine of the emergency escape system.

The sealed crew compartment contained a stationary couch in which the astronaut sat in a space suit. It also contained the consoles and manual controls, apparatus of the automatic attitude control system; apparatus for radio communications, telemetry, and monitoring of the orbit; program and clock controlled and switching instruments; life support system equipment; the thermal regulation system; and power sources. Heat was dissipated through evaporation of water. The heat from the cabin air was removed by an evaporative heat exchanger. Carbon dioxide was removed from the cabin atmosphere with lithium absorbers. The astronauts were supplied with oxygen from pressurized cylinders. The atmosphere inside the sealed module was pure oxygen at a pressure of 0.36 atmospheres.

The exterior of the pressurized module contained optical horizon scanners operating in the infrared region, two sets of jet engines of the attitude control system, a tank, compressed gas cylinders, and equipment for delivering propellant to the control engines. The propulsion system used a single-component propellant: hydrogen peroxide at a high concentration.

The retrorocket system consisted of three solid propellant engines mounted on the forward heat shield of the spacecraft with metal tie rods. The thrust of each engine was approximately 450 kg. After the retrothrust, the solid propellant system separated from the spacecraft.

The Mercury spacecraft was inserted into orbit by the Atlas rocket, while suborbital flights used the Redstone rocket.

Descent from orbit was effected by the joint operation of the attitude control system and the retrorocket system. There were two attitude control systems on board, one automatic, the other manual.

The forward heat shield was made of material sublimated under high temperature, similar to the material used in the heat shield of the Vostok. The protective casing of the surface was made of titanium.

In case of an emergency during launch or flight, there was an emergency escape system. In the event of an emergency, the connection between the rocket and spacecraft would be broken, the solid propellant engine of the escape system would be fired, and the spacecraft would be carried up and to the side of the booster. This system became a model for future escape systems.

The parachute landing system was deployed when the spacecraft approached the surface of the Earth, or rather water, since the spacecraft landed in the ocean. The parachute was

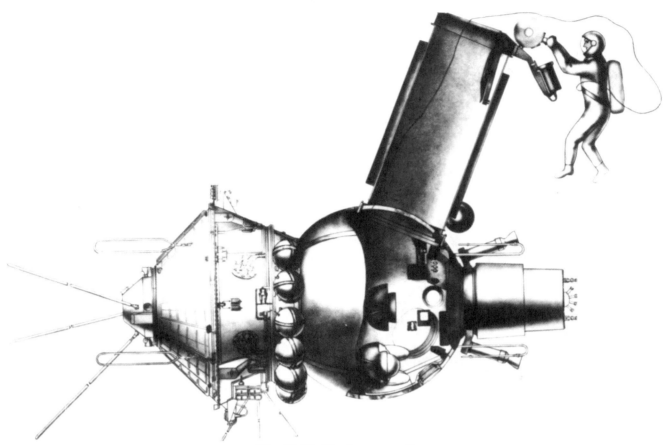

Fig. 15 Voskhod spacecraft

released at about 13 km.

After the main parachute had filled, the forward heat shield separated. Its downward movement caused a perforated canopy skirt of rubberized fabric to emerge. The forward shield moved away to a distance of 1.2 m and along with the canopy skirt formed a shock absorber which upon landing in the water reduced acceleration to an acceptable level. The splashdown velocity was approximately 9 m/s.

An advantage of this design configuration is that the maximum temperature on the forward heat shield during descent into the atmosphere did not exceed approximately 1650° due to ablation of its material. The maximum deceleration on descent was approximately 8-g.

The lift-off mass, including the tower and emergency escape system was approximately 2000 kg, while orbital weight was approximately 1350 kg. The total height, including the emergency escape system, was approximately 8 m. The maximum diameter was approximately 1.9 m and the length of the descent module was approximately 3 m.

In 1962-1963, there were four Mercury orbital flights with durations ranging from 5 hours to 1 1/2 days.

C. Voskhod

The design of the Voskhod spacecraft was based on and very similar to the design configuration of the Vostok (Fig. 15).

It consisted of three modules: an instrument-equipment module with the main propulsion system, a descent module, and a back-up solid propellant propulsion system. The instrument-equipment module was taken virtually unaltered from Vostok. The dimensions and design of the body and thermal shield of the descent module were similar to those of Vostok, although the interior was significantly altered. The ejection seat was removed, the internal configuration of the equipment was different, and three cosmonauts were seated on contoured couches. Each couch was custom-contoured to conform to the body of an individual cosmonaut. The couch design was intended to provide optimal endurance of force at the moment of landing. Experiments performed during ground-based development confirmed this design. In addition, the descent module housed a new parachute-jet landing system. When the major canopies (with an area of approximately 1150 m²) of the parachute were deployed, a solid propellant landing engine emerged from the parachute container. The parachute cords were attached to its top, and the cables linking it to the suspension unit of the parachute-jet system on the hull of the descent module were attached to its other side. The descent module approached the Earth at a velocity of approximately 7-8 m/s on the main canopies. After the main canopies filled, a hatch opened in the forward portion of the descent module and a 1 1/2 m probe was ejected. When the end of this probe touched the ground, the retrorocket engine was fired and the

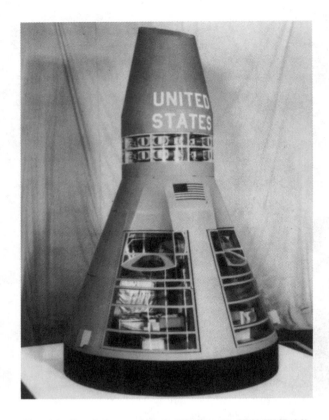

Fig. 16 Gemini spacecraft (NASA 62-GEMINI-11)

velocity of approach to the ground decreased to 3-5 m/s. Air pressure and composition in the descent module were that of the normal atmosphere, and the cosmonauts did not wear suits in the spacecraft. The back-up solid propellant propulsion system was added to the design of the spacecraft to provide redundancy for the main propulsion system.

The spacecraft was inserted into orbit by a three-stage modified R7 rocket. It had a new third stage, which made it possible to increase the mass of the spacecraft to 5.3 metric tons.

Stores of oxygen, food, and water were provided for the 3 days of the flight. The spacecraft flew in 1964.

The Voskhod 2 was intended for the first experimental extravehicular activity (EVA). It differed from the first Voskhod in that, instead of three cosmonauts, it carried two cosmonauts wearing space suits. To make the EVA possible, there was a folded inflatable airlock instead of the ejection hatch. After the spacecraft was inserted into orbit, the airlock was inflated. The walls of the lock formed a double rubberized envelope enclosing a cylindrical space. When a pin was removed, compressed gas entered the space between the envelope, and the airlock became a rigid structure with two hatches on either end—one for leaving the lock to go into space and the other for entering the lock from the spacecraft cabin. During an EVA the cosmonaut was tethered to the spacecraft with a line and cables. After completion of the EVA, the cosmonaut returned to the airlock and then entered the spacecraft, closed the hatch between the spacecraft and

airlock. Before descent, the airlock separated from the spacecraft.

The successful flight of Voskhod 2 took place in 1965. The first EVA demonstrated that humans retain spatial orientation and sound judgement even encased in a space suit face to face with the void of space.

D. Gemini

Gemini was a two-man spacecraft designed for final testing of certain operations, procedures, and equipment for the future lunar mission. The goals of this project were:
- long-term flights continuing up to 14 days
- flight testing of the life support system
- final testing and improvement of the rendezvous and docking process for spacecraft in orbit
- final testing of EVA equipment and procedures
- testing of an electric power supply system using electrochemical generators in weightlessness
- testing and further development of a new system for controlling descent in the atmosphere using aerodynamic lift.

The spacecraft consisted of three modules: the descent module, the retrorocket module, and an equipment module (Fig. 16).

The descent module was shaped like a truncated cone; the large end (as was the case for Mercury) was covered with a heat shield in the form of a spherical segment. Through a shift of the center of mass from the axis of symmetry, a spacecraft of this shape could achieve aerodynamic lift while moving through the atmosphere. In the air stream, the shift in the center of mass caused the spacecraft to tilt slightly, resulting in lift. When the bank of the spacecraft was changed, it altered the vertical component of the lift, and thus the descent trajectory could be controlled, making landing more accurate.

The upper portion of the descent module contained a compartment housing the rendezvous radar, the parachute system, the docking unit, and the reentry attitude control system that operated during descent. That system used nitrogen tetroxide and monomethylhydrazine. Aside from the engines, the system included propellant tanks, compressed gas cylinders for pressurization, and an automatic pneumohydraulic device for control and delivery of propellant to the engines.

Inside the descent module, there were ejection seats for two astronauts in space suits; a console and manual controls, apparatus to control attitude and rendezvous; apparatus to control descent, communications, and life support and thermal regulation systems; and chemical batteries for the instruments and equipment of the module during descent from orbit.

The atmosphere was pure oxygen pressurized at 0.36 atmospheres. The diameter of the descent module was approximately 2.3 m, the length was approximately 3.5 m, the volume of the pressurized cabin was about 2 m^3.

In the conical retrorocket module were four solid propellant engines, each having thrust of about a metric ton, for use during descent from orbit, and six liquid-propellant jet en-

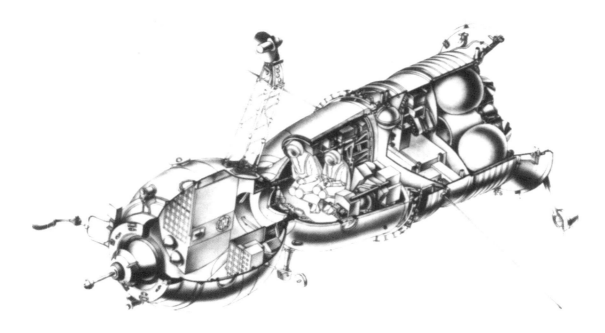

Fig. 17 Soyuz spacecraft

gines for attitude and translation control, arranged so that the retrothrust would be along the lateral axes of the spacecraft for maneuvering in orbit and during rendezvous and docking.

The nonpressurized equipment module contained instruments and equipment used only during orbital flight: radio apparatus for communications, control of orbital parameters, transmission of commands and instructions, and telemetry; two engines used for output of boosting impulses (during maneuvering in orbit and for rendezvous and docking), eight engines used for attitude control during the orbital portion of flight, tanks containing propellant, pneumohydraulic apparatus, a tank containing liquid oxygen for the life support system, tanks with liquid hydrogen and liquid oxygen for the electrochemical generators to power on-board apparatus and equipment (starting with Gemini 5), water tanks, thermal regulation systems and its radiators. The propulsion systems in the equipment and descent modules ran on nitrogen tetroxide and monomethylhydrazine. The equipment module separated from the spacecraft before reentry.

The rendezvous operations were generally performed using a specially developed rocket stage of the Agena, which was inserted into orbit as part of the Atlas-Agena rocket. To control rendezvous and docking, a radar, a gyroscope platform with acceleration meters, and an on-board computer were used. A radio transponder, working with the spacecraft radar, was installed on the target. The radar measured distance, radial velocity, and angle of sighting. Radio communications and, thus, measurement began at a distance of approximately 300 km and ended at 1-2 m.

The ejection seat was intended for use in case of an emergency at launch, during the active portion of the flight, or during parachute descent. The escape system (as with Vostok)

had the disadvantage that, after a certain point in the rocket flight it could not save the crew in an emergency. This point was determined by the flight velocity at which the temperature generated on the surface of the space suit after the astronaut had entered the air stream was high enough to destroy the suit. This method would work if there were a heatproof suit. But without such a suit, at the most critical portion of the rocket's flight during insertion of the spacecraft into orbit (in the area of maximum velocity), the astronauts were unprotected in the event of a rocket emergency.

As was the case with Mercury, the astronauts landed in the water. Deployment of the parachute system began at an altitude of approximately 13 km. The maximal acceleration during deployment of the parachute system was approximately 3-3.5 g. Rate at splashdown was approximately 9 m/s.

The mass of the spacecraft remained approximately 3.8 metric tons. The full length was approximately 3 m.

In 1965-1966, there were 10 flights of Gemini spacecraft, of up to 14 days in duration. During these flights, a number of problems were solved and the experience necessary for performance of the lunar mission was obtained.

E. Soyuz

The Soyuz spacecraft was initially created for autonomous orbital flights, conducting specific research and experiments, and final testing of the then new processes of rendezvous and docking in orbit, and control of the reentry modules during descent from orbit using aerodynamic lift. After these goals were achieved, during the stage of construction of orbital stations, the spacecraft was further improved and developed in order to convert it into a transport spacecraft to deliver cosmonauts to orbital stations and return them to Earth after completion of their stays on the station.

The spacecraft consists of three modules: the reentry module, the orbital module, and the instrument-equipment module (Fig. 17).

The reentry module was used to return cosmonauts to Earth. Its lateral surface was conical in shape with the angle of inclusion of the cone equal to 14. The large base is covered with a heat shield in the form of spherical segment. The upper portion of the reentry module was shaped like a portion of a sphere. Thus, the reentry module was asymmetrical in shape. The design of the body and the configuration of the equipment caused the center of mass to be displaced relative to the axis of symmetry. This caused the spacecraft to tilt slightly as it moved in the airstream, producing aerodynamic lift and making it possible to control the descent trajectory, decrease acceleration during descent, and increase landing accuracy. The reentry module's diameter was 2.2 m.

The exterior of the reentry module was protected from the effect of hot plasma by a heat shield coating. The forward shield was made from ablative material of the asbotextolite type, similar to the heat shield used on Vostok. The sides and rear portion of the reentry module were covered with glass-textolite material over fibrous thermal insulation material.

The reentry module contained:
• two or three cosmonauts in space suits
• contoured couches
• life support equipment
• control console and levers for manual control of attitude and the spacecraft's coordinates
• a visual orientation instrument, which makes it possible for a cosmonaut to orient the spacecraft in the orbital coordinate system from a visual picture of the horizon and the flow of terrain in the central field of vision
• apparatus for communications and to produce a direction-finding signal to be used by search parties after the module has landed
• instruments for automatic and manual control of descent
• programmed and switching instruments for controlling on-board apparatus
• devices for automatic control of parachute deployment and landing
• parachutes
• eight solid propellant rocket engines mounted on the bottom and used immediately before touchdown to decrease velocity
• chemical batteries for electric power to module equipment during descent
• rocket engines for controlling the reentry module's attitude during descent, utilizing single-component propellant (hydrogen peroxide) with tanks and automatic pneumohydraulic delivery of propellant to the engines.

The available internal volume of the reentry module was about 2 m^3. The reentry module weighed about 3 metric tons. The maximum deceleration was 3-4 g.

The orbital module provided a second working and living area where the crew conducted research and experiments; slept; donned, and removed their space suits; and performed natural functions. The orbital module housed the life support system, thermal regulation, flight control instruments, and apparatus for measuring parameters of the relative motion of the approaching spacecraft. The antennae of this system were mounted on the exterior surfaces of the spacecraft. In the upper portion of the module was a docking port of the probe-cone type, which provided a mechanically strong connection of the spacecraft with the station, pressurization of the joint, and connections for electrical and hydraulic lines.

Normal Earth atmospheric composition and pressure was maintained in both inhabited modules.

The instrument module consisted essentially of the instrument, equipment, and transfer compartments.

The instrument compartment contained computers, the attitude control system, radio equipment for command and programmed radio links, orbit monitor, telemetry, the main equipment for the thermal regulation system, the electric power system, and other control equipment.

The equipment compartment housed two propulsion systems that operate with self-igniting components. It contained the main and standby cruise engines, attitude control engines, engines for changing coordinates and for stabilization of the spacecraft when the main cruise engine was operating, tanks of propellant, cylinders for pressurizing tanks, and an automatic propulsion system device.

The transfer compartment was a ring-shaped girder structure connecting the reentry and instrument modules. It contained cylinders with oxygen for the life support system and some of the attitude control engines (for motion along the lateral axis and deceleration).

Power supply to the instruments and equipment was provided through the combined use of solar panels and chemical batteries. Deployed after insertion into orbit, the solar panels were mounted on the equipment compartment. On the lower flare of this compartment were the batteries.

On the exterior of the spacecraft were an infrared local horizon sensor, a solar sensor, the radiator of the thermoregulation system, radio system antennae, and the vacuum screening thermal insulation that covered the orbital and reentry modules, the transfer and instrument modules, and the equipment compartment.

The length of the spacecraft was about 7 m. The available volume in the inhabited modules was about 6 m^3. The mass of the spacecraft was about 7 metric tons. The maximal acceleration at insertion was approximately 4 g.

The main problem in the construction of the Soyuz spacecraft was that of docking. On the first Soyuz spacecraft the method of parallel approach was used, although the best method uses free trajectories. In the latter method, the parameters of relative motion of the approaching objects are used to compute the required magnitude and direction of velocity change that must be imparted to the active spacecraft in order to connect with the other one. This operation must be repeated two or three times. It is critical that the process converge for the docking process to occur. For this method to be used there must be a computer on board. However, in the early 1960s, when the first Soyuz spacecraft were being designed, the U.S.S.R. did not yet produce small on-board computers (they existed only as experimental prototypes). A different method had to be used—the method of parallel approaches. The idea behind this method is that firing of the engine of the active spacecraft damps the angular velocity of the line of sight (the line between the two spacecraft) and approach occurs along this line. The angular velocity along the line of sight may be measured using a gyrostabilized radar vectoring head to track the passive spacecraft, which carries a transponder radar. The same radar measures the distance and radial velocity between two approaching spacecraft. This computation turns out to be relatively simple, and can be accomplished by analog computing devices. It is appropriate to use the method of parallel approaches with relatively small distances, starting at 20 km, and before that to have the approach controlled by ground-based radio measurements and computer calculations. The radar set needed was relatively easy to produce. A configuration was adopted in which the process of approach and docking was completely automated, with the option of switching to manual control of docking starting at a distance of 200-300 m, if necessary.

After small on-board computers began to be produced, they were installed on the next version of the spacecraft (Soyuz T and Soyuz TM). This made it possible to return to the method of free trajectories, as a more economical and accurate method, that required the least number of firings of the rendezvous engines.

The Soyuz used a probe-type docking port, which had the disadvantage that spacecraft with that probe port could dock only with a spacecraft or station equipped with the appropriate cone adapter. Under normal circumstances this characteristic does not lead to major problems. However, in unforeseen circumstances and emergencies, especially when rescue operations are called for, this characteristic can lead to major problems. In the 1970s, during the Soviet-American cooperation, an androgynous docking port was developed to enable any spacecraft to dock with any other. However, this port was more massive and demanded considerably more accuracy in spacecraft approach for docking to occur. For this reason this kind of docking port was not put into the Soyuz at that time; however, it is evidently the port of the future.

The Soyuz reentry module landed with the aid of two parachute systems, solid propellant landing retrorockets, instruments measuring altitude and velocity of the descending spacecraft, and instruments of the landing computer for processing these measurements and issuing commands. During descent, at a height of approximately 10 km and spacecraft velocity of approximately 200 m/s, the parachute system began to deploy. The hatch of the container for the main parachute system was blasted open, deploying the auxiliary parachute. The auxiliary parachute drew the drogue parachute after it and it in turn decreased the velocity of the spacecraft to 80-90 m/s. Then the cord of the brake canopy

separated from the suspension unit, and as the brake canopy fell it drew the main parachute canopy out of the container behind it and the latter began to fill. After the main canopy filled, a diagnostic procedure determined whether the process of parachute descent was proceeding normally: the velocity of descent over a distance of 1 kilometer was measured. If the descent velocity was high, the landing computer designated the process as abnormal (for example, due to tearing of the main canopy) and issued a command to separate the canopy of the main parachute system from the suspension point. After separation of the main system, the computer issued a command for deployment of the standby parachute system: its hatch was blasted open, the auxiliary parachute was deployed, then the drogue parachute, and then the main canopy of the standby parachute system was deployed and filled. After filling of the main canopy of the main or standby systems and designation of a normal landing by the computer, the suspension system was adjusted so that the parachute was suspended symmetrically. The forward heat shield separated, to clear the solid propellant landing retrorocket for operation. At an altitude of 1-1.5 m, the engines were fired in response to a command from a gamma-altimeter. Before their firing, the rate of descent was approximately 7 m/s if the main system was being used and about 8 m/s if the standby system was used. The landing rockets damped the spacecraft's velocity to 2-4 m/s.

The principle underlying the emergency escape system on Soyuz was the same as that on Mercury. However, some difficulties were encountered implementing this principle on Soyuz. The orbital module was above the reentry module, and during the atmospheric portion of insertion, the spacecraft was covered by the nose fairing. The orbital module was located in front of the reentry module, because if this were not the case, there would have to be a hatch in the nose of the reentry module (so cosmonauts could enter the orbital module from it), and the couches and equipment under them would have to be removable during the flight, which would be unacceptable and unsafe.

Given the design configuration of the spacecraft, the emergency rescue engine could not be installed on the reentry module. In order to rescue the crew by distancing the spacecraft from the launch vehicle using a very powerful rocket engine, the rescue system had to be very complicated in design and operation.

The nose fairing was divided into sections by two cuts. One, passing through the axis of the fairing, made it possible to divide it into two flaps, which could be opened after the rocket left the dense layers of the atmosphere during normal flight. The other cut, running laterally, was used in an emergency situation. This cut was located in the area of the joint between the reentry module and the escape tower. The engine of the emergency escape system was located on the upper portion of the fairing. There were devices coupling the orbital and reentry modules with the nose fairing, that were put into operation if an emergency arose. In normal flight there was no rigid coupling between the spacecraft and the fairing.

In an emergency at launch or during the active leg of flight, the following sequence of actions would have taken place:

• The rocket engines would have shut down.

• The connection between the reentry module and the tower of the instrument-equipment compartment would have broken, and the lateral joint of the nose fairing opened.

• The upper portion of the fairing and the reentry and orbital module connector would have connected (the connector would have seized the nose fairing by the "waist," the place where the reentry module and orbital module are joined).

• The engine of the emergency rescue system would have fired.

• The spacecraft within the upper portion of the fairing would have moved up and to the side from the emergency booster.

• The connection between the orbital module and the reentry module would have broken and the latter would have begun to fall.

• At a command generated automatically by the emergency rescue system an automatic landing controller would have begun to operate in accordance with a program corresponding to this leg of flight, and commands are would have been given to deploy the parachute system.

• The landing process of the reentry module would have been completed.

The Soyuz spacecraft was developed in the early 1960s. Work to modernize the spacecraft was begun in the early 1970s and was completed with the development of the modified Soyuz T. The following features distinguished the modified Soyuz T from the previous Soyuz:

• The on-board equipment included a digital computer.

• The flight control system did not include gyroplatforms; it operated by using angular velocity sensors and constructed a system of coordinates relative to which it displayed the axis of the spacecraft by integrating equations describing the movement of the spacecraft around the Earth and around the center of mass of the spacecraft.

• There was a new system to control descent utilizing the digital computer.

• There was a unified propulsion system in which the cruise, attitude control, and the maneuvering engines had the same components and were powered from the same tanks.

• On-board systems were modernized (the parachute system, the landing retrorockets, standby bank control engines added to the descent control system, consoles, a command program radio link, a system for controlling the on-board equipment, a landing computer, a television, and elements of the thermoregulation and electric power systems).

As early as the mid-1980s, another phase in the modernization of the Soyuz spacecraft was undertaken, which culminated in the development of Soyuz TM. Improvements included parachutes made of a new material that was stronger and lighter, a lighter engine for the emergency rescue system, introduction of segmentation in the system for delivering propellant to the unified propulsion system, and improvement of a number of on-board systems.

There were two tragic accidents associated with Soyuz flights. In the first, V. Komarov was killed during landing after performing the first manned test flight of the Soyuz spacecraft. After release of the drogue parachute canopy of the main parachute system, the main canopy failed to emerge from the parachute container and the reentry module continued its descent on the drogue canopy. The landing computer detected excessive descent velocity and issued a command to deploy the standby system. However, the main canopy of the standby system did not fill because its harness got tangled with the harness of the drogue canopy of the main system. Analysis of this fatality failed to reveal unambiguously the reason for the failure of the main canopy to emerge from the parachute container. On the basis of possible reasons, the parachute system and supporting structures were improved and additional tests of the landing system were conducted. These improvements had a positive result—there were no other cases of failure of the main parachute canopy to emerge from the parachute container, nor of any other dangerous failures of the parachute landing system.

In the second accident, G. Dobrovolskiy, V. Volkov, and V. Patsayev were killed returning from the first mission to the Salyut space station. At an altitude of about 150 km, during separation of the orbital and reentry modules, the valves of the reentry module ventilation system suddenly opened (this was supposed to happen at an altitude of 5 km). Experiments performed to analyze the causes of this disaster did not reveal a clear picture of what occurred. The accident was most likely associated with the mechanical stresses occurring after breaking of the connection between the modules, since the ventilation valve is on the frame of the reentry module, through which the reentry module is attached to the orbital module. As a result of this analysis, improvements were made in the structure connecting the modules (in order to decrease dynamic stresses when the modules separate), and in the valves (in order to eliminate even the theoretical possibility that the valves would open as a result of mechanical stress). No further cases of depressurization have occurred.

F. Apollo

The Apollo spacecraft, designed for lunar missions, consisted, in essence, of two separate spacecraft: an orbital spacecraft (also called Apollo) module and the Lunar Module (Fig. 18).

The following sequence of operations occurred during the lunar mission:

• insertion of the spacecraft on a relatively low near-Earth orbit using the Saturn 5 rocket, involving operation of the first, second, and partially the third stage

• translunar insertion using the third stage of the rocket

• docking of the two spacecraft (which had been separated when carried by the booster) by reconfiguring of the third stage of the rocket, the lunar module, and the orbital spacecraft, during which the orbital spacecraft separated, moved away, rotated 180° and docked with the lunar module; the

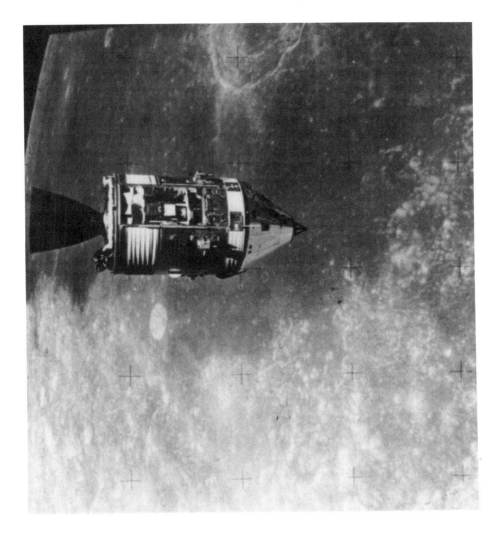

Fig. 18 Apollo command and service modules above the Moon (NASA 71-H-1417)

lunar module had been prepared for docking by opening the flaps of the transfer compartment within which it had been mounted

• separation of the two-spacecraft complex from the third stage of the rocket

• midcourse correction of lunar trajectory by the engine of the orbital spacecraft

• insertion of the spacecraft complex into translunar satellite orbit by the engine of the orbital spacecraft

• development of an orbit from which the lunar module could land on the Moon (minimum altitude was approximately 30 km)

• transfer of two of the astronauts from the orbiter to the lunar module

• separation of the lunar module from the orbiter, firing of the engines of the lunar module landing stage, and landing on the surface of the Moon

• correction of orbit of the orbiter to increase minimum altitude to approximately 100 km

• performance of work on the surface of the Moon

• take-off of the lunar module (without the lander, which was no longer necessary) into satellite orbit, where the orbiter awaited it

• docking and transfer of the crew to the orbiter

• separation of the orbiter from the lunar module

• trans-Earth insertion through operation of the propulsion system of the orbiter

• midcourse correction of the trajectory to Earth to ensure necessary conditions for the reentry of the orbital spacecraft into the atmosphere

• separation of the command module from the service module of the orbiter and reentry into the Earth's atmosphere with escape velocity

• deceleration of the command module and splashdown in the ocean.

This mission profile illustrates the role of the separate portions of the Apollo spacecraft and explains their functional purpose.

The orbiter consisted of two parts: the command module and the service module.

The command module was shaped like a cone with a divergent angle of 66°. The base of the cone was covered with a forward heat shield, in the shape of a spherical segment. The diameter of the spacecraft was 3.85 m, its length was about 3.5 m. The center of mass was displaced relative to the axis of symmetry, tilting it with respect to the velocity vector to create aerodynamic lift during atmospheric flight. The ratio of aerodynamic lift to aerodynamic resistance of the Apollo command module was approximately 0.4.

During the atmospheric leg of orbital insertion, a four-sided escape tower with a solid propellant emergency rescue engine was mounted on the command module in case of a rocket accident. The emergency rescue system worked like the one used on Mercury. For protection from air flow during the insertion phase, the command module was covered with a protective heat cap.

The command module contained:
- three astronauts in space suits sitting in individual impact-attenuated couches
- life support system equipment and food supplies
- control consoles, instrument panels, and manual control levers
- apparatus of the navigation, control, attitude control and stabilization systems, radio communications apparatus, and landing control equipment
- three chemical batteries for powering apparatus after separation of the command module from the service module and two for circuits of the explosive hatch opening devices
- a probe-type docking unit in the upper portion of the module
- a parachute system
- jet engines operating on monomethylhydrazine and nitrogen tetroxide, for controlling the movement of the command module after it separated from the service module tanks with propellant, pressurization cylinders, and an automatic pneumohydraulic system for delivering propellant to the engines.

The atmosphere inside the module was oxygen at a pressure of approximately 0.4 atmospheres. The weight of the command module was approximately 5.5 metric tons.
The service module was cylindrical, with a diameter of about 3.9 meters and length of about 7.5 m. It contained:
- the propulsion system of the orbiter, including a cruise engine, tanks, pressurization cylinders, and automatic pneumohydraulic propellant delivery system
- oxygen bottles for the crew's air supply system and the associated automatic pneumohydraulic device
- antennae.

To control spacecraft attitude and motion during operation of the propulsion and navigation systems, the following were employed: an on-board digital computer, a gyrostabilized platform with acceleration meters, angular velocity sensors, integrating gyroscopes, an accelerometer oriented along the long axis, optical instruments for navigation measurements of the altitude of stars above the horizon of the Earth and Moon, a radar transponder and control levers.

This equipment ensured control during the translunar insertion stage of the flight, navigational measurements and midcourse corrections during flight to the Moon, insertion into stable orbit around the Moon, rendezvous and docking, trans-Earth insertion, and reentry into the atmosphere. It enabled a shift to manual control during rendezvous, midcourse correction, descent, and in emergencies.

The cruise propulsion system operated on self-igniting reactants: Aerozine-50 and nitrogen tetroxide. The thrust of the cruise engine was 9.3 metric tons. To provide high reliability, a propellant-pressured feed system was used for delivering propellant to the engine.

The engines for attitude control, stabilization, and motion control operated on self-igniting reactants: monomethylhydrazine and nitrogen tetroxide.

The radio equipment of the orbital spacecraft provided telephone contact, telemetry, measurement of orbital parameters, transmission of commands and program information from the Earth, and transmission of television images to the Earth.

The electrical power for the on-board apparatus and equipment came from three oxygen/hydrogen electrochemical generators; the flight program could be performed even if one of them failed.

Heat was released through a heat transfer fluid to the radiator on the external surface of the service module.

A byproduct of the fuel cells was water, which was used by the crew. The crew was provided with oxygen from a tank where it was stored in supercritical state.

The parachute system contained a brake canopy, three auxiliary canopies, and three main canopies. When the command module attained an altitude of about 7.5 km, the drogue canopy was deployed. After the velocity had been damped somewhat by the drogue canopy, it separated and the three auxiliary canopies were deployed, and these dragged the three main canopies into the air flow. This system ensured safe splashdown even if one of the main canopies failed to fill. The normal splashdown velocity was approximately 8 m/s. If one of the canopies failed, this velocity could have reached 10.5 m/s.

The launch weight of the orbital spacecraft was approximately 29 metric tons.

The lunar module consisted of the spacecraft cabin with an ascent propulsion system and a descent stage with landing gear.

The pressurized cabin contained:
- two astronauts in space suits
- a harness system for restraining them while they worked (couches were not provided; this saved space and there seemed to be no real need for them in the lunar module)
- control consoles and panels
- levers to control attitude, descent to the Moon, landing, approach, and docking with the orbital spacecraft
- a ventilation system for the space suits with absorbers of water vapor, carbon dioxide, and harmful contaminants in the cabin atmosphere

• a space suit backpack, worn by the astronauts when they left the module, including a self-contained life support system
  • food supplies
  • research equipment.

The cabin atmosphere was pure oxygen with pressure of 0.3-0.4 atmospheres. Even when the cabin was pressurized the astronauts did not remove their space suits; they were permitted only to open their helmets. Before the astronauts went out onto the lunar surface, the cabin was depressurized; after they returned and the egress hatch was closed, the cabin was pressurized. The available volume of the cabin was approximately 4.5 m^3.

The pressurized cabin had two hatches. One was for passing through the docking port into the orbital spacecraft, and the other was for egress onto the surface of the Moon.

The following equipment was mounted on the exterior surface of the pressurized crew cabin:

  • cone-type docking adapter
  • apparatus for controlling attitude, the descent and landing, rendezvous, and docking, including a radar set for measuring the altitude and velocity of descent during landing, a radar for measuring distance, rate of approach, and angles of view of the orbiter spacecraft during approach; an inertial measurement system; angular velocity sensors; acceleration meters; an on-board computer, etc.
    • communications radar for monitoring orbit and telemetry
    • current source
    • antennae for radio communications and radar
    • flashing beacon
    • propulsion system, including cruise engine, tanks of propellant, cylinders for pressurizing them (the ascent propulsion system also used a propellant-pressured feed system for propellant delivery), and a pneumohydraulic system
      • tank containing water for the crew
      • thermal regulation system.

The cruise engine had a thrust of about 1.6 metric tons. It operated on self-igniting reactants: Aerozine-50 and nitrogen tetroxide. The control engines also used these propellants.

The thrust of the engine of the descent stage could change during the process of landing in response to commands of the control system from a maximum of about 4.5 metric tons to a value of approximately 10 percent of the maximum value. It also operated on self-igniting components: Aerozine-50 and nitrogen tetroxide. The system for feeding propellant components to the engine was propellant-pressured, and included tanks, pressurization cylinders, and a pneumohydraulic system.

Aside from the propulsion system the descent stage was fitted with a four-footed lander with impact absorbers and dish-shaped landing pads, each of which contained a mechanical landing probe for sensing contact with the surface (at a signal from these probes the engines were shut off). It also was fitted with isotope generators, a ladder for descent to the lunar surface, research equipment, and a lunar rover to allow the astronauts to move around on the surface on the Moon (on Apollo 15, 16, 17).

The landing engine was fired at an altitude of approximately 3 km. The velocity vector of the spacecraft at this moment was directed almost parallel to the surface of the Moon and the programmed value of thrust was approximately 2.7 metric tons. At the beginning of the landing process the velocity vector was directed almost vertically, at a velocity of approximately 8 m/s, and altitude of 150 m. During this operation, before the spacecraft approached the surface, the velocity was damped to 1 m/s.

The mass of the descent stage was approximately 10 metric tons.

The lunar rover was a self-propelled, four-wheel cart. Each wheel had its own drive with an electric motor. To protect against the high heat of the Sun on the lunar surface and to attenuate impact, the rim of each wheel was made of braided wire. The electric motors were powered by chemical batteries attached to the vehicle. The rover had two seats for the astronauts, equipment and antennas for communications and transmission of television images, a console, and controls. The rover weighed approximately 200 kg (without passengers or cargo). The loaded weight could reach 750 kg. The length was approximately 3 m, the wheel spacing was 1.8 m, clearance was 0.35 m. The lunar rover could reach a speed of up to 14 km/hr.

On the surface of the Moon, the astronauts used space suits with self-contained, backpack-mounted devices containing a control console, supplies of oxygen, absorbers of carbon dioxide and water vapor, a thermal regulation system, communications and telemetry apparatus, and a power source.

The following equipment was used to conduct research on the surface of the Moon:

  • seismometers
  • gravimeters
  • a magnetometer
  • ion and charged particle detectors
  • a spectrometer for study of the solar wind
  • a roll of foil as a trap for particles of solar wind
  • a television camera for taking panoramic images of the lunar surface
  • a laser reflector for measuring the distance between the Earth and the Moon.

Humans will probably return to the Moon around the turn of the century to establish one or more bases for further lunar exploration, to establish a new generation of space observatories, and for the purpose of learning how to live on another planetary body for an extended time.

Although a quite satisfying general picture of the Moon's origin and evolution has emerged as a result of the intensive research that followed the Apollo Program, there are, inevitably, many loose ends and uncertainties that make the description of the Moon in Chapter 3 of this volume still only tentative. Thus, the planetary scientist still has much unfin-

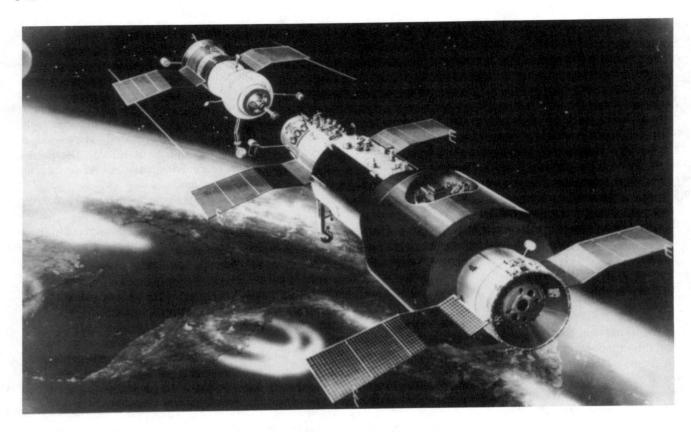

Fig. 19 Salyut orbital station

ished business for further lunar exploration. The agenda calls for the acquisition of a definitive global map of the Moon (not acquired in the 1960s in the rushed space race of that era) in terms of the distribution of many physical and chemical attributes—surface figure, chemical elements, mineralogy, magnetic field, gravity field—and, also, for more field geology on the Moon including the collection of selected surface samples. With such new data planetary scientists can seek definitive answers to many open questions about the different phases of the evolution of the Moon.

Astronomers also look toward the Moon as a potentially ideal location to establish the most powerful observatories of the next century, provided that an answer can be found to the costly logistics needed to build and operate telescopes there.

G. Salyut

The Salyut space stations were designed as orbital laboratories to empirically test existing ideas about the operation of orbital stations; to investigate human tolerance of relatively long-term exposure to weightlessness (up to 1-2 months); and to conduct research, experiments, and observations using existing apparatus and the capabilities of the orbital station.

The dimensions, configuration, and weight of the station were determined by the capacities of the Proton rocket, which the U.S.S.R. had developed at that time.

The Salyut station consisted of four modules (Fig. 19): the

work and transfer modules and the equipment and scientific instrument bays. The shell of the work module had the form of two cylinders linked by a conical connector, with spherical ends. The diameter of the larger cylinder was 4.15 m, while the diameter of the smaller one was 2.9 m. At one end of the smaller cylinder was a pressurized hatch for entering the work module from the transfer module.

The shell of the transfer module (cylinder and cone) was connected to the work module at one end and to the docking port for the transport spacecraft at the other end. The nonpressurized cylindrical equipment bay was attached to the other end of the work module.

Two solar panels deployed during flight were mounted on the exterior surface of the transfer module and equipment bay. The radiator of the thermal regulation system, about 20 m^2 in area, was mounted on the smaller work module cylinders. In addition, optical instruments of the attitude control system, radio antennas, and scientific instruments that required a nonpressurized environment were mounted on the exterior of the station.

The work module was the main working and living quarters of the station. It contained the major station equipment and the systems for its control. This is where the cosmonauts worked, ate, and slept. The instruments and equipment were generally located in special areas. The crew's living and working areas were separated from the instrument areas by removable panels. Mounted along the left and right walls at the larger end were chemical batteries and other equipment for the electrical power system, the system for controlling on-board equipment, radio communications radio devices, radio equipment for measuring trajectory parameters and receiving commands, and apparatus for controlling the attitude and translational motion of the station.

The smaller end housed the regenerators and absorbing cartridges of the system that maintained the station atmosphere.

Gyroscopic instruments of the attitude control and control systems were mounted on a special rigid frame in the forward portion of the work module, near the hatch connecting the transfer and work modules. This was the central control post of the station and contained the main control consoles and warning devices for controlling major station systems, station attitude, and the operation of the propulsion system. In front of the main post was a kind of periscope, which was partly within and partly outside the pressurized cabin. This instrument allowed the crew to see along the station axis and perpendicular to it, permitting the cosmonauts to orient the station in the orbital system of coordinates on the basis of an annular representation of the horizon and from the direction of terrain flow in the central visual field of the device. In addition, the small diameter section contained a conical connecter and, near the scientific instrument bay, consoles for control of scientific apparatus and experimental set-ups.

All the control posts and cosmonaut work stations were provided with equipment for telephonic communication and lamps. Other lamps illuminated the remainder of the work module. Additional light sources were used for taking photographs and movies.

Behind the central control post was the dining area: a small table, on the surface of which were devices for anchoring objects (Velcro, suction cups). This table could be used as a surface for repair of the instruments and equipment. Adjacent to the dining area was the kitchen, containing a food heating unit and a set of eating utensils. The cupboard for storing food and the refrigerator were located in the large diameter end. Water was stored in spherical containers that were divided into two sections: one filled with water and one with gas, separated by an internal membrane. Water was pumped out of the container by exerting pressure on the gas-filled area. The cosmonauts generally slept in the large diameter area, off the floor along the side panels. The commode was located at the rear of the work module.

Since the station was intended for long-term flights, it was provided with exercise machines for compulsory daily physical exercise sessions to prevent deconditioning.

The transfer compartment contained control consoles for astro-orientation and the Orion apparatus for astrophysical research. The latter was located in an unpressurized niche in the transfer module. The transfer compartment also contained levers for controlling orientation and communications equipment. The windows of the transfer module faced in different directions for observing the Earth, the horizon, etc. To conduct observations in the shadow of the Earth, the hatches could be closed in the spacecraft and the station, and the illumination turned off.

The equipment bay contained two propulsion systems: a cruise engine for midcourse correction, and a system for control of attitude and stabilization of engines. Both propulsion systems ran on self-igniting propellant. The cruise propulsion system had a main engine and a standby. The main engine had a single chamber, while the standby engine two chambers. Both had turbopump systems for feeding propellant into the combustion chamber. The cruise (orbital maneuvering) propulsion system ran on nitric acid and hydrazine-type fuel. The propulsion systems included tanks of propellant, gas cylinders for pressurizing the tanks, and automatic pneumohydraulic supply devices. The thrust of both the main and the standby engines was about 400 kg each.

The scientific instrument bay was a conical niche in the work module. It contained scientific instruments pointed out at the void of space.

The systems for control of attitude and translational motion (including optical and gyroscopic sensors, radar, visual instruments for orientation, and computers) oriented the station during approach and docking (when the longitudinal axis of the station is aligned with the approaching transport vehicle), as well as orienting the orbital and inertial systems of coordinates perpendicular to the plane of the solar panel, toward the Sun, and turning the station around this axis. With this arrangement, when the work being performed did not require a specific station orientation, the solar batteries could be charged without wasting propellant on keeping the panels oriented to the Sun (the solar panels were attached rigidly to the station hull and could not be rotated).

The thermal regulation system maintained air temperature in the living quarters of the station and whatever spacecraft was docked with it within a range of 15-25 °C, and maintained humidity within a range of 10-70 percent. The cooling and dehumidifying unit facilitated condensation and collection of moisture, and stored excess heat in the air in a heat-transfer medium. The heat-transfer medium was pumped through the ducts of the thermal regulation system, and the heat was transferred to the radiator, which released it into space. Air temperature in the instrument areas was maintained within a range of 10-30 °C. To ensure reliability of the system's operation, there were back-ups for all key components (the cooling and dehumidifying unit, pumps, regulators, etc.).

The cone-shaped docking unit mounted on the transfer module, along with a probe-type docking unit on the transport vehicle, ensured mechanical capture during docking, aligned the axes of the spacecraft and station, tightened the connection until it was airtight, and connected the electrical and hydraulic lines.

Ensuring reliability and supporting long-term operations are the principal problems for orbital stations designed to function for a relatively long period using hundreds of instruments, units and systems. The standard solution of backing up all components cannot solve the problem completely. It would have been natural to take advantage of the human presence on the station to increase its reliability and safety; in other words, to have the cosmonauts themselves repair or replace malfunctioning instruments or units. In practice, this would have required access to all instruments and equipment within the pressurized cabins as well as on its outer surfaces, in the equipment bay, and scientific instrument bay. On the first Salyut station and all the other first generation stations (up to Salyut 6), this idea was not taken seriously enough and was not adequately implemented in the design, although a start was made.

An analogous problem of fire hazard was foreseen by designers and cosmonauts, since this complex machine was crammed with electrical instruments, including many kilometers of electrical wire. Aside from the simplest measures that had already been taken on unmanned and manned spacecraft (as well as in aircraft and automobile designs), such as using low voltages in electrical circuits and installing fire extinguishers on board, there was a need for new heat-stable electrical cables that did not ignite, even in response to substantial increases in temperature, new electrical insulation material that did not emit toxic substances into the atmosphere at high temperatures or when burning, and new supplementary tests of already developed structures and electrical circuits for fire hazard and fire resistance. These problems were not solved on the first generation orbital stations, but experience with developing, producing and testing electrical components and utilizing these stations permitted designers to understand the problem.

The Salyut station was inserted into orbit in April 1971 and operated in orbit for 175 days, after which it was put into a reentry trajectory. The components that did not burn up in the atmosphere fell into the Pacific Ocean in October 1971.

Noteworthy among the first generation stations was Salyut 4, inserted into orbit in late 1974. The major differences between Salyut 4 and Salyut were:

• additional scientific instruments, experimental facilities, and the associated expansion of the research program

• increase in the efficiency and output of power supply systems for on-board apparatus and equipment, through replacement of the fixed solar panels with three panels that could be adjusted to face the Sun, each with an area of about 20 m^2

• inclusion of an experimental system for regenerating water from humidity condensate collected by the cooling and dehumidifying units of the crew life support system.

Noteworthy research projects on Salyut 4 included the study of the Sun using an on-board solar telescope operating in the ultraviolet wave band, systematic photographing of the surface of the Earth to study natural resources, and medical and biological studies.

Salyut 4 operated alternately in unmanned and manned mode for 2 years. Two space crews worked on it for periods of 1 and 2 months.

Salyut, Salyut 4, and the subsequent Salyut 6, Salyut 7, and Mir were developed by the design bureau formerly headed by S.P. Korolyov.

Salyut 2, 3, and 5 were developed in V.N. Chelomey's design bureau. In principle, these were also first generation stations with only one docking port and the same limited potential duration of operation in orbit. Salyut 2, inserted into orbit in 1973, operated for only 22 days and was unmanned. Salyut 3, inserted into orbit in 1974, was inhabited by one crew for 16 days. Two crews lived on Salyut 5, which was inserted into orbit in 1976. Their missions lasted 49 and 17 days. Crews were transported to these stations and returned to Earth in the first modification of the Soyuz transport vehicles.

H. Skylab

The American space station, Skylab, was designed as a large orbital laboratory to study the physiological effects of long-term space flight on humans, to conduct scientific and materials processing experiments, and to obtain experience in developing and utilizing long-duration space stations.

Skylab (Fig. 20) consisted of an orbital workshop, instrument unit, airlock module, multiple docking adapter, and the Apollo telescope mount (ATM).

The orbital workshop was based on the third stage of the Saturn 5 rocket. It consisted of a laboratory and living quarters located within the redesigned hydrogen tank of the stage, and a waste compartment located in the redesigned oxygen tank.

The laboratory and living quarters were the major living and working areas for the three-man crew. Both areas were also used to house various storage containers for food, water, and clothing, and spacecraft systems.

Ventilators circulated the air through the orbital workshop, driving air between the pressure bulkhead and the inner wall and through the interior areas. This circulation thermally stabilized the pressure bulkhead, which was important for reducing temperature differentials that could result in condensation and subsequent corrosion.

Handholds, handrails, and foot restraints were mounted in the interior to facilitate the astronauts efforts in microgravity.

The living quarters were located in the lower portion of the hydrogen tank (aft compartment). There were separate quarters for sleeping, leisure activities, food preparation and dining, personal hygiene, and medical research. The living quarters were separated from the laboratory by a nonpressurized wall. The medical research area also contained a collapsible shower stall, exercise machines, and equipment for medical studies. The living and dining area held a dining table, cupboards, and refrigerators with food supplies, and a window facing away from the Sun (when the telescope was focused on the Sun).

The laboratory compartment (forward compartment) was intended mainly for research and experiments requiring a relatively large area and to provide access to airlocks in order to place scientific apparatus in the vacuum of space. There were two small airlocks in the wall. One pointed toward the Sun and the other pointed in the opposite direction.

The laboratory compartment contained the experimental astronaut maneuvering unit (although experiments were con-

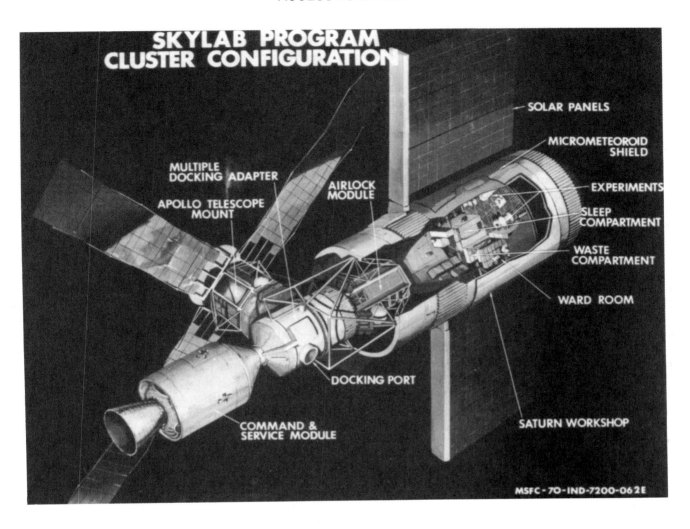

Fig. 20 Skylab (NASA-71-H-943)

ducted only inside the laboratory compartment), water tanks, refrigerators, food cabinets, crew life support and thermal regulation equipment, and control and communications consoles.

An airlock connected the laboratory and living quarters with the waste storage unit through an airlock. The upper part of the laboratory compartment had a trapdoor hatch for entering the airlock.

Within pressurized areas, atmospheric pressure was maintained at 0.35 atmospheres. The atmosphere was 74 percent oxygen and 26 percent nitrogen.

The diameter of the orbital workshop was 6.6 m. The interior volume of the laboratory and living quarters was approximately 270 m^3. Below the waste compartment were cylinders with compressed nitrogen for the attitude control engines and the radiator of the thermal regulation system.

Above the laboratory compartment was the nonpressurized instrument unit, in the form of a cylindrical ring with the same diameter as the hydrogen tank. It contained chemical batteries, on-board computers, and telemetric measurement apparatus.

The mass of the orbital workshop was approximately 35 metric tons. It was approximately 15 m in length.

The radiator of the thermal regulation system was mounted on the lower portion of the exterior of the laboratory compartment. A meteor shield covered the remaining portion of the cylindrical surface of the laboratory; it also served, along with insulation, to minimize uncontrolled heat exchange with the environment, protecting against solar overheating. In addition, there were two rotatable solar array panels, each one about 110 m^2 in area.

During orbital insertion, when the atmospheric friction of the inrushing air flow reached a maximum, one solar array wing and a portion of the antimeteor shield were ripped off. The second solar array wing did not deploy after orbital insertion because it was jammed by a fragment of metal. All this created a significant problem at the start of the station's operations. However, the bold and persistent efforts of the first crew, mission control center and the companies that manufactured the special repair tools, corrected this problem.

The airlock module, with two airtight hatches connected the orbital laboratory and the docking adapter; and was the airlock used by the astronauts to perform EVAs. The airlock volume was approximately 6 m^3. Oxygen and nitrogen tanks and chemical batteries were mounted on the exterior of the airlock.

The multiple docking adapter was a cylinder about 3 m in diameter, and about 5.2 m in length. The working volume of the airlock was about 30 m^3. It had two cone-type docking ports for docking with the manned transport spacecraft. The axial nose port was the primary docking adapter, with the lateral port acting as a back-up. The adapter housed a control and attitude control console for the station, a video tape machine, control consoles for the ATM instruments and study of the natural resources of the Earth, supplies of movie and photographic film, equipment for technological experiments, electrical and television equipment, storage for spare parts and exposed film, a carbon dioxide absorber, etc.

The ATM astrophysical observation module, designed mainly for study of the Sun, was mounted above the docking adapter. The axis of the ATM unit, which had to be pointed at the Sun during solar observation, was perpendicular to the longitudinal axis of the station.

The ATM module consisted of two major parts: a truss structure and, within it, the solar telescope block. Four solar array panels, each 110 m^2 in area, were mounted on the truss structure perpendicular to the axis of the ATM. In addition to the solar panels, chemical batteries working in tandem with the solar panels, optical attitude sensors, powered gyroscopes for the station attitude control system, and other equipment were mounted on the truss structure. The powered gyroscopes were used not only to eliminate consumption of propellant for maintaining orientation, but, more importantly, to provide a clean area around the station, eliminating potential exhaust during attitude control. The clean area around that station was an important condition for the operation of the ATM optical instruments.

The solar telescope block was placed in a gimbal mount, so it could be aimed and oriented with greater accuracy. The ring (pivoting) joint suspension of the solar telescope block made it possible to rotate it by up to 120°. The solar telescope block was rotated relative to the station with electrical drives.

A thermal shield was installed at the end of the block with openings for telescopes and solar sensors. Covers were controlled from the console in the docking structure.

The telescope block was shielded with a cylindrical covering, 3 m long and about 2 m in diameter, inside which the temperature was maintained at 21 °C.

The total length of the station was about 36 m and the internal volume (including the cabin of the Apollo descent module) was about 330 m^3. The station weighed about 70 metric tons.

The operation of the on-board equipment and scientific apparatus and station attitude were controlled with the aid of two on-board computers.

Sensing elements for attitude control included infrared horizon sensors, an inertial measurement block, and a radar transponder used during rendezvous with the transport spacecraft.

Three powered gyroscopes and jet engines running on compressed nitrogen acted as servo elements. The jet engines were used to damp disturbances of the station after separation from the second stage of the booster, for initial orientation, and for damping the kinetic moment of the powered gyroscopes. The system provided accuracy of orientation of about 3 angular minutes. The attitude control system of the ATM block supported accuracy of axis orientation of about 2.5 angular seconds in pitch and yaw and about 10 angular seconds in roll.

The radio apparatus of the station provided radiotelephone and teletype communications with the Earth, intra-station communication, communication with the station and with Earth during EVA, transmission of programs and instructions for the on-board computer, transmission of television images, video recording, radio measurement of orbital parameters, and telemetry.

Electric power for the on-board apparatus and equipment was provided by tandem operation of the solar arrays and chemical batteries. The voltage of the on-board circuit was 28 volts, which is standard for spacecraft. The total mean electric power when the solar panels were facing the Sun was about 18 kilowatts.

The thermal regulation system included a gas-to-fluid heat exchanger for transmission of excess heat from the air of the pressurized compartments to a liquid cooling agent, pumps for pumping the cooling agent through the ducts of the system, heaters, a radiator to receive the heat from the cooling agent, an automated control device, regulators, fans, thermal insulation, and a heat shield. In its normal mode, the thermal regulation system maintained air temperature within the station at about 21 °C.

The station's life support system included a system for feeding oxygen to the pressurized compartments of the station; absorbers of carbon dioxide, water vapor, and toxic gaseous contaminants; supplies of water and food; food preparation devices; personal hygiene facilities, including a shower and devices for collecting and disposing of human wastes; underwear; clothing; exercise equipment for maintaining conditioning in weightlessness (bicycle ergometer, lower body negative pressure device); and equipment for medical monitoring and diagnosis.

Oxygen was stored in the instrument unit, whereas water, food, clothing, etc., were stored in the laboratory compartment. The exercise machines were located in the living compartment.

The shower, a small folding stall with flexible walls, was also located in the aft compartment. Heated water was fed into the stall at low pressure through a sprayer, and a ventilator sucked the water-air mixture out of the shower stall.

Approximately 900 kg of food, packed mainly in cans, was needed to support the planned mission on the station. In addition, there were frozen, dehydrated, and freeze-dried products.

A total of 210 pairs of underwear, 60 changes of clothing,

and 30 athletic suits were stored, allowing the astronauts to change their outer garments once a week and underwear several times a week.

Space suits with self-contained life support systems were used for EVA.

The nature of the scientific and experimental equipment was determined by the research program. In astrophysics this included instruments for studying the Sun and solar corona in the X-ray, ultraviolet, and visible wave bands of solar radiation; mapping X-ray radiation sources; recording radiation from stars and galaxies in the ultraviolet portion of the spectrum; obtaining panoramas of the celestial sphere in ultraviolet radiation; and studying the comet Kohotek.

The research program on the Earth's natural resources included survey and targeted photography of the Earth, and observations in a variety of spectral wave bands.

The materials processing research program entailed study of a range of processes of melting, soldering, welding, crystallization, and cutting of various metals with different LASERS, MASERS, etc., as well as the production of composite materials.

The medical research program focussed on the study of human physiology under space-flight conditions.

In addition, there was an attempt to test the astronaut EVA maneuvering unit within the laboratory compartment.

Two telescopes for photographing the Sun in the H-a line, a coronograph for photographing the solar corona, a spectrograph, a spectroheliometer, and two X-ray telescopes were mounted in the ATM. The program of solar observations included study of the structure of the chromosphere and supergranulation; study of active areas and their development; observation of solar flares, prominences, and plumes; study of areas on the disk with depressed activity; and observation of phenomena developing slowly over a period of days or weeks.

The set of instruments for the study of Earth's natural resources included six cassette television cameras, an infrared spectrometer, a multiband scanning television camera, a radar set, and a radiometer.

The materials processing research equipment included devices for growing crystals, for soldering and welding metals, etc.

The Skylab station was inserted into orbit in 1973 by a Saturn 5 rocket. Three crews worked on the station for 28, 59, and 84 days, respectively. The crews were transported to the station and returned to Earth after completion of their mission by Apollo spacecraft.

The major results of research on Skylab included:

• a demonstration that humans can work safely and productively in space under conditions of weightlessness for up to 3 months

• evidence of the great potential for repair and troubleshooting in weightlessness and in the vacuum of space

• information about the biological, chemical and physical processes taking place in the human body during long-term space flight

• an effective program of solar research.

I. Salyut 6, 7

Salyut 6 and 7 were second generation orbital stations. During the habitation of orbital stations, resources were expended to provide life support for the crew (oxygen, water, food, clothing, etc.). Propellant was expended to compensate for the decelerating effect of the atmosphere and for attitude control. A crew of three men working on the station continually for 1 year required expenditure of approximately 10 metric tons of various materials. The supplies necessary for the operation of all first generation stations were inserted into orbit along with the station.

Second generation stations differed from first generation ones mainly because their operation was not limited by the supplies carried into orbit with them. Rather, additional cargo and propellant were supplied by cargo transport vehicles after the stations were in orbit. Of course, unloading the cargo and propellant could be completely automated, but today it is practical to assign this work to the on-board crew. In practice, this entailed the mounting of two docking ports on the station so that it can be docked simultaneously with a manned spacecraft and a cargo spacecraft.

Thus, aside from the station itself, the space station complex had to include a manned transport vehicle and a cargo vehicle.

The dimensions and configuration of Salyut 6 and 7 were similar to the dimensions and configuration of the first Salyuts, since they were also largely determined by the capacity of the Proton rocket that inserted them into orbit. These stations had five modular components: the work module, transfer module, intermediate chamber, equipment module, and scientific instrument module (Fig. 21).

During the flight, the crew spent most of their time in the work module. This module housed the major station equipment, which was generally installed along the right and left sides of the station, as well as under the floor. The instrument areas were separated from the living areas by removable panels. The rear area contained equipment for control of attitude and translational movement, control of the station systems, electric power, communications, program and command radio links, telemetry, and trajectory measurement. Food storage cabinets and water tanks were also located there. Near the rear wall, at the entrance to the intermediate chamber, was the sanitary facility containing a commode with forced suction ventilation, separator filters, and collectors of liquid and solid wastes. In the center was a collapsible shower stall with walls of flexible translucent material. Close to the rear wall were two airlocks for disposing of waste containers. One of the airlocks was also used for experiments requiring a vacuum.

The smaller end of the work module housed atmosphere recycling units, including a CO_2 processing unit that absorbed carbon dioxide and water vapor and emitted oxygen. The remaining portion of the water vapor emitted by the crews

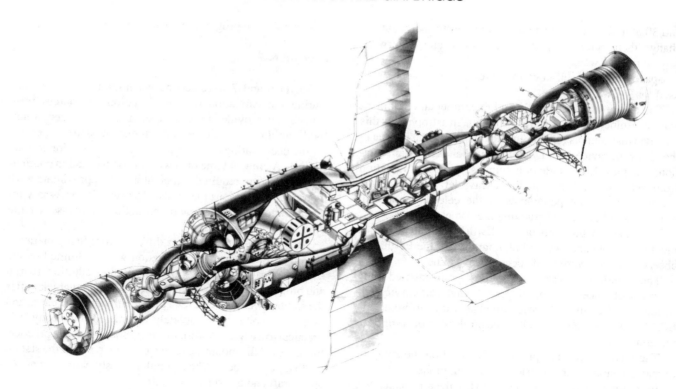

Fig. 21 Salyut 6 orbital station

during respiration was collected by the cooling and dehumidifying units of the thermal regulation system. Gyroscopic wicks and scavenger pumps then conveyed the vapor into the condensation collectors. The collectors fed the water into the water regeneration system, where it was cleaned in ion exchange columns and filters, disinfected, warmed, and prepared for use for drinking and preparation of dehydrated food products. In the middle section of the module were exercise machines: a bicycle ergometer, treadmill, and negative pressure device. Near the transfer module was the main work station of the crew—the central control post—with instruments for visual orientation, the main console, a management information system, and consoles for individual systems. In addition, there were control posts for astro-orientation, astrophysical instruments, and biomedical equipment.

On the exterior of the small diameter section of the module were three solar panels, which could be rotated along an axis perpendicular to the longitudinal axis of the station. During flight, each of these was oriented to obtain the greatest amount of energy from the Sun for any given station orientation. The area of each panel was 20 m². Also mounted on the exterior were the radiator of the thermal regulation system, an infrared local horizon finder, a solar sensor, some of the sensors for orienting the solar panels, instruments for visual orientation, antennae for the rendezvous guidance system, a television camera for monitoring berthing during docking with an approaching spacecraft, etc. To protect the solar panels and optical sensors from the effects of the onrushing air stream during launch the small cylinder of the work module (with the solar panels furled) was covered by a nose fairing. The nose

fairing was jettisoned during insertion into orbit after passing through the dense layers of the atmosphere.

There were two more control posts in the transfer module. This module also housed two EVA space suits and their onboard ventilation system, an EVA control console, levers for controlling attitude, and radio communications equipment.

The transfer module adjoined the front wall of the work module and could be entered through a connecting hatch. One of the two station docking ports, and the port used by manned transport vehicles, was mounted on this module. The transfer module was used for visual observations through windows and for EVA, in which case it acted as an airlock.

The nonpressurized equipment bay was mounted on one side of the back wall of the work module. Its diameter was 4.15 m, and its length 2.2 m. It housed the integrated propulsion system, antennae, sensors for orienting the solar panels, antennae for the rendezvous guidance system, and a television camera for monitoring the docking of the spacecraft with the side of the equipment bay.

The propulsion system was composed of two cruise jet engines with thrust of 300 kg each, 32 control engines, 6 propellant tanks (with metal bellows-type separators) of pressurization gas and propellant, cylinders with pressurization gas for the tanks, pumps for pumping gas from the tanks to the cylinder before refueling them with propellant, and an automated pneumohydraulic device. The reactants used in the propulsion system were unsymmetrical dimethylhydrazine and nitrogen tetroxide.

Thermostability of the hull of the equipment bay, like that of the work and transfer modules, was maintained by the heat-transfer fluid of the thermal regulation system pumped through pipes welded to the skin.

Along the axis of the equipment bay and inside it was the intermediate chamber. On one side it was welded to the lower end of the work module, on the other was the second docking port. Both manned and unmanned transport vehicles docked there. There were two hydraulic connectors on the docking port through which propellant was pumped from the cargo vehicle into the propulsion system.

The scientific instrument bay was a conical niche in the large diameter section of the work module. On the hull of this area was a cover that opened during observations.

The major differences between Salyut 6 and preceding Salyut stations were:
- introduction of the second docking port
- adoption of a new integrated propulsion system, which could be refuelled repeatedly in space
- additional guidance equipment for rendezvous and docking, enabling automatic rendezvous and docking of spacecraft with the side of the equipment bay
- development of the Progress cargo vehicle for regular delivery of life support supplies, propellant, supplementary research equipment, instruments, and equipment for station repair to the station.

The design of the unmanned Progress cargo transport vehicle was based on Soyuz (see Fig. 17). It consisted of three compartments: cargo, propellant, and instrument-equipment. A docking port was mounted on the cargo compartment so that after docking its interior volume could be combined with the interior volume of the station. It was used for dry cargo. After docking and opening of the hatches, the crew had access to the cargo that had been delivered. The lower portion of the cargo compartment was attached to the propellant compartment. There were two hydraulic connectors on the intermediate chamber docking port. These connectors were linked by a system of pipes to the tanks in the cargo vehicle propellant compartment. In addition to the tanks, this compartment contained pressurization cylinders for the tanks, an automatic pneumohydraulic device, and a water tank. The propellant compartment occupied the place of the descent module in the cargo vehicle.

The instrument-equipment module was similar in design and equipment to the corresponding Soyuz module.

Refuelling of the station took place after docking of the cargo vehicle through a sequence of operations:
- verification that the docking lines were airtight
- pumping gas from the tanks of the station propulsion system using compressors in its equipment bay (to prevent resistance to feeding propellant from the cargo vehicle into the station tanks); the gas was held in the pressurization cylinders of the station propulsion system
- transfer of propellant and then oxidant from the tanks of the propellant compartment of the cargo vehicle to the tanks of the station propulsion system
- closing the valves on the pipelines in the vicinity of the docking ports that separate the fuelling lines from the remain-

der of the hydraulic lines of the cargo vehicle propellant compartment, and flushing the pipelines.

This sequence was conducted so that when the spacecraft undocked with the station, the reactant remaining in the lines did not fall on the surface of the station docking port, from where, when the hatch was opened during subsequent docking, it could enter the living quarters of the station.

Long-duration use of the Salyut station led to identification of new problems characteristic of orbital stations, such as dust, toxic gaseous contaminants, microbial contamination, noise, and the meteor hazard.

Experience with crew life support in a relatively small closed area showed that, despite daily and weekly cleaning, dust accumulated in the atmosphere of the living quarters, interfering with operation of the ventilators and causing the crew discomfort.

The station had a large number of instruments and pieces of equipment in constant operation as well as kilometers of electrical wires with various types of insulation. Starting on the first day of use of the station, moisture was absorbed on the electrical wire insulation and on the sides of the instruments, corrosion occurred, and gas was emitted.

Moreover, the habitation of such a small space by various individuals (members of the prime and visiting crews) for several years created the problem of microbial contamination of the station atmosphere, walls, panels, and instruments.

To combat these adverse consequences of station operation, the living quarters were cleaned and disinfected with a hydrogen peroxide solution, and bactericidal lamps were used. In addition, air and interior surface samples were returned to Earth regularly for monitoring. However, it is obvious that these problems must be dealt with through regular use of various filters and other specialized equipment. It is also necessary to develop and use various automatic techniques for monitoring and eliminating dust, harmful gas contaminants, microflora, and microfauna.

The use of powered gyroscopes and the continuous running of the many ventilators used in the thermal regulation, life support, and other systems, along with the regular operation of all sorts of remote switches, leads to a rather high level of noise within the living quarters. When a crew works on the station for many months and is exposed to this noise for 24 hours a day, it becomes a notable adverse flight factor. At present, a mean level of noise approximately 55-60 decibels is considered acceptable for a station. However, on one hand, a noise level this low is difficult to attain, while on the other hand the acceptability of this level of noise is open to question and requires additional research.

The multiyear operation of orbital stations intensifies the problem of meteor hazard. The probability of puncture of the pressure bulkhead of a station or spacecraft may be evaluated using the function:

$$p = 1 - e^{-ast}$$

where p is the probability of a puncture; a is a coefficient determined by the characteristics of the meteor cloud in the vicinity of Earth, and the thickness, material, and structure of the hull; s is the area of the exterior pressurized modules of the spacecraft; and t is time in orbit.

Calculations using this formula show that for small spacecraft with a pressurized module surface area approximately tens of square meters and short-duration flights of approximately several days, the probability of puncture by micrometeors (and thus the probability of depressurization) is rather low (measured in hundredths of a percent). But when the size of the spacecraft increases (the exterior surface of the core module of Salyut or Mir are already 10 times greater than the above area, for example), and especially when flight time increases to a year, then the probability of depressurization (if special measures are not taken) becomes not only considerable, but unacceptable. If we take 10 years to be the estimated duration of station flight, then depressurization is almost guaranteed. Methods for protecting the pressurized modules of orbital stations from micrometeors have been developed and are being used. These involve increasing the thickness of walls and installing antimeteor shields, which are associated with increases in structural weight.

The problem with regard to manned transport vehicles, which have thin-walled modules (the orbital module of Soyuz), is somewhat more complicated. During flight, as part of the station for a year, the probability of puncture of a manned transport vehicle is considerable (approximately a fraction of a percent). That is enough to prompt consideration of additional measures for antimeteor protection.

But is it appropriate to estimate danger of depressurization in this way? After all, some types of spacecraft may be used for 10 and even 20 years. Several spacecraft of this type are sequentially and sometimes simultaneously in orbit. From the point of view of a specific crew, a probability of depressurization approximately a fraction of a percent may be acceptable. However, from the standpoint of the spacecraft developers, or of those directing the flight program of the orbital station, this method of calculating probability of depressurization is inappropriate. The calculation must use the total expected time of flight for all spacecraft of this type, i.e., 10-20 years. Once such calculations are performed, it will be unambiguously demonstrated that manned transport craft that will be used regularly for orbital stations must have antimeteor protection.

Salyut 6 was inserted into orbit in 1977. It was inhabited by 15 crews, of which 5 were prime crews, remaining in orbit for periods of 96, 140, 175, 185, and 75 days.

Salyut 7 was inserted into orbit in 1982. It was inhabited by 10 crews, of which 5 were prime crews working for periods of 211, 149, 236, 168, and 64 days.

The major results of work on these stations were:

• performance of long-term human flights with duration of up to 236 days

• performance of a broad program of biomedical, astrophysical, technological, and geophysical research and experiments.

J. Mir

Space station Mir was the next stage in the development of orbital stations. Its core module (Fig. 22) was inserted into orbit in 1986.

The main difference between Mir and previous stations is Mir's capacity to expand by taking on additional structures, on-board systems, and research capacities while in operation. The transfer compartment of the station's core module has five docking ports. One, the axial port, is for docking with transport vehicles, while the four lateral ports are for incorporating new modules weighing 10-20 metric tons. Thus, it is possible for five new modules to dock with the core module: four at the lateral ports of the transfer compartment and the fifth at the axial port of the equipment bay. The modules intended for docking with the transfer compartment first approach the station and dock with the axial port of the transfer compartment and are then transferred by a manipulator to one of the lateral ports.

At the end of 1990, three modules were docked with the core: the astrophysical Kvant module, the Kvant 2 module, and the Kristall module for materials processing research.

The body of the core module of Mir is similar to that of the Salyut station. The major differences in configuration are the five docking ports, new solar panels, and the instrumentation that must be accommodated. The mass of the core module is approximately 21 metric tons.

The Kvant module is docked to the axial port on the equipment module. It was inserted into orbit along with a special-purpose module by the Proton rocket. The special-purpose module was designed to perform maneuvering operations in orbit and to facilitate rendezvous between the Kvant and itself with the space station. After rendezvous, berthing, and docking of the complex with the Mir core module, the special-purpose module separated from the station. The Kvant module has two docking ports. One (the active port, of the probe type) is docked with the core module of the station. The other, on the opposite end, is designed for docking with cargo and manned transport vehicles, and thus with the station as a whole. The major purpose of the Kvant module is astrophysical research. A number of X-ray and ultraviolet telescopes are mounted on it. The module's weight is about 20 metric tons.

The Kvant 2 and Kristall modules are docked at the side ports of the transfer compartment of the core module. Their configuration is substantially different from that of Kvant. In these modules, which like Kvant were inserted into orbit by the Proton rocket, the special section used for maneuvering in orbit, rendezvous, and docking with the station is an integral part of the section that remains docked with the station, substantially increasing the weight of the scientific apparatus that can be accommodated.

The Kvant 2 module contains additional life support equipment, an EVA airlock, a special unit for allowing the cosmonauts to maneuver in space, and a remotely controlled platform for observing the surface of the Earth.

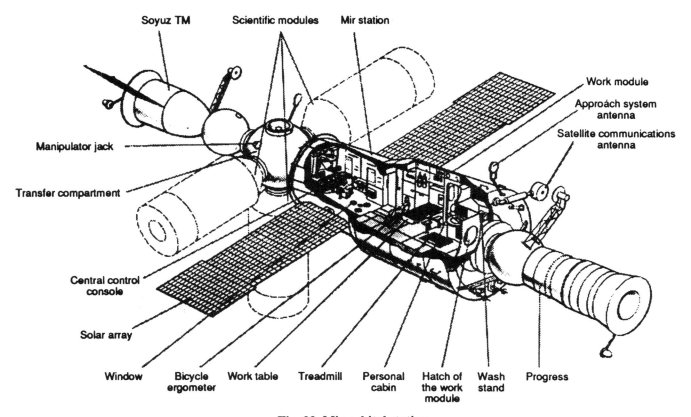

Fig. 22 Mir orbital station

The Kristall module was designed for research on technological processes in weightlessness.

The mass of the Kvant 2 and Kristall modules is approximately 21 metric tons each.

Almost all the on-board systems used on the core and other Mir modules are new. The "brain" of the station is the system of on-board computers that controls virtually all processes on the station.

The most important new feature of the attitude control system is that, in addition to using standard propellant-powered jet engines for attitude control, it also uses single-axis powered gyroscopes mounted on the Kvant and Kvant 2 modules, making it possible to orient the station without expending propellant. In addition, there is a new system for measuring the relative motion of the spacecraft and station, which makes it possible for the station to remain motionless during rendezvous and not have to align its longitudinal axis to the approaching spacecraft.

The power of the electrical system was increased by adding significantly larger solar array panels to the core, Kvant 2, and Kristall modules. A voltage stabilization system was also added.

In addition to the types of radio communication systems used on Salyut, a new system was introduced to connect the station with the ground control center through retranslator satellites.

Several crews have already worked on this station. The longest mission lasted 1 year.

K. Space Shuttle Orbiter

The American Space Shuttle Orbiter was the first attempt to create a reusable transport spacecraft. It was designed for inserting various payloads into orbit, for autonomous flight in orbit for specific one-time missions, and eventually for delivering crews and cargo to orbital stations.

It is a hypersonic aircraft (see Fig. 4) with a deltoid wing, which at hypersonic speed has an aerodynamic ratio of up to 1.3, with an angle of attack of 34°. This ensures relatively low heat loadings on the structure of the aircraft.

At subsonic speed, the shape selected for the aircraft ensures an aerodynamic ratio of about 4.4, at an angle of incidence of 18°. To support these characteristics, the wing has a double sweep with angles of 81° and 45° to the forward edge. The length of the aircraft is approximately 37 m and the wingspan is about 24 m. The launch weight is 110-115 metric tons, and the landing weight 85 metric tons. The standard size crew is seven or eight astronauts.

The fuselage consists of forward, central, and aft sections. In the forward section is the pressurized crew cabin, the forward reaction control system, and the forward undercarriage leg. The central section houses the nonpressurized payload bay. The aft section holds the three main engines, the orbital maneuvering system, descent engines, the tail portion of the reaction control system engines, and the keel. The main undercarriage legs are located in the wings.

The pressurized crew cabin has an upper deck and a

middeck. Some of the astronauts work in the upper flight deck, which contains consoles, instrument panels, displays, manual flight controls, and astronaut seating. The others work in the middeck, containing electronic equipment, the kitchen, supplies of food, a lavatory, sleeping accommodations and astronaut couches, etc.

All the windows (aside from the one overlooking the payload bay) have three panes: an outer thermal protective pane, a central pane, and an inner pressurized one. To decrease heat flow between the bulkhead and the cabin, the bulkhead is attached to the hull at only four points. The available volume in the pressurized cabin is about 30 m^3.

The payload bay is about 18 m in length and 4.6 m in diameter. The available volume of the bay is about 340 m^3. During orbital insertion and descent, the bay is covered by two flaps under which are two deployable panels of the thermal regulation system radiator. Under the floor of the bay is the equipment of the electric power system. On the bay's left side is a manipulator, remotely controlled from the cabin. When the spacecraft docks with space stations or other spacecraft, a special docking module with a docking port connected to the crew cabin may be mounted in the payload bay. The payload bay can accommodate a payload weighing approximately 30 metric tons.

To protect the structure from the effects of high thermal flux of the incandescent plasma surrounding it on reentry, the entire surface of the spacecraft is covered with a thermal protective coating. The nose of the fuselage and the edges of the wings, which are most subject to overheating in flight (up to a temperature approximately 1500 °C), are covered with tiles made of a carbon-carbon composite material that withstands such temperatures. The lower surface of the wings, the fuselage, and the rudder are protected with quartz fiber tiles. The remaining surface is covered with tiles made from material capable of withstanding the effects of temperatures of up to 600-700 °C.

The main engines operate only during orbital insertion and are fed with propellant from the central hydrogen-oxygen tank of the second stage, which is jettisoned at the end of orbital insertion.

There are three propulsion systems: the main propulsion system, the orbital maneuvering and reentry system, and the reaction control system (attitude and translational motion control). The main propulsion system supports the operation of the forward group of control engines. The other two are located in the tail section. They include two cruise engines with thrust of 2.7 metric tons each, control engines, tanks, gas cylinders for tank pressurization, and an automatic pneumohydraulic device. The propulsion system uses monomethylhydyrazine and nitrogen tetroxide.

The life support system provides the crew with oxygen from the liquid oxygen tanks also used by the electric power system. It also cleans the cabin atmosphere of carbon dioxide and water vapor, provides water (a small portion from stores, with the majority generated by the fuel cells of the electric power system) and food, etc. The composition of the atmo-

sphere is 21 percent oxygen and 79 percent nitrogen at normal atmospheric pressure.

The thermal regulation system delivers heat to panels of the radiator, which deploy after insertion into orbit and after the payload bay doors are opened.

Five on-board computers control orientation, navigation, translational motion, and other processes of the spacecraft.

The attitude control, navigation, and control systems include three inertial measurement blocks, three gyroscope blocks, three accelerometer blocks, radar for supporting landing, apparatus of the radio navigation system, radio-altimeters, instruments displaying information about the environment, and manual controls. It should be noted that the reentry velocity of the spacecraft is approximately 335 km/hour, which complicates the task of the pilot on return from space, since the major mode of control during landing is manual (there are plans to fully automate).

The communications apparatus supports communication with the Earth through direct contact with ground observation points or through retranslator satellites, communication with astronauts on EVA, measurement of orbital parameters, transmission of computer commands, and telemetry.

The maximal acceleration on orbital insertion is about 3 g, and on reentry about 1.5 g.

The typical duration of a flight is 4-7 days. In the future, flights are planned to last up to 30 days.

The spacecraft began to fly regularly in 1981. The creation of the Space Shuttle was an outstanding engineering achievement and an important stage in the development of space technology and aviation. The main facets of this achievement are:

• the reusable nature of the spacecraft

• the development of a hypersonic aircraft capable of entering the atmosphere of the Earth with orbital velocity, performing maneuvers during atmospheric flight and landing normally on a runway.

The shortcomings include:

• the absence of an emergency rescue system for the most dangerous leg of the flight of the rocket system in the atmosphere, which was the main reason for the tragic outcome of the flight in 1986

• the excessive cost of inserting a payload into orbit, significantly greater than with even old, nonreusable rockets.

L. Buran

Like the Space Shuttle, the Soviet reusable orbital spacecraft, Buran, is designed for orbital insertion of various payloads, autonomous flight, return of spacecraft from orbit, and delivery of crews and cargoes to orbital stations. The estimated weight of the payload for insertion into an orbit of 220-240 km is 30 metric tons, and for delivery to an orbital station is 12-15 metric tons. The Buran spacecraft is inserted into orbit by the Energiya rocket. In configuration, dimensions, and specifications, the buran is similar to the Space Shuttle.

The first flight of Buran took place in 1988 in unmanned mode. The flight was controlled from Earth. Descent and landing in an airport were performed on automatic pilot.

VI. Space Flight Control

Modern unmanned and manned spacecraft are able to fly only with the participation of ground facilities. In other words, they are all remotely controlled. Ground personnel utilize facilities on Earth, in the ocean, and in orbit, as well as radio communications between the spacecraft and ground stations, and on-board measurement systems that monitor the orbit of the spacecraft, operation of its systems, and the status of the apparatus (pressurization, thermal conditions, mechanical device operation, etc.) and the crew, transmit commands, digital information, and recommendations to the crew on the spacecraft.

The ground and orbital facilities supporting space flight include flight control centers; ground-based monitoring and control points for reception of telemetric measurements, radio monitoring of the orbit, transmission to the spacecraft of instructions and commands, machine-machine communications from the spacecraft to the Earth and radio communications with the crew; floating (ocean vessels) monitoring and control points and flight control centers; ground-based means of communications between monitoring and control points and flight control centers; communications satellites; and navigation system satellites.

During the flight of a spacecraft, a large number of ground-based personnel work with all of these facilities to coordinate the hardware being used, monitor their operations, analyze the incoming information, develop programs and recommendations, etc. On the whole, this is very complicated and expensive. Thus, one of the important objectives in the development of space technology is the creation of spacecraft that can complete flights virtually autonomously, without support from the Earth. With hard work and research, this objective is completely achievable.

Bibliography

Booster Rockets, Moscow, Voyennoye Izdatelstvo, 1981 (in Russian).

Gatland, K., *The Illustrated Encyclopedia of Space Technology: A Comprehensive History of Space Exploration*, London, Salamander Books, Ltd., 1981.

Keldysh M.V., Marov M.Ya. *Space Research*, Moscow, Nauka, 1981 (in Russian).

McElroy, J.H. *Space Sciences and Applications: Progress and Potential*. Piscataway, New Jersey, IEEE Press, 1986.

Spacecraft, Moscow, Voyennoye Izdatelstvo, 1983 (in Russian).

Wood, J.A. *The Solar System.*, Englewood Cliffs, New Jersey, Prentice Hall, 1979.

Appendix: Astronomical and Physical Quantities

Physical Constants:
Speed of light: $c = 2.998 \times 10^{10}$ cm/s
Gravitational constant: $G = 6.67 \times 10^{-8}$ dyn $\cdot$ m^2/g^2
Planck's constant: h (i.e. $h/2\pi$) $= 1.054 \times 10^{-27}$ erg $\cdot$ s
Boltzmann constant: $k = 1.3809 \times 10^{-16}$ erg $\cdot$ K^{-1}

Mass:
Mass of the Sun: 1 $M_{SOL} = 1.989 \times 10^{33}$ g
Mass of the Earth: 1 $M_\oplus = 5.9676 \times 10^{27}$ g
Mass of the galaxy (without the corona): $M_g = 2 \times 10^{11}$ M_{SOL}

Time:
Age of the universe and galaxy: $T_g \approx T_u \approx (1\text{-}1.5) \times 10^{10}$ years
Age of the solar system: $T_{ss} \approx 4.6 \times 10^9$ years
Duration of life on Earth: $T_L \approx 3.5 \times 10^9$ years

Distance:
Astronomical unit: 1 AU $= 1.4967 \times 10^{13}$ cm
Parsec: 1 pc $= 3.08 \times 10^{18}$ cm
Kiloparsec: 1 kpc $= 10^3$ pc
Megaparsec: 1 mpc $= 10^6$ pc
Light year: 9.4695×10^{17} cm
Mean distance between the Earth and Moon: $= 3.84 \times 10^{10}$ cm

Physical Properties of the Sun and Solar System:
Sun's radius $R_{SOL} = 6.96 \times 10^{10}$ cm
Effective temperature of the surface of the Sun $T_{eff} = 5770$ °C
Wave length of radiation corresponding to maximum intensity in the spectrum at T_{eff} $\lambda = 5.1993 \times 10^3$ Å
Total solar luminosity $L_{SOL} = 3.9 \times 10^{33}$ erg/s
Mean time for electromagnetic radiation to travel between the Sun and the Earth $t = 498.2$ s
Inclination of ecliptic to equator $= 23° 27'$

Units of Nuclear Physics:
Electron mass $m_e = 9.1 \times 10^{-28}$ g
Proton mass $M_p = 1.67 \times 10^{-24}$ g
Electron-volt energy unit for nuclear reactions:
    1 ev $= 1.602 \times 10^{-12}$ erg
    1 kev $= 10^3$ ev
    1Mev $= 10^6$ ev
    Energy of nuclear reactions is often expressed in units of mass of 1 atomic mass
      (MI) $= 1.49 \times 10^{-3}$ erg $= 931.8$ mev

Ratios Between Energy Units:
Energy in ergs corresponding to:
    1 j $= 10^7$ erg
    1 W $= 1$ j/s $= 10^7$ erg/s
    1 cal $= 4.18 \times 10^7$ erg
Photon energy corresponding to radiation wave length:
    1Å $= 12.6$ kev
    0.1Å$=126$ kev
    (1Å$=10^{-10}$m$=10^{-8}$cm)
      (1μm$=10^{-6}$m)

Afterword

Future Directions in Space Exploration

From our perspective in the 1990s, we face a universe of possibilities in the future utilization and exploration of space. The Earth faces the prospect of accelerated environmental change, including climate warming, deforestation, desertification, ozone depletion, and a reduction in biodiversity. However, new capabilities in the use of space remote sensing provide us with an exciting new way of understanding and contending with these problems. Looking outward, the exploration and eventual colonization of the solar system present other exciting challenges for the human race. By extending the duration that humans can remain safely in that environment, humans leaving the Earth in the 21st century will be capable of working for long periods in space and successfully readapting to the Earth's gravity upon return. Enabling a permanent human presence in space will also require the continued development of an array of new technologies. Life support systems, power systems, robotics, transportation systems, information systems, and planetary habitats are only a few examples of the capabilities that engineers and scientists must provide. These two space thrusts will form the basis of national and international programs in the 21st century. For the purposes of discussion, we will call one such program a "Mission to Planet Earth," and another a "Mission from Planet Earth." A myriad of space activities can be carried out within the context of these two missions.

Mission to Planet Earth

In the 1990s and the early 21st century, the U.S. and other spacefaring nations will pursue the Mission to Planet Earth. Using spaceborne remote-sensing instruments, this effort will enable a wide range of investigations to examine, understand, and predict changes in Earth's environment.

There are two base research components of the Mission to Planet Earth. The first focuses on deploying advanced remote sensing capabilities to gain a better understanding of the global processes that maintain the Earth's global environmental balance, and the variables, including human activity, that are affecting that balance. The United States program will be composed of three new space program elements: the Earth Observing System (EOS), the Earth Probes program, and eventually a Geostationary Platforms program. These three elements will form a constellation of satellites in a variety of orbits around the Earth. Other elements will be launched by Japan and Europe, and Russian space assets will also contribute. A second component of the mission will be the development of global scale interactive models, built upon an understanding of system processes and validated against the long-term data sets residing in the EOS Data Information System (EOSDIS). EOSDIS will enable efficient use of remote-sensing data from EOS, the Earth Probes, and from a variety of other remote-sensing sources.

Mission from Planet Earth

Humans engaged in the missions envisioned by a Mission from Planet Earth will venture out into environments more harsh and inhospitable than any encountered on Earth. Basic differences between space and Earth, such as the lack of gravity, inadequate atmospheres, deep cold, and radiation hazards challenge our ability to protect, nurture, and sustain the individuals who will pioneer the solar system.

The U.S. participation in a Mission from Planet Earth is expected to be an evolutionary program, proceeding in a series of steps: Space Station Freedom, a base on the Moon, and then a manned flight to Mars. The attainment of these goals will depend on the political climate and on economics—the availability of funding. Nevertheless, we have a strong base from which to proceed. In addition, each step on the exploration pathway—Space Station Freedom, the Moon, and Mars— offers discrete opportunities for space science. These opportunities include studying the effects of gravity (and microgravity) on life, comparing the evolution of Earth and the other planets, and further characterizing the physical universe through astronomical observations.

Science and operations conducted at a manned lunar base in the early 21st century can greatly increase our knowledge of Earth's nearest neighbor in space, and provide critical preparatory experience for later operations on more distant and less accessible Mars. Economically useful activity would be initiated, including the investigation of the possibility and desirability of lunar mining. At first glance at least, the construction of an astrophysical observatory appears to offer certain important advantages over ground-based and orbital telescopes.

Both manned and unmanned mission elements will be needed for the exploration of the solar system. Unmanned robotic precursor missions to the Moon and Mars will aid in outpost site selection and resource identification, and will support the engineering design process for the transportation vehicles and hardware to be used on planetary surfaces. Unmanned missions will also emplace the hardware to support subsequent human activity, and demonstrate key mission capabilities and system concepts. Mars precursor missions may include planetary observers, communications orbiters, global stationary surface data network, rovers, and sample return vehicles.

Human exploration and settlement of Mars will build directly on the technologies proven during the lunar missions and robotic phases of Mars exploration. For all mission systems and elements, a major challenge for human settlement of the Moon and Mars is to minimize the total mass that must be launched into low Earth orbit and transported to the planetary surfaces.

The eventual establishment of permanent colonies on the Moon, and later, Mars, will require an extensive program of research and technology development aimed at overcoming the limitations to extended human presence in space. For example, the space radiation environment is not well understood. There is scant information on the long-term effects (e.g., carcinogenesis) of exposure to solar flares and galactic cosmic rays, potential hazards for a lunar base and an interplanetary flight to Mars. To ensure performance and safe readaptation to Earth's gravity, physiological changes in a microgravity environment and the extent to which they can be counteracted are a driving concern. Although two cosmonauts have spent over a year on the space station Mir, much additional research—in space and on the ground—will be needed to characterize thoroughly the effects of long-term space flight on bone, muscle, and other body systems, and to develop effective countermeasures. Life support systems for exploration and planetary habitation must provide the basic necessities of human life and meet a range of challenges, including absolute reliability far from Earth. Given the high costs and difficult logistics of resupply, these closed-loop systems eventually will have to incorporate bioregenerative techniques; their development will follow an incremental course, extrapolating the knowledge gained from one phase of exploration to the next. Finally, mission success in the isolated and confined settings associated with exploration will depend on the psychological health of crew members and sustained positive interaction within the crew.

And Beyond

If we can succeed in reaching Mars, then our future may find a focus there. The possibility of using Mars as a habitat for terrestrial life is no longer solely the realm of science fiction. As it happens, many of the environmental factors that are unfavorable for the establishment of life on Mars would be ameliorated by modifying the planet's temperature. The surface temperatures of Mars could be increased, and the diurnal temperature variations reduced, if a way could be found for increasing the atmospheric mass of Mars by vaporizing the martian polar caps. Increasing the amount of carbon dioxide, water vapor, or certain other gases in the atmosphere would increase the surface temperature of Mars. This warming, known as "the greenhouse effect," occurs because certain gases absorb some of the thermal radiation from the surface of the planet so that not all of the radiation is lost to space. Modification of the martian climate by means of greenhouse heating would increase enormously the area of the planet available for growth of organisms that could be adapted from Earth environments, and would optimize the conditions under which such growth would occur.

It is interesting to speculate upon the possibility of creating novel species of photosynthetic organisms better adapted to growth in a modified martian environment, in effect, transforming currently available "best fit" organisms into "ideal" organisms. Earth organisms may be able to further transform Mars into a habitable environment for Earth's life forms. This terraforming, or greening, of the red planet would be the most ambitious scientific and engineering project in human history. It could create a new home for humankind out of what was once an inhospitable, cold, and barren neighbor, and assure our future in space.

The Editors

Addresses of Contributors to Volume I

U.S. Contributors

David S. Bartlett, Ph.D.
Associate Director, Institute for the
    Study of Earth, Oceans, and Space
University of New Hampshire
Science and Engineering Research Building
Durham, NH 03824-3525

John Billingham, Ph.D.
Chief, SETI Office
Mail Stop 244-11
NASA Ames Research Center
Moffett Field, CA 94035

Geoff Briggs, Ph.D.
Science Director
Center for Mars Exploration
Mail Stop 260-1
NASA Ames Research Center
Moffett Field, CA 94035-1000

Berrian Moore III, Ph.D.
Director, Institute for the
    Study of Earth, Oceans, and Space
University of New Hampshire
Science and Engineering Research Building
Durham, NH 03824-3525

David Morrison, Ph.D.
Chief, Space Science Division
Mail Stop 245-1
NASA Ames Research Center
Moffett Field, CA 94035-1000

Tobias Owen, Ph.D.
Institute for Astronomy
University of Hawaii
Honolulu, HI 96822

John D. Rummel, Ph.D.
Manager, Exobiology Program
Solar System Exploration Division
Code SLC
NASA Headquarters
Washington, DC 20546

Jill Tarter, Ph.D.
HRMS Project Scientist
Mail Stop 244-11
NASA Ames Research Center
Moffett Field, CA 94035

Russian Contributors

Konstantin Petrovich Feoktistov
N.E. Bauman Moscow State Technical University
d. 5, 2-aya Baumanskaya Ulitsa
107005 Moscow-B-5
Russia

Academician Albert Abubakirovich Galeev
Director, Institute of Space Research, Russian
    Academy of Sciences
84/32 Profsoyuznaya Ulitsa
Moscow, V-485, GSP-7, 117810
Russia

Armen Aramovich Gurjian
Institute of Biomedical Problem, Russian Federation
Ministry of Health
76a Khoroshevskoye Shosse
Moscow D-7, 123007
Russia

Academician Mikhail Vladimirovich Ivanov
Director, Institute of Microbiology, Russian Academy of
Sciences
7 korp 2, 60-letiya Oktyabrya Prospekt
Moscow, GSP-7, 117811
Russia

Academician Vladimir Aleksandrovich Kotelnikov
Chairman, Interkosmos Council
14 Leninskiy Prospekt
Moscow V-71, GSP-1, 117901
Russia

Viktoriya Gdalevna Kurt
Scientific Research Institute of Nuclear Physics,
    Moscow State University
Leninskiye Gory
Moscow, V-324, 117234
Russia

Yuriy Ivanovich Logachev
Scientific Research Institute of Nuclear Physics,
    Moscow State University
Leninskiye Gory
Moscow, V-324, 117234
Russia

Mikhail Yakovlevich Marov
M.V. Keldysh Institute of Applied Mathematics,
    Russian Academy of Sciences
D-4 Miusskaya Ploshchad
Moscow 125047
Russia

Novomir Fedorovich Pisarenko
Institute of Space Research, Russian Academy of Sciences
84/32 Profsoyuznaya Ulitsa
Moscow, V-485, GSP-7, 117810
Russia

Academician Boris Viktorovich Rauschenbach
Institute of the History of Science and Technology,
    Russian Academy of Sciences
1/5 Staropanskiy Pereulok
Moscow K-12, 103012
Russia

Viktor Nikolayevich Sokolskiy
Institute of the History of Science and Technology,
    Russian Academy of Sciences
1/5 Staropanskiy Pereulok
Moscow K-12, 103012
Russia

Index